Fundamentals of Family Medicine

Second Edition

Springer
New York
Berlin
Heidelberg
Barcelona
Budapest
Hong Kong
London
Milan
Paris
Singapore
Tokyo

Robert B. Taylor
Editor

Fundamentals of Family Medicine

The Family Medicine Clerkship Textbook

Second Edition

Associate Editors

Alan K. David   Thomas A. Johnson, Jr.
D. Melessa Phillips   Joseph E. Scherger

With 55 Illustrations

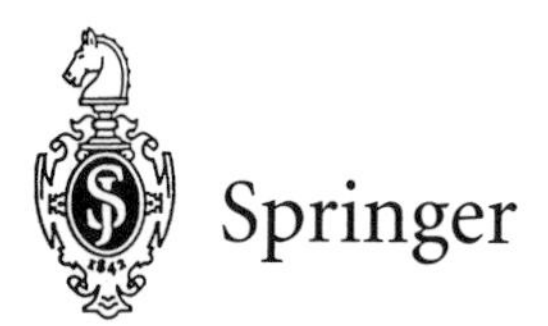

Springer

Robert B. Taylor, M.D.
Professor and Chairman
Department of Family Medicine
Oregon Health Sciences University
School of Medicine
Portland, OR 97201, USA

Alan K. David, M.D.
The Fred Lazarus Jr. Professor and Director
Department of Family Medicine
University of Cincinnati College of Medicine
Cincinnati, OH 45267, USA

D. Melessa Phillips, M.D.
Professor and Chairman
Department of Family Medicine
University of Mississippi School of Medicine
Jackson, MS 39216, USA

Thomas A. Johnson, Jr., M.D.
Chairman
Department of Family Medicine
St. John's Mercy Medical Center
St. Louis, MO 63141, USA

Joseph E. Scherger, M.D., M.P.H.
Associate Dean for Clinical Affairs
Professor and Chairman
Department of Family Medicine
University of California, Irvine
College of Medicine
Irvine, CA 92697, USA

Library of Congress Cataloging-in-Publication Data
Fundamentals of family medicine : the family medicine clerkship textbook /
Robert B. Taylor . . . [et al.]. — 2nd ed.
p. cm.
"Consists of an overview of the principles of generalist health care followed by 25 . . . chapters from the fifth edition of Family medicine"—Pref.
Includes bibliographical references and index.
ISBN 0-387-98445-3 (softcover : alk. paper)
1. Family medicine. I. Taylor, Robert B. II. Family medicine.

[DNLM: 1. Family Practice. 2. Primary Health Care. 3. Education, Medical. WB 110 F981 1998]
RA418.5.F3F86 1998
616—dc21

98-2746

Printed on acid-free paper.

Production managed by Princeton Editorial Associates, Inc., and supervised by Terry Kornak and Karina Mikhli; manufacturing supervised by Jacqui Ashri.
Typeset by Princeton Editorial Associates, Inc., Roosevelt, NJ.
Printed and bound by Edwards Brothers, Inc., Ann Arbor, MI.
Printed in the United States of America.

9 8 7 6 5 4 3 2 1

ISBN 0-387-98445-3 Springer-Verlag New York Berlin Heidelberg SPIN 10662935

This book is dedicated:

To the medical student in the clinical years

Who wishes to understand a specialty not limited to one organ, system, or technology,

That is based on relationships with people, their families, and their communities.

Preface

This Second Edition of *Fundamentals of Family Medicine* is designed to be the course text for family medicine/primary care clerkships in medical schools. The chapters that follow are intended to present the clinical approach to common problems in generalist practice, to describe the process by which family physicians provide high quality comprehensive care for their patients, and to serve as the basis for small group discussions by students and faculty.

The book consists of an overview of the Principles of Generalist Health Care followed by 25 all new chapters from the Fifth Edition of *Family Medicine: Principles and Practice.*[1] I selected chapter topics based on the content of general and family practice as recorded in the National Ambulatory Medical Care Survey (see Chapter 1, Table 1) and on patient problems seen by medical students in our own Family Medicine Clerkship over the past nine years.

Preparing medical students to manage different types of uncertainty has been identified as an important goal of medical schools.[2] One key to developing this vital competency is understanding *process*—how the family physician can define, prioritize, and manage the diverse problems of many patients in time-limited visits. The *how* is the generalist approach, described in an updated Chapter 1. This approach, which emphasizes patient-centered concepts and focused clinical questions, is reinforced through the case presentations and discussion topics at the end of each clinical chapter. The patients in the 25 case scenarios are all members of one extended family, affording the reader a sense of continuity of care and an awareness of the effects of illness on various family members. The Nelson family and the case presentations are explained in Notes for the Reader.

I appreciate the contributions of the authors and the four associate editors for the Fifth Edition: Alan K. David, M.D.; D. Melessa Phillips, M.D.; Thomas A. Johnson, M.D.; and Joseph E. Scherger, M.D., M.P.H. I also thank Coelleda O'Neil, Laretta Borg, Dawn Vredenburg, and Laurie Charron for assistance in manuscript preparation.

In preparing this Second Edition, I have spoken with many medical students and family medicine educators, and some of their thoughts are found in the pages that follow. I continue to encourage suggestions from readers in North America and around the world.

Robert B. Taylor, M.D.
Portland, Oregon

References

1. Taylor RB. editor. Family medicine: principles and practice, fifth edition. New York: Springer Verlag, 1998.
2. Fargason CA, Evans HH, Ashworth CS, Capper SA. The importance of preparing medical students to manage different types of uncertainty. Academic Med 1997; 72:668–92.

Contents

Contents

Notes for the Reader

To the Student

Your time on the family medicine/primary care clerkship may be the most important of all in medical school.[1] Here you will encounter concepts that will shape your future patient care—whether or not you choose a generalist speciality as a career: concepts such as personal care, longitudinal care, the meaning of illness, and the investment of self in the therapeutic relationship. This book presents these and other principles of generalist health care plus factual data regarding selected clinical problems, supplemented by case presentations that involve members of a single family.

The discussion questions are not intended to be post-tests of the factual content of each chapter and the answers to some questions may not actually be in the chapter, but in your own reasoning abilities and personal experiences. The questions are designed to stimulate thought about the issues, encourage discussion, and even inspire a quest for more information.

To the Faculty

This book, intended to be a single source text for your clerkship, has been prepared to meet the General Guidelines for a Third-Year Family Medicine Clerkship as developed by the Society of Teachers of Family Medicine (Table 1).[1] The 26 clinical chapters present a broad spectrum of family practice problems. The case presentations and questions that follow each chapter are intended to be the basis of small group discussions, including both traditional questions about medical history, physical examination, diagnosis, and management, as well as psychosocial issues such as the reason for the visit, the impact of illness on the family, the patient's adaptation to illness, and the resources used in management. The case discussions have been "field-tested" with third-year medical students, and they work. Try them.

TABLE 1. General guidelines for a third-year family medicine clerkship

By the completion of a third-year family medicine clerkship, the medical student is expected to possess, at a level appropriate for a third-year student, the knowledge, attitudes, and skills needed to:

1. Provide personal care for individuals and families as the physician of first contact and continuing care in health as well as in illness
2. Assess and manage acute and chronic medical problems frequently encountered in the community
3. Provide anticipatory health care using education, risk reduction, and health enhancement strategies
4. Provide continuous as well as episodic health care, not limited by a specific disease, patient characteristics, or setting of the patient encounter
5. Provide and coordinate comprehensive care of complex and severe problems using biomedical, social, personal, economic, and community resources, including consultation and referral
6. Establish effective physician–patient relationships by using appropriate interpersonal communication skills to provide quality health care

Source: Working Committee to Develop Curricular Guidelines for a Third-Year Family Medicine Clerkship. Curricular Guidelines for a Third-Year Family Medicine Clerkship. Kansas City, MO: The Society of Teachers of Family Medicine. With permission.

About the Case Discussions in this Book: The Nelson Family

Each chapter is followed by a case presentation with discussion questions, all involving members of a single extended family: the Nelsons. The Nelson family genogram is shown in Figure 1. During a period of 12 months, various members of the Nelson family come to the office for care, some making two or three visits during the year. The reader will find that the problems of various family members are interconnected and that they evolve over time.

The following introduces the four-generation Nelson family, some of whom have been your patients for more than a decade and who look to you as their personal physician. You and your patients live in a community of 40,000 people.

Harold and Mary Nelson

The senior family members are Harold and Mary Nelson, both in their 70s. Harold Nelson retired from his job as a welder at age 61. He now leads a quiet life and seldom leaves the house. He has had type 2 diabetes mellitus for 24 years and osteoarthritis of the hands for 20 years, both of which were considerations in his early retirement.

Mary Nelson, aged 71, is a retired nursery school teacher. She has been hypertensive, taking medication, for 10 years. Also, she has episodes of

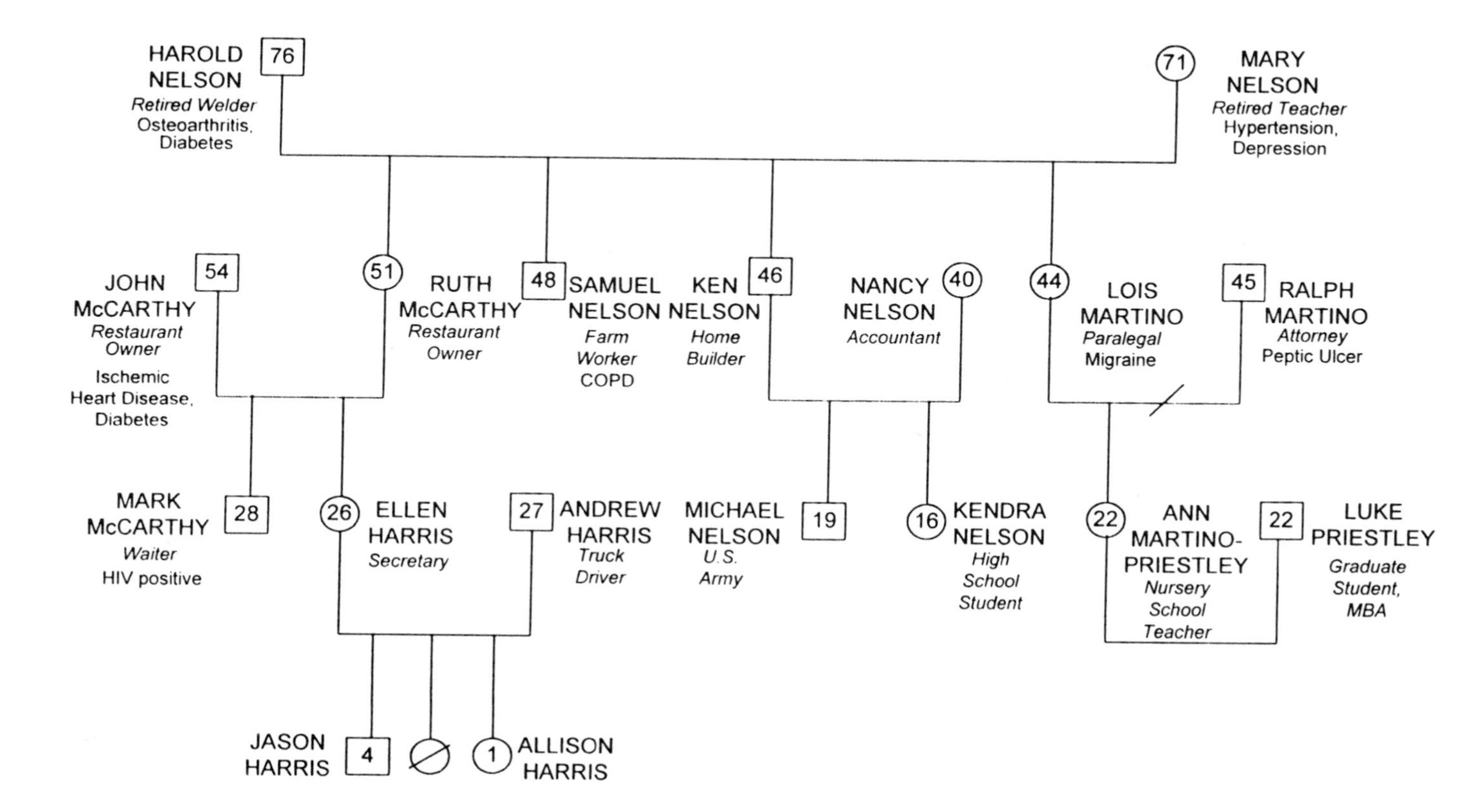

Nelson family genogram: family members, occupations, chronic health problems. Symbols used: [76], male, age 76; (71), female, age 71; □—○, marriage; □—/—○, divorce; ∅, deceased.

depression that require treatment. She wishes that she and Harold were "doing more" in their retirement and worries about what will happen to their son Samuel when they die.

Harold and Mary Nelson have four children: Ruth, Samuel, Ken, and Lois—all in their 40s and 50s.

John and Ruth McCarthy

Ruth, the oldest Nelson daughter, is married to John McCarthy. Together they own and operate a small delicatessen-style restaurant. Their restaurant business struggles financially, and Ruth and John sometimes seek "loans" from her parents during lean times. Both work long hours in the restaurant. Ruth enjoys good health, but John has coronary artery disease with angina pectoris for which he had been treated by an internist who retired recently, and John has decided to transfer his care to you.

John and Ruth McCarthy have two children. Their oldest son is Mark, aged 28, who dropped out of college to organize a rock group that disbanded about 2 years ago. Mark now works as a waiter in his parents' restaurant. John and Ruth openly disapprove of Mark's life style, which includes cigarette smoking, marijuana use, and many sexual contacts. Recently, Mark was found to be human immunodeficiency virus (HIV)-positive.

The McCarthys' second child is Ellen, aged 26, who works as a secretary in a business office. Ellen is married to Andrew Harris, a truck driver who is on the road a good deal of the time. Ellen and Andrew Harris have two children: Jason, aged 4, and Allison, aged 1. A third child, who would have been 3 years old this year, died in infancy of meningitis.

Samuel Nelson

Samuel Nelson, aged 48, is the second child of Harold and Mary Nelson. Samuel was a high school dropout at age 16 when he began work at a nearby orchard. Today, he lives with his parents and has no close friends. He has kept the same job as a farm worker for 32 years and spends his spare time watching television. Samuel has been a heavy smoker since his teens and now has chronic obstructive pulmonary disease.

Ken and Nancy Nelson

The third son is Kenneth Nelson, aged 46, who works as a contractor, building new homes in middle-class neighborhoods. Ken is married to Nancy, who has an accounting degree and works part-time for a public accounting firm. Nancy has always described herself as "nervous," which has limited her ability to take a full-time job.

Ken and Nancy Nelson have two children. The oldest is Michael Nelson, aged 19, a U.S. Army paratrooper stationed at Fort Bragg, North Carolina. Still living at home is their 16-year-old daughter, Kendra, a high school sophomore. Kendra is an above-average student and a varsity athlete. She has had her first serious relationship with a boyfriend for the past year.

Lois and Ralph Martino

The fourth child is Lois, aged 44, who has training as a paralegal and works in a large law firm. Ten years ago, Lois separated from her husband, Ralph Martino, an attorney previously employed in the same law firm as Lois and now in solo practice. Although Ralph's relationship with Lois and the Nelson family is strained, he has continued to consider you his personal physician.

Lois and Ralph have one child, Ann, aged 22, who works mornings as a nursery school teacher. A year ago, Ann married Luke Priestley, a graduate student now working on his Masters of Business Administration degree. Ann's parents secretly worry about Ann's marriage because Luke seems very distant and moody.

Reference

1. Senf JH, Campos-Outcalt D. The effect of a required third-year family medicine clerkship on medical students' attitudes: value indoctrination and value clarification. Acad Med 1995;70:142–8.

Contributors

Adelman, Alan M., M.D. M.S., Professor, Department of Family and Community Medicine, Penn State University College of Medicine, Hershey, PA

Ambuel, Bruce, Ph.D., M.S., Assistant Professor, Department of Family and Community Medicine, Medical College of Wisconsin, Milwaukee, WI; Behavioral Science Coordinator and Research Director, Waukesha Family Practice Residency, Waukesha Memorial Hospital, Waukesha, WI

Bailey, Boyd L., Jr., M.D., Associate Professor, Department of Family Medicine, University of Alabama School of Medicine at Birmingham, AL; Clinic Director, Selma Family Medicine Residency Program, Selma, AL

Breuner Cora Collette, M.D., Clinical Assistant Professor, Department of Family Medicine, University of Washington School of Medicine; Faculty, Swedish Family Medicine Residency, Swedish Medical Center, Seattle, WA

Brunton, Stephen A., M.D., Director. Family Medicine Residency Program, Long Beach Memorial Medical Center, Long Beach, CA; Clinical Professor, Department of Family Medicine, University of California-Irvine College of Medicine, Irvine, CA

Calmbach, Walter L., M.D., Assistant Professor, Department of Family Practice, The University of Texas Health Science Center; Director, Sports Medicine Training Program, University Hospital, San Antonio, TX

Campbell, Bryan, M.D., Assistant Professor, Department of Family and Preventive Medicine, University of Utah School of Medicine, Salt Lake City, UT: McKay-Dee Hospital, Ogden, UT

Carden, Ann, Ph.D., Staff Psychologist, Clinical Supervisor, Child and Family Intervention Team, Medina, OH

Celestino, Frank, M.D., Associate Professor, Department of Family and Community Medicine, Director of Geriatrics, Bowman Gray School of Medicine; North Carolina Baptist Hospital, Winston-Salem, NC

Clarity, Greg, M.D., Assistant Professor, Department of Family Medicine, East Tennessee State University, James H. Quillen College of Medicine, Johnson, TN

Edwards, Rita K., Pharm. D., Pharmacist, Long Beach Memorial Medical Center, Long Beach, CA

Elizondo, Margaret V., M.D., Director, Perinatal Education, Sharp Grossmont Family Practice Residency, La Mesa, CA

Evans, Paul, D.O., Clinical Associate Professor, Department of Family Medicine, University of Washington School of Medicine, Seattle, WA; Chief, Department of Family Practice, Madigan Army Medical Center, Tacoma, WA

Fields, Scott A., M.D., Associate Professor, Department of Family Medicine, Oregon Health Sciences University School of Medicine, Portland, OR

Gilchrist, Valerie J., M.D., Professor, Department of Family Medicine, Northeastern Ohio Universities College of Medicine, Rootstown, OH; Associate Director, Family Practice Residency Program, Aultman Hospital, Canton, OH

Goetz, Rupert R., M.D., Assistant Professor, Department of Psychiatry, Oregon Health Sciences University School of Medicine, Portland, OR

Goldschmidt, Ronald H., M.D., Professor and Vice Chair, Department of Family and Community Medicine, University of California, San Francisco School of Medicine; Director, Family Practice Inpatient Service, San Francisco General Hospital, San Francisco, CA

Hale, Frank A., Ph.D., Professor, Department of Family and Community Medicine, Director, Faculty Development Program, University of Arizona, College of Medicine, Tucson, AZ

Katerndahl, David A., M.D., M.A., Professor, Department of Family Practice, University of Texas Health Science Center at San Antonio; Director of Family Practice Research and Education; University Hospital, San Antonio, TX

Kirkpatrick, George L., M.D., Associate Professor, Department of Family Practice, University of South Alabama School of Medicine, Mobile, AL

Kligman, Evan W., M.D., Professor and Head, Department of Family Medicine, University of Iowa College of Medicine, Iowa City, IA

Knight, Aubrey L., M.D., Associate Professor, Department of Clinical Family Medicine, University of Virginia School of Medicine, Charlottesville, VA; Associate Director of Family Practice Education, Roanoke Memorial Hospitals, Roanoke, VA

Legg, Jill J., M.D., Assistant Clinical Professor, Department of Family and Community Medicine, University of California, San Francisco School of Medicine, San Francisco, CA

Lewan, Richard B., M.D., Assistant Professor, Department of Family and Community Medicine, Medical College of Wisconsin, Milwaukee, WI; Director, Waukesha Family Practice Residency Program, Waukesha Memorial Hospital, Waukesha, WI

Miser, William F., M.D., Clinical Associate Professor, Department of Family Medicine, University of Washington School of Medicine, Seattle, WA; Director, Faculty Development Fellowship, Madigan Army Medical Center, Tacoma, WA

Monroe, Alicia D., M.D., Assistant Professor, Department of Family Medicine, Brown University School of Medicine; Memorial Hospital of Rhode Island/Brown University, Pawtucket, RI

Murphy, John B., M.D., Associate Professor, Department of Family Medicine, Brown University School of Medicine; Director of Residency Training, Memorial Hospital of Rhode Island/Brown University, Pawtucket, RI

Nuovo, Jim, M.D., Assistant Professor, Department of Family Practice; Director of Family Practice Residency Training, University of California, Davis School of Medicine, Sacramento, CA

Richardson, James P., M.D., M.P.H., Clinical Associate Professor, Department of Family Medicine and Department of Epidemiology and Preventive Medicine, University of Maryland School of Medicine; Director, Division of Geriatric Medicine, Good Samaritan Hospital, Baltimore, MD

Rosenfeld, Jo Ann, M.D., Associate Professor, Department of Family Medicine, East Tennessee State University School of Medicine, Bristol, TN

Sander, Robert W., M.D., Assistant Professor, Department of Family and Community Medicine, Medical College of Wisconsin, Milwaukee, WI; Associate Director, Waukesha Family Practice Residency Program, Waukesha Memorial Hospital, Waukesha, WI

Scherger, Joseph E., M.D., M.P.H., Professor and Chairman, Department of Family Medicine; Associate Dean for Clinical Affairs, University of California, Irvine College of Medicine, Irvine, CA

Sheehan, John P., M.D., Associate Clinical Professor, Department of Medicine, Case Western Reserve University, Cleveland, OH; Medical Director, North Coast Institute of Diabetes and Endocrinology, Inc., Westlake, OH

Smith, Charles Kent, M.D., Professor and Chairman, Department of Family Medicine, Case Western Reserve University School of Medicine, Cleveland, OH

Snell, George F., M.D., Associate Professor, Department of Family and Preventive Medicine, University of Utah School of Medicine, Salt Lake City, UT; Director of Residency Training-Retired, McKay-Dee Hospital, Ogden UT

Sweha, Amir, M.D., Assistant Clinical Professor, Department of Family Practice, Family Practice Clinic Director, University of California, Davis School of Medicine, Sacramento, CA

Taylor, Robert B., M.D., Professor and Chairman, Department of Family Medicine, Oregon Health Sciences University School of Medicine, Portland, OR

Toffler, William L., M.D., Professor, Department of Family Medicine, Oregon Health Sciences University School of Medicine, Portland, OR

Tuggy, Michael L., M.D., Clinical Assistant Professor, Department of Family Medicine, University of Washington School of Medicine; Faculty, Swedish Family Medicine Residency, Swedish Medical Center, Seattle, WA

Ulchaker, Margaret M., M.S.N., R.N., C.D.E., N.P.-C., Clinical Instructor, Medical/Surgical Nursing, Case Western Reserve University, Cleveland, OH; Director of Patient Education/Research Coordinator, North Coast Institute of Diabetes and Endocrinology, Inc., Westlake, OH

Van Durme, Daniel J., M.D., Associate Professor, Department of Family Medicine, University of South Florida College of Medicine, Tampa, FL

Walling, Anne D., M.B., ChB, FFPHM, Professor, Department of Family Medicine, University of Kansas School of Medicine, Wichita, KS

Weinberg, Howard, M.D., Private Practice, Virginia Beach, VA; Sentara Hospitals, Norfolk, VA

Willard, Mary, M.D., Department of Family Medicine, University of Medicine and Dentistry of New Jersey, Robert Wood Johnson School of Medicine, New Brunswick, NJ; Director, West Jersey Family Practice Residency, West Jersey Health System, Voorhees, NJ

1

Principles of Generalist Health Care

ROBERT B. TAYLOR

This first chapter is about caring for *patients*—as distinct from diseases or organs—and the generalists who provide personal health care. It is about the baby with a fever, the teenager with concerns about sexually transmitted disease, the laborer with back pain, and the manager with heartburn. It is about home visits to the paraplegic young man with the flu and nursing home care of the elderly woman with a stroke—and about how these illnesses affect their lives and the lives of those close to them. Because such care is, to a great degree, characteristic of the individual physician, I have written this chapter in the first person.

I was a general practitioner before family practice existed as a specialty. In 1969, when general practice became family practice, I began to think of myself as a family physician, and then I became a board-certified family physician in 1971. In the 1980s the term "primary care" became popular and has recently been redefined by the Institute of Medicine as "the provision of integrated, accessible health care services by clinicians who are accountable for addressing a large majority of personal health care needs, developing a sustained partnership with patients, and practicing in the context of family and community."[1]

We—my colleagues in family practice, general internal medicine, and general pediatrics, and I—are also called generalists. I have practiced in the United States Public Health Service and in a small town group practice. I spent 10 years in rural solo practice before entering academic medicine. Although I am currently chairman of a Family Medicine department in an academic medical center, I still think of myself as a rural family physician and what follows reflects that practice-oriented viewpoint.

In this book, I have decided to use the term generalist, which seems to be the favored designation for the foreseeable future.

What Is Generalist Health Care and Who Provides It?

Generalist health care is continuing, comprehensive, and coordinated medical care provided to a population undifferentiated by gender, disease, or organ system.[2] This type of care is also called primary care and the terms are often used interchangeably. Generalists offer first-contact and longitudinal care for persons with diverse problems such as earache, chest pain, fracture, or cancer. They provide care that is not problem or technology specific. They coordinate the patient's health care, whether provided in the generalist's own office or in the emergency department, consultant's office, or hospital. The spectrum of generalist care varies with the setting—suburban, rural, inner city, community health clinic, or academic medical center—and melds into a continuum in which some generalists, in fact, include tertiary care activities as part of their practice.[3] My current practice is in an academic medical center, and hence my patients tend to have much more complicated problems than did those I saw in private practice.

The U.S. Department of Health and Human Services describes four primary care/generalist competencies[4]:

Health promotion and disease prevention
Assessment and diagnosis of common symptoms and physical signs
Management of common acute and chronic medical conditions
Identification of and appropriate referral for other needed health services

Persons who choose careers in the generalist specialties are those who, like me, want to do it all. We worked hard to learn the full spectrum of medicine and do not want to give anything up. By offering a broad range of services, I can offer truly comprehensive care to my patients. If Mrs. Jones, for example, has migraine headaches, a skin rash, and irregular menstrual periods, I can provide care for all these complaints, often in a single office visit and without referrals. What is more, with each encounter the patient and I add to a cumulative fund of medical and personal knowledge, what Balint called the "mutual investment company," that allows increasingly effective health care.[5] As I learn more and more about Mrs. Jones and her stress at work, her problems with her teenage son, and her concern about her husband's alcohol use, she and I can better manage her various problems; but these data are never fully elucidated in one visit or two.

Exactly what does the generalist do? Most generalist practice is office practice and the variety of problems is reflected in the top 20 principal diagnoses in office visits as recorded in the National Ambulatory Medical Care Survey (see Table 1.1).[6] This list covers family and general practice, and thus contains the broadest scope of generalist health care.

TABLE 1.1. Office visits to general and family physicians: most frequent principal diagnoses: United States 1993

Rank	Principal diagnosis for visit of patient	Number of visits (in thousands)
	Total (all visits)	197,605
1	Essential hypertension	13,363
2	General medical examination	7,627
3	Upper respiratory infections	7,534
4	Bronchitis	6,196
5	Sinusitis	5,577
6	Otitis media	5,210
7	Diabetes mellitus	4,940
8	Pharyngitis	4,796
9	Health supervision of infant or child	3,961
10	Back strain	3,486
11	Asthma	3,284
12	Normal pregnancy	3,044
13	Special investigation or examination	2,616
14	Urinary tract infection	2,521
15	Influenza	2,413

Source: U.S. Department of Health and Human Services, Public Health Service, Centers for Disease Control and Prevention, National Center for Health Statistics; 1993 data.

Generalists provide a wide spectrum of care: This includes *anticipatory care,* counseling the teenager on avoidance of injury or unplanned pregnancy, and *symptomatic care* to relieve the pain of a back strain. There are *therapeutic care* of acute asthma or chronic ulcerative colitis and the *palliative care* of the person with terminal cancer or late-stage acquired immunodeficiency syndrome (AIDS). All of these types of care are provided in the setting of the clinical encounter, which has been identified as "the procedure" of the family physician.[7]

Generalist care occurs in many sites in addition to the physician's office. Most generalists provide hospital and nursing home services for their patients.[8] Home care is an important part of care in many communities, allowing the physician to visit the patient in his or her own "habitat." Other generalists work in schools, community health centers, the military, or government service.

Some generalists develop special areas of expertise such as care of the elderly, adolescent medicine, sports medicine, occupational medicine, or administrative medicine. At times, the focus may be on the community—community-oriented primary care—an expression of generalism in which the target is a community and the health problems that affect it (e.g., preventing cervical cancer by increasing the number of women screened with Pap smears) rather than concentrating exclusively on health problems at the level of the individual patient.

We are in the midst of profound changes in the United States medical workforce. "As a policy, the Association of American Medical Colleges (AAMC) advocates an overall national goal that a majority of graduating medical students be committed to generalist careers (family medicine, general internal medicine, or general pediatrics) and that appropriate efforts be made by all schools so that this goal can be reached within the shortest possible time."[9] In its Fourth Report to Congress and the Department of Health and Human Services Secretary, the Council on Graduate Medical Education (COGME) recommended in 1994 that "at least 50% of residency graduates should enter practice as generalist physicians (family physicians, general internists, and general pediatricians)."[10] But most significant is the tremendous need of managed care organizations for generalists. We are in the "managed care era," which calls for some 50% generalists and 50% limited specialists. The medical work force is now only about 30% generalists, and the current imbalance only emphasizes the value of the primary care physician and underscores the need to balance the ratio of generalists to specialists in the United States.

Of course, the AAMC, COGME, and managed care organizations are important considerations, but the key to the future is the people who receive health care. Family practice arose in the 1960s as a social movement to combat the fragmentation in medicine, to put medicine back together again, and to deliver it to the people. This same evangelical spirit continues today. Generalism is about the public need for personal health care, for a physician about whom one can say, "That's my doctor." It is about the physician who will make the commitment inherent in saying, "I am your personal physician. I will be there when you need me."

How to Provide Generalist Health Care: Asking the High Payoff Questions

How do we do it? How do I as a generalist stay current with all of medicine and see 25 patients per day? First of all, as a generalist, it is not my responsibility to know "all of medicine;" instead, I aspire to maintain current clinical knowledge and skills pertinent to the *common problems* of the patient population I serve. If knowledge could be weighed, my fund of knowledge would "weigh" about the same as that of an endocrinologist, neurologist, or any other limited specialist. It is just that my fund of knowledge and my competencies are broad based, whereas those of the more limited specialists are concerned with an organ, system, or technology. Their in-depth knowledge of uncommon problems—the pheochromocytoma or myasthenia gravis—allows me to identify these "zebras" and refer them to the subspecialist for definitive care, while I maintain a supportive role with the patient and family.

The added value that I bring to the clinical encounter is my knowledge of the patient. Family practice is, first of all, a specialty grounded in the principles of relationship-based health care. Thus I aspire to know everything possible about the patient and family, including all the personal concerns that may influence health and illness. In a sense, I become "a member of the family." I have a longitudinal view of the health problems of a small group of people with a committed relationship. Also, on a practical basis, I already know the past medical history, family history, social history, and habits of most patients I see. Thus I can direct my attention, knowledge, and competencies to the key issues that require attention today.

I apply the generalist fund of knowledge and competencies to help a relatively large number of patients daily by efficient application of the most commonly performed generalist procedure: *the focused clinical encounter.* Typically compressed into a 15-minute time slot, the focused clinical encounter flows seamlessly through five phases: offering of the problem, elucidation of key issues, a targeted physical examination, explanation of the diagnosis, and negotiation of plans for management and follow-up. In less than a quarter hour, I can elicit a history of epigastric distress and what makes it better and worse, explore life stresses, examine the abdomen, explain my findings, and work with the patient to plan for dietary change, stress management, and appropriate use of antacids or an H_2-receptor blocker.

Of necessity, the time-limited visit targets the high-probability diagnosis (e.g., gastritis, duodenitis) while considering the possibility of the "must-never-miss" diagnoses (e.g., gastric cancer). The focused clinical encounter will include exploration of psychosocial topics, such as the patient's need to take a second job to cover credit card debt or concerns about a child in trouble at school. The experienced physician knows how often these nonphysical issues hold the key to understanding the patient's illness.

High-yield questions are how the skilled generalist focuses the time-limited clinical encounter. These questions are open-ended and can often begin with, "Tell me about . . ." They can be phrased in ways that are most comfortable to each physician and in complexity appropriate to the patient's understanding. The high-yield questions are used along with standard queries about: "How long have you had chest pain?" "Does the pain radiate anywhere?" and "Have you taken any medicine for the chest pain?" The full scope of the problem may finally become clear with the response to the open-ended query: "Tell me about what's been going on lately." or "Let's talk about what's most stressful in your life right now."

The following are six areas of high-yield questions. For each I have described a rationale, with some examples. Specific questions are listed, in varying levels of specificity, for both the patient and for you or me, the physician.

What Is the Reason for the Visit?

Patients visit physicians for many reasons, which are not always self-evident. A 65-year-old man came on a first visit, requesting a "complete physical examination." In response to a question, "Why?", I learned that the patient was planning a second marriage, that there had been a question of a prostate nodule in the past, and that he needed to know more about his health outlook to make some financial decisions. If I had not dug deeper, I would have failed to meet the patient's needs for the encounter.

The reasons for a visit may be classified under five headings (see Table 1.2). Most new-problem visits are for the diagnosis and treatment of physical problems, such as earache. The next most common category, concern about the meaning of a sign or symptom, includes many instances in which the patient with a problem is less bothered by the discomfort than by what the discomfort might *mean*. For example, in Chapter 17, Andrew Harris comes to the physician with back pain that began while lifting boxes at work; there is some radiation of pain to the right leg and foot. Is Mr. Harris in the office for relief of his pain so that he can sleep at night and return to work soon? Is he here because he is concerned about the possibility of a herniated disc necessitating back surgery, as happened to his brother? Or is the visit for an administrative purpose—to establish a workers' compensation claim?

Patients sometimes identify their problems as social or emotional, but more often such problems are offered as physical complaints, sometimes referred to as a "ticket of admission" (to health care). One young married woman visited my office repeatedly complaining of lower abdominal pains. She and her husband had three small children and their income was limited. The chief problem seemed to be that he spent most evenings playing softball and drinking with his friends, leaving her alone at home with the children. Although the patient continued to offer a physical complaint, her "reason for the visit" was, in my opinion, a social problem.

TABLE 1.2. Why patients visit physicians: problems and needs that prompt patients to initiate medical encounters

Reason	Example
Physical problem	Ankle sprain
Worry or concern	Coughed up sputum with flecks of blood
Administrative purpose	Insurance medical examination
Emotional problem	Anxiety
Social problem	Loneliness

Questions for the patient:

- What do we need to accomplish on this visit?
- Is there anything you are concerned (or worried) about?
- Tell me why you are here with this problem *at this time.*
- How can I help you at this visit?

Questions for the physician to consider:

- Does the patient's stated problem seem "not quite right?"
- Might the patient, for some reason, have misled the receptionist or nurse (or me) about the complaint?
- Have I possibly made an incorrect assumption about the patient's objectives?
- Is the reason for the patient's visit here today someone else's?

Am I Listening Carefully to What the Patient Is Trying to Tell Me?

There is an old clinical aphorism: Listen to the patient; he (or she) is telling you the diagnosis.

This need to listen carefully extends to all phases of the clinical encounter. It begins with thinking about why the patient came (and perhaps why he or she came *today*) complaining of, for example, abdominal pain, the response to a remark by a family member in the room, a comment about some part of the physical examination, or the objection to a suggested therapeutic intervention. The phrase "listening with the third ear" is sometimes used to describe this type of active listening.

In the lexicon of decision analysis, all the above are defined as "cues." The following are some examples from my practice: One patient was a 14-year-old girl who asked if birth control pills might help her acne. What she really sought was a prescription for oral contraceptives because of an emerging sexual relationship with her boyfriend. In another instance, I watched as a patient's neck muscles tightened and he crossed his arms when I asked casually, "How are things at home?" In this instance, his response, "Okay," turned out to be evasive, and on further inquiry I was able to link his chest pains and the repeated arguments with his wife about his perceived need to work long hours overtime. A 4-year-old girl who had always been lively was noted to be withdrawn and avoiding eye contact; this turned out to be the tip-off to childhood sexual abuse.

In Chapter 25, high-school basketball player Kendra Nelson visits the physician with the second ankle sprain in 4 months. Although she cannot bear weight and must hop rather than walk, she insists that the pain is "not really bad." Is Kendra minimizing the pain so that she can get an early release to return to her basketball team? Is she under peer or parental pressure to return to sports? Is she concerned that the physician may apply a cast that would interfere with a planned social activity?

Following the path of a clinical cue is often accomplished over several visits. A 42-year-old school teacher with migraine headaches insisted on her first two visits that everything in her life "couldn't be better." The reportedly "perfect" life proved to be a cue, and on the third visit we discussed her threatened layoff at work, her husband's drinking problem, and the concerns about their 15-year-old son's suspected drug use. In such instances, a sense of uncertainty can be a useful diagnostic tool.[11]

The ongoing attention—and revisiting—of clinical cues leads to the *continuing evolving diagnosis.* The clinician begins to generate hypotheses upon learning the chief complaint, or perhaps even before. Diagnostic possibilities are rejected, validated, or set aside for future consideration. The complex origins of the patient's symptoms and their interrelatedness to life events is most often clarified over time.

The awareness of the evolutionary nature of diagnosis helps the generalist deal with undifferentiated health care problems, such as fatigue and dizziness. It also helps the clinician tolerate the diagnostic ambiguity and complexity often found in primary care. This comfort with sometimes murky health problems actually characterizes those who choose family practice and other primary care specialties.[12] It also helps explain why generalists as a group tend to be those who can see possibilities, can think in patterns, and are intrigued by the process of clinical reasoning.

Questions for the patient:

- Is there some aspect of today's problem that we should discuss further?
- Events in a person's life can affect health. What is going on in your life that might be affecting your health?
- Is any part of the physical examination causing you concern?
- Are there ways that you and your family could improve your health that we should discuss?

Questions for the physician to consider:

- Has the patient seemed reluctant to discuss certain issues?
- Does there seem to be a part of the problem that I do not yet understand?
- Does the patient seem inappropriately sensitive to some part of the physical examination?
- Is there some apparently obvious resource—such as family support, time, or money—that the patient seems reluctant to use? If so, why?

What Is the Meaning of the Illness to the Patient?

Think back to the last time you had the flu, with high fever, achiness, and fatigue. Along with the need to stay in bed for a few days to get well, what did the flu mean to you? Did it mean that you would miss class or a sports event? Might it have meant that you would be absent for an important examination or that you might perform poorly on the test? Could it be that you were not prepared for the examination, and were, in fact, happy for a delay? Perhaps the chief concern was the economic impact of the flu—the cost of care or the loss of a weekend job. Did the chills and fever remind you of the first stages of pneumonia that ended with the death of a grandparent? Or did the flu symptoms have some other special meaning for you?

Disease and illness are not synonymous. Disease refers to a biomechanical, physiologic, or psychologic dysfunction. Illness includes the patient's disease—with all its pain, worry, inconvenience, or loss—and places it in the context of the life, family, community, and society of the affected individual. Ellen Harris (Chapter 16) visits your office with a complaint of vaginal discharge. She is married and works as a secretary. A straightforward problem? Probably, but not necessarily. Could the symptom mean loss of sexual relations with her husband for a week or more? Does this mean he will be angry? Could she have passed an infection to him? Could the infection have been caught from him? Could that mean that he acquired it someone?

The physician must never neglect the patient's unspoken concerns: Will I be able to return to work after my heart attack? Will my husband still love me after my mastectomy? Might I pass my chest cold (or infectious mononucleosis, or skin rash, or chlamydia infection) to my partner?

Another example: In Chapter 5, Harold Nelson, age 76, develops urinary incontinence. What might this mean to him? "Will I have to go to the hospital?" "Will I need an operation?" "Will I need to go to a nursing home?" Although Mr. Nelson may be hesitant to ask these questions, it is likely that they have occurred to him.

It is important to understand the meaning of the sick role and the legitimization of illness. When you or I are sick, we are excused from our usual duties, and others offer medicine, food, and support. That is, we are allowed to assume *the sick role.* Part of the contract, however, is that we will make every effort to get well—and no longer assume the sick role. Of course the sick role has definite advantages, not the least of which are reduced responsibility and increased service by others. Not surprisingly, some persons would prefer to prolong the sick role, and the physician may become involved. Many office visits are concerned with legitimization of the sick role, whether explicitly by signing an excuse for work or implicitly by writing a prescription for a cough or renewing a physical therapy order for a painful neck.

If you overlook the contextual meaning of the illness to patients such as Mrs. Harris or Mr. Nelson, has your clinical encounter—your "procedure"—been successful?

Questions for the patient:

- What do you believe is the cause of the illness?
- Tell me how you feel about this illness.
- How does this illness affect your activities at home or at work?
- What would getting well mean to you?

Questions for the physician to consider:

- How might this illness be affecting the patient's self-image?
- What are the implications of the patient assuming the sick role?
- Might this illness remind the patient of something that happened to a family member or friend?
- Might you—the physician—have personal experience or feelings that are affecting your judgment about this patient's illness?

What Is the Impact of the Illness on the Family?

If you have any doubt that illness is a family affair, ask any child, sibling, or parent of a person with a chronic problem such as asthma, diabetes mellitus, or cerebral palsy. Resources and attention that should be equally shared are diverted to the identified "patient." The patient's sick role eventually becomes a family burden, and other family members come to think of themselves as caretakers. Anger begets guilt and the illness permeates all family relationships. Eventually, the illness becomes part of the family lore.

Describing the legacy of migraine in her own family, Anne Walling, M.D. (author of Chapter 7) writes, "My father's severe attacks were part of our family's normal pattern of life. Like spells of bad weather, they were unpredictable, significant events that appeared to take a perverse delight in disrupting the most intricately planned and eagerly anticipated events." And then, "My mother abhorred migraine and grimly warned us against developing even remotely migrainous symptoms."[13]

The effect of illness on a family is not predictable. Chronic, recurrent childhood illness such as renal failure or hyperactivity can be the stress that results in disruption of a young family, and many parents of leukemic children see their marriages end in divorce. On the other hand, I have cared for a family with a child whose asthma attacks seemed to occur at just the times needed to divert the parents' attention to the child and away from their own arguments.

In Chapter 3, you will meet Ann Martino-Priestley, age 22, and her husband Luke. Ann is pregnant with their first child. Of course, pregnancy is not an illness, but it will have an impact on the couple/family. How does each feel about the pregnancy? How will a child affect their relationship? Can they afford to have a baby at this time? Will Ann be able to continue to work? What about Luke's studies for his MBA degree? How might all of these issues affect health care decisions?

Questions for the patient:

- How is your spouse (or children, parents, partner, etc.) affected by this illness?
- What are you hearing from others about your illness?
- Tell me what has changed in your relationships since the illness began.
- How would things be different at home if you were well?

Questions for the physician to consider:

- Who, besides the patient, is affected by this illness?
- What emotions might the patient's family be experiencing: sorrow, anger, abandonment, frustration, guilt?
- Have I, as physician, spoken with key people in my patient's life?
- By engaging in the care of this patient's illness, what might be the effect on me and my family?

What Is the Appropriate Locus of Care for this Person's Illness?

The seminal work on the locus of care was the 1961 paper by White et al.[14] showing that of 1000 adults "at risk," each month: 750 reported one or more illnesses or injuries; 250 of these persons consulted a physician one or more times; 9 of these patients were admitted to hospital; 5 patients were referred to another physician; and 1 patient was referred to a university medical center.

Some thoughts about this study and what it means today: Note that although 75% of adults reported an illness or injury during a month, only one illness/injury in three resulted in a medical encounter; fully two-thirds of care was home care in which the physician was not directly involved. The consultation rate was 2%, less than the 7% to 10% generalist consultation rates of today, but, of course, the White study recorded contact with any physician, which necessarily included a large number of self-referrals to specialists. Finally, there was only one academic medical center admission among the 1000 at-risk adults, a key finding considering that research data and therapeutic guidelines tend to come from academic medical centers and thus are based on 0.1% of the population.

A current issue in managed care centers around appropriate use of consultation and referral. The following family practice approach to locus of care was presented in the first edition of *Family Medicine: Principles and Practice*[15]:

Definitive Care: The physician provides independent care, perhaps with the participation of ancillary personnel, but without subspecialist consultation or referral. Examples include depression, type 2 diabetes mellitus, and an undisplaced fracture of the fibular malleolus. The residency trained family practice generalist should be competent to manage 85% to 90% of Definitive Care problems without need for consultation or referral.

Shared Care: These problems generally necessitate consultation for some aspect of diagnosis or therapy. Care is thus shared by the generalist and subspecialist for problems such as thyroid mass or active pulmonary tuberculosis. Some 7% to 10% of problems will be best managed by Shared Care.

Supportive Care: These are clearly subspecialty problems such as extensive third degree burns or retinal detachment. The generalist has the responsibility to direct the patient to appropriate care and to maintain educational and emotional support for the patient and family.

The physician's decisions in locus of care options will be guided by individual choices in interest, competence, and comfort levels. In our Family Practice Center, some physicians perform colposcopy (as a Definitive Care procedure); others refer patients needing colposcopy (for them, it is thereby a Shared Care procedure). Of course, physicians are responsible for only part of the decision making. Patient preferences play a role, as do practice guidelines of the health care organization or hospital.

In Chapter 21, we encounter an increasingly common locus-of-care decision: Mark McCarthy, age 28, is human immunodeficiency virus (HIV) positive and for 3 weeks has had a fever and cough productive of yellow-gray sputum. His parents ask, "Is it safe for him to stay at home, or should he be in the hospital? Should he have a consultation with a specialist? Should a specialist be in charge of his care? By having him living at home, are we—his parents—at risk?" Answers to these and related questions are often complex, and may be clouded by misinformation, fear, protection of turf, and concerns about maintaining practice volume.

Questions for the patient:

- Have you had this problem before, and how was it managed?
- Tell me your view of the treatment needed today.
- What concerns do you have about our plans for management and follow-up?
- Tell me your understanding of the reason we are seeking consultation and the questions we are hoping to answer.

Questions for the physician to consider:

- Is the problem within my area of competence and comfort?
- Does the patient expect a consultation and, if so, is it medically appropriate?

- Is there an administrative need that would call for a consultation or referral: insurance, litigation, disability determination, or other?
- Am I making my consultation/referral recommendation for the right reasons?

What Resources Are Available to Help in Managing the Illness?

The rise in managed care in the United States is a reflection of what families have known all along: health care resources are not limitless. Individuals and families have always had to face limits on care that can be given in the home, cost of medication purchased, and nursing home care provided. Recognition of resources that are available—and those that are not available—is important in assuring optimal care for patients.

The categories of resources are listed in Table 1.3. Financial resources include the direct ability to pay and also medical insurance, emergency assistance in times of disaster, and loans or gifts from family. Care by family members, visiting nurses, community health workers, nurses, physicians, and other providers all constitute medical care resources. The time and energy resources may come from the patient, the family, medical personnel, and volunteers such as neighbors or church members. Patient and family knowledge of medicine, community contacts, and funding sources can affect the quality of care ultimately received, as can the availability of medical equipment and supplies.

In Chapter 4, Allison Harris is brought to your office by her mother "for her 1-year-old check-up and shots." There are resource implications even in this routine visit: Mrs. Harris missed several hours of work to bring Allison to the appointment. There is a cost to the Harris family for the check-up that is not covered by their health insurance. There is a vaccine cost that, although covered by a state-subsidized program, is inflated by the hidden cost of vaccine-related litigation.

Generalists work together with patients, families, community agencies, hospitals, and others to help ensure the appropriate and cost-effective

TABLE 1.3. Resources used to manage patients' health care problems

Resource	Example
Financial	Health insurance
Medical care	Office visit to physician
Time and energy	Middle-aged person stays at home caring for elderly parent
Knowledge	Information from medical reference book
Equipment and supplies	Wheelchair from community loan program

deployment of resources. The higher priced prescription is not necessarily better, and not every patient with pneumonia needs hospitalization. The Medical Outcomes Study demonstrated that, even when data are controlled for patient mix, generalists use fewer health care resources than subspecialists. Among the generalist specialties, family physicians use the fewest resources of all.[16]

Questions for the patient:

- Who is your most important support person, and how is he or she involved in caring for this illness?
- Are you now a client of any community agencies that could help today?
- Tell me about family or friends that could help us at this time.
- Is there some special way you deal with problems—reading about them, meditation, pastoral counseling—and how can we put this to work now?

Questions for the physician to consider:

- What are the patient's personal and family resources that can be used?
- What community resources might be useful in management?
- Does the illness have public health or community implications?
- Have I appropriately involved the patient and family in resource use decisions?

Why Is Generalist Care Important?

Writing on his own decision to become a general practitioner, British physician Robin Hull recalls, "I began to look at patients not as a means of locomotion of interesting pathology, but as people who were quite fascinating in their own right."[17] Dr. Hull's comment provides insight into why technological medicine is unsatisfying to many. Patients are people, not machines with broken parts, and their illnesses have diverse origins which include the family, the community, the workplace, and the complex relationships of a lifetime.

Generalist health care is not a substitute for scientifically oriented and research-based clinical activity; actually generalist care expands the dimensions of disease-oriented clinical practice by adding the contextual basis through which both physician and patient come to understand the *illness.* Is there a clinical payoff to such patient-centered behavior? Certainly the diagnosis of acute myocardial infarction—documented on the electrocardiogram—is enhanced by understanding the patient's high fat diet, which began in childhood at the family dining room table, the cigarette smoking started with friends in high school, the long hours at work, and the recent concern about the company takeover that may cost his job at age 56. Is all this reflected on the ECG tracing? No. Is the context important? Definitely!

Generalist health care calls for a committed investment of self. As a family physician I become, in a sense, a member of the family; on home visits I see my name and telephone number posted on the refrigerator door along with those of other family members and the clergy. The generalist physician is a member of the community; he or she is active in clubs, civic groups, and church—and enjoys dealing with patients in these settings.

Most of all, generalist health care means *being there* for the patient and family. This has been called accessibility, but it's more. It is making the follow-up telephone call. It is asking the patient about the disabled parent at home. It is showing the patient that you care. Almost 30 years ago I cared for an elderly man dying at home of the multiple complications of a hard life and a poor genetic endowment. He and his wife lived in a trailer in the woods about 40 minutes from my office, and I visited him every Wednesday afternoon—my day for house calls for my practice group. One Monday morning the patient died at home, somewhat unexpectedly. My schedule was overbooked and the waiting room was full of patients. I did the logical thing. I sent my partner to pronounce the patient dead, sign the death certificate, and comfort the widow. After all, it was my partner's day to do the house calls. I next saw the widow at the viewing (yes, many generalists make a final visit to their patients). Here she quietly let me know that she had expected *me* to come when he died. I had failed to *be there* when she needed me. She taught me a lesson about being a physician that I still remember.

Family practice and today's generalist physicians are the current expression of the "horse and buggy" doctors of early America.[18] We have assumed the role of maintaining patient-centered values while providing state-of-the-art health care in an increasingly technical age. We have aspired to be the standard-bearers of, as Pellegrino has described, medicine as a "moral enterprise grounded in a covenant of trust."[19] Changing health care economics predict that the health care systems of the next few decades will be based on a primary care centered model.

The secret of keeping our commitment to patients and yet achieving the universally accessible, affordable new care model will be to remain true to our first principles—offering our patients competent medical care that includes consideration of how their acute or chronic illness is part of the fabric of their lives.

References

1. Vanselow NA, Donaldson MS, Yordy KD. A new definition of primary care. JAMA 1995;273:192–4.

2. A statement on the generalist physician from the American Boards of Family Practice and Internal Medicine. JAMA 1994;271:315–6.
3. Wartman SA, Wilson M, Kahn N. The generalist health work force: issues and goals. J Gen Intern Med 1994;9 supplement 1 (April):S7–S13.
4. Rivo ML. Division of Medicine Update. Washington DC: USPHS Health Resources and Services Administration, Bureau of Health Professions. Summer, 1992.
5. Balint M. The doctor, his patient and the illness. New York: International Universities Press, 1957.
6. National Ambulatory Medical Care Survey: U.S. Department of Health and Human Services, Public Health Service, National Center for Health Statistics, 1993.
7. Taylor RB. The clinical encounter as the family physician's procedure: looking ahead to the new millenium. In press.
8. Stadler DS, Zyzanski SJ, Stange KC. Family physicians and current inpatient practice. J Am Board Fam Pract 1997;10:357–62.
9. AAMC policy on the generalist physician. Acad Med. 1993; 68:1–6.
10. Council on Graduate Medical Education: Fourth report to Congress and the Department of Health & Human Services Secretary. Washington DC: USPHS Public Health Services, Health Resources and Services Administration, 1994.
11. Fargason CA, Evans HH, Ashworth CS, Capper SA. The importance of preparing medical students to manage different types of uncertainty. Acad Med 1997;72:688–92.
12. Taylor AD. How to choose a medical specialty, third edition. Philadelphia: Saunders, 1999.
13. Walling AD. The legacy of migraine. J Fam Pract 1994;38:629–30.
14. White KL, Williams F, Greenberg B. Ecology of medical care. N Engl J Med 1961;265:885–91.
15. Taylor RB, Family Medicine: Principles and practice, first edition. New York: Springer Verlag, 1978.
16. Tarlov AR, Ware JE, Greenfield S. The medical outcomes study: an application of methods for monitoring the results of medical care. JAMA 1989; 262:925–30.
17. Hull R. Just a GP. Oxford, England: Radcliff, 1994.
18. Stanard JR. Caring for America: the story of Family Practice. Virginia Beach, VA: Donning, 1997.
19. Pellegrino ED. Dismembering the Hippocratic oath. Boston: Boston University Alumni Report, Fall, 1995:11–17.

Assignments for Small Group Discussion

The following are assignments for class discussion. They are based on the model of a 6-week Family Practice/Primary Care Clerkship in the clinical years of medical school. The assignments further assume that students are spending part of their time each week in the offices of practicing physicians.

Week 1

Present a case that illustrates the significance of *The Reason for the Visit.* The case presented may, for example, show how a psychosocial problem was presented as a physical complaint, or how the identification of the true reason for the visit was the key to understanding a puzzling clinical problem.

Week 2

Present a case that highlights the importance of *Listening to What the Patient Is Trying to Tell.* An example might be an instance when you or your doctor used an open-ended question to clarify a complex clinical presentation. Or, perhaps tell about an instance when you overlooked a key clinical issue because you missed a cue offered by the patient.

Week 3

Describe a case that exemplifies the importance of *The Meaning of the Illness to the Patient.* Perhaps describe an instance in which the disease actually offered a special benefit to the patient, or tell about a patient whose symptom held some special meaning that was revealed only later in the encounter.

Week 4

Present a case that highlights *The Impact of Illness on the Family.* This may be an instance of one person's illness having an unfavorable impact on the life of one or more family members. Another approach might be identifying an instance in which disease advantaged someone in the family and how this might influence the outcome of care.

Week 5

Describe an instance that illustrates the importance of the *Appropriate Locus of Care for a Person's Illness.* You might tell of an instance of planned, timely consultation or referral, and how this might have been valuable in care. An alternative might be a time in which a patient or family member insisted on a consultation or referral that your physician believed inappropriate, and how the physician dealt with the request.

Week 6

Tell about a clinical case in which the *Resources Available to Help in Managing Illness* were important in the outcome of care. You may choose an instance in which your physician referred the patient to a social service agency, and tell how this influenced care. On the other hand, you may present an instance in which the lack of access to resources had a profound impact on the clinical outcome, and what might be done in the future to help patients gain access to needed resources.

2

Clinical Prevention

EVAN W. KLIGMAN AND FRANK A. HALE

Clinical prevention is the connecting link between public health and primary care. Health education and health promotion counseling skills are among the most important tools in the family physician's medical bag. A major challenge facing the family physician is how to bridge the gap between clinical prevention knowledge and practice, recognizing the impact of personal behaviors on health. The traditional biomedical approach to the diagnosis and treatment of disease is only a partial response to addressing the health care needs of patients. Americans want preventive care; according to national polls, most adults would change their doctor if they believed they were not getting appropriate clinical preventive services.[1] Patient care must encompass a prospective preventive approach toward helping individuals and families assume major responsibility for their own health-related behaviors.[2,3]

Background

Family Physician's Office

Many factors affecting preventive care can be modified by the physician: office hours, convenience, location, private dressing rooms to prepare for procedures and screening tests, flow charts and checklists, colored chart stickers to flag certain risk factors, and follow-up protocols for behavior change counseling or screening tests initiated.[4] Modifications in the reception area, examination rooms, and patient flow alterations are environmental strategies that can enhance the delivery of preventive services.[4] The office should have a system of continuous improvement and monitoring, inclusive of self-audits, to promote a high level of patient satisfaction and acceptance of clinical preventive services.[5] Organizational and leadership commitment is essential to elicit policy change when necessary and provide necessary resources (e.g., patient educators and materials). Given limited resources, the clinical setting must provide effective, efficient use of appointment time. Procedures must be established to emphasize the importance of patients returning for follow-up visits when undergoing behavioral change or for repeat screening.[6]

Physician–Patient Encounter

Family physicians must incorporate a preventive attitude in the context of each patient encounter. The *Guide to Clinical Preventive Services*[5] of the U.S. Preventive Services Task Force places great emphasis on integrating clinical prevention into patient care, noting that counseling and patient education may be the most valuable clinical prevention activities, that preventive services are an appropriate part of all visits, and that all patients should be counseled. Each acute or chronic problem cared for in the family physician's office should have a prevention component. Indeed, the primary care physician is expected to deliver a range of preventive services, including health enhancement, risk avoidance, risk reduction, early identification, and complication reduction.

The concept of offering clinical prevention to all patients based on their age, sex, and risk level is important for the family physician. Clinical preventive services identified by the U.S. Preventive Services Task Force[5] encompass four categories: counseling, screening, immunizations, and chemoprophylactic agents. The Task Force's report, when combined with the preventive recommendations for asymptomatic adults generated by other groups[7,8] and the work of individual clinicians, provides a database to justify the selection of appropriate preventive clinical services for individuals and families.

Preventable Factors Contributing to Premature Death

Although the role of the family physician is critical to the management of disease and acute care, the overwhelming threat to health for most people is related to nonmedical factors,[9] including health-related life style behaviors, the environment, and genetic background. Family physicians must base clinical prevention strategies on a spectrum of influences. McGinnis and Foege have identified the top 10 "actual" causes of death in the United States, illustrating the fact that more than 1 million deaths in 1990 could have been postponed or averted by the delivery of appropriate clinical preventive services[10] (Table 2.1).

About 10% of premature deaths result from inadequate access to health care services. Shorter life expectancy is associated with lower educational and income levels. Common life style risk factors, such as smoking, obesity, stress, poor nutrition, and alcohol and drug use, contribute to more than 50% of premature deaths. Environmental factors, such as

TABLE 2.1. Actual causes of death in the United States in 1990

Cause of death	Estimated no. of deaths	Percent of total deaths
Tobacco use	400,000	19
Diet/activity patterns	300,000	14
Alcohol	100,000	5
Microbial agents	90,000	4
Toxic agents	60,000	3
Firearms	35,000	2
Sexual behavior	30,000	1
Motor vehicles	25,000	1
Illicit use of drugs	20,000	<1
Total	1,060,000	50

Source: McGinnis and Foege.[10] With permission.

sanitation, food safety, pollution, toxic exposures, and occupational risks and hazards, contribute to about 20% of premature deaths. Family history, genetic influence, and inherited susceptibility to certain diseases are believed to be responsible for another 20% of premature deaths.[9] For instance, the relative risk related to genetic susceptibility for many adult-onset disorders may range from 2 to 180.

Selection of Clinical Preventive Services for Individuals and Families

General Guidelines for Developing Protocols

Clinical preventive services are an integral part of the patient care process. The traditional concept of the annual physical examination has been replaced by the practice of conducting selective health maintenance procedures at periodic intervals based on rational guidelines. Practice guidelines have been developed to reduce inappropriate services, control geographic variations in practice patterns, and encourage more efficient and effective use of resources. Efficient delivery of clinical preventive services means that not all patients need every clinical intervention. Identification of high risk patients (see Tables 2.2, 2.4–2.7, 2.9–2.11, below), whether based on personal or family medical history (or both), a particular life style behavior, or "physiologic" rather than "chronologic" age, is important when customizing clinical prevention.

This process of "risk assessment" involves collection of data from various sources on the patient's risk factors (personal characteristics, physiologic parameters, symptoms, or preclinical disease states) that increase his or her chances of developing a disease.[6] The accuracy of preventive intervention (e.g., screening test) and effectiveness of intervention (e.g., early detection) must also be taken into consideration when selecting the conditions to target with preventive services. For instance, the accuracy of a screening test is determined by its sensitivity and specificity. Sensitivity is a measurement of the proportion of persons with a condition who test positive. Conversely, specificity is a measurement of the proportion of persons without a condition who test negative. If sensitivity is low or poor, there is a high percentage of false-negative test results. If specificity is low or poor, there is a high percentage of false-positive test results. Additional evaluation of a screening test includes the proportion of patients with a positive test result who have the disease, or the positive predictive value of the test. Conversely, the proportion of patients with negative test results who do not have a condition is known as the negative predictive value.

Determining the effectiveness of early detection is another criterion for measuring the value of a screening test. It is determined by evaluating treatment efficacy, lead time, and length bias and assessing population benefits. Potential adverse effects must also be considered. In addition to a screening test being effective for detecting asymptomatic disease, the condition to be screened for must be a significant public health problem with respect to morbidity and mortality; its natural history must be understood; adequate treatment for the disease should be available; and the costs of screening and treatment must be reasonable and acceptable to the patient and provider.

Other criteria for determining the effectiveness of other preventive interventions have been established by the U.S. Preventive Services Task Force. There must be evidence of: efficacious vaccines when selecting immunizations; effective counseling strategies and known risk reduction efficacy when selecting counseling interventions; and proved efficacy and counseling effectiveness when selecting chemoprophylactic agents. Guidebooks are available to assist the clinician in implementing selected preventive interventions once risks have been assessed.[11]

Periodic Health Examination

The periodic health examination is the centerpiece of prevention in the office setting. Such visits should be targeted to the patient's risk profile and include a review of screening needs, health promotion counseling, and identification of immunization and chemoprophylaxis needs. It is now customary to include clinical prevention as a component of any acute or chronic care visit. For most patients and most family physicians caring for patients in managed care plans, these visits provide the only opportunity for receiving preventive services. These visits may, in fact, provide both appropriate and timely opportunities for physicians to counsel patients. Thus one or two preventive interventions should be delivered at all patient encounters. The discovery of a pregnancy may become a "teachable moment" to counsel the mother-to-be on the hazards of smoking, or knowledge of a family history of breast cancer may be the basis for recommending that a patient undergo mammography.

Revising and Updating Protocols

Because guidelines and recommendations may change as new data become available, it is important for family physicians to stay abreast of current information. The field of clinical prevention is rapidly advancing. A number of large group practices and health maintenance organizations (HMOs) have standing committees to update their prevention protocols, taking into consideration such factors as costs, effectiveness, efficacy, and the unique profile and needs of their enrollees.

Delivery of Preventive Services to Special or High-Risk Populations

Populations at risk pose important health challenges to our society owing to higher rates of death and disability based on environmental, cultural, or economic risk factors and life style practices. Special populations include low-income groups, minorities, and people with disabilities.[2] For each of these subgroups, special clinical prevention efforts may be indicated. They must frequently compensate for economic, racial, or linguistic barriers. Many underserved populations are cared for on an acute-need basis, and the clinical preventive needs ordinarily available to the mainstream population are not as readily available.

Special training in understanding other cultural perspectives is necessary to be effective at prevention with special populations. The physician must develop sensitivity toward individual perspectives on health and well-being as well as be familiar with particular health beliefs of culturally or ethnically defined populations. Ethnosensitivity can enhance communication, patient satisfaction, and willingness to modify behaviors.[12]

Family practice training is increasingly recognized as providing physicians with the necessary skill to practice population-based medicine. Indeed, a number of governmental strategic plans and directives indicate that family physicians are expected to play an increasing role in improving the well-being of underserved Americans and take the lead in designing preventive health care strategies and personal health promotion activities.[2] One of these efforts comprises linkages between family medicine education programs and Public Health Service clinics established to provide community-based, comprehensive, prevention-oriented primary care services. The delivery of preventive services in these settings is based on a team approach involving health educators, mid-level health providers, and often volunteer lay health promoters from the community.

Clinical Preventive Services Guidelines

The most effective way to develop and maintain a preventive-oriented attitude is to care for patients utilizing a framework of specific guidelines and strategies for implementing preventive services. When focusing the preventive interventions, physicians should take into consideration the leading causes of death and disability for the patient's age group. The life cycle presented in this chapter is divided into nine stages. Providers should develop a stage system that most clearly reflects the age distribution of patients in their practice.

The system that follows is oriented toward a balanced family practice population. The age-specific Tables 2.2, 2.4, 2.6, and 2.9 are based on the second edition of *The Guide to Clinical Preventive Services* by the U.S. Preventive Services Task Force[5] and are recommendations of minimum preventive interventions.

General recommendations made by the AAFP Subcommittee on Periodic Health Intervention include the following:[8]

1. All new patients should undergo a comprehensive history and physical examination, have a database/health risk appraisal completed, and be exposed to various preventive services based on the recommended guidelines (outlined below).
2. Previous health records should be obtained to avoid duplication of services (e.g., pneumonia vaccine).
3. Additional services may be added routinely based on (1) protocols developed by each physician or practice or (2) the individual patient's risk profile.
4. Physicians must update their protocols as new scientific findings become available.

Birth to Ten Years

After preconception care and the prenatal period (see Chapter 3), the first 18 months of life remain the most formidable for establishing health patterns for years to come. During the first week, a number of screening interventions are recommended (Table 2.2). Counseling topics during the first year and a half include nutritional intake and injury prevention. Other preventive services include immunizations and chemoprophylaxis to prevent infectious diseases. Flow sheets and tracking forms are most useful

Table 2.2. Interventions considered and recommended for periodic health examination and leading causes of death: birth to 10 years

Leading causes of death

- Conditions originating in perinatal period
- Congenital anomalies
- Sudden infant death syndrome (SIDS)

Interventions for general population

SCREENING

- Height and weight
- Blood pressure
- Vision screen (age 3–4 years)
- Hemoglobinopathy screen (birth)[a]
- Phenylalanine level (birth)[b]
- T_4 and/or TSH (birth)[c]

COUNSELING

Injury Prevention

- Child safety car seats (age < 5 years)
- Lap-shoulder belts (age ≥ 5 years)
- Bicycle helmet, avoid bicycling near traffic
- Smoke detector, flame-retardant sleepwear
- Hot water heater temperature < 120°–130°F
- Window/stair guards, pool fence
- Safe storage of drugs, toxic substances, firearms, matches
- Syrup of ipecac, poison control phone number
- CPR training for parents/caretakers

Diet and exercise

- Breast-feeding, iron-enriched formula and foods (infants and toddlers)
- Limit fat and cholesterol, maintain caloric balance, emphasize grains, fruits, vegetables (age 2 years)
- Regular physical activity[d]

Substance use

- Effects of passive smoking[d]
- Antitobacco message[d]

Dental health

- Regular visits to dental care provider[d]
- Advice about baby bottle tooth decay[d]

IMMUNIZATIONS

- Diphtheria-tetanus-pertussis (DTP)[e]
- Oral poliovirus (OPV)[f]
- Measles/mumps/rubella (MMR)[g]
- *H. influenzae* type b (Hib) conjugate[h]
- Hepatitis B[i]
- Varicella[j]

CHEMOPROPHYLAXIS

- Ocular prophylaxis (birth)

Interventions for high-risk populations

POPULATION	POTENTIAL INTERVENTIONS[k] [see detailed high risk (HR) definitions in footnotes]
Preterm or low birth weight	Hemoglobin/hematocrit (HR1)
Infants of mothers at risk for HIV	HIV testing (HR2)
Low-income; immigrants	Hemoglobin/hematocrit (HR1); PPD (HR3)
TB contacts	PPD (HR3)
Native Americans/Alaska natives	Hemoglobin/hematocrit (HR1); PPD (HR3); hepatitis A vaccine (HR4); pneumococcal vaccine (HR5)
Travelers to developing countries	Hepatitis A vaccine (HR4)
Residents of long-term care facilities	PPD (HR3); hepatitis A vaccine (HR4); influenza vaccine (HR6)
Certain chronic medical conditions	PPD (HR3); pneumococcal vaccine (HR5); influenza vaccine (HR6)
Increased individual or community lead exposure	Blood lead level (HR7)
Inadequate water fluoridation	Daily fluoride supplement (HR8)
Family history of skin cancer; nevi/fair skin, eyes, hair	Avoid excess/midday sun, use protective clothing[d] (HR9)

[a]Whether screening should be universal or targeted to high-risk groups depends on the proportion of high-risk individuals in the screening area and other considerations.
[b]If done during first 24 hours of life, repeat by age 2 weeks.
[c]Optimally between days 2 and 6 but in all cases before newborn nursery discharge.
[d]The ability of clinician counseling to influence this behavior is unproved.

TABLE 2.2 (*continued*)

[e]At 2, 4, 6, and 12–18 months; once between ages 4–6 years (DTaP may be used at 15 months and older).
[f]At 2, 4, 6–18 months; once between ages 4–6 years.
[g]At 12–15 months and 4–6 years.
[h]At 2, 4, 6, and 12–15 months; no dose needed at 6 months if PRP-OMP vaccine is used for first two doses.
[i]At birth and 1 and 6 months; or 0–2 months, 1–2 months later, and 6–18 months. If not done during infancy: current visit and 1 and 6 months later.
[j]At 12–18 months; or older child without history of chickenpox or previous immunization. Include information on risk during adulthood, duration of immunity, and potential need for booster doses.
[k]*HR1* = infants age 6–12 months who are living in poverty, Blacks, Native Americans, and Alaska natives; immigrants from developing countries; preterm or low birth weight infants; or infants whose principal dietary intake is unfortified cow's milk. *HR2* = infants born to high-risk mothers whose HIV status is unknown. Women at high risk include those with past or present injection drug use; persons who exchange sex for money or drugs and their sex partners; injection drug-using, bisexual, or HIV-positive sex partners currently or in past; persons seeking treatment for sexually transmitted diseases (STDs); blood transfusion during 1978–1985. *HR3* = persons infected with HIV, close contacts of persons with known or suspected tuberculosis (TB), persons with medical risk factors associated with TB, immigrants from countries with high TB prevalence, medically underserved low-income populations (including homeless), residents of long-term care facilities. *HR4* = persons ≥ 2 years of living in or traveling to areas where the disease is endemic and where periodic outbreaks occur (e.g., those in countries with high or intermediate endemicity; certain Alaska natives, Pacific islanders, Native Americans, and religious communities). Consider for institutionalized children aged ≥ 2 years. Clinicians should also consider local epidemiology. *HR5* = immunocompetent persons ≥ 2 years with certain medical conditions, including chronic cardiac or pulmonary disease, diabetes mellitus, and anatomic asplenia; immunocompetent persons ≥ 2 years living in high-risk environments or social settings (e.g., certain Native American and Alaska native populations). *HR6* = annual vaccination of children ≥ 6 months who are residents of chronic care facilities or who have chronic cardiopulmonary disorders, metabolic diseases (including diabetes mellitus), hemoglobinopathies, immunosuppression, or renal dysfunction. *HR7* = children about age 12 months who (1) live in communities in which the prevalence of lead levels requiring individual intervention, including residential lead hazard control or chelation, is high or undefined; (2) live in or frequently visit a home built before 1950 with dilapidated paint or with recent or ongoing renovation or remodeling; (3) have close contact with a person who has an elevated lead level; (4) live near a lead industry or heavy traffic; (5) live with someone whose job or hobby involves lead exposure; (6) use lead-based pottery; or (7) take traditional ethnic remedies that contain lead. *HR8* = children living in areas with inadequate water fluoridation (< 0.6 ppm). *HR9* = persons with a family history of skin cancer, a large number of moles, atypical moles, poor tanning ability, or light skin, hair, and eye color.

during infancy and early childhood given the number of recommended interventions at each visit (Table 2.2; see also Table 2.4).

Universal immunization over the past 40 years has eliminated the threat of major infectious diseases to many children, a significant cause of mortality and morbidity in this age group. With the decrease in immunization rates among some groups of young children in the United States, there are regions with sporadic outbreaks of pertussis, measles, and other preventable communicable infectious diseases. Thus a second measles/mumps/rubella (MMR) immunization is now recommended at 4 to 6 years (Table 2.3).

Unintentional injuries are the major health problem for children in this age group. Periodic preventive interventions during this life period should focus on injury prevention. Environmental and socioeconomic factors are also significant determinants of health and illness in this age group. Poor children have a higher prevalence of learning disorders, mental retardation, vision and speech impairments, and emotional and behavioral problems. One serious cause of such developmental problems is lead exposure. More than 3 million children between age 6 months and 5 years showed high levels of serum lead (about 15 μg/dl) in 1984. By 1989 that number was reduced to 503,000 through implementation of national objectives.[3] Respiratory problems such as influenza and asthma are the chief illness-related reasons young children miss school. The role of parental smoking and passive smoking exposure, a major trigger of these illnesses, should be addressed periodically during this age period (Table 2.2; see also Table 2.4). Healthy child development depends on establishing healthy behaviors during this age period to avoid smoking and alcohol abuse and develop good nutrition and physical activity.

Screening for hypercholesterolemia in all children over age 2 is controversial. The U.S. Preventive Services Task Force has concluded there is insufficient evidence to recommend for or against routine screening of children and adolescents for cholesterol and other lipid disorders. Without data on the costs, risk, and benefits of intervention strategies for children with high cholesterol concentrations, general screening of all children for total cholesterol values must be considered carefully.[13] Many children with high cholesterol levels have normal levels during young adulthood in the absence of prescribed individual interventions.

The controversy regarding universal cholesterol screening in children was addressed by the National Cholesterol Education Program.[14] It calls for a dietary approach aimed at lowering the average cholesterol levels of all Americans above age 2[14] by consuming less than 30% of total calories from fat (with no more than 10% from saturated fatty acids) and less than 300 mg of dietary cholesterol intake per day. Selective screening is also recommended for children and adolescents at greatest risk of having high cholesterol as adults: (1) those whose parents or grandparents had coronary atherosclerosis or angiography before age 56; (2) those whose parents or grandparents had a myocardial infarction, angina, peripheral vascular disease, or sudden cardiac death before age 56; and (3) those whose parents' blood cholesterol level is above 240 mg/dl.

Other important interventions to promote cardiovascular health in children include counseling about obesity and smoking. Routine updating of the family history of cardiovascular disease during well-child visits is also important. Physicians should practice targeted screening to be effective in this area[15] (Table 2.2).

TABLE 2.3. Childhood immunization schedule

Vaccine	Age										
	Birth	1 mo	2 mo	4 mo	6 mo	12 mo	15 mo	18 mo	4–6 yr	11–12 yr	14–16 yr
Hepatitis B	HepB-1	HepB-2			HepB-3					Hep B	
Diphtheria/tetanus/pertussis (DPT)			DTaP or DTP	DTaP or DTP	DTaP or DTP		DTP or DTaP		DTP or DTaP	Td	
Haemophilus influenzae type B			Hib	Hib	Hib	Hib					
Polio			Polio	Polio		Polio			Polio		
Measles/mumps/rubella (MMR)						MMR			MMR or	MMR	
Varicella/zoster virus (Var)							Var			Var	

This schedule is approved by the CDC Advisory Committee on Immunization Practices, American Academy of Pediatrics, and American Academy of Family Physicians.

Hepatitis B: (1) Infants born to mothers who are negative for hepatitis B surface antigen (HBsAg) should receive 2.5 μg of Merck vaccine (Recombivax HB) or 10 μg of SmithKline Beecham vaccine (Engerix-B). The second dose should be administered ≥ 1 month after the first dose. (2) Infants born to HBsAg-positive mothers should receive 0.5 ml of hepatitis B immune globulin within 12 hours of birth and either 5 μg of Recombivax HB or 10 μg of Engerix-B at a separate site. The second dose is recommended at 1–2 months of age and the third dose at 6 months of age. (3) Infants born to mothers whose HbsAg status is unknown should receive either 5 μg of Recombivax HB or 10 μg of Engerix-B within 12 hours of birth. The second dose of vaccine is recommended at 1 month of age and the third dose at 6 months of age. (4) Adolescents who have not previously received three doses of hepatitis B vaccine should initiate or complete the series at the 11- to 12-year old visit. The second dose should be administered at least 1 month after the first dose and the third dose at least 4 months after the first dose and at least 2 months after the second dose.

Diphtheria/tetanus/pertussis: The fourth dose of DTP may be administered at 12 months of age if at least 6 months have elapsed since the third dose. DTaP (diphtheria and tetanus toxoids and acellular pertussis vaccine) is licensed for the fourth and/or fifth vaccine dose(s) for children aged ≥ 15 months and may be preferred for these doses in this age group. Td (tetanus and diphtheria toxoids, absorbed, for adult use) is recommended at 11–12 years of age if at least 5 years have elapsed since the last dose of DTP, DTaP, or DT.

Haemophilus influenzae type B: Three *H. influenzae* type B (Hib) conjugate vaccines are licensed for infant use. If the Merck vaccine (Pedvax- HIB) is administered at 2 and 4 months of age, a dose at 6 months is not required. After completing the primary series, any Hib conjugate vaccine may be used as a booster.

Polio: Providers may choose among 3 schedules: (1) Inactivated poliovirus vaccine (IPV) at 2 and 4 months; oral poliovirus (OPV) at 12 months and 4–6 years; (2) IPV at 2 and 4 months, 12 months, and 4–6 years; or (3) OPV at 2 and 4 months, 6–18 months, and 4–6 years. Oral poliovirus vaccine is recommended for routine infant vaccination. Inactivated poliovirus vaccine (IPV) is recommended for persons with a congenital or acquired immunodeficiency disease or an altered immune status as a result of disease or immunosuppressive therapy, as well as for their household contacts, and is an acceptable alternative for other persons. The primary three-dose series for IPV should be given with a minimum interval of 4 weeks between the first and second doses and 6 months between the second and third doses.

Measles/mumps/rubella: The second dose of MMR is routinely recommended at 4–6 years of age or at 11–12 years but may be administered at any visit, provided at least 1 month has elapsed since receipt of the first dose.

Varicella/zoster virus: Varicella-zoster virus vaccine can be administered to susceptible children any time after 12 months of age. Unvaccinated children who lack a reliable history of chickenpox should be vaccinated at the 11- to 12-year-old visit.

TABLE 2.4. Interventions considered and recommended for the periodic health examination and leading causes of death: ages 11–24 years

Leading causes of death	
Motor vehicle/other unintentional injuries	Malignant neoplasms
Homicide	Heart diseases
Suicide	
Interventions for general population	
SCREENING	*Diet and exercise*
Height and weight	Limit fat and cholesterol; maintain caloric balance; emphasize grains, fruits, vegetables
Blood pressure[a]	Adequate calcium intake (females)
Papanicolaou (Pap) test[b] (females)	Regular physical activity[e]
Chlamydia screen[c] (females > 20 years)	*Dental health*
Rubella serology or vaccination history[d] (females > 12 years)	Regular visits to dental care provider[e]
Assess for problem drinking	Floss; brush with fluoride toothpaste daily[e]
COUNSELING	IMMUNIZATIONS
Injury prevention	Tetanus/diphtheria (Td) boosters (11–16 years)
Lap/shoulder belts	Hepatitis B[f]
Bicycle/motorcycle/ATV helmets[e]	MMR (11–12 years)[g]
Smoke detector[e]	Varicella (11–12 years)[h]
Safe storage/removal of firearms[e]	Rubella[d] (females > 12 years)
Substance use	CHEMOPROPHYLAXIS
Avoid tobacco use	Multivitamin with folic acid (females planning/capable of pregnancy)
Avoid underage drinking and illicit drug use[e]	
Avoid alcohol/drug use while driving, swimming, boating[e]	
Sexual behavior	
STD prevention[e]: abstinence, avoid high-risk behavior; condoms/female barrier with spermicide	
Unintended pregnancy: contraception	
Interventions for high-risk populations	
POPULATION	POTENTIAL INTERVENTIONS (see detailed high risk definitions)
High-risk sexual behavior	RPR/VDRL (HR1); screen for gonorrhea (female) (HR2), HIV (HR3), *Chlamydia* (female) (HR4); hepatitis A vaccine (HR5)
Injection or street drug use	RPR/VDRL (HR1); HIV screen (HR3); hepatitis A vaccine (HR5); PPD (HR6); advice to reduce infection risk (HR7)
TB contacts; immigrants, low income	PPD (HR6)
Native Americans/Alaska natives	Hepatitis A vaccine (HR5): PPD (HR6); pneumococcal vaccine (HR8)
Travelers to developing countries	Hepatitis A vaccine (HR5)
Certain chronic medical conditions	PPD (HR6); pneumococcal vaccine (HR8); influenza vaccine (HR9)
Settings where adolescents and young adults congregate	Second MMR (HR10)
Susceptible to varicella, measles, mumps	Varicella vaccine (HR11); MMR (HR12)
Blood tranfusion between 1978–1985	HIV screen (HR3)
Institutionalized persons; health care/laboratory workers	Hepatitis A vaccine (HR5); PPD (HR6); influenza vaccine (HR9)
Family history of skin cancer; nevi/fair skin, eyes, hair	Avoid excess/midday sun, use protective clothing[e] (HR13)
Prior pregnancy with neural tube defect	Folic acid 4.0 mg (HR14)
Inadequate water fluoridation	Daily fluoride supplement (HR15)

[a]Periodic BP for persons aged ≥ 21 years.
[b]If sexually active at present or in the past: q≤3 years. If sexual history is unreliable, begin Pap tests at age 18 years.

TABLE 2.4. (*continued*)

[c]If sexually active.
[d]Serologic testing, documented vaccination history, and routine vaccination against rubella (preferably with MMR) are equally acceptable alternatives.
[e]The ability of clinician counseling to influence this behavior is unproved.
[f]If not previously immunized: current visit and 1 and 6 months later.
[g]If no previous second dose of MMR.
[h]If susceptible to chickenpox.
[i]*HR1* = persons who exchange sex for money or drugs and their sex partners; persons with other STDs (including HIV); and sexual contacts of persons with active syphilis. Clinicians should also consider local epidemiology. *HR2* = females who have had two or more sex partners during the last year; a sex partner with multiple sexual contacts; exchanged sex for money or drugs; or a history of repeated episodes of gonorrhea. Clinicians should also consider local epidemiology. *HR3* = males who had sex with males after 1975; past or present injection drug use; persons who exchange sex for money or drugs and their sex partners; injection drug-using, bisexual, or HIV-positive sex partners currently or in the past; blood transfusion during 1978–1985; persons seeking treatment for STDs. Clinicians should also consider local epidemiology. *HR4* = sexually active females with multiple risk factors including a history of prior STD; new or multiple sex partners; age under 25; nonuse or inconsistent use of barrier contraceptives; cervical ectopy. Clinicians should also consider local epidemiology of the disease when identifying other high-risk groups. *HR5* = persons living in, traveling to, r working in areas where the disease is endemic and where periodic outbreaks occur (e.g., countries with high or intermediate endemicity; certain Alaskan native, Pacific Island, Native American, and religious communities); men who have sex with men; injection or street drug users. Vaccine may be considered for institutionalized persons and workers in these institutions, military personnel, and day-care, hospital, and laboratory workers. Clinicians should also consider local epidemiology. *HR6* = HIV-positive, close contacts of persons with known or suspected TB, health care workers, persons with medical risk factors associated with TB, immigrants from countries with high TB prevalence, medically underserved low-income populations (including homeless), alcoholics, injection drug users, and residents of long-term care facilities. *HR7* = persons who continue to inject drugs. *HR8* = immunocompetent persons with certain medical conditions, including chronic cardiac or pulmonary disease, diabetes mellitus, and anatomic asplenia. Immunocompetent persons who live in high-risk environments or social settings (e.g., certain Native American and Alaskan native populations). *HR9* = annual vaccination of residents of chronic care facilities; persons with chronic cardiopulmonary disorders, metabolic diseases (including diabetes mellitus), hemoglobinopathies, immunosuppression, or renal dysfunction; and health care providers for high-risk patients. *HR10* = adolescents and young adults in settings where such individuals congregate (e.g., high schools and colleges), if they have not previously received a second dose. *HR11* = healthy persons aged ≥ 13 years without a history of chickenpox or previous immunizations. Consider serologic testing for presumed susceptible persons aged ≥ 13 years. *HR12* = persons born after 1956 who lack evidence of immunity to measles or mumps (e.g., documented receipt of live vaccine on or after the first birthday, laboratory, evidence of immunity, or a history of physician-diagnosed measles or mumps). *HR13* = persons with a family or personal history of skin cancer, a larger number of moles, atypical moles, poor tanning ability, or light skin, hair, and eye color. *HR14* = women with prior pregnancy affected by a neural tube defect who are planning pregnancy. *HR15* = persons aged ≤ 17 years living in areas with inadequate water fluoridation (< 0.06 ppm).

Eleven to Twenty-Four Years

Adolescence through early adulthood represents a time of changing health hazards. Major health impediments to screen for and counsel about include injuries, violence, tobacco use and substance abuse, school failure, delinquency, suicide, unwanted pregnancy, and sexually transmitted diseases (Table 2.4).

TABLE 2.5. Adolescent preventive services

Health topics	Health guidance	Screening	Immunizations
Parenting and family adjustment	•		
Psychosocial adjustment	•		
Intentional and unintentional injury	•		
Dietary habits, eating disorders, and obesity	•	•	
Physical fitness	•		
Sexual development and the adverse consequences of sexual intercourse	•	•	•
Hypertension		•	
Hyperlipidemia		•	
Use of tobacco products	•	•	
Use of alcohol, other drugs, and anabolic steroids	•	•	
Severe or recurrent depression and suicide		•	
Physical, sexual, and emotional abuse		•	
Learning and school problems		•	
Infectious diseases		•	•

Source: AMA.[16] With permission.

Three-fourths of children have smoked their first cigarette by grade 9, and the average age of first use of alcohol and marijuana is age 13.[2] Important screening and counseling topics include fat in diet, cholesterol/lipoprotein analysis as indicated, selection of an exercise program, sex education, maintenance of dental health, and injury prevention. The AMA Guidelines for Adolescent Preventive Services identifies 14 health topics that require health guidance, screening, or immunization recommendations[16] (Table 2.5).

Twenty-Five to Sixty-Four Years

Young adults have an opportunity to assume personal responsibility for their health and life expectancy; most of the leading causes of mortality during this age period (Table 2.6) are preventable through adoption of healthy behaviors. Important screening recommendations cover identification of infectious and sexually transmitted diseases; clinical and personal examinations for the early detection of breast, testicular, and skin cancer; and tests to identify coronary heart disease risk factors, as heart disease is the leading cause of mortality beyond age 40. Topics of concern for counseling include diet and exercise, substance abuse, sexual practices, and injury prevention. It is important to remember to offer immunizations (e.g., tetanus-diphtheria toxoid boosters) and initiate preconception care routinely to women prior to pregnancy (Table 2.7).

Heart disease, cancer, stroke, and chronic lung disease are the leading causes of mortality from age 40 to 64 years. Each entity is associated with

TABLE 2.6. Interventions considered and recommended for the periodic health examination and leading causes of death: ages 25–64 years

Leading causes of death	
Malignant neoplasms	Human immunodeficiency virus (HIV) infection
Heart diseases	Suicide and homicide
Motor vehicle and other unintentional injuries	
Interventions for the general population	
SCREENING	*Injury prevention*
Blood pressure	Lap/shoulder belts
Height and weight	Motorcycle/bicycle/ATV helmets[e]
Total blood cholesterol (men ages 35–65, women ages 45–65)	Smoke detector[e]
	Safe storage/removal of firearms[e]
Papanicolaou (Pap) test (women)[a]	*Sexual behavior*
Fecal occult blood test[b] and/or sigmoidoscopy (≥ 50 years)	STD prevention; avoid high-risk behavior;[e] condoms/female barrier with spermicide[e]
Mammogram ± clinical breast examination[c] (women age 50–69 years)	Unintended pregnancy; contraception
	Dental health
Assess for problem drinking	Regular visits to dental care provider[e]
Rubella serology or vaccination history[d] (women of childbearing age)	Floss; brush with fluoride toothpaste daily[e]
COUNSELING	IMMUNIZATIONS
Substance use	Tetanus/diphtheria (Td) boosters
Tobacco cessation	Rubella[d] (women of childbearing age)
Avoid alcohol/drug use while driving, swimming, boating[e]	CHEMOPROPHYLAXIS
Diet and exercise	Multivitamin with folic acid (women planning or capable of pregnancy)
Limit fat and cholesterol; maintain caloric balance; emphasize grains, fruits, vegetables	Discuss hormone prophylaxis (peri- and postmenopausal women)
Adequate calcium intake (women)	
Regular physical activity[e]	
Interventions for high-risk population	
POPULATION	POTENTIAL INTERVENTIONS[f] [see detailed high-risk (HR) definitions in footnotes]
High-risk sexual behavior	RPR/VDRL (HR1); screen for gonorrhea (female (HR2), HIV (HR3), *Chlamydia* (female) (HR4); hepatitis B vaccine (HR5); hepatitis A vaccine (HR6)
Injection or street drug use	RPR/VDRL (HR1); HIV screen (HR3); hepatitis B vaccine (HR5); hepatitis A vaccine (HR6); PPD (HR7); advice to reduce infection risk (HR8)
Low income; TB contacts; immigrants; alcoholics	PPD (HR7)
Native Americans/Alaskan natives	Hepatitis A vaccine (HR6); PPD (HR7); pneumococcal vaccine (HR9)
Travelers to developing countries	Hepatitis B vaccine (HR5); hepatitis A vaccine (HR6)
Certain chronic medical conditions	PPD (HR7); pneumococcal vaccine (HR9); influenza vaccine (HR10)
Blood product recipients	HIV screen (HR3); hepatitis B vaccine (HR5)
Susceptible to measles, mumps, or varicella	MMR (HR11); varicella vaccine (HR12)
Institutionalized persons	Hepatitis A vaccine (HR6); PPD (HR7); pneumococcal vaccine (HR9); influenza vaccine (HR10)
Health care/laboratory workers	Hepatitis B vaccine (HR5); hepatitis A vaccine (HR6); PPD (HR7); influenza vaccine (HR10)
Family history of skin cancer; fair skin, eyes, hair	Avoid excess/midday sun, use protective clothing[e] (HR13)
Previous pregnancy with neural tube defect	Folic acid 4.0 mg (HR14)

TABLE 2.6. (*continued*)

[a]Women who are or have been sexually active and who have a cervix: q $\leq$ 3 years.
[b]Annually.
[c]Mammogram q1–2 years, or mammogram q1–2 years with annual clinical breast examination. Other groups recommend mammography q1–2 years between ages 40–50 and beyond age 69.
[d]Serologic testing, documented vaccination history, and routine vaccination (preferably with MMR) are equally acceptable alternatives.
[e]The ability of clinician counseling to influence this behavior is unproved.
[f]*HR1* = persons who exchange sex for money or drugs, and their sex partners; persons with other STDs (including HIV); and sexual contacts of persons with active syphilis. Clinicians should also consider local epidemiology. *HR2* = women who exchange sex for money or drugs or who have had repeated episodes of gonorrhea. Clinicians should also consider local epidemiology. *HR3* = men who had sex with men after 1975; past or present injection drug; persons who exchange sex for money or drugs and their sex partners; injection drug-using, bisexual, or HIV-positive sex partner currently or in the past; blood transfusion during 1978–1985; persons seeking treatment for STDs. Clinicians should also consider local epidemiology. *HR4* = sexually active women with multiple risk factors, including history of STD, new or multiple sex partners; nonuse or inconsistent use of barrier contraceptives; cervical ectopy. Clinicians should also consider local epidemiology. *HR5* = blood product recipients (including hemodialysis patients), persons with frequent occupational exposure to blood or blood products, men who have sex with men, injection drug users and their sex partners, persons with multiple recent sex partners, persons with others STDs (including HIV), travelers to countries with endemic hepatitis B. *HR6* = persons living in, traveling to, or working in areas where the disease is endemic and where periodic outbreaks occur (e.g., countries with high or intermediate endemicity; certain Alaska native, Pacific Island, Native American, and religious communities); men who have sex with men; injection or street drug users. Consider for institutionalized persons and workers in these institutions, military personnel, and day-care, hospital, and laboratory workers. Clinicians should also consider local epidemiology. *HR7* = HIV-positive, close contacts of persons with known or suspected TB, health care workers, persons with medical risk factors associated with TB, immigrants from countries with high TB prevalence, medically underserved low-income populations (including homeless), alcoholics, injection drug users, and residents of long-term care facilities. *HR8* = persons who continue to inject drugs. *HR9* = immunocompetent institutionalized persons aged $\geq$ 50 years and immunocompetent persons with certain medical conditions, including chronic cardiac or pulmonary disease, diabetes mellitus, and anatomic asplenia. Immunocompetent persons who live in high risk environments or social settings (e.g., certain Native American and Alaska native populations). *HR10* = annual vaccination of residents or chronic care facilities; persons with chronic cardiopulmonary disorders, metabolic diseases (including diabetes mellitus), hemoglobinopathies, immunosuppression, or renal dysfunction; and health care providers for high risk patients. *HR11* = persons born after 1956 who lack evidence of immunity to measles or mumps (e.g., documented receipt of live vaccine on or after the first birthday, laboratory evidence of immunity, or a history of physician-diagnosed measles or mumps). *HR12* = healthy adults without a history of chickenpox or previous immunization. Consider serologic testing for presumed susceptible adults. *HR13* = persons with a family or personal history of skin cancer, a large number of moles, atypical moles, poor tanning ability, or light skin, hair, and eye color. *HR14* = women with previous pregnancy affected by neural tube defect who are planning pregnancy.

precursor health behaviors that are totally preventable or modifiable through effective physician intervention.

CORONARY HEART DISEASE

More than 20% of persons who die from heart disease fall into this age group. The following interventions are recommended for primary prevention of myocardial infarction[17]: smoking cessation, lower choles-

TABLE 2.7. Interventions considered and recommended for the periodic health examination: Pregnant women

Interventions for general population

SCREENING

First Visit

- Blood pressure
- Hemoglobin/hematocrit
- Hepatitis B surface antigen (HBsAg)
- RPR/VDRL
- *Chlamydia* screen (< 25 years)
- Rubella serology or vaccination history
- D(Rh) typing, antibody screen
- Offer CVS (< 13 weeks)[a] or amniocentesis (15–18 weeks)[a] (age ≥ 35 years)
- Offer hemoglobinopathy screening
- Assess for problem or risk drinking
- Offer HIV screening[b]

Follow-up visits

- Blood pressure
- Urine culture (2–16 weeks)
- Offer amniocentesis (15–18 weeks)[a] (age ≥ 35 years)
- Offer multiple marker testing[a] (15–18 weeks)
- Offer serum α-fetoprotein[a] (16–18 weeks)

COUNSELING

- Tobacco cessation; effects of passive smoking
- Alcohol/other drug use
- Nutrition, including adequate calcium intake
- Encourage breast-feeding
- Lap/shoulder belts
- Infant safety car seats
- STD prevention: avoid high-risk sexual behavior,[c] use condoms[c]

CHEMOPROPHYLAXIS

- Multivitamin with folic acid[d]

Interventions for high-risk populations

POPULATION	POTENTIAL INTERVENTIONS[e] (see detailed high-risk definitions)
High-risk sexual behavior	Screen for *Chlamydia* (1st visit) (HR1), gonorrhea (1st visit) (HR2), HIV (1st visit) (HR3); HBsAg (3rd trimester) (HR4); RPR/VDRL (3rd trimester) (HR5)
Blood transfusion 1978–1985	HIV screen (1st visit (HR3)
Injection drug use	HIV screen (HR3); HBsAg (3rd trimester) (HR4); advice to reduce infection risk (HR6)
Unsensitized D-negative women	D(Rh) antibody testing (24–28 weeks) (HR7)
Risk factors for Down syndrome	Offer CVS[a] (1st trimester), amniocentesis[a] (15–18 weeks) (HR8)
Prior pregnancy with neural tube defect	Folic acid 4.0 mg,[d] offer amniocentesis[a] (15–18 weeks) (HR9)

See Tables 2.4 and 2.6 for other preventive services recommended for women of childbearing age.

[a]Women with access to counseling and follow-up services, reliable standardized laboratories, skilled high-resolution ultrasound scans, and, for those receiving serum marker testing, amniocentesis capabilities.

[b]Universal screening is recommended for areas (states, counties, or cities) with an increased prevalence of HIV infection among pregnant women. In low-prevalence areas, the choice between universal and targeted screening may depend on other considerations.

[c]The ability of clinician counseling to influence this behavior is unproved.

[d]Beginning at least 1 month before conception and continuing through the first trimester.

[e]*HR1* = women with history of STD or new or multiple sex partners. Clinicians should also consider local epidemiology. *Chlamydia* screen should be repeated during third trimester if at continued risk. *HR2* = women under age 25 with two or more sex partners during the last year or whose sex partner has multiple sexual contacts; women who exchange sex for money or drugs; and women with a history of repeated episodes of gonorrhea. Clinicians should also consider local epidemiology. Gonorrhea screen should be repeated during the third trimester if at continued risk. *HR3* = in areas where universal screening is not performed because of low prevalence of HIV infection, pregnant women with the following individual risk factors should be screened: past or present injection drug use; women who exchange sex for money or drugs; injection drug-using, bisexual, or HIV-positive sex partner currently or in the past; blood transfusion during 1978–1985; persons seeking treatment for STDs. *HR4* = women who are initially HBsAg-negative who are at high risk due to injection drug use

TABLE 2.7 (*continued*)

suspected exposure to hepatitis B during pregnancy, multiple sex partners. *HR5* = women who exchange sex for money or drugs, women with other STDs (including HIV), and sexual contacts of persons with active syphilis. Clinicians should also consider local epidemiology. *HR6* = women who continue to inject drugs. *HR7* = unsensitized D-negative women. *HR8* = prior pregnancy affected by Down syndrome, advanced maternal age (≥ 35 years), known carriage of chromosome re-arrangement. *HR9* = women with previous pregnancy affected by neural tube defect.

terol level, treatment of hypertension, maintenance of a physically active life style, avoidance of obesity, maintenance of normal glucose tolerance, postmenopausal estrogen-replacement therapy, mild to moderate consumption of alcohol, and prophylactic low-dose aspirin (Table 2.8). Individual lifetime excess risks of heart disease death due to environmental tobacco smoke are 1 to 3 per 100.[18] Exercise stress testing is available to screen for ischemic heart disease in asymptomatic men at risk, determine functional capacity, and generate an exercise prescription[19] (see Chapter 12).

CANCER

More than 30% of cancer deaths are linked to smoking, and about 35% are associated with diet. Many primary and secondary prevention interventions are recommended by the National Cancer Institute and Healthy People 2000. Counseling regarding tobacco use with an integrated office-based program best supports physician activities[20]: organized identification, progress records, brief physician messages, follow-up assistance, and a focus on those most interested in quitting. Passive smoking ex-

TABLE 2.8. Primary prevention of myocardial infarction

Intervention	Estimated mean risk reduction[a]	Efficacy of strategies to modify risk
Smoking cessation	50–70% ⇓ if stop within 5 years	Fair
⇓ Serum cholesterol	2–3% ⇓ per 1% ⇓ in level	Fair to good
Hypertension treatment	2–3% ⇓ per 1 mm ⇓ in DBP	Good
Exercise	45% ⇓ if maintain active life style	Fair
Ideal body weight	35–55% ⇓ if within 20% of IBW	Poor
Normoglycemia in diabetics	Insufficient data	Fair to poor
Postmenopausal ERT	44% ⇓ with estrogen alone	NA
Mild to moderate ETOH use	25–45% ⇓ compared with nondrinkers	NA
Aspirin	35% ⇓ compared with nonusers	NA

Source: Adapted from Manson et al.[17] With permission.
DBP = diastolic blood pressure; IBW = ideal body weight; ERT = estrogen replacement therapy; NA = not applicable; ETOH = alcohol.
[a]Estimated reductions in risk refer to the independent contribution of each risk factor to myocardial infarction.

posure is responsible for 3000 lung cancer cases each year in the United States among never-smokers.

Breast Cancer. Breast cancer is the most commonly diagnosed cancer and the second leading cause of mortality due to cancer.[21] Although there has been an increased incidence in recent years, perhaps because of improved screening, the death rate remains stable. Unalterable risk factors include family history and age at menarche and menopause. Other factors, such as parity and age at first pregnancy, are not easily modifiable. Thus primary prevention interventions such as maintaining a low-fat diet and secondary prevention screening by mammography are essential. In 1990 only 58% of women aged 40 or older had had a mammogram within the preceding 2 years.[22]

Colon Cancer. Screening for colon cancer is controversial. The U.S. Preventive Services Task Force in 1995 recommended for all persons age 50 and older annual fecal occult blood testing (FOBT), sigmoidoscopy (periodicity undefined), or both.[5] If the FOBT is positive, follow-up examination with either colonoscopy or flexible sigmoidoscopy plus air-contrast barium enema (ACBE) should be ordered. Persons with a family history of hereditary syndromes associated with a high risk of colon cancer should undergo colonoscopy before the age of 50.

There were 140,000 new cases of colon cancer diagnosed in 1994 with more than 55,000 related deaths.[21] The percent of lesions detected by each method and relative cost of the tests are estimated to be as follows:[23]

FOBT	20–50%	$5
Flexible sigmoidoscopy	40%	$100–200
ACBE	66–92%	$200
Colonoscopy	95%	$300–500

One study found that screening with rigid sigmoidoscopy can lead to a 60% to 70% reduction in risk of death due to rectal or distal colon cancer.[24] In patients with a history of colon or rectal cancer in one or more first-degree relatives, screening colonoscopy should be performed at age 40 to 50 years, especially if the cancer was diagnosed when the relative was younger than age 40.[23]

Prostate Cancer. Diagnosed in more than 244,000 men each year, prostate cancer kills more than 40,400 annually, making it the second leading cause of cancer death of men over age 55.[21] One in eleven men develop this cancer in their lifetime, one in nine if African American. The U.S. Preventive Services Task Force[5] does not recommend screening with digital rectal examination, serum prostate-specific antigen (PSA), or transrectal ultrasonography, citing that the benefits of these types of screening are still unknown whereas the risks resulting from screening are quantifiable and substantial.

The median age at diagnosis is 72. An annual digital rectal examination (DRE) is recommended by the American Cancer Society to begin at age 40.[21] They further recommend a serum PSA measurement annually, beginning at age 50 or age 40 for African American men and those with a family history of prostate cancer. If a PSA test is performed and is significantly elevated (> 10.0 ng/ml), the likelihood of a malignancy is significantly increased, and an ultrasound-guided biopsy is indicated. The PSA at present is the most accurate diagnostic marker available for prostate cancer, although it lacks adequate sensitivity and specificity to recommend for generalized screening. Following the rate of change in serum PSA over time may be helpful for detecting a greater percentage of curable prostate cancer lesions. DRE probably has no clinically important effect on the PSA level[25]; but urinary tract infection, urinary tract manipulations, and prostate biopsy can cause spurious elevations in PSA levels. Thus if serum PSA levels are determined, they should be obtained prior to DRE or at a minimum of 6 weeks after any urinary infection or manipulation.

Osteoporosis

Osteoporosis is another major public health problem, affecting 24 million Americans including 50% of women over age 45 and 90% of women over age 75 (see Chapter 18). Three groups of women are most likely to benefit from increased risk-reduction strategies: premenopausal women, perimenopausal or postmenopausal women without previous estrogen supplementation, and women with multiple risk factors[26] (Table 2.6).

Chemoprophylaxis

The U.S. Preventive Services Task Force noted that there is insufficient evidence to recommend for or against routine aspirin prophylaxis for the primary prevention of myocardial infarction, citing uncertainty when weighing the risks against the benefits. If aspirin administration is considered for the prevention of coronary heart disease, and possibly colon cancer,[27] the potential risks and benefits should be discussed before beginning its use.

Adults who take aspirin 16 times a month for at least a year reduce their risk of dying from colon cancer by 40% compared with nonaspirin users. Regular use of nonsteroidal antiinflammatory drugs is associated with a 50% reduction in combined risk of colon and rectal cancer. Estrogen, calcium, vitamin D, and exercise for osteoporosis prevention and estrogen for heart disease prevention in postmenopausal women have been recommended. Other recommendations include sunscreen with sun-protection factor (SPF) 16 or higher and active against both ultraviolet A and B (UVA and UVB) rays and specific antioxidant vitamins to inhibit cancer promotion and atherosclerosis. Low plasma levels of selenium, vitamins A, C, and E, and β-carotene may be associated with an increased risk of cancer mortality late in life.[2] The evidence is particularly strong for men over age 60. Low vitamin C intake is associated with increased gastrointestinal and stomach cancer. Vitamins A and E may inhibit cancer promotion. In addition, vitamins C and E and β-carotene may protect older persons against cataract formation, and vitamin E may have a protective role as an antioxidant in reversing or retarding atherosclerosis.[28]

Age Sixty-five and Older

People who reach age 65 can expect to live into their eighties. Many seniors have successfully "postponed" chronic conditions to later periods of their life through previous successful risk reduction behaviors (Table 2.9). The quality and quantity of life remaining are important considerations for the family physician when selecting preventive interventions for this age group. The elderly are not a homogeneous population, a point that must be taken into consideration when customizing a package of prevention services for each patient. Older individuals may be more vulnerable to adverse effects of preventive services, so the relative value for certain interventions may be questionable. Cognitive function is impaired in many elderly, which represents a significant health problem in that it may place the individual or others in physical danger. One of the most important considerations for the healthy older adult is sustaining a physically active life style to reduce the incidence of coronary disease, hypertension, diabetes, colon cancer, depression, and anxiety; increase bone mineral content; maintain appropriate body weight; and improve balance, coordination, and strength to reduce falls.

Other counseling topics include review of medication use and the importance of social support networks. Valuable clinical preventive services that are clearly effective in the elderly include identification and control of hypertension; screening for cancers, early signs or symptoms of dementia, depression, reversible sensory deficits, and urinary incontinence; and immunization against pneumonia and influenza.[29] Chemoprophylaxis with aspirin, estrogen, calcium, vitamins, and sunscreen is also recommended.

Indicators of poor nutritional status include physical signs and specific symptoms or sets of symptoms: significant weight loss over time, significant low or high weight for height, significant reduction in serum albumin to less than 3.5 mg/dl, significant reduction in midarm circumference, significant increase or decrease in skinfold measurement, significant obesity, inappropriate food intake, and selected nutrition-related disorders.[30]

TABLE 2.9. Interventions considered and recommended for periodic health examination and leading causes of death: Age 65 and older

Leading causes of death	
Heart diseases	Chronic obstructive pulmonary disease
Malignant neoplasms (lung, colorectal, breast)	Pneumonia and influenza
Cerebrovascular disease	
Interventions for general population	
SCREENING	Lap/shoulder belts
Blood pressure	Motorcycle and bicycle helmets[d]
Height and weight	Fall prevention[d]
Fecal occult blood test[a] and/or sigmoidoscopy	Safe storage/removal of firearms[d]
Mammogram ± clinical breast examination[b] (women ≤ 69 years)	Smoke detector[d]
Papanicolaou (Pap) test (women)[c]	Set hot water heater to < 120–130°F[d]
Vision screen (age 3–4 years)	CPR training for household members
Assess for hearing impairment	Dental health
Assess for problem drinking	Regular visits to dental care provider[d]
COUNSELING	Floss; brush with fluoride toothpaste daily[d]
Substance use	Sexual behavior
Tobacco cessation	STD prevention: Avoid high-risk sexual behavior[d]; use condoms[d]
Avoid alcohol/drug use while driving, swimming,boating[d]	IMMUNIZATIONS
Diet and exercise	Pneumococcal vaccine
Limit fat and cholesterol; maintain caloric balance; emphasize grains, fruits, vegetables	Influenza[a]
Adequate calcium intake (women)	Tetanus/diphtheria (Td) boosters
Regular physical activity[d]	CHEMOPROPHYLAXIS
Injury prevention	Discuss hormone prophylaxis (women)
Interventions for high-risk populations	
POPULATION	POTENTIAL INTERVENTIONS[e] [see detailed high-risk (HR) definitions in footnotes]
Institutionalized persons	PPD (HR1); hepatitis A vaccine (HR2); amantadine/ rimantadine (HR4)
Chronic medical conditions: TB contacts; low income, immigrants; alcoholics	PPD (HR1)
Persons ≥ 75 years or ≥ 70 years with risk factors for falls	Fall prevention intervention (HR5)
Cardiovascular disease risk factors	Consider cholesterol screening (HR6)
Family history of skin cancer; nevi; fair skin, eyes, hair	Avoid excess/midday sun, use protective clothing[d] (HR7)
Native Americans/Alaskan natives	PPD (HR1); hepatitis A vaccine (HR2)
Travelers to developing countries	Hepatitis A vaccine (HR2); hepatitis B vaccine (HR8)
Blood product recipients	HIV screen (HR3); hepatitis B vaccine (HR8)
High-risk sexual behavior	Hepatitis A vaccine (HR2); HIV screen (HR3); hepatitis B vaccine (HR8); RPR/VDRL (HR9)
Injection or street drug use	PPD (HR1); hepatitis A vaccine (HR2); HIV screen (HR3); hepatitis B vaccine (HR8); RPR/ VDRL (HR9); advice to reduce infection risk (HR10)
Health care/laboratory workers	PPD (HR1); hepatitis A vaccine (HR2); amantadine/ rimantadine (HR4); hepatitis B vaccine (HR8)
Persons susceptible to varicella	Varicella vaccine (HR11)

[a]Annually.
[b]Mammogram q1–2 years or mammogram q1–2 years with annual clinical breast examination.

TABLE 2.9 (*continued*)

[c]All women who are or have been sexually active and who have a cervix: q ≤ 3 years. Consider discontinuation of testing after age 65 years if previous regular screening with consistently normal results.
[d]The ability of clinician counseling to influence this behavior is unproved.
[e]*HR1* = HIV-positive, close contacts of persons with known or suspected tuberculosis (TB), health care workers, persons with medical risk factors associated with TB, immigrants from countries with high TB prevalence, medically underserved low-income populations (including homeless), alcoholics, injection drug users, and residents of long-term care facilities. *HR2* = persons living in, traveling to, or working in areas where the disease is endemic and where periodic outbreaks occur (e.g., countries with high or intermediate endemicity; certain Alaskan native, Pacific Island, Native American, and religious communities); men who have sex with men; injection or street drug users. Consider for institutionalized persons and workers in these institutions, and day-care, hospital, and laboratory workers. Clinicians should also consider local epidemiology. *HR3* = men who had sex with men after 1975; past or present injection drug use; persons who exchange sex for money or drugs and their sex partners; injection drug-using, bisexual, or HIV-positive sex partner currently or in the past; blood transfusion during 1978–1985; persons seeking treatment for STDs. Clinicians should also consider local epidemiology. *HR4* = consider for persons who have not received influenza vaccine or are vaccinated late: when the vaccine may be ineffective due to major antigenic changes in the virus; for unvaccinated persons who provide home care for high-risk persons; to supplement protection provided by vaccine in persons who are expected to have a poor antibody response; and for high-risk persons in whom the vaccine is contraindicated. *HR5* = persons aged 75 years and older or aged 70–74 with one or more additional risk factors including: use of certain psychoactive and cardiac medications (e.g., benzodiazepines, antihypertensives): use of four or more prescription medications; impaired cognition, strength, balance, or gait. Intensive individualized home-based multifactorial fall prevention intervention is recommended in settings where adequate resources are available to deliver such services. *HR6* = insufficient evidence to recommend routine screening in elderly persons, but clinicians should consider cholesterol screening on a case-by-case basis for persons ages 65–75 with additional risk factors (e.g., smoking, diabetes, or hypertension). *HR7* = persons with a family or personal history of skin cancer, a larger number of moles, atypical moles, poor tanning ability, or light skin, hair, and eye color. *HR8* = blood product recipients (including hemodialysis patients), persons with frequent occupational exposure to blood or blood products, men who have sex with men, injection drug users and their sex partners, persons with multiple recent sex partners, persons with other STDs (including HIV); travelers to countries with endemic hepatitis B. *HR9* = persons who exchange sex for money or drugs and their sex partners; persons with other STDs (including HIV); and sexual contacts of persons with active syphilis. Clinicians should also consider local epidemiology. *HR10* = persons who continue to inject drugs. *HR11* = healthy adults with no history of chickenpox or previous immunization. Consider serologic testing for presumed susceptible adults.

The most rapid population increase during the 1990s is occurring among those over age 85. This age group is composed of a substantial number of persons not independent in terms of physical functioning. Thus the focus for clinical preventive services in this age group should be on maintaining function physically, socially, and emotionally. Table 2.10 lists specific preventive services that have improved or diminished effectiveness in the elderly (> age 85).[29] In this age group, the family physician should change orientation from the prevention of conditions to monitoring and decreasing the impact of chronic conditions on quality of life (see Chapter 5).

TABLE 2.10. Periodic health examination ages ≥ 85 years (preventive services that have improved or diminished effectiveness): Scheduled annually

Preventive service	Improved effectiveness	Diminished effectiveness
History		
Accidents		
Falls prevention; particularly with a history of previous falls	X	
Motor vehicle		X
Mobility: ADL/IADL assessment	X	
Nutrition (undernutrition) screening or counseling	X	
Podiatry care	X	
Polypharmacy identification	X	
Dementia screening	X	
Urinary incontinence screening	X	
Physical examination		
Blood pressure		X
Cancer screening		
Breast		X
Cervix		X
Hearing screening	X	
Visual acuity screening	X	
Laboratory evaluation		
Cholesterol		X
Interventions		
Advance directives counseling	X	
Vaccinations		
Influenza immunization	X	

Source: Adapted from Zazove et al.[29] With permission.
ADL = activities of daily living; IADL = instrumental activities of daily living.

Health Maintenance Strategies for Integrating Clinical Preventive Services into the Family Practice Office

Clinical prevention is best delivered by following protocols and guidelines, and it is enhanced by practice aids such as flow sheets and reminder systems. The health maintenance strategies that follow are tools and competencies that may enhance the ability of physicians to change patient behaviors so as to reduce health risks. They are central to the physician–patient relationship and parallel the strategies traditionally employed for the care of individuals with acute and chronic problems. Effective physician counseling skills lead to empowering and motivating patients to make changes in health behavior.

It is helpful to audit charts to determine baseline rates when performing various preventive interventions, such as immunizations, counseling, identifying smokers, and recommending mammograms. Physicians should establish reasonable goals for an office-based, age-specific prevention program, given existing resources and patient population needs. The goals include profiling patients based on risk factors and membership in high-risk groups.

Development and use of a "prevention-friendly" patient record and charting system can improve adherence to preventive service guidelines and recommendations. This system should permit effective organization and management of prevention information longitudinally on both patient and practice population levels. It may include problem lists with risk factors identified, flow sheets, patient-held minirecords, tracking forms, manual and computerized reminders, and health risk appraisals.

1. *Flow sheets* for health maintenance are the most commonly used tracking tool.[31] Studies have shown that they improve physician record-keeping; yet physicians do not always record all interventions on such sheets. Flow sheets should be in examination rooms as posters and on patient charts. They are especially useful in group practices to maintain continuity in the delivery of preventive services when different providers may be involved. Qualities of a good flow sheet include all information on one page per age group to facilitate the ease of seeing dates of procedures done; limited writing and codes or initials; prominent location in the chart near the front cover; adequate staff and physician training to use the sheets; and a system of periodic prompts or reminders.[31] Prompts or reminders seem to increase health risk behavior counseling and the efficacy of behavioral prescriptions.[32] Improved physician compliance over a 5-year period (from 71% to 85%) has been shown to occur with a "package" of major, noncontroversial, screening interventions (blood pressure, smoking history, alcohol use history, fecal occult blood test, Papanicolaou smear, and clinical breast examination), with systematic placement of a health maintenance flow sheet (age appropriate) on all adult charts.[33]

2. *Patient-held minirecords* have been successfully used to promote preventive care.[34] In one study their use was well accepted by providers and led to improvements in compliance with guidelines. They can help build cooperation between patient, providers, and nursing staff. The pocket-sized booklets allow patients to keep track of their health histories and the preventive services they need or have received.

3. *Tracking forms,* such as those often mandated for Medicaid populations to deliver early periodic screening and developmental testing (EPSDT) services, are also useful for prompting and "memory-jogging." Use of these tracking forms at the University of Arizona Family Practice Office has led to completion of 91% of all possible clinical prevention interventions (e.g., nutritional assessment of 95% of children seen for

well-child care, 89% with developmental assessments, 76% with age-appropriate completed physical examinations, 96% with immunizations up to date, and 88% receiving counseling on anticipatory guidance topics identified on the forms).

4. *Reminder/prompting systems* involve the generation of compliance reminders, either manually or by computer, as a systematic approach to tracking patients in need of routine preventive care. Generating an updated report on health care maintenance needs for each visit and distributing the report to the patient is also helpful. Manual prompts include routine charting, a tickler file, or stickers on the charts of patients with life style risks. Messages can be stamped onto progress notes periodically to remind physicians to update problem lists or flow sheets—ask patients about their physical activity level, whether they use seat belts, and so on. Postcard reminder systems may prompt patients who do not have appointments for acute problems to return for health care maintenance.[31] Mailed influenza vaccine reminders have increased the percentage of patients who obtain immunizations in 1 year from 11.1% to 45.5%.[35] A meta-analysis of randomized clinical trials studying the effect of physician reminders found significant increases in cervical cancer screening and tetanus immunizations.[36] The main weaknesses of manual reminder systems are their dependence on physician motivation and inadequate outreach to inactive patients.

5. *Computer-generated systems* range from offering a status report for the physician at each visit (e.g., listing the preventive services that should be delivered to the patient) to programs for recalling inactive patients. Cost-effective programs are linked to the practice's billing system to eliminate duplicate demographic data gathering. Such prompting reports often identify office educational/counseling resources or list appropriate community referrals to streamline physician actions. Often programs generate letters to patients on their birthdays reminding them of recommended annual preventive services. Computer-generated physician and patient reminders have been shown to improve adherence to preventive services. The best results occur when the reminders are applied to both groups, using a population-based approach. In one study[37] use of reminders increased the percentage of patients with cholesterol screening, an annual FOBT, a mammogram, and current tetanus vaccination. Computer reminders to obtain an influenza vaccine may promote independent action among young patients but engender dependence on the reminder among older patients who have more frequent visits. To improve pneumococcal vaccine delivery, active approaches using either a nurse-directed vaccine algorithm or computer-generated physician reminders were determined to be effective interventions (2.4 times and 1.9 times control, respectively).[38]

The "Put Prevention into Practice" (PPIP) program of the U.S. Public Health Service[1] is an excellent example of a bundled information management system, with kits for physicians that include an updated clinician's handbook[11] on selecting and administering preventive services, flow sheets for patient charts, a set of colored chart stickers to alert physicians to patients who require periodic services (e.g., tobacco use counseling or flu vaccines), postcards to notify patients when preventive services are needed, and pocket-sized, patient-held minirecords in Spanish and English.

Barriers to the delivery of clinical preventive services most often cited by office-based clinicians include (1) uncertainty and confusion about selecting preventive interventions and their frequency of application; (2) inadequate or lack of reimbursement for the interventions and the time required to deliver them; (3) insufficient clinician knowledge about the importance of preventive services and how best to deliver them; (4) lack of patient understanding and confusion from conflicting information in the media; and (5) lack of office or clinic systems to integrate these services into routine patient care. Whereas the first barrier is addressed by the U.S. Preventive Services Task Force guide,[5] the latter three are targeted by the PPIP program.[1] Kits with patient minirecords are available by contacting the American Academy of Family Physicians' Order Department at 816-333-9700, ext. 5510 or 1-800-944-0000 (Kit E-1999, $60). A PPIP Home Page can be reviewed on the Internet: http://www.os.dhhs.gov:81/PPIP/.

6. *Health risk appraisals* (HRAs) can add impact to initial risk evaluation using flow sheets.[39] These instruments determine an individual's risk from preventable death or chronic illness on the basis of health history, life style, physiologic test findings, age, and gender. The patient's profile is compared to a database of epidemiologic and mortality statistics. They can be used by physicians to motivate and educate patients, encourage them to take greater responsibility for their health, make healthy life style decisions, and make appropriate use of medical services. They are intended to be used with persons who are free from chronic illnesses, and their use has been mostly with middle-class, middle-aged, white populations. Health risk appraisals should be used only in conjunction with risk reduction counseling or programs. For more information, contact the Society of Prospective Medicine at 412-749-1177. A directory has been prepared by the Society to assist providers in selecting the instrument most appropriate for their practice population. Conversational microcomputer-based HRAs seem cost-effective with older users.[40] There have been few controlled trials of HRAs in primary care practice.

Availability of Quality Patient Education Materials

Patient education can be streamlined by providing easy-to-read handouts with large print (especially important for the elderly and those with visual impairment) at the literacy level appropriate to a given patient population. Literacy levels usually range from fourth to eighth grade in diverse urban practice settings. Simple tests (e.g., Fog test) are available to determine literacy level. Often comic book formats are effective. If a significant portion of a practice is Spanish-speaking, materials should be available in Spanish.

The patient education newsletter can be an effective tool in family practice, allowing the physician to communicate information on preventive services and health promotion recommendations.[41] Staff should participate in its preparation. Information from a variety of sources can be assimilated. Monthly practice themes with attractive posters and buttons for patients and staff can be rotated periodically. Educational videotapes to view in the waiting room can save time and serve to supplement physician advice. Magazines should exclude tobacco advertising. Explicit and implicit prevention messages should be delivered in the simplest format possible.

Special kits are available for specific types of interventions. For example, the American Academy of Family Physicians (AAFP) Stop Smoking Kit includes a variety of clinical tools, patient materials, chart forms, and staff/physician manuals. The AAFP also has immunization record cards and chart stickers available. In addition to this kit, a series of patient education brochures, *Health Notes from Your Family Doctor,* is available as a free sample package from the AAFP at 1-800-944-0000.

Linkages with the Community

Linkages are recommended in *Healthy People 2000,* where it is suggested that physicians become involved with local groups to develop county-wide or state-wide prevention plans and incorporate the objectives of Healthy Older Adults 2000 or Healthy Youth 2000 into practice plans. Physicians can serve as catalysts within their communities to encourage establishment of local objectives and priorities and implementation of innovative methods to achieve them.[2] Family physicians often provide clinical prevention information to community groups and local media. Family physician involvement with schools can effectively lead to important preventive health changes. For example, in one study family physicians volunteered time at six public schools and doubled helmet ownership among bicycle riders (they provided 15-minute talks at each school during a 1-week educational intervention).[42]

Office Team Approach to Manage Time Efficiently

All available office personnel can be included in a team effort to promote and reinforce a healthy environment and life style for patients and staff alike. Office personnel have a vital role in implementing practice prevention policies. Staff and the office setting should reinforce prevention messages.[32] Assigning an office staff member the responsibility of coordinating specific prevention activities can be effective.

Offering group classes as an alternative to well-child care visits can be a time-efficient method of discussing such health issues as feeding, immunizations, and home safety. Such group parent education classes are successful with as many as 40 parents at once. They drastically reduce the number of times the physician or other providers must give the same preventive advice.

The nursing staff can be trained to track preventive care delivered and prompt physicians to recommend interventions. After nurses clipped reminder slips to the front of patient charts, the administration of FOBTs was increased from 32% to 47%, physician clinical breast examination from 29% to 46%, and influenza vaccination from 18% to 40%.[43] It is also important to involve patients in screening and preventive activities. A number of studies have reported the benefit of simply using preprinted sticky notes on patient charts.[44] Furthermore, distributing self-administered FOBT slide kits to patients at clinic registration increased screening to 57% and was more successful than reminder cards on patient charts and training programs.[45]

Developing "Minicounseling" Topics

Physicians can develop five to ten minicounseling topics, each about 3 to 10 minutes in duration. Topics are selected based on the risks and needs of the physician's practice population. A sample list for a practice might be physical activity, nutrition, stress reduction, cancer prevention, tobacco use, injury prevention, discipline and parenting skills, preventing heart disease, midlife challenges, and family health promotion.

Accountability for Clinical Preventive Services

The integration of health care delivery during the 1990s, propelled by marketplace forces, has led to increasing accountability and cost-efficiency requirements in clinician practice patterns. At least four models have been developed to evaluate preventive services: (1) Health Plan Employer Data and Information Set (HEDIS) report cards where four of nine quality indicators concern preventive services (childhood immunizations, cholesterol screening, mammography, and Papanicolaou smears); (2) Passports, as described in the PPIP program; (3) the HCFA-initiated Developing and Evaluating Methods to Promote Ambulatory Care Quality (DEMPAQ) project, using the following preventive service interventions as quality indicators for the Medicare population: blood pressure every 2 years, flu vaccine at least once in 2 years, breast examination within 2 years, and mammogram within 2 years for women under 75 years old; and (4) the AHCPR-funded Patients Reports on System Performance (PROSPER) now being tested in HMOs.[46] As these models become more commonplace in primary care practice, it is important for data systems to identify the population (e.g., the denominator) being served by a clinician or practice.[47]

Reimbursement Issues and the Economics of Prevention

Thousands of years ago, Chinese physicians were reimbursed for their services only when their patients maintained their health. Today prepaid capitated HMO plans are expected to provide routine preventive services, yet access to and payment for preventive services continue as major issues. Despite a growing body of research demonstrating the health benefits and cost-effectiveness of preventive services, physicians remain appropriately frustrated by the current reimbursement system, which for the most part denies payment for preventive screening, counseling, and immunizations.[48]

Included in the nation's health priorities for the year 2000, as elucidated in *Healthy People 2000,* is the important goal to "improve the financing and delivery of clinical preventive services so virtually no American has a financial barrier to receiving, at a minimum, the screening, counseling, and immunization services recommended by the U.S. Preventive Services Task Force."[2]

Use of preventive strategies has been strongly linked with insurance.[49] For instance, poor women with Medicaid are less likely to be referred for mammography.[50] Even enrollees in health insurance plans who are required to share costs made significantly less use of preventive services than did those who received free care.[51] In HMOs and in settings where care is not billed to the patient, there is greater utilization of preventive services. There is significant variation in the specific items covered on various insurance plans. Point of service and HMO plans provide broader coverage than conventional indemnity and preferred provider organization plans.

In general, uninsured and underinsured patients are not likely to have the financial resources to invest in preventive services, especially when the benefits of such interventions are not immediately apparent. However, public insurance plans (Medicare and Medicaid) cover selected preventive services, as determined by state or federal mandate. All Medicaid-eligible children under 21, for instance, must receive a comprehensive package of preventive services, known as the Early and Periodic Screening, Diagnostic, and Treatment Program (EPSDT).

Other barriers exist to the reimbursement for and financing of clinical preventive services. Historically, health insurance was established to cover unpredictable and catastrophic medical problems, rather than prospective, preventive care. Third-party payors tend to apply a more rigorous "cost-effectiveness" test to preventive versus diagnostic and treatment interventions.

It is important for physicians to charge appropriately for the time and resources used when delivering preventive care, based on the length of visit. Such documentation is also important for future reimbursement schedules. Fortunately, efforts among private insurers and Medicare suggest that improvements in coverage are occurring rapidly during the 1990s. Medicare's resource-based relative value scale (RBRVS) codes allow physicians to include their counseling services as "contributory components" in both inpatient and outpatient settings. Typical areas related to preventive services include discussion with patient, family, or both (the very young and very old) concerning diagnostic results from screening tests and recommended diagnostic studies, the importance of compliance with management options, risk factor reduction, and patient and family education.

It has been estimated that comprehensive implementation of a basic prevention package for all Americans would boost the nation's net health care bill by an estimated $1 billion to $3 billion annually. Nevertheless, the average cost of preventive services benefits would only be about $7.50 per month for family coverage. Other estimates for total lifetime preventive costs incurred by age 85 years range from $2900 to $4300 for men and from $4700 to $6600 for women.[51] In 1992 dollars, other estimates of lifetime annual costs are $78 a year for females and $55 a year for males. The Office of Disease Prevention and Health Promotion estimates a cost of $46 per adult per year for preventive services, or around 1% of the nation's annual health spending.

Prevention may not save money; it usually adds to medical expenditures. Thus when assessing preventive interventions, a cost-effective analysis (how much health is obtained by spending money on medical care) is more appropriate than cost-benefit analysis (how much money is saved by spending some). The cost of success is often the price of longer life. Two potential "costs" to society are the cost of diseases that the aged live to develop and the added cost of old-age pensions, including Social Security payments.

Future Trends

Family physicians increasingly practice in settings driven by large-scale computerized database systems to control costs and analyze the quality of clinical care and types of clinical prevention activities being delivered.

Group practice environments with sophisticated database systems require that tomorrow's family physicians be recognized for their health promotion expertise. Thus the professional education of family physicians will be more oriented toward health promotion, disease prevention, and patient counseling activities. These clinical preventive foci will, in turn, reflect the rapidly advancing knowledge base regarding clinical prevention. Thus a critical competence for the family physician is the ability to absorb new information regarding clinical prevention in a rapid manner and to translate that information into prevention-oriented patient care.

Evidence-based recommendations on the selection of clinical preventive services, such as the second edition of the *Guide to Clinical Preventive Services* by the U.S. Preventive Services Task Force[5] set standards for family physicians. These standards are periodically revised and strategies modified as research in the area of clinical prevention yields new information on which to base improved practice guidelines.

The challenge for the family physician is to implement practical, simple, reproducible clinical prevention strategies in the office setting to address the existing barriers to clinical prevention that arise from the health system, patient behaviors, and traditional physician practice styles. Guidelines, outcomes research, randomized controlled studies, and model practices are needed to increase our understanding about how clinical prevention can become more effective. Physicians and health care organizations will inevitably be offering preventive services as a strategy to increase market share.

Based on current state-of-the-art programs, clinical prevention efforts in the primary care settings of the future can be characterized in the following ways:

1. They will become more widespread as more physicians, especially during their years of training, are exposed to concepts of preventive medicine.
2. As evidence supporting the cost-effectiveness of comprehensive health promotion and disease prevention packages mounts, such services will be mandated by employers, insurance companies, and federal and state regulatory agencies, who will also pay for the delivery of such services.
3. They will be delivered by "teams" creatively using mid-level practitioners to decrease the physicians' time and operating costs.
4. Group practices will identify one physician as their clinical preventive medicine specialist or an interdisciplinary committee of staff members to develop and periodically review their comprehensive health promotion package (assessment instruments, screening procedures, resources for counseling and education, data collection to describe population) and to help initiate targeted campaigns based on their practice population needs.

5. The quality of care delivered and reimbursement received by physicians will be determined in part on their ability to provide health promotion services and to affect the morbidity and mortality of their defined practice populations.
6. National standards with respect to the quality of clinical prevention activities in primary care will be developed and monitored by regulatory agencies.
7. Health assessment technologic advances will allow physicians to individualize health risk trends more accurately and produce risk profiles for much earlier identification of cancer and cardiovascular disease. Most importantly, impetus for the continued delivery of clinical prevention activities should be documented proof of their impact on improving quality of life and compressing morbidity,[52] rather than on reducing health care dollar expenditures alone.

References

1. McGinnis JM. Put prevention into practice. Arch Intern Med 1996;156: 130–2.
2. US DHHS. Healthy people 2000: national health promotion and disease prevention objectives. PHS 91-50212. Washington, DC: Government Printing Office, 1991.
3. US DHHS. Healthy people 2000: midcourse review and 1995 revisions. Washington, DC: Government Printing Office, 1995.
4. Pommerenke FA, Dietrich AD. Improving and maintaining preventive services. 2. Practical principles for primary care. J Fam Pract 1992;34:92–7.
5. US Preventive Services Task Force. Guide to clinical preventive services: an assessment of the effectiveness of 169 interventions. Baltimore: Williams & Wilkins, 1996.
6. Thompson RS, Woolf SH, Taplin SH, et al. How to organize a practice for the development and delivery of preventive services. In: Woolf SH, Jonas S, Lawrence RS, editors. Health promotion and disease prevention in clinical practice. Baltimore: Williams & Wilkins, 1996:483–504.
7. Canadian Medical Association. The role of physicians in prevention and health promotion. Can Med Assoc J 1995; 153:208A–B.
8. AAFP Subcommittee on Periodic Health Intervention. Age charts for periodic health examination. Reprint No. 510. Kansas City, MO: American Academy of Family Physicians, 1996.
9. Healthy people: the Surgeon General's report on health promotion and disease prevention. Washington, DC: Government Printing Office, 1979. DHEW pub. No. (PHS) 79-55071.
10. McGinnis JM, Foege WH. Actual causes of death in the United States. JAMA 1993;270:2207–12.
11. US DHHS. Clinician's handbook of preventive services. Washington, DC: Government Printing Office, 1994.
12. Borkan JM, Neher JO. A developmental model of ethnosensitivity in family practice training. Fam Med 1991;23: 212–17.

13. Clarke WR, Lauer RM. The predictive value of childhood cholesterol screening. JAMA 1992;267:101–2.
14. National Cholesterol Education Program. Highlights of the report of the expert panel on blood cholesterol levels in children and adolescents. Am Fam Physician 1992;45:2127–36.
15. Kluger CZ, Morrison JA, Daniels SR. Preventive practices for adult cardiovascular disease in children. J Fam Pract 1991;33:65–72.
16. American Medical Association. AMA guidelines for adolescent preventive services: recommendations and rationale. Baltimore: Williams & Wilkins, 1994.
17. Manson JE, Tosteson H, Satterfield S, et al. The primary prevention of myocardial infarction. N Engl J Med 1992; 326:1406–16.
18. Steenland K. Passive smoking and the risk of heart disease. JAMA 1992; 267:94–9.
19. Evans CH, Karunaratne HB. Exercise stress testing for the family physician. I. Performing the test. Am Fam Physician 1991;45:121–32.
20. Solberg LI, Maxwell PL, Kottke TE, et al. A systematic primary care office-based smoking cessation program. J Fam Pract 1990;30:647–54.
21. Wingo PA, Tong T, Boloden S. Cancer statistics, 1995. CA 1995;45:8–30.
22. Public Health Focus: Mammography. MMWR 1992;41:454–9.
23. Levine R, Tenner S, Fromm H. Prevention and early detection of colorectal cancer. Am Fam Physician 1992;45:663–8.
24. Selby JV, Friedman GD, Quesenberry CD, et al. A case-control study of screening sigmoidoscopy and mortality for colorectal cancer. N Engl J Med 1992;326:653–7.
25. Crawford ED, Schutz MJ, Clejan S, et al. The effect of a digital rectal examination on prostate specific antigen levels. JAMA 1992;267:2227–8.
26. Bourguet CC, Hamrick GA, Gilchrist VJ. The prevalence of osteoporosis risk factors and physician intervention. J Fam Pract 1991;32:265–71.
27. Thun MJ, Namboodiri MM, Health CW. Aspirin use and reduced risk of fatal colon cancer. N Engl J Med 1991;325: 1593–6.
28. Cooper KH. Antioxidant revolution. Nashville: Thomas Nelson, 1994.
29. Zazove P, Mehr DR, Riffin MT, et al. A criterion-based review of preventive health care in the elderly. 2. A geriatric health maintenance program. J Fam Pract 1992;34:320–47.
30. Ham RJ. Indicators of poor nutritional status in older Americans. Am Fam Physician 1992;45:219–28.
31. Frame PS. Health maintenance in clinical practice: strategies and barriers. Am Fam Physician 1992;45:1192–1200.
32. Johns MB, Howell MF, Drastal CA, et al. Promoting preventive services in primary care: a controlled trial. Am J Prev Med 1992;8:135–40.
33. Shank JC, Powell T, Llewelyn J. A five-year demonstration project associated with improvement in physician health maintenance behavior. Fam Med 1989;21:273–8.
34. Dickey LL, Petitti D. A patient-held minirecord to promote preventive care. J Fam Pract 1992;34:457–63.
35. McDowell I, Newell C, Rosser W. A follow-up study of patients advised to obtain influenza immunizations. Fam Med 1990;22:303–6.

36. Austin SM, Balas EA, Mitchell JA, et al. Effect of physician reminders on preventive care: meta-analysis of randomized clinical trials. Proceedings of the Annual Symposium on Computer Applications in Medical Care: 121–4, 1994.
37. Garr DR, Ornstein SM, Jenkins RG, et al. The effect of routine use of computer-generated preventive reminders in a clinical practice. Am J Prev Med 1993;9:55–61.
38. Lebuhn CB, Flanagan JR, Helms CM, et al. Comparison of interventions to improve pneumococcal vaccine delivery in ambulatory care. Poster presented at the Infectious Disease Society of America, September, 1996.
39. Peterson KW, Hilles SB, editors. SPM handbook of health risk appraisals. Charlottesville, VA: Society of Prospective Medicine, 1996.
40. Ellis LBM, Joo H, Gross CR. Use of a computer-based health risk appraisal by older adults. J Fam Pract 1991;33:390–4.
41. Aukerman GF. Developing a patient education newsletter. J Fam Pract 1991;33:304–5.
42. Towner P, Marvel MK. A school-based intervention to increase the use of bicycle helmets. Fam Med 1992;24:156–8.
43. McDonald CJ, Hui SL, Smith DM, et al. Reminders to physicians from an interactive computer medical record. Ann Intern Med 1984;100:130–8.
44. Konen JC. Systems to improve clinical prevention. Arch Fam Med 1994; 3:223–4.
45. Struewing JP, Pape DM, Snow DA. Improving colorectal cancer screening in a medical resident's primary care clinic. Am J Prev Med 1991;7:75–81.
46. Cooper JK. Accountability for clinical preventive services. Milit Med 1995;160:297–9.
47. Frame PS. Clinical prevention in primary care; everyone talks about it, why aren't we doing it? J Am Board Fam Pract 1994;7:449–50.
48. Parkinson MD. Paying for prevention: recent developments and future strategies. J Fam Pract 1991;33:529–30.
49. Woolhandler S, Himmelstein DU. Reverse targeting of preventive care due to lack of health insurance. JAMA 1988;259: 2872–4.
50. Hamblin JE. Physician recommendations for screening mammography: results of a survey using clinical vignettes. J Fam Pract 1991;32:472–7.
51. Davis K, Bialek R, Parkinson M, et al. Paying for preventive care: moving the debate forward. Am J Prev Med 1990;6:32.
52. Fries JF. Aging, natural death, and a compression of morbidity. N Engl J Med 1980;303:130–6.

CASE PRESENTATION

Subjective

PATIENT PROFILE

Ruth Nelson McCarthy is a 51-year-old married white female restaurant owner.

PRESENTING PROBLEM

"Here for my pap smear."

PRESENT ILLNESS

Mrs. McCarthy has a periodic examination every 2 years. Her menses ceased 3 years ago, and she has not used estrogen replacement. She has no other medical complaints.

PAST MEDICAL HISTORY

Asthma in childhood.

SOCIAL HISTORY

She and her husband have owned and operated a small restaurant for 11 years. She works long hours 6 days per week.

HABITS

She uses no tobacco, alcohol, or drugs.

FAMILY HISTORY

Her father, aged 76, has diabetes mellitus and "arthritis." Her mother is 71 years old and has high blood pressure. She and her husband have two children. Her daughter is living and well at age 26. Their son, aged 28, has recently been diagnosed as HIV-positive.

REVIEW OF SYSTEMS

She reports an occasional mild rash on her hands that becomes red and itching but is not present at this time.

- What other historical information would be useful for this periodic health maintenance examination?
- What are common areas of concern for patients of this age group, and how would you approach these possibilities?
- What else would you like to know regarding her menopausal symptoms?
- What might be the meaning of her health status to the patient, and what unspoken reasons might be bringing her to the physician today?

Objective

VITAL SIGNS

Height, 5 ft 4 in; weight, 182 lb; blood pressure, 138/90; pulse, 72; temperature, 37.2°C.

EXAMINATION

The patient is overweight for height. The eyes, ears, nose, and throat are normal. The neck and thyroid glands are unremarkable. Examination of the chest, heart, and breasts is normal. There is no mass, tenderness, or organ enlargement in the abdomen. The vaginal introitus is mildly atrophic; the cervix, fundus, adnexa, and rectal examination are normal. The neurologic examination and peripheral pulses are normal. Examination of the skin, including the hands, reveals no abnormalities.

LABORATORY

A pap smear is performed today.

- What more—if anything—should be included in this health maintenance examination? Why?
- What might point to a physical cause for obesity?
- What—if any—laboratory tests would you order today, and why?
- What—if any—diagnostic imaging would you order today, and why?

Assessment

- What is your diagnosis regarding Mrs. McCarthy's menopausal status, and how would you describe this to the patient?
- What is the patient's ideal weight, and how would you initiate a discussion regarding weight control?
- How might decreased estrogen and increased weight influence the patient's relationship with her husband? How might you address this issue?
- What are likely to be key stressors in the patient's life, and how might these affect her future health status?

Plan

- What are the disease prevention and health promotion opportunities for this visit?
- Describe your recommendation regarding weight control.
- Describe your recommendation regarding estrogen use.
- What continuing care would you advise for Mrs. McCarthy?

3

Normal Pregnancy, Labor, and Delivery

JOSEPH E. SCHERGER AND MARGARET V. ELIZONDO

Pregnancy and birth are normal physiologic processes for most women. The current cesarean delivery rate of nearly 25% in the United States is a reflection of a higher than expected rate of medical intervention in the birth process. Unfortunately, modern medicine has been guilty of using a disease model for the management of pregnancy and birth, resulting in higher than expected rates of complications. At least 90% of women should have a normal birth outcome without medical intervention.[1]

The disease model for pregnancy and birth took hold during the 1920s, led by a Chicago obstetrician, Joseph DeLee, who questioned what is normal and pioneered efforts to improve medically on the "cruelty of nature."[2] During this period, childbirth in America went from the home to the hospital, and the legacy of hospital interventions in the birth process began. Much good has come from modern hospital obstetric care, with maternal mortality having decreased to low levels; moreover, infant mortality has steadily declined for populations having access to perinatal care. Modern prenatal care also developed during the first half of the twentieth century; and with a focus on good nutrition and screening for problems during pregnancy it has improved birth outcome.[3]

A renewed respect for normal childbirth came about as a reaction to hospital interventions, led by Dick-Read during the 1930s and 1940s,[4] La Maze during the 1950s,[5] Kitzinger during the 1960s,[6] and eventually a social movement in America during the 1970s with the widespread development of childbirth education. Odent's *Birth Reborn* represents a culmination of the effort to rediscover normal pregnancy and birth.[1]

Technologic obstetrics, with its steady focus on improving the uncertainty of nature and sparing women the pain of childbirth, continues to march onward. Prenatal care has become preoccupied with serial ultrasound evaluations and screening for α-fetoprotein abnormalities, gestational diabetes, genetic disorders, and every potentially infectious agent. Continuous electronic fetal monitoring, developed during the early 1970s, quickly became the standard of care in most American hospitals, despite little evidence of benefit and cumulative evidence that it causes unnecessary cesarean interventions.[7,8] Epidural anesthesia has become so commonplace in some hospitals that labor units are quiet and nurses have little experience helping women through natural labor.

Approximately 30% of U.S. family physicians provide maternity care. The current lack of access to prenatal care for many women in both rural and urban areas is a compelling reason for more family physicians to deliver these services. Knowledgeable about scientific medicine, yet with a humanistic approach to pregnancy and birth similar to that of midwives, the family physician is well suited to provide a balance between nature and technology and may be a guiding force to appropriate maternity care.[9]

This chapter focuses on normal pregnancy and delivery from a perspective of family-centered care. Family-centered maternity care has been defined by the International Childbirth Association as care that focuses on how the birth of a child affects the entire family. A woman who gives birth forms new relationships with those close to her, and all family members take on new responsibilities to each other, the baby, and the community. Family-centered maternity care recognizes the importance of these new relationships and responsibilities and has as its goal the best possible outcome for all family members. Family-centered maternity care is an attitude rather than a specific program. It respects the woman's individuality and need for autonomy and requires that a woman be guided, not directed, and that she be allowed to make her own decisions in accordance with her goals.[10] The family physician, as physician for the woman, the father, and the children, is well suited to provide family-centered maternity care.

This chapter reviews the principles and practice of normal pregnancy, labor, and delivery. Some of this material has been published in a paper by members of the Working Group on Teaching Family-Centered Perinatal Care of the Society of Teachers of Family Medicine [reprinted with permission].[11]

Prenatal Care

Current prenatal care begins before conception. Prenatal care after conception should begin as early as possible, as health screening and intervention early during pregnancy may improve birth outcome. For example, taking folic acid in doses present in multivitamins during the first 6 weeks of pregnancy provides a three- to fourfold reduction in the chance of neural tube defects in the offspring.[12] Early screening and intervention may also help in glucose control of diabetes, genetic screening, changing teratogenic drugs such as phenytoin (Dilantin), treating infections, and life style modifications of such factors as smoking, alcohol use, recreational drugs, and maternal nutrition.

The traditional approach to prenatal care, developed early during the twentieth century, has been modified by an expert panel convened by the U.S. Public Health Service.[13] Rather than a single comprehensive initial visit followed by monthly visits until the third trimester, this panel recommended more intensive intervention early in pregnancy if risk factors exist that can be modified. For example, women who smoke, have poor nutrition, or have a high-risk home environment may benefit from frequent visits and a multidisciplinary team approach early in pregnancy. Women at low risk may require fewer visits than are scheduled with the traditional protocol.

Prenatal care in the normal or healthy woman is part of preventive medicine. A biopsychosocial approach with a family perspective should be used, with an emphasis on advocacy for the pregnant woman.[14] Prenatal care encompasses both primary prevention, such as proper nutrition to enhance birth outcome, and secondary prevention through screening for conditions that can be modified or that alter patient management.

Health Promotion

All those who care for childbearing women should approach pregnancy as an opportunity to promote the health and well-being of the family. Counseling to reinforce healthful behaviors and education about pregnancy, childbirth, and parenting are crucial parts of perinatal care—not "extras."

In a family practice, education about pregnancy, birth, and parenting begins prior to the first conception and continues throughout the parenting years. Pregnancy is an opportunity for more intensive involvement. Table 3.1 is an outline of topics to be covered in the education of all pregnant women and their support persons.[15] Experienced parents require only an abbreviated program, focusing on selected areas of interest to them. Preparation for natural childbirth (birth without regional or systemic analgesic drugs) and for vaginal birth after a previous cesarean section can reduce maternal anxiety and the rates of operative delivery and associated complications.[16] Childbirth preparation classes, often run by hospitals, clinics, or private childbirth educators, fulfill this function well. In addition, during pregnancy care it is important that the practitioner spend time discussing with the woman recommendations specific to her care, such as the purpose of tests and

TABLE 3.1. Sample topics for birth and parenting classes

Early pregnancy

- Nutrition; optimum weight gain; iron, calcium, vitamin supplements
- Exercise and sex during pregnancy
- Common symptoms and remedies: fatigue, nausea/ vomiting, backache, round ligament pain, syncope, constipation
- Danger signs: bleeding, contractions, dysuria, vaginitis, weight loss
- Psychology of pregnancy: body image, libido; need for security: education for self-help; changing family roles; acceptance of pregnancy
- Fevers, hot tubs, saunas
- Environmental and occupational hazards and how to mitigate them; stress management
- Exposure to infectious agents (e.g., toxoplasmosis, rubella, HIV, varicella)
- Avoidance of tobacco, alcohol, x-rays, other drugs
- Resources available for pregnant and parenting families

Late pregnancy

- Common symptoms and remedies: heartburn, backache, "loose joints," hemorrhoids, edema, insomnia
- Nutrition/fetal growth
- Avoidance of tobacco and other drugs
- Potentially serious symptoms: edema, bleeding, headache, meconium-stained fluid, decreased fetal movements
- Exercise (e.g., Kegel's, pelvic tilt), sex, travel (avoid prolonged sitting because of risk of deep vein thrombosis)
- Occupational adjustments (avoid excessive exertion, prolonged standing, stress) and postpartum plans
- Breast-feeding
- Signs of labor
- Stages of labor
- Techniques for pain control (and practice relaxation, visualization)
- Cesarean section, vaginal birth after cesarean, other potential interventions
- Birth plan; importance of labor companion and early parent–infant contact
- Positions for labor and birth
- Seat belt use; infant car seats
- Circumcision
- Sibling preparation

Postpartum/parenting

- Care of the perineum, Kegel's exercises
- Practical support for breast-feeding
- Reasons to contact provider (e.g., maternal hemorrhage, fever, increased pain; infant jaundice, respiratory distress)
- Postpartum exercises
- Nutrition, especially calcium and iron
- Rest and sleep
- Return to work
- Sex, contraception
- Sibling adjustment
- Infant immunizations and preventive care schedule
- Infant growth and development: normal expectations and parenting issues at each age

procedures and the steps to follow when labor begins. The benefits of breast-feeding for baby and mother should be discussed with women and their family members prior to or early during pregnancy and then modeled at delivery. The effectiveness of education on preventing low birth weight has not been proved; however, information about smoking, alcohol and drug use, prevention of sexually transmitted infection, and mobilizing family supports and social services in the community are likely to be beneficial. Health education may have a profound effect on the problem of low birth weight if it is undertaken during preconception, pregnancy, and postpartum, even though the gains may not be noticed until subsequent pregnancies.

Motivation to adopt more healthy behaviors is probably stronger during pregnancy than at most other times. On the other hand, pregnancy may intensify the pressure on close relationships, increasing the pregnant woman's dependence on them. Many women are motivated to stop smoking during pregnancy but may resume after delivery. During pregnancy the couple may be involved, and the benefits of a nonsmoking household for children should be emphasized.

Abstention from alcohol and recreational drugs is also important. Alcohol exposure during gestation is now a more common cause of mental retardation than Down syndrome.[17] The prevalence of cocaine use during pregnancy is as high as 17% in some populations but often is not admitted to the physician.[18] With a paucity of research on substance use by women and few treatment programs accepting pregnant women, this area is a challenge to professionals caring for them.

Physicians are often in a position to counsel women about work during perinatal care. The physician should review the effects of physical exertion and prolonged standing during pregnancy, occupational and environmental hazards (e.g., heat, heavy metals, anesthetic gases, x-rays, possibly cathode ray tubes), legal rights of pregnant workers, child care, and breast-feeding.

Physical fitness may improve pregnancy and childbirth. Prescription and occasionally proscription of exercise during pregnancy and discussion of sexuality during perinatal care are appropriate.

Nutrition and weight should be closely monitored during prenatal care. Physicians must be knowledgeable about nutritional requirements and concerning practical suggestions regarding management of nausea and vomiting, reflux esophagitis, constipation, obesity, anticipatory guidance about body image changes, and ways of modifying the diet within various constraints (e.g., vegetarianism, lactose intolerance). Optimal weight gain during pregnancy varies depending on the prepregnancy weight. A thin woman may benefit from gaining 40 pounds, whereas an obese woman might do well gaining 10 pounds. The normal weight gain of 25 to 30 pounds is often exceeded without harm to the fetus. Nutritional advice to pregnant women should focus on a high quality, high protein diet with a steady, gradual weight gain profiled to the woman's size and eating habits. Pregnant women should be instructed to avoid the presence of cat feces and eating raw meat (toxoplasmosis).

Pregnancy is an opportunity to assess family supports and liabilities and to intervene with the potential of an improved perinatal outcome. If there is a history of maternal deprivation, postpartum depression, physical abuse, or substance use by significant others, interventions can be begun during pregnancy and continued during care of the parent(s) and child. The physician must ask explicitly about these issues, which often are not spontaneously mentioned by women. Finally, physicians should be knowledgeable and able to recommend the public social service programs available to aid and support the pregnant patient and family.

Prenatal Screening

The purpose of prenatal screening is to identify problems that could affect the outcome of pregnancy and for which effective interventions are available. The number of conditions for which screening is available seems limitless. Therefore the choice of items should be based on a rational assessment of the current literature, legislation, medicolegal climate, cost-effectiveness, and treatment effectiveness. Screening means that the search for the presence of a specific condition is not based on signs or symptoms but is carried out for the prenatal population as a whole or for those with historic or demographic risk factors. Each screening test should be evaluated to ensure that the benefits of the test and the planned intervention outweigh the risks and complications. Unfortunately, not all currently recommended screening techniques have been so rigorously evaluated.

Screening may include identification of conditions of the mother or fetus that require monitoring during the pregnancy or that may be treatable during the pregnancy or after delivery. Prenatal screening should be discussed with each patient at the first prenatal visit. Elective screening items should be recommended and pursued based on a joint decision between doctor and patient. It may be helpful to provide written materials for patients to review at home. Screening tests should be scheduled so as to minimize blood drawing and number of visits.

Traditional medical teaching focuses on screening for medical conditions using blood tests, ultrasonography, amniocentesis, and physical examination. A comprehensive approach would also include screening through questioning about family and social dysfunction, such as single parent status, a history of child abuse, economic hardship, and work-related stresses. The relation between psychosocial stress and outcome of pregnancy is now well established.[19,20]

Medical conditions appropriate for prenatal screening can be divided into three groups: those that are universal, selective, and elective. Universal screening tests include the Papanicolaou smear, urinalysis, urine culture, complete blood count, blood type and Rh factor, indirect Coombs' test, and tests for syphilis, rubella immunity, *Chlamydia,* gonorrhea, hepatitis B surface antigen, and blood glucose. All of these tests are appropriately performed at preconception or at the first prenatal visit, except that for blood glucose, which should be done at 24 to 28 weeks' gestation in low-risk patients. Genital culture for group B β-hemolytic streptococcus (group B strep) is routinely done at 34 to 36 weeks' gestation.[21] A hemoglobin or hematocrit should be rechecked during the third trimester. The physical examination routinely screens for weight gain or loss, blood pressure, edema, fundal growth, fetal heart sounds, and fetal position.

Screening for gestational diabetes is still controversial, and screening based on risk factors is advocated by some. The currently recommended test is the use of an oral 50-g glucose solution with a 1-hour blood glucose assay, regardless of earlier food intake. This test has a high false-positive rate.[22] One- or two-hour postprandial blood glucose assays may also be used for screening. Positive screening tests are followed by a standard glucose tolerance test before a diagnosis of gestational diabetes is made.

Selective screening tests are chosen for patients who fit a particular risk category. If indicated, tests for sickle cell disease, toxoplasmosis, and human immunodeficiency virus (HIV) should be carried out at the first prenatal visit. All pregnant women should be offered HIV testing and counseled about risk factors and safe sex practices. If indicated by the history, the patient should undergo tests for HIV, *Chlamydia,* gonorrhea, and syphilis again at 36 weeks. Herpes screening remains controversial, and screening by culture those women with a history of herpes fails to prevent most cases of neonatal herpes. Screening is best done by questioning and by examination early during labor for possible herpes lesions. Rh-negative patients should be screened for Rh antibodies at 28 weeks and given antenatal RhoGAM if these tests are negative. Amniocentesis or chorionic villous sampling, if indicated by maternal age or a previous chromosomal abnormality, is performed during the first trimester or early second trimester.

Elective screening tests include maternal serum α-fetoprotein assay (msAFP) and ultrasonography. Some states require that the msAFP assay be offered to all pregnant women. This assay can be used as a screening test to detect fetal abnormalities, particularly neural tube defects. In some states, screening for msAFP is offered to all pregnant women despite its low positive predictive value (1.9% for spina bifida) and relatively low sensitivity (90% for spina bifida).[23] An "expanded α-fetoprotein screening program" is available in some states that use levels of human chorionic gonadotropin (hCG) and unconjugated estriol (uE_3) in addition to msAFP to increase detection rates for Down syndrome and trisomy 18. Down syndrome is associated with decreased levels of msAFP and uE_3 and an increased level of hCG. Trisomy 18 is associated with low levels of all three of these substances. An elevated msAFP level may be found in patients with inaccurate dates, multiple gestation, neural tube defects, abdominal wall defects, congenital nephrotic syndrome, fetal demise, fetomaternal hemorrhage, and normal pregnancy. A low level may be found with inaccurate dates, chromosomal trisomy (e.g., Down syndrome), fetal demise, molar pregnancy, and normal pregnancy. If the initial AFP screening is abnormal, it may be necessary to repeat the test or to order a diagnostic ultrasound scan to confirm gestational age and evaluate for fetal abnormalities. Amniocentesis may be indicated to measure amniotic fluid AFP and acetylcholine esterase and for chromosome evaluation. Because AFP screening is widely available and is considered standard by some, the test should be discussed with all patients, with a mutual agreement of patient and practitioner regarding its use. The screening is done between 15 and 20 weeks' gestation, optimally at 16 to 18 weeks.

Routine ultrasonography currently falls into a gray area. In the United States, a National Institutes of Health (NIH) Consensus Conference recognized 27 indications for prenatal ultrasonography that result in examinations in most pregnancies.[24] The American College of Obstetricians and Gynecologists recommended adherence to these guidelines.[25] In most of western Europe, ultrasonography is done routinely at 16 to 18 weeks. The benefits and cost-effectiveness of universal screening are still controversial and are the subject of ongoing study.[26,27]

Risk Assessment

The outcome of screening is identification of patients at risk for complications during pregnancy. Conventional risk assessment divides patients into low-, medium-, and high-risk categories. Because most family physicians are trained to care for low and medium risk patients, and to refer or share the care of high-risk patients with perinatal specialists, proper risk assessment is crucial. Complex risk scoring mechanisms have been developed but have failed to cause any improvement over simpler clinical identification of known risk factors.[28] Table 3.2 indicates well-established risk factors recognized by the American Board of Family Practice and the American College of Obstetricians and Gynecologists.[29] Family physicians in some areas and with appropriate training provide high risk obstetric care, but the classification of risk status remains

TABLE 3.2. Obstetric risk criteria

Category I: high-risk factors
Initial prenatal factors
Age ≥ 40 or < 16
Multiple pregnancy
Insulin-dependent diabetes
Chronic hypertension
Renal failure
Heart disease, class 2 or greater
Hyperthyroidism
Rh isoimmunization
Chronic active hepatitis
Convulsive disorder
Isoimmune thrombocytopenia
Subsequent prenatal and intrapartum factors
Vaginal bleeding, second or third trimester
Pregnancy-induced hypertension (or toxemia), moderate or severe
Fetal malformation, by α-fetoprotein (AFP) screening, ultrasonography, or amniocentesis
Abnormal presentation: breech, face, brow, transverse
Intrauterine growth retardation
Polyhydramnios
Pregnancy > 43 weeks or < 35 weeks
Abnormal fetal/placental tests
Persistent severe variable or late decelerations
Macrosomia
Cord prolapse
Mid-forceps delivery
Category II: medium-risk factors
Initial prenatal factors
Ages 35–39, 16–17
Drug dependence
High-risk family—lack of family/social support
Uterine or cervical malformation or incompetence
Contracted pelvis
Previous cesarean section
Multiple spontaneous abortions (>3)
Grand multiparity (> 8)
History of gestational diabetes
Previous fetal or neonatal demise
Hypothyroidism
Heart disease, class I
Severe anemia (unresponsive to iron)
Pelvic mass or neoplasia
Subsequent prenatal and intrapartum factors
Gestational diabetes
Pregnancy-induced hypertension (toxemia), mild
Pregnancy at 42 weeks, obtain appropriate fetal/placental tests
Active genital herpes
Positive high or low AFP screen
Estimated fetal weight > 10 pounds (5.5 kg) or < 6 pounds (2.7 kg)
Abnormal nonstress test
Arrest of normal labor curve
Persistent moderate variable decelerations or poor baseline variability
Ruptured membranes beyond 24 hours
Second stage beyond 2 hours
Induction of labor

important for guiding clinical care. The prenatal record should conveniently assist in the evaluation and indication of risk status.

High-risk categories should not be absolute contraindications to care by family physicians. For example, family physicians may be the best qualified to handle high-risk social situations and substance abuse. Because of broad medical training, family physicians may have more experience than some obstetricians in an area dealing with medical problems, such as thyroid or pulmonary disease. Consultation does not preclude shared care. Many high-risk problems resolve during the pregnancy, and the birth may be a low-risk event. The family physician should be encouraged to stay in contact with the patient after consultation or referral. The woman with a high-risk pregnancy and her family continue to benefit from a comprehensive, biopsychosocial approach.

Prenatal Visits

The schedule of prenatal visits has traditionally been every 4 weeks through the 28th week of pregnancy, every 2 weeks until the 36th week of pregnancy, and then weekly until delivery. A U.S. Public Health Service report suggested that low-risk patients require fewer visits, whereas patients with risk factors may need modified or intensive care.[13] For example, risk factors identified early in pregnancy, such as smoking, alcohol or drug use, family dysfunction, or lack of social support, should be aggressively managed with frequent visits early during pregnancy. Subsequent risk factors, such as elevated blood pressure or preterm labor, require more frequent visits beginning as soon as the condition develops.

The initial prenatal visit consists of a detailed history, physical examination, and laboratory assessment. A complete physical examination is performed as early as possible. The pelvic assessment, which includes a bimanual examination, is helpful for dating the pregnancy and evaluating the pelvic structure. Screening laboratory investigations are undertaken as stated above. Accurate dating of the pregnancy is critically important for prenatal care, the proper performance and interpretation of screening tests, and avoiding unnecessary testing due to a misdiagnosis of prematurity or postdates. If the dates are not clear from the initial visit, an ultrasound scan should be performed during the first or second trimester.

First trimester prenatal care (up to 14 weeks) includes a determination of the patient's well-being during pregnancy, a review of family and life style issues, and a reevaluation of the risk status. A clinical assessment would include measuring uterine growth and maternal weight gain, detecting fetal heart tones by Doppler ultrasonography, and counseling patients toward a healthy pregnancy. Genetic prenatal diagnostic tests that may be performed during the first trimester include chorionic villous sampling and early amniocentesis.

Second trimester prenatal care (14–28 weeks) includes confirmation of the estimated date of delivery by quickening at 18 to 20 weeks or earlier, the uterus being at the umbilicus at 20 weeks, and fetal heart tones being heard using a stethoscope. The fetus may be evaluated by ultrasonography if fetal age is in doubt. Health education during the second trimester includes planning for labor and delivery through childbirth education classes, initial discussion of infant feeding including encouragement of breast-feeding, and planning for parenting by recommending reading or classes. Mothers should be instructed to report symptoms that would indicate a pregnancy risk, such as vaginal bleeding, swelling of the face or fingers, continuous headache, blurring of vision, abdominal pain, persistent vomiting, chills, fever, dysuria, escape of fluids per vagina, or change in frequency or intensity of fetal movements.

Third trimester prenatal care (28 weeks to delivery) includes screening for anemia, gestational diabetes, and sexually transmitted diseases if risk is present. Culture for group B streptococcus is also done during this time (34–36 weeks). More frequent visits are generally made during the third trimester to evaluate for elevated blood pressure and other signs of preeclampsia. Labor signs are taught to the patient with careful attention to the possibility of preterm labor. Labor and delivery preferences of the mother and father should be clarified; and a completed prenatal record, including documentation of the parent's birth request, should be given to the patient or sent to the hospital.

Fetal Assessment

Methods have been developed to assess the well-being of the fetus during pregnancy, including fetal movement counting, the nonstress test (NST), nipple stimulation or oxytocin contraction stress test (CST), and ultrasonography for amniotic fluid evaluation. The biophysical profile is a quantitative score that combines fetal heart rate testing with ultrasound evaluation of the fetus and amniotic fluid.[30] This test is time-consuming and requires special training of the ultrasonographer. A combination of fetal heart rate testing (NST or CST) and amniotic fluid evaluation is an alternative to the biophysical profile. These methods are used according to accepted protocols when risk factors are present that may jeopardize the fetus. They are routinely applied when a pregnancy becomes postdates (42 weeks from the last menstrual period) or earlier for certain conditions, such as intrauterine growth retardation (IUGR), diabetes during pregnancy, chronic hypertension or renal disease, pregnancy-induced hypertension, previous unexplained stillbirth, Rh sensitization, oligohydramnios, multiple gestation, or maternal perception of decreased

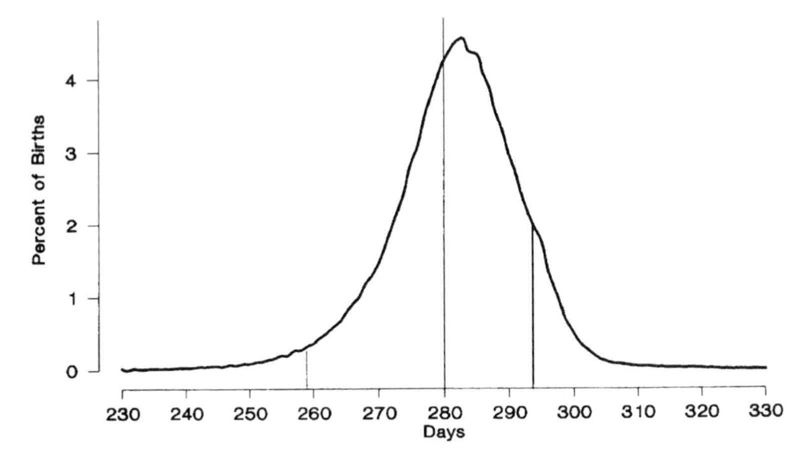

FIGURE. 3.1. Distribution of duration of pregnancy, in days from last menstrual period to birth, among 383,484 singleton, noncesarean births with certain menstrual dates in Sweden, 1976–1980. Vertical lines are drawn at 259, 280, and 294 completed days. The line has been drawn between day-to-day percentage values, without any smoothing of the curve ("raw data"). (From Bergsjo P, Denman DW III, Hoffman HY, et al. *Acta Obstet Gynecol Scand* 1990;69:197–207. With permission.)

fetal movement. Some authorities recommend that women monitor fetal movements regularly during the third trimester of pregnancy. Family physicians should understand these methods and be aware of their relative usefulness, including their sensitivity, specificity, and predictive values.[31]

Duration of Pregnancy

The normal duration of human pregnancy has considerable variation. The "bell-shaped curve" of human pregnancy is illustrated in Figure 3.1. The median is just past 280 days, or 40 weeks, from the last menstrual period. Two standard deviations from the mean would be 37 to 43 weeks. About 10% of pregnancies reach 42 weeks, confirming the normalcy of postdates pregnancy for many women. However, as pregnancies extend beyond 42 weeks, conditions such as oligohydramnios, passage of meconium into the amniotic fluid, macrosomia, and dysmaturity with potential IUGR can cause significant risk for the fetus.

Labor and Delivery

Labor

Labor in the first stage is defined as progressive dilation of the cervix with uterine contractions. The early (latent) phase of labor occurs up to 4 cm dilation and is variable in duration. Progress during this phase is often slow because of the time needed for effacement of the cervix.

The active phase of labor is more rapid and predictable, yet there is still considerable individual variation. With frequent, regular contractions, the average is 1.2 cm dilation per hour in primigravidas and 1.5 cm per hour in multigravidas, but flexibility is important. Friedman attempted to describe labor, not to define parameters women must follow.[32] Arrest of labor is present where there has been no cervical dilation for 2 hours during this active phase.

When the pregnant patient presents in labor, her prenatal record must be carefully reviewed and risk assessment done. Decisions regarding need for antibiotics (e.g., mitral valve prolapse with regurgitation or positive group B streptococcus screening with prolonged rupture of membranes) should be made early.

Support and observation are the hallmarks of managing normal labor. Women in labor should be given as much freedom of movement as possible. The dorsal supine (lithotomy) position is avoided, as the gravid uterus may compress the inferior vena cava and cause maternal hypotension and fetal distress. Upright women in labor report less pain and have greater intrauterine pressure through the cervix.[33] Fatigued women may want to rest on their sides.

During the first stage of labor the blood pressure and the frequency and duration of contractions are measured every 15 to 30 minutes. The fetal heart rate should be monitored during and immediately after a contraction every 30 minutes during the first stage by whatever method is most convenient (electronically, Doppler ultrasonography, or fetoscopic auscultation). Intermittent fetal heart rate monitoring is preferable to continuous monitoring in normal or low-risk patients, as continuous monitoring interferes with freedom of movement and has a high false-positive rate.[7,8] Continuous electronic fetal monitoring in low-risk patients has resulted in three times the diagnosis of fetal distress and twice the frequency of cesarean sections without improving birth outcome.[34]

Women succeed best during the second stage of labor (expulsion of the fetus) when they are allowed and encouraged to use their instincts about pushing. Prolonged breath-holding and Valsalva maneuvers should be avoided, as they may result in decreased oxygenation of the placenta and fetal hypoxia. Women push more effectively and are in less pain when upright: sitting, squatting, kneeling, or standing.[35] Fatigued or hypotensive women may push while lying on their side. Again, the lithotomy position should be avoided to prevent inferior vena cava compression and fetal distress. The fetal heart rate should be monitored every 15 minutes during the second stage in low-risk patients.[36]

SUPPORT DURING LABOR

Continuous emotional support of the woman during labor enhances the birth process. It may be provided by a "labor support team" consisting of the nurse, the delivering physician or midwife, the father, and any other person close to the mother. A "doula" is a lay person trained to provide continuous support to the woman in labor and may be provided by the hospital to ensure that all women in labor receive optimal emotional support for labor and birth. Support during labor may reduce the need for intrapartum medication and technologic intervention.[37]

INTRAPARTUM ANALGESIA AND ANESTHESIA

Because all medications given during labor have side effects for both the mother and fetus, none is given routinely. Pain during labor may be managed by nonpharmacologic methods primarily, such as support from labor attendants, change of position, rest, physical contact, ambulation, and a warm shower or bath. Labor and birth without medication may be satisfying for the woman and her partner.

Some women benefit from pain medication during labor. A short-acting narcotic given parenterally during the first stage of labor may help the woman cope, and it may even facilitate dilation of the cervix.

Lumbar epidural anesthesia has become increasingly common and provides effective pain relief. It has a place in the management of dystocia and is of benefit for cesarean section. Its use during labor should be carefully considered, not elective. Studies in Europe and North America have shown that elective use of epidural anesthesia during labor increases the need for oxytocin augmentation and may increase the cesarean rate.[32,38] Documented effects of epidural anesthesia on labor include decreased uterine activity, prolongation of the first stage of labor, relaxation of the pelvic diaphragm predisposing to minor malpresentation, decreased maternal urge and ability to push, prolonged second stage of labor, and increased use of instrumental vaginal delivery.[39]

Despite these effects, epidural anesthesia has become almost routine in many hospitals, including hospitals with residency programs, and is requested by many women. If women and their birth attendants hope to avoid epidural anesthesia, prenatal education, support during labor, and management of the birthing environment must receive high priority. Low-dose epidural anesthesia, perhaps self-administered, may decrease some of the problems associated with its use.[40]

Delivery

Normal delivery of the infant should occur in whatever position is comfortable for the woman, and the physician should be as flexible as possible with birth positions. The infant's head should remain flexed during delivery to decrease the diameter presenting to the perineum. An episiotomy is avoided unless the infant is large or delivery must occur quickly. Sometimes delivery of the head can be more controlled by gently pushing between contractions. After the head is delivered the physician should not rush to deliver the shoulders. He or she should assess for shoulder dystocia (Is the infant's head tightly retracted to the perineum?), check for a nuchal cord and reduce or clamp and cut it if necessary, dry off the baby's head, and allow spontaneous delivery of the shoulders. The anterior and posterior shoulders should be delivered during a contraction with limited traction. Patience and gentleness result in fewer perineal lacerations.

The delivered infant is assessed immediately for color, tone, and respiratory effort. If no resuscitation efforts are necessary, the infant is placed against the mother for bonding, warming, and drying. Clamping and cutting the cord and assigning of Apgar scores may follow these initial steps.

Delivery of the placenta (third stage of labor) should not be attempted until separation from the uterus has occurred (up to 20 minutes). Placental separation is likely when there is a sudden gush of blood, the uterus becomes globular or firm and rises in the abdomen, and the cord protrudes farther out of the vagina. Gentle traction on the cord and suprapubic pressure to avoid uterine inversion spontaneously delivers the placenta. The placenta is examined for completeness, number of vessels, and abnormalities. The mother is examined for cervical, vaginal, or perineal lacerations. Most first-degree lacerations (skin or mucosal tears) do not require suturing. Conditions that require action immediately postpartum include hepatitis immunization of infants from mothers with positive hepatitis B surface antigen, rubella vaccine for susceptible women, and RhoGAM for Rh-negative women.

Summary

The family physician may be skillful in the management of normal pregnancy, labor, and delivery. Inclusion of this joyous part of the family life cycle in the physician's practice has numerous benefits for diversifying the practice and bonding the family with the physician. The family physician may play an important role in advocating the proper support and management of normal pregnancy, labor, and delivery in an environment filled with extensive technology.

References

1. Odent M. Birth reborn. New York: Pantheon, 1984.
2. Wertz RW, Wertz DC. Lying-in: a history of childbirth in America. New Haven: Yale University Press, 1989.

3. Gortmaker SL. The effects of prenatal care on the health of the newborn. Am J Public Health 1979;69:653–60.
4. Dick-Read G. Childbirth without fear, second edition. New York: Harper & Row, 1959.
5. Karmel M. Thank you, Dr. Lamaze. Philadelphia: Lippincott, 1959.
6. Kitzinger S. The experience of childbirth. New York: Pelican, 1967.
7. Freeman R. Intrapartum fetal monitoring—a disappointing story. N Engl J Med 1990;322:624–6.
8. Banta HD, Thacker SB. The case for reassessment of health care technology. JAMA 1990;264:235–40.
9. Larimore WL, Reynolds JL. Family practice maternity care in America: ruminations on reproducing an endangered species—family physicians who deliver babies. J Am Board Fam Pract 1994;7:478–88.
10. International Childbirth Education Association. Definition of family-centered maternity care. Int J Childbirth Educ 1987;2(1):4.
11. Scherger JE, Levitt C, Acheson LS, et al. Teaching family centered perinatal care in family medicine. Parts 1 and 2. Fam Med 1992;24:288–98, 368–74.
12. Willett WC. Folic acid and neural tube defect: can't we come to closure? Am J Public Health 1992;82:666–8.
13. Expert panel on the content of prenatal care: The content of prenatal care. Washington, DC: US Public Health Service, 1989.
14. Midmer OK. Does family-centered maternity care empower women? The development of woman-centered childbirth model. Fam Med 1992;24: 216–21.
15. Nichols FH, Humenick SS. Childbirth education: practice, research and theory. Philadelphia: Saunders, 1988.
16. Scott JR, Rose NB. Effect of psychoprophylaxis (Lamaze preparation) on labor and delivery in primiparas. N Engl J Med 1976;294:1205–7.
17. US Preventive Services Task Force. Guide to clinical preventive services. Baltimore: Williams & Wilkins, 1989:289–95.
18. Volpe JJ. Effect of cocaine use on the fetus. N Engl J Med 1992;327:399–404.
19. Gjerdingen DK, Froberg DG, Fontaine P. The effects of social support on women's health during pregnancy, labor and delivery, and the postpartum period. Fam Med 1991; 23:370–5.
20. Williamson HA, LeFevre M, Hector M. Association between life stress and serious perinatal complications. J Fam Pract 1989;29:489–96.
21. Rouse DJ, Goldenberg RL, Cliver SP, et al. Strategies for the prevention of early-onset neonatal group B streptococcal sepsis: a decision analysis. Obstet Gynecol 1994;83:483–94.
22. Sacks DA, Abu-Fadil S, Greenspoon JS, et al. How reliable is the fifty-gram, one-hour glucose screening test? Am J Obstet Gynecol 1989;161:642–5.
23. Cunningham FG, Gilstrap LC. Maternal serum alpha-fetoprotein screening. N Engl J Med 1991;325:55–6.
24. US Department of Health and Human Services, Public Health Service, National Institutes of Health: Diagnostic ultrasound imaging in pregnancy. Washington, DC: Government Printing Office, 1984. NIH Publ No. 84-667.

25. American College of Obstetricians and Gynecologists: Ultrasonography in pregnancy. Washington, DC: ACOG, 1993. ACOG Technical Bulletin No. 187.
26. Bucher H, Schmidt JG. Does routine ultrasound scanning improve outcome in pregnancy? Meta-analysis of various outcome measures. BMJ 1993;307:13–7.
27. Ewigman BG, Crane JP, Frigoletto FD, et al. Effect of prenatal ultrasound screening on perinatal outcome. N Engl J Med 1993;329:821–7.
28. Alexander S, Keirse JNC. Formal risk scoring during pregnancy. In: Chalmers I, Enkins M, Keirse JNC, editors. Effective care in pregnancy and childbirth. New York: Oxford University Press, 1989:345–64.
29. American Board of Family Practice. Normal pregnancy: reference guide 17. Lexington, KY: American Board of Family Practice, 1983.
30. Norman LA, Karp LE. Biophysical profile for antepartum fetal assessment. Am Fam Physician 1986;34(4):83–9.
31. American College of Obstetricians and Gynecologists. Antepartum Fetal Surveillance. Washington, DC: ACOG, 1994. ACOG Technical Bulletin No. 188.
32. Friedman EA. Disordered labor: objective evaluation and management. J Fam Pract 1975;2:167–72.
33. McKay S, Mahan CS. Laboring patients need more freedom to move. Contemp Obstet Gynecol 1984;24(1):90–119.
34. Neilson JP. Electronic fetal heart rate monitoring during labor: information from randomized trials. Birth 1994;21(2):101–4.
35. Olsen R, Olsen C, Cox NS. Maternal birthing positions and perineal injury. J Fam Pract 1990;30:553–7.
36. American College of Obstetricians and Gynecologists. Intrapartum fetal heart rate monitoring. Washington, DC: ACOG, 1995. ACOG Technical Bulletin No. 207.
37. Kennell J, Klaus M, McGrath S, et al. Continuous emotional support during labor in a U.S. hospital. JAMA 1991;265: 2197–201.
38. Ramin SM, Grambling DR, Lucas MJ, et al. Randomized trial of epidural versus intravenous analgesia during labor. Obstet Gynecol 1995;86:783–9.
39. Johnson S, Rosenfeld JA. The effect of epidural anesthesia on the length of labor. J Fam Pract 1995;40:244–7.
40. Viscome C, Eisenach JC. Patient-controlled epidural analgesia during labor. Obstet Gynecol 1991;77:348–51.

CASE PRESENTATION

Subjective

PATIENT PROFILE

Ann Martino-Priestley is a 22-year-old married white female nursery school teacher.

PRESENTING PROBLEM

"Possible pregnancy."

PRESENT ILLNESS

Mrs. Martino-Priestley, who has never been pregnant in the past, reports that her last normal period was 7 weeks ago. She has had morning nausea and urinary frequency, and an over-the-counter pregnancy test was positive. She has had a few episodes of spotting over the past week.

PAST MEDICAL HISTORY

No serious illnesses or hospitalization.

SOCIAL HISTORY

Mrs. Martino-Priestley graduated from college a few months ago and is working part-time as a nursery school teacher. She has been married for 1 year to Luke, who is a graduate student in an MBA program.

HABITS

She does not smoke, she takes alcohol occasionally on weekends, and she uses no drugs.

FAMILY HISTORY

Her parents are divorced. Her biological father, aged 45, has peptic ulcer disease. Her mother has migraine headaches. She has no siblings.

REVIEW OF SYSTEMS

Her only other symptom is occasional heartburn if she is under stress and drinks too much coffee.

- What other information about her current health status would you like to know? Why?
- What more would you like to know about her social history? Explain.
- What might be the meaning of pregnancy to Ann and Luke at this time, and how would you approach this issue?
- Is there anything in the patient's history that might concern you at this time? Why?

Objective

VITAL SIGNS

Height, 5 ft 5 in; weight, 130 lb; blood pressure, 130/88; pulse, 70; temperature, 37.3°C.

EXAMINATION

The head, eyes, ears, nose, and throat are normal. The neck and thyroid glands are normal. The chest and heart are unremarkable. There are no breast masses. The abdomen has no tenderness or mass palpable. On pelvic examination, there is a thin vaginal discharge. The cervical isthmus is soft. The fundus is enlarged to a 6- to 8-week pregnancy size and is nontender. The adnexa and the rectal examination are normal.

LABORATORY

An office pregnancy test is positive.

- What more—if anything—would you include in the physical examination, and why?
- What—if anything—would you do today to evaluate the blood pressure reading of 130/88?
- What are your concerns regarding the vaginal discharge, and what would you do to further evaluate this finding?
- What laboratory studies would you order on this first prenatal visit?

Assessment

- How would you describe your conclusions and prognosis to Mrs. Martino-Priestley?
- What are your concerns regarding this pregnancy?
- What might be the impact of this pregnancy on the patient as an individual? How might you address this topic?
- What changes are this pregnancy likely to cause in Ann and Luke's life as a couple, and how should these issues be addressed?

Plan

- What advice would you offer the patient at this time regarding diet, vitamins, medications, and activity?
- If the patient is found to have a trichomonas vaginitis, how would you explain this to the patient, and what therapy would you recommend?
- What community agencies might be helpful to Ann and Luke, and how might these agencies be contacted?
- Describe your plans for continuing care of this patient and her pregnancy.

4

Problems of the Newborn and Infant

RICHARD B. LEWAN, BRUCE AMBUEL, AND
ROBERT W. SANDER

Family-centered care offers diverse opportunities for reducing risk and improving the health of newborns and infants. Premarital, preconception, and prenatal visits allow assessment for genetic disorders, ensure healthy life style changes (e.g., nutrition), provide preconception vitamins, manage chronic diseases such as diabetes, and intervene when prenatal disorders such as toxemia threaten. Optimal care requires preparation for emergencies (e.g., neonatal resuscitation, sepsis), management of common problems, timely referral for complicated conditions, and prevention through early identification of feeding, growth and developmental problems, and family violence. Full family involvement prepares each member for new roles, recruits participation in healthy habits, and maintains cohesiveness when problems arise.

Newborn Care

Newborn Resuscitation

Skillful resuscitation can prevent lifelong complications of common neonatal emergencies. Proper preparation for the distressed newborn begins with a search for risk factors with each delivery. Participation in a resuscitation course[1] or hospital-based practice sessions promotes teamwork and leadership. Then team members can develop and maintain skills using an organized plan of assessment and intervention. Figure 4.1 outlines an intervention protocol based on meconium, respiratory effort, heart rate, and color. This figure can be posted with a list of tested equipment in a visible location in the resuscitation area. Ready access to the equipment must be provided and medications listed. When time permits, all equipment is laid out and tested. Prior to obtaining intravenous access, epinephrine and naloxone can be given by endotracheal tube followed by 1 to 2 ml of saline if necessary. Basic resuscitation skills for a depressed newborn include (1) controlling the *thermal environment* with proper use of a radiant warmer and rapid, thorough drying; (2) *positioning, suction-*

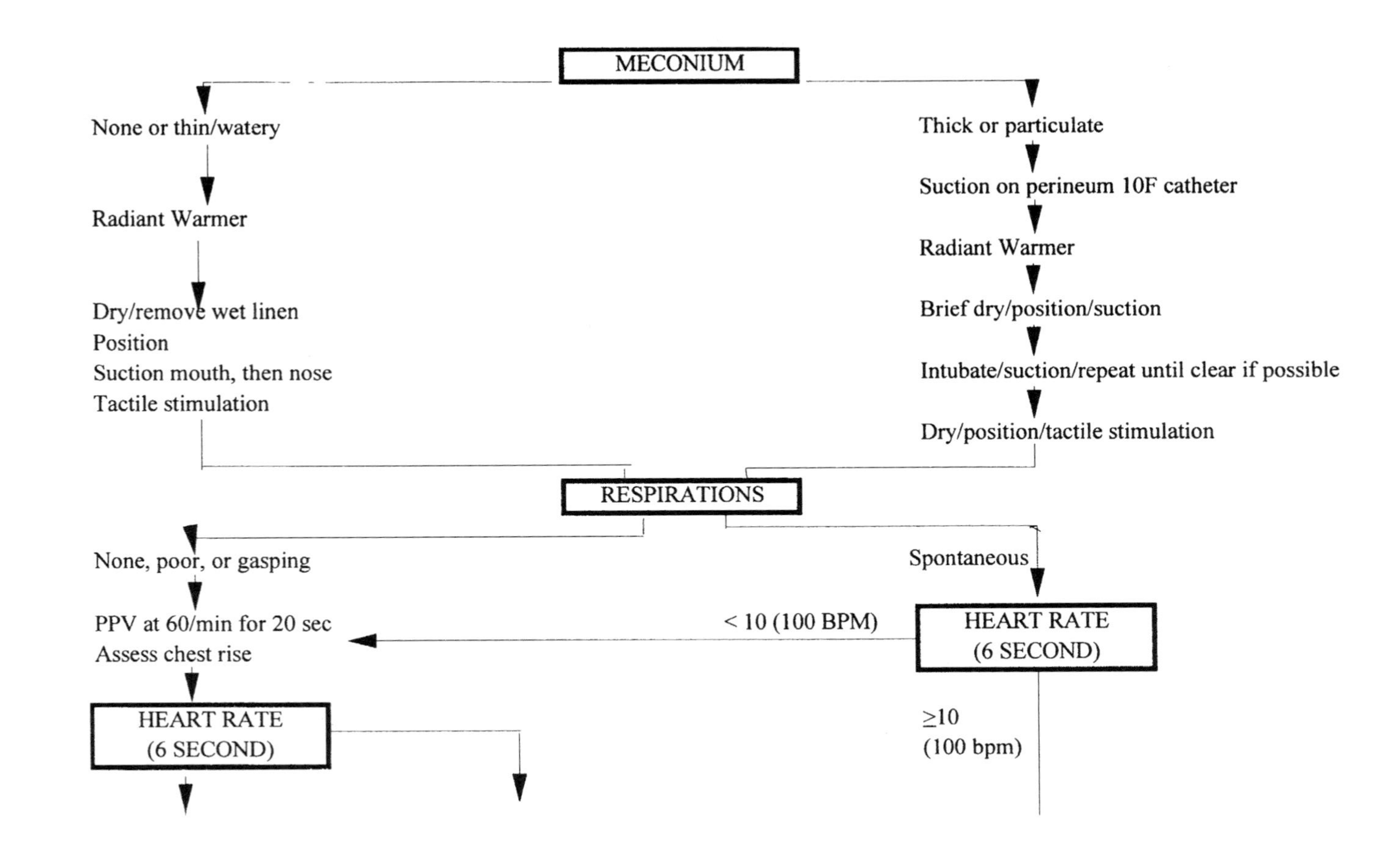
MECONIUM
None or thin/watery
Radiant Warmer
Dry/remove wet linen
Position
Suction mouth, then nose
Tactile stimulation
Thick or particulate
Suction on perineum 10F catheter
Radiant Warmer
Brief dry/position/suction
Intubate/suction/repeat until clear if possible
Dry/position/tactile stimulation
RESPIRATIONS
None, poor, or gasping
PPV at 60/min for 20 sec
Assess chest rise
HEART RATE
(6 SECOND)
Spontaneous
HEART RATE
(6 SECOND)
< 10 (100 BPM)
≥10
(100 bpm)

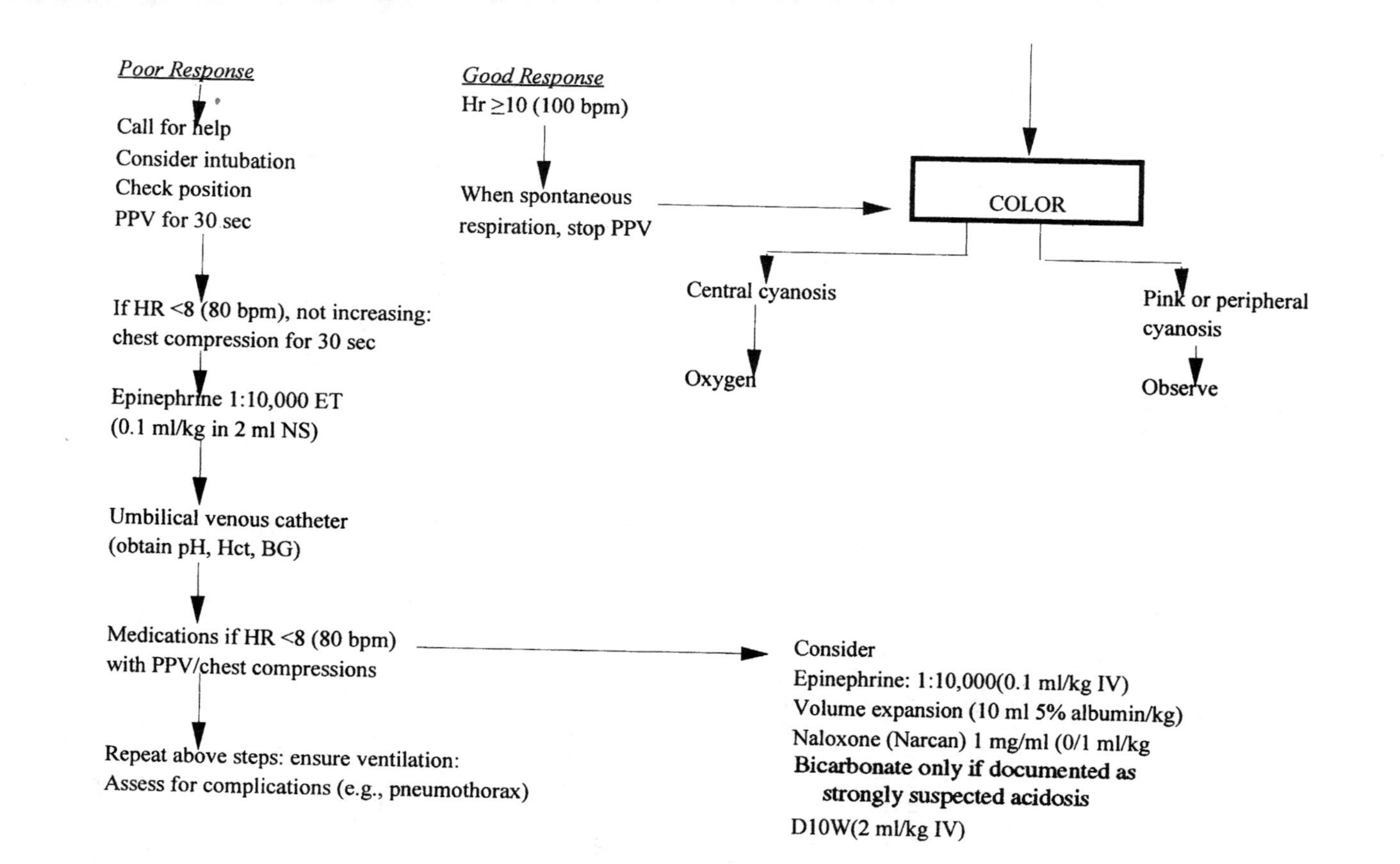

FIGURE. 4.1. Neonatal resuscitation. bpm = breaths per minute; HR = heart rate; PPV = positive-pressure ventilation; ET = endotracheal; NS = normal saline; Hct = hematocrit; BG = blood glucose.

ing, and gentle *tactile stimulation;* (3) *catheter suctioning of meconium* from the airway or the perineum followed by gentle bulb syringe suctioning after delivery, as well as tracheal suctioning of thick or particulate meconium through an endotracheal tube (repeat until clear unless the neonate is overly distressed); and (4) providing immediate *bag and mask ventilation* for newborns with apnea or poor respiratory effort. Effective positioning and skillful assisted ventilation revive most distressed neonates. Short delays greatly prolong recovery time.

Advanced skills for those without immediate consultation include (1) *endotracheal tube placement* with ventilation for those not responding or requiring more prolonged bag and mask ventilation; (2) *chest compressions* at 120 per minute for a sustained heart rate of less than 80 beats per minute (bpm); (3) *central circulation access* through the umbilical venous catheter because peripheral intravenous access is often unsuccessful; and (4) *chest puncture* at the second intercostal space in the mid-clavicular line with a 20-gauge angiocatheter for tension pneumothorax.

Stabilization for Transfer to the Nursery or Transport to Intensive Care

Postresuscitation priorities include assessment for emergent anomalies, maintenance of basic needs, effective communication with and support of the family, and deciding on the level of care required. Pulse oximetry and a cardiorespiratory monitor are used to monitor ongoing success. Oxygen saturations should be kept at 88% to 92% for preterm newborns and 92% to 95% for term newborns. Baseline tests for unstable newborns include a chest radiograph, complete blood count (CBC), glucose, and blood gases (arterial if possible, otherwise capillary). A sepsis workup and other laboratory tests may then be considered. Ventilatory support is needed for persistent respiratory distress, apnea, or deteriorating blood gases (especially $P_{CO_2} > 60$ with acidosis). Feedings should then be avoided and a nasogastric tube placed. Intravenous fluids are started with 10% dextrose in water ($D_{10}W$) at 65 to 80 ml/kg/day for the first 24 hours. Timely transport of unstable or high risk neonates for tertiary care enhances outcome (e.g., early surfactant therapy for hyaline membrane disease).

Common Problems in the Nursery

LOW-BIRTH-WEIGHT NEWBORNS

Every hospital should provide a standard graph that allows plotting of weight to gestational age (by dates and examination) to identify newborns who are premature (< 37 weeks), small for gestational age (SGA; weight < 10th percentile), or both. Once classified, problems unique to each can be prevented or anticipated. For example, prematurity is associated with hyaline membrane disease, apnea, jaundice, and intracranial hemorrhage. Asymmetric SGA newborns (small trunk relative to head size, caused by uteroplacental insufficiency) are at risk for asphyxia, meconium aspiration, hypoglycemia, hypothermia, and polycythemia. Symmetric SGA (small head and body, caused by genetic or TORCH syndromes) adds risk for congenital malformations and poor subsequent catch-up growth. All may be at risk for sepsis.

Those newborns cared for in a low-risk nursery are ready for discharge when: (1) medically stable; (2) feeding well (100 kcal/kg/day); (3) more than 2 kg with consistent weight gain; (4) able to maintain stable body temperature in an open crib; (5) apnea-free (or home monitoring and parental instruction is complete); and (6) parents are able to cope with the infant at home.

POSTTERM NEWBORNS

After 42 weeks' gestation there may be absent lanugo and vernix, long nails, scaly skin, abundant scalp hair, and increased alertness. Some are large and at risk for birth trauma and asphyxia; others are SGA due to placental insufficiency with risks as described above.

NEONATAL SEPSIS

Sepsis is often accompanied by nonspecific signs and symptoms, making early detection difficult: 2/1000 neonates have bacterial sepsis. Risk increases with preterm labor, premature rupture of membranes, or intrapartum fever. Group B streptococcus (GBS) and *Escherichia coli* are responsible for 70% of the infections and *Listeria monocytogenes,* enterococcus, *Staphylococcus aureus,* and *Haemophilus influenzae* for the rest. Early manifestations include temperature instability, lethargy, and poor feeding. Only about 50% have a temperature higher than 37.8°C (100°F axillary). Prompt evaluation and careful observation every few hours can clarify when a thorough workup is needed. Hepatosplenomegaly, jaundice, petechiae, seizures, stiff neck, and bulging fontanel occur late and denote a poor prognosis.

Group B streptococcal infection is associated with 20% mortality and often presents at or just after birth with rapid deterioration, unexplained apnea, tachypnea, respiratory distress, or shock. Late-onset disease (mean 24 days), usually presents as meningitis. Intrapartum chemoprophylaxis based on a 1996 Centers for Disease Control (CDC) recommendation[2] may reduce morbidity and mortality of neonatal GBS infections.

Diagnosis. Helpful studies include CBC, chest radiography, and cultures of blood, cerebrospinal fluid (CSF), and urine. Catheterization or suprapubic aspiration are preferable for culture and the rapid antigen test of urine. The CSF may contain up to 32 white blood cells (WBC)/mm^3 during the first few days, so a Gram stain and protein and glucose levels in the CSF should be checked. Surface cultures are no longer recommended.

Treatment. Antibiotics should be initiated quickly with a combination of ampicillin (200 mg/kg/day IV or IM *divided* bid for infants during the first week of life, tid thereafter) plus gentamicin (2.5 mg/kg per dose bid for the first week, tid thereafter). Dosages are reduced for low-birth-weight infants or if meningitis is excluded. Antibiotics can be stopped at 48 hours with sterile cultures unless the suspicion for infection was high; treatment is then continued intravenously at least 7 days while monitoring gentamicin levels.[3] If the latter assay is not available, cefotaxime can be used instead of gentamicin. Methicillin should replace ampicillin when starting antibiotics after 3 days of life. Bacteremia is treated for 7 to 10 days depending on the response. Meningitis requires at least 14 days of therapy.

RESPIRATORY DISTRESS

Tachypnea, grunting, nasal flaring, retractions, cyanosis, apnea, or stridor should be evaluated with a chest radiograph, blood gases, glucose, and hematocrit. Early onset causes include *hyaline membrane disease* (HMD), *meconium aspiration, transient tachypnea of the newborn* (TTN), or "wet lung" and less commonly in utero acquired pneumonia or congenital defects compromising the respiratory tract. At several hours after birth sepsis, metabolic abnormalities, cardiac failure, and intraventricular hemorrhage become more likely.

Hyaline membrane disease affects preterm newborns, who manifest "stiff" lungs, hypercarbia, hypoxia, and a "ground-glass" radiograph with air bronchograms. Rapid stabilization and early surfactant therapy improves outcome. Meconium aspiration usually occurs after 34 weeks, causing airway obstruction and edema. Radiography reveals hyperinflation and possibly pneumothorax. After resuscitation, aggressive support with ventilation and oxygen should maintain the Po_2 above 80 mm Hg. Sepsis workup and antibiotic coverage are indicated for HMD and meconium aspiration because the risk of pneumonia is increased.

Transient tachypnea of the newborn presents just after birth in term or preterm newborns and improves significantly within 24 hours. Tachypnea, less severe hypoxia, and radiographic findings of perihilar streaking and fluid in the fissures are common. Oxygen requirements gradually decrease after the first few hours. If the course is atypical or there is risk of sepsis, other causes including *neonatal pneumonia* must be considered.

APNEA

A respiratory pause of 20 seconds (shorter if associated with cyanosis or bradycardia) should prompt a complete history about the event including respiratory effort, color, tone, relation to feeding, and unusual movement. A careful cardiorespiratory and neurologic examination, CBC, and calcium, magnesium, and electrolyte levels are assessed. If apnea occurs during the first 24 hours of life, sepsis must be excluded. Based on the suspicion, an electrocardiogram (ECG), echocardiogram, arterial blood gases, electroencephalogram (EEG), head computed tomography scan (CT), or reflux studies may be needed. A 24-hour breathing study (pneumogram) may support the need for home monitoring in preterm infants for usually 2 to 3 months. All underlying problems should be corrected or managed.

Cyanosis

Blue hands and feet are sometimes normal or may be due to slowed circulation. Trunk and mucous membrane involvement (i.e., central cyanosis) after the first 20 minutes of life requires rapid evaluation. If hypothermia, hypoglycemia, narcotic respiratory depression, hypotension, and choanal atresia are not found, causes may include pulmonary, cardiac, neurologic, and metabolic disorders as well as polycythemia, sepsis, and acidosis. Intermittent cyanosis with alternating "spells" of apnea and periods of normal breathing suggests a neurologic disorder. Involvement in the upper or lower part of the body or continuous cyanosis without respiratory signs strongly suggests a cardiac cause, especially if a Po_2 of 100 mm Hg is not achieved when the infant is placed in 100% oxygen for 20 minutes. Hypoxia should be reversed with oxygenation and assisted ventilation in preparation for rapid referral.

Hypotension and Shock

After quick assessment including repeated vital signs and obtaining essential laboratory tests (i.e., CBC, coagulation studies, glucose, electrolytes and pH, calcium, cultures, and if fetal hemorrhage is suspected the Kleihauer-Betke test), volume expansion with 5% albumin (10 ml/kg over 30 minutes) should be undertaken promptly for suspected hypovolemia, sepsis, or neurogenic causes. Once stabilized, the history and physical examination can direct further study. Any suggestion of sepsis requires a workup and antibiotic coverage. If cardiogenic causes are likely, inotropic agents may be indicated and should be considered when volume expansion is ineffective.

Cardiac Murmurs

Soft, benign murmurs are common during the first 24 hours of life, but loud murmurs suggest valvular stenosis or regurgitation. Murmurs of cardiac shunts may be heard at 72 hours but more often at 2 to 3 weeks. Loud murmurs, abnormal heart sounds, or findings suggesting cardiac disease (i.e., cyanosis, poor color or feeding, tachycardia, bradycardia, abnormal blood pressure, respiratory distress, or hepatomegaly) necessitate a prompt ECG, chest radiograph, and, if pathology is suspected, cardiology consultation. All neonates require careful auscultation at the 2 week visit.

JAUNDICE

Jaundice is noted in at least 50% of Caucasian newborns, with 6% having total serum bilirubin (TSB) levels more than 12.9 mg/dl. Higher levels are noted in Asian and American Indian newborns. Kernicterus leading to death or severe neurologic handicap is preventable if bilirubin levels do not exceed 25 to 30 mg/dl (lower in sick premature neonates). Early discharge may contribute to delayed recognition of high TSB levels and a resurgence of kernicterus.

Diagnosis. Icterus, best detected by blanching blood from the skin, is first noted in the face and progresses to the feet as TSB levels rise. Transcutaneous bilirubinometry estimates TSB but is inaccurate with rapid progression, after phototherapy, or with dark skin. TSB levels are necessary for severe or rapid-onset jaundice. They may be inaccurate by ± 1 mg/dl.

Physiologic jaundice is common with a typical pattern of unconjugated hyperbilirubinemia, reaching an average peak of 6 mg/dl by day 3 and resolution within 1 week in term infants and within 2 weeks in preterm infants. A search for pathologic jaundice is needed with (1) icterus during the first 24 hours (assess *quickly* for hemolysis); (2) TSB rising more than 5 mg/dl per day; (3) TSB exceeding 15 mg/dl in term infants and 10 mg/dl in preterm infants; (4) icterus lasting longer than 10 days in term infants and 21 days in preterm infants; and (5) a direct bilirubin level exceeding 1.5 mg/dl. Review the maternal and perinatal history for risk factors, reexamine, determine the infant's blood type and Rh, and perform a direct Coombs' test (if possible, on cord blood saved from the delivery). If these tests are normal, an exaggerated physiologic jaundice pattern is likely. If hemolysis is present a hematocrit, blood smear, and enzyme assay [e.g., glucose-6-phosphate dehydrogenase (G6PD)] may be indicated. The direct bilirubin level should be checked if jaundice persists or cholestasis is suspected (light stool, dark urine, jaundice with a green tinge).

Treatment. Despite the recent trend of high TSB levels before treatment, earlier treatment is needed for those at risk of kernicterus (i.e., hemolysis, asphyxia, and prematurity). *Jaundice during the first 24 hours* of life requires prompt evaluation and consideration for exchange transfusion if hemolysis is found.

To encourage clinical judgment, TSB ranges are recommended for starting phototherapy in *healthy term newborns* as follows: TSB of 12 to 15 mg/dl at 24 to 48 hours, 15 to 18 mg/dl at 48 to 72 hours, and 17 to 20 mg/dl at more than 72 hours.[4] Increasing or high TSB levels (i.e., 20 mg/dl at 24 to 48 hours, 25 mg/dl at more than 48 hours) require intensive (double or special lights) phototherapy. If TBS levels do not decline 1 to 2 mg/dl within 6 hours or higher levels are encountered at any time (i.e., 25 mg/dl at 25 to 48 hours and 30 mg/dl at any time), exchange transfusion should be added. Phototherapy precautions include increasing fluids by 15 mg/kg/day, patching eyes, and monitoring for temperature instability. A transient rash, green stools, lethargy, irritability, and abdominal distension may occur. Phototherapy can be stopped when the TSB falls below 14 mg/dl. A small rebound may occur. If jaundice persists or bronze discoloration is noted, fractionate the bilirubin to search for cholestasis. Home phototherapy (using a fiberoptic panel) with uncomplicated jaundice and a reliable family allows breast-feeding and bonding to proceed with minimal interruption.

Breast-feeding is associated with elevated bilirubin levels beginning on the third day. More frequent feeding (i.e., 10 times in 24 hours without supplements unless milk production is low) reduces TSB levels. "Breast milk jaundice" is a delayed, sometimes alarming, common form of jaundice. It begins after the third day, peaks by the end of the second week, and gradually resolves over 1 to 4 months. If the evaluation previously described reveals no pathologic cause, parental preference should strongly influence whether to breast-feed frequently (formula supplement if low output), begin phototherapy, or interrupt breast-feeding. Interruption of breast-feeding for 48 hours, while confirming the diagnosis with an abrupt decline in TSB, increases the risk of breast-feeding failure significantly and should be used infrequently.

Hypoglycemia

Blood glucose levels should be higher than 40 mg/dl for all newborns. Hypoglycemia can occur without risk factors and be asymptomatic. The most common symptoms are "jitteriness," cyanosis, convulsions, apnea, apathy, abnormal cry, limpness, and poor feeding. A capillary glucose strip from a warmed heel allows screening of high-risk or symptomatic infants. Any value less than 45 mg/dl must be confirmed by venipuncture. Hypoglycemia is prevented by keeping newborns warm, providing early caloric support if high risk, and then monitoring every 30 minutes initially. If symptomatic, a bolus of $D_{10}W$ (2 ml/ kg) over 2 to 3 minutes is followed by an infusion of 8 mg/kg/min. The glucose strip is rechecked at 15 minutes and again hourly until three consecutive normal values occur.

Metabolic Disorders

Unexplained poor feeding, vomiting, lethargy, convulsion, or coma in a previously healthy newborn suggests an inborn error of metabolism even during the first few hours of life. After excluding hypoglycemia and hypocalcemia, plasma ammonia, bicarbonate, and pH should be checked. Early consultation and treatment avoids severe metabolic and neurologic disturbances.

ANEMIA

A central venous hematocrit less than 45% in newborns delivered after 34 weeks is often caused by blood loss and less often by hemolysis or congenital anemias. Careful review of the history, physical examination, red blood cell (RBC) indices, and peripheral smear can guide further evaluation. Coombs' test, reticulocyte count, and Kleihauer-Betke stain of maternal blood to look for fetomaternal transfusion may be needed. Shock requires repeated 5 ml/kg infusions over 5 minutes of crossmatched or O-negative blood until symptoms are alleviated. Severe hemolysis may require exchange transfusion.

POLYCYTHEMIA

A hematocrit of more than 65% venous or 70% capillary may cause plethora, subsequent jaundice, and hyperviscosity. If the infant is symptomatic (lethargy, apnea, irritability, seizures, feeding difficulties, respiratory distress, cyanosis, hypoglycemia) and after confirming the hematocrit elevation, a partial exchange transfusion should be given to lower the hematocrit to 50%.

BIRTH INJURIES

Head injuries include soft tissue swelling of the scalp resulting from vertex delivery (caput succedaneum), slow subperiosteal hemorrhage limited to the surface of one cranial bone and not crossing the midline (cephalohematoma), and skull fracture that requires treatment only if depressed. Clavicle fracture, the most common fracture, manifests as limited arm movement and crepitus over the injury. Immobilization of the affected arm and shoulder may be considered.

Erb's palsy (neuritis of C5–C6 roots due to delivery trauma) causes arm adduction and internal rotation, elbow extension and pronation, and wrist flexion ("waiter's tip" posture). Five to nine percent have diaphragm paralysis. Early improvement of hand grasp suggests a favorable prognosis. Recovery should be complete within 3 to 6 months. If no shoulder, arm, or clavicle fractures exist, the infant's sleeve can be pinned in a functional position for 1 week followed by gentle passive exercises.

HUMAN IMMUNODEFICIENCY VIRUS INFECTION IN NEONATES AND INFANTS

In 1993 an estimated 1630 human immunodeficiency virus (HIV)-infected infants were born in the United States. Fortunately, the AIDS Clinical Trials

Group (ACTG) Protocol 076 demonstrated that if previously untreated HIV-positive pregnant women with CD4 counts less than 200/mm^3 are treated with zidovudine (ZDV or AZT), the risk of vertical HIV transmission drops from 25.5% to 8.3%. Such women should be started on oral ZDV (100 mg 5 times daily) as early as 14 weeks' gestation. It is continued through delivery (loading dose of 2 mg/kg over 1 hour and then continuous infusion of 1 mg/kg/hr) and given to the newborn during the first 6 weeks of life (2 mg/kg q6h beginning 8–12 hours after birth).[5] In addition, because 35% of HIV-positive women report unprotected heterosexual intercourse as their only risk factor, physicians should screen all pregnant women for HIV.[6]

In utero infection causes 30% to 50% of the cases of vertical transmission. These infants typically have a more virulent infection, with laboratory evidence of infection at birth. Most of the other cases of vertical transmission occur intrapartum through exposure to infected cervical and vaginal secretions. The rate of such transmission is almost doubled when delivery follows rupture of membranes of more than 4 hours duration. It is unclear whether using cesarean section to minimize exposure to secretions reduces transmission.[7] Transmission is significantly reduced, though, even in women who have not received antepartum ZDV, by the use of the intrapartum and neonatal portions of the ACTG Protocol 076. Laboratory evidence of intrapartum infection is generally not found until 1 to 12 weeks of life.

The final route of transmission is through breast milk. HIV-positive mothers should be urged to use formula.[8]

Newborns of HIV-positive mothers who did not receive antepartum or intrapartum ZDV should be started on the neonatal arm of the ACTG Protocol 076 within 24 hours of birth. If a woman at high risk for acquiring HIV delivers with an unknown HIV status, the CDC recommends that both mother and infant should be screened for HIV.[6]

Diagnosis. It is imperative that infants infected with HIV be identified as rapidly as possible to ensure early use of therapies to reduce HIV replication and to prevent opportunistic infections. Physical examination at birth is usually normal, and the presenting symptoms are often subtle. Symptoms include failure to thrive, lymphadenopathy and hepatosplenomegaly, chronic or recurrent diarrhea, interstitial pneumonia, and persistent oral thrush. Diagnosis depends on laboratory testing. Any infant exhibiting these symptoms who is born to a mother at high risk or who exhibits other signs of immune compromise, should be tested. Certainly all infants born to HIV-positive mothers should be tested immediately after birth. Historically, the initial screen should be the DNA polymerase chain reaction (PCR). If negative, it should be repeated weekly during the first month of life and again at four months of age or until positive. Two negative PCRs performed at ≥1 month of age, with at least one at ≥ 4 months of age, reasonably excludes HIV infection. Any positive PCR should be immediately confirmed by HIV culture. Treatment, though, can be started while the culture is pending[8,9]. One study indicates that HIV-1 RNA levels may be a more sensitive method for detecting infection, allowing earlier initiation of treatment and better prediction of the rate of progression of the disease[10].

Treatment. Owing to often complex and changing recommendations, management of the HIV-infected infant should be done in conjunction with a consultant. A detailed discussion of management is therefore not offered here, although a few general concepts are helpful. Close attention should be paid to nutritional status. Development is monitored closely so any needed supplemental physical or occupational therapy can be started in a timely manner. Prevention of *Pneumocystis carinii* pneumonia (PCP) is one of the most important goals of HIV management. Thus all infants 6 weeks to 1 year of age born to HIV-positive mothers or who prove to be HIV-infected themselves should receive prophylaxis with 150 mg of trimethoprim plus 750 mg of sulfamethoxazole per square meter body surface per day divided twice daily and given 3 days weekly. If HIV infection can later be reasonably excluded, PCP prophylaxis can be discontinued.[8] See Chapter 21 for additional information on management of the HIV-infected child.

Approaches to Common Neonatal Anomalies

Table 4.1 provides a brief overview of common anomalies encountered by those caring for newborns.

Guidelines for Early Hospital Discharge of the Newborn

Resurgence of kernicterus demonstrates the risk of early discharge in a changing health care environment. Careful assessment of medical risk and stability, completed education of parents on proper care and warning signs, and secured early medical follow-up are essential components of care prior to discharge between 6 and 24 hours. Examples of eligibility criteria are adequate prenatal care, uncomplicated and low-risk pregnancy and delivery, 1-minute Apgar score over 6, weight over 2500 g, gestational age 38 weeks or more, normal vital signs, stable medical condition including jaundice, completed physician examination, normal glucose, at least two successful feedings, voiding of urine, appropriate parent–newborn interaction, and ability of the parents to verbalize instructions and complete their education. A home visit at 2 to 3 days of life by a physician or trained nurse improves infant assessment, early identification of problems, and ongoing educational efforts.

TABLE 4.1. Approaches to common neonatal anomalies

Abnormality	Causes	Evaluation/treatment
Head		
Macrocephaly (head size > 97%)	May be normal; hydrocephalus; metabolic disorders	Check for neurologic impairment; consider ultrasonography (US), head computed tomography (CT)
Microcephaly (head size < 3%)	Cerebral dysgenesis; prenatal insults	Head US, CT
Large fontanels	Skeletal disorders; chromosomal anomalies; hypothyroidism; high intracranial pressure,	Check for neurologic impairment
Small fontanels	Hyperthyroidism; microcephaly; craniosynostosis	Check for neurologic impairment
Craniotabes (softening of cranial bones, giving a "ping-pong ball" sensation)	If local, benign bone demineralization. If generalized, syphilis or osteogenesis imperfecta	Recalcifies and hardens over 3 months, VDRL; check for blue sclera and fractures
Eyes		
Abnormal red reflex ("white pupil")	Half (50%) of patients have cataracts	Ophthalmologic evaluation
Nasolacrimal duct obstruction (5% of newborns; overflow tearing or mucopurulent drainage; erythema)	Incomplete canalization of duct with residual membrane near nasal cavity	Nasolacrimal massage qid; topical antibiotics for mucopurulent drainage; duct dilatation if persistent
Ears		
Any significant ear anomaly and preauricular pits/fistulas		Check for hearing impairment and possible renal abnormalities
Mouth/palate		
Long philtrum, thin upper lip, small jaw, large tongue		Check for genetic abnormalities
Epstein's pearls (2- to 3-mm white papules on the gums or palate)	Keratogenous cysts	Spontaneous resolution in weeks; reassurance
Short lingual frenulum ("tongue-tied")	Normal	Clip if feeding impaired, tip of tongue notches when extruded, or tongue cannot touch upper gums
Cleft lip or palate	Isolated variant; some genetic anomalies	Feeding assessment; lip repair usually at 2 months, palate by 1 year; revision of repair at 4–5 years
Neck		
Fistulas, sinuses, or cysts midline or anterior to the sternocleidomastoid (SCM); may retract with swallow	Branchial cleft anomalies; thyroglossal duct cysts	Nonemergent surgical referral
Cystic hygroma (soft mass of variable size in the neck or axilla)	Dilated lymphatic spaces	Semiurgent surgical referral as lesion can expand rapidly

TABLE 4.1. (*continued*)

Abnormality	Causes	Evaluation/treatment
Congenital torticollis (tilting of the infant's head due to SCM spasm)	Isolated abnormality from muscular hematoma that appears at 2 weeks	Early physical therapy
Skin		
Café au lait spots (flat, light brown macules usually < 2 cm)	Consider neurofibromatosis if more than six spots or large lesions	No treatment
Hemangiomas (often raised, red, vascular nodules, deeper lesions appear blue; usually < 4 cm; onset during first 3–4 weeks, increases over 6–12 months)	Multiple lesions suggest possible dissemination involving internal organs	Most involute and disappear by 7–9 years of age; observe without treatment unless involving vital structures, ulceration, or infection; evaluate further if multiple
Mongolian spots (gray-blue plaques, up to several centimeters, often lumbosacral, may appear elsewhere)	Hyperpigmentation, seen in up to 70% of nonwhite infants	Benign; most fade over first year; document location
Nevi (variably sized light to dark brown macules; some congenital; others appear later during infancy)	Congenital giant (> 20 cm) may undergo malignant degeneration	No treatment needed, although some advise removal of congenital nevi at puberty; refer giant nevi for evaluation
Petechiae (normal only on head or upper body after vaginal births)	Infection or hematologic problem if abnormal	If abnormal, look for signs of TORCH syndrome
Port-wine stains (permanent vascular macules)	Possible associated ocular or CNS abnormalities	Cosmetic problem only, unless other abnormalities
Subcutaneous fat necrosis (hard, purplish, defined areas on cheeks, back, buttocks, arms, or thighs; appear during the first week)	Necrosis of fat from trauma or asphyxia	Spontaneous resolution over several weeks; rare complication of fluctuance or ulceration
Abdomen/gastrointestinal tract		
Mass	Genitourinary (GU) in 50% (either kidney or bladder)	Emergent ultrasonography of urinary tract
Single umbilical artery	Other congenital defects in 6%	Careful examination for other defects
Intestinal atresia (bilious vomiting with variable degrees of distension)	If duodenal, resorption of lumen; if jejunoileal, mesenteric vascular accident	Nasogastric tube, laboratory tests, chest and supine/upright abdominal films; contrast enema; surgery
Meconium ileus (distended at birth, radiograph shows distended loops and bubbly picture of air and stool in right lower quadrant; absent air–fluid levels)	Abnormal meconium trapping resulting in small bowel obstruction	Supine/upright abdominal films; treat with hyperosmolar gastrografin enema (successful in two-thirds), otherwise surgery

Genitourinary tract		
Ambiguous genitalia (if gonads are palpable, likely to be male)	Due to virilization of genetic female (especially congenital 21-hydroxylase deficiency) or undermasculinized male	Obtain karyotype and 17α-hydroxyprogesterone level quickly; withhold diagnosis of sex until karyotype complete
Hypospadias (urethral opening proximal to tip of glans; may be associated chordee: abnormal penile curvature)	Isolated defect unless other GU anomalies; suspected genetic basis	Avoid circumsion; repair before 18 months of age by experienced surgeon; check for cryptorchidism and hernia; siblings at increased risk
Cryptorchidism (failure of testicular descent; 30% bilateral; long-term complications of infertility and cancer if left untreated)	May be normal: seen in 33% of preterm, 3% of term; if bilateral, consider ambiguous genitalia; if hypospadias and bilateral, consider urologic or endocrine problems	Observe for descent by 3 months; if not, treatment by age 2 years; if bilateral, obtain karyotype; if also hypospadias, do full urologic and endocrine evaluation
Hydrocele (scrotal swelling that transilluminates)	Communication of testicular tunic with abdominal cavity	If no hernia, observe for spontaneous resolution in 3–12 months; surgical referral if hernia, increasing size, or persistence
Musculoskeletal system		
Syndactyly (fusion of two or more digits)	Autosomal dominant with varying expressivity	Surgery during first year of life
Polydactyly (more than five digits)		If no cartilage or bone, remove early; otherwise delay surgery per consultant
Metatarsus adductus (forefoot supinated and adducted; may be flexible or rigid; ankle range of motion must be normal)	Hereditary "tendency" but often due to uterine crowding; minor association with hip dysplasia	If flexible and overcorrects into abduction, no treatment; if corrects only to neutral, use corrective shoe for 4–6 weeks and reassess; if rigid, needs early casting
Talipes equinovarus (clubfoot; variably rigid foot, calf atrophy, hypoplasia of tibia, fibula, and foot bones)	Multifactorial with autosomal dominant component; 3% risk in siblings and 20–30% for offspring of affected parent	Anteroposterior and lateral standing radiograph; early serial casting; if persists, surgery by 6–12 months
Nervous system		
Spina bifida occulta (spinal defect with cutaneous signs: patch of abnormal hair, dimple, lipoma, hemangioma)	Nonfusion of posterior arches of spine; may be tethering of cord or sinus connecting to intraspinal space	Examine for neurologic deficits; nonemergent referral to neurosurgeon if dermal sinus or tethering suspected or if deficits present

Source: Adapted from Judith A. Pauwels in Lewan et al. In: Taylor RB, editor. Family Medicine, 4th ed. New York: Springer-Verlag, 1994. With permission.

Infant Care

Well-Child Care and Normal Development

Well-infant visits, with an emphasis on answering parents' questions and providing anticipatory guidance, are critical during this period of rapid transitions. They facilitate the accommodation of the family to its newest member while building a relationship of trust with the physician. Cultural and socioeconomic issues, familial expectations and stresses, and an assessment of the infant's physical environment should be addressed, preferably starting prenatally. To allow early treatment of disabilities, each visit should include a systematic age-appropriate physical examination and assessment of fine and gross motor development, sensory function, language expression and comprehension, and social behavior. These visits also provide an opportunity to administer immunizations and obtain screening tests, as discussed in Chapter 2. Performing this variety of tasks is simplified by using standardized forms.

Nutrition, Feeding, and Associated Problems

Future mothers typically decide by the second trimester of their pregnancy whether they will breast-feed or bottle-feed. Whenever possible, discussion about the advantages and disadvantages of these two forms of nutrition should occur early in pregnancy.

BREAST MILK FEEDING

Breast milk is the preferred form of sustenance for newborns and young infants because of its better digestibility and enhancement of infant immunity. Breast-feeding allows the infant to share the mother's immunity to the pathogens present in the community at any given time. It also results in significant reductions in the incidence of gastrointestinal infections and otitis media as well as perhaps other respiratory infections. Although two of the principal immunologic factors have their highest concentrations in the colostrum, the immunologic protection increases with the duration of breast-feeding and is greatest for serious and persistent infections.[11,12]

Infection and Chemicals. Breast milk, unfortunately, can transmit pathogens from the mother to the infant. Thus in developed countries the presence of maternal HIV, septicemia, active tuberculosis, or typhoid fever is an absolute contraindication to breast-feeding, and the presence of hepatitis B and cytomegalovirus are relative contraindications.

When seeking to explain any unexpected change in the behavior of a breast-fed infant, it is always important to examine the diet and drug history of the mother. Nicotine can cause infant irritability and reduces both the amount of milk produced and the let-down. Alcohol should be avoided for 1 to 2 hours prior to breast-feeding for each drink consumed. Marijuana is excreted for several hours after even occasional use, and cocaine is excreted for 24 to 36 hours.[11]

Vitamin Supplementation. Vitamin D supplementation (400 IU) is needed by mothers who receive little sunlight and possibly those whose skin is darkly pigmented. Because the fluoride content of breast milk is low, the totally breast-fed baby is supplemented with 0.25 mg of fluoride daily starting at 6 months of age. A term totally breast-fed infant should receive supplemental iron (2 mg/kg up to 15 mg/day) after 4 months of age and a preterm infant from birth.[11]

Supporting Breast-Feeding. Physician support is often critical to successful breast-feeding. Mothers must be reassured that it is rare not to be able to provide adequate milk for their infants and that infants often require 3 to 4 days to become good nursers. Mothers are advised that breast-fed infants often feed every 2 to 4 hours, and that developing a feeding routine is often a compromise between the infant's spontaneous pattern and the mother's schedule. When problems arise the assistance of a lactation specialist can be invaluable.

Formula Feeding

Most infants thrive on cows' milk-based formula. For those who cannot breast-feed long term, a good compromise may be to encourage breast-feeding for the initial few weeks after birth and then to primarily use formula while breast-feeding only a couple of times daily. In most cases such part-time breast-feeding can be accomplished so long as a nipple with a small hole is used so the formula feeding more closely reproduces breast-feeding.

Differences between the brands of formula are generally insignificant. True infant intolerance to cows' milk-based formulas is unusual, and soy protein formulas are of value only if lactose intolerance is strongly suspected, such as after a prolonged episode of diarrhea. Even then intolerance is usually transient and a trial of cow's milk-based formula should be attempted every 2 to 4 weeks. Because formulas do not contain fluoride the use of powdered forms mixed with fluoridated water is suggested. Low-iron formulas offer no advantages over regular iron fortification, as constipation from iron is rare.

Advancing Infant Diet

Infants should remain on either breast milk or formula until 12 months of age because the introduction of whole cows' milk before this age increases the risk of occult gastrointestinal bleeding and iron deficiency anemia. At 12 months of age a child is generally placed on whole or 2% milk to provide the extra calories available from the milk fat and then gradually switched to skim milk by 2 or 3 years of age in those eating well (30% of calories from fat).

Introducing nonmilk foods into the diet prior to age 4 to 6 months neither benefits the infant nor increases the likelihood of the infant sleeping through the night. On the other hand, as infants approach 12 months of age, introducing such foods can avoid making the diet too protein-dense, especially if there is a focus on whole cereals, green vegetables, legumes, and fruits. This practice accustoms children at a young age to nutritionally balanced high fiber diets.

Some generally accepted guidelines for introducing nonmilk foods are (1) separate the introduction of new foods by at least 3 days to more easily determine the cause of any food intolerance; (2) start with easily digested foods such as cereals, especially rice, and yellow vegetables; (3) postpone such potential allergens as citrus fruits and eggs until 9 to 12 months of age; and (4) minimize the risk of airway obstruction by avoiding spongy foods (e.g., hot dogs and grapes) and foods with kernels (e.g., corn, and nuts) until at least 2 years of age. Once a child is eating a balanced diet there is no need for supplemental vitamins and iron. Fluoride, though, continues to be supplemented if the supply in the water system is less than 0.6 ppm.

OBESITY

The significance of being overweight as an infant is unclear, with up to three-fourths of such infants becoming normal-weight adults and most obese adults not being obese as infants. However, when there is a genetic predisposition to obesity, especially if associated with a strong family history of cardiovascular disease, hypercholesterolemia, and diabetes, it is reasonable to encourage primary prevention. It can include breast-feeding and delayed introduction of solids, avoiding overfeeding by not using the bottle as a pacifier, and using only a small spoon to feed solids. However, restriction of fat prior to the age of 2 years can result in failure to consume adequate calories and other nutrients.[13]

COLIC

The syndrome of colic is most commonly defined as paroxysms of irritability, fussing, or crying with the infant seeming to be in pain and difficult to console without apparent cause. Episodes typically last for a total of more than 3 hours a day but rarely occur daily. They most often appear in the afternoon or evening and between the ages of 2 weeks and 4 months. Because up to 49% of all infants can present with this picture, the other factor that seems to define these babies is that one or both parents have difficulty dealing with this facet of the infant's behavior. Parental behavior does not seem to be a cause of the colic, however, only a response.

Before infants are diagnosed as having colic they should have a thorough physical examination to identify any acute processes, such as infection or intussusception, especially if the onset is sudden.

A principal focus of treatment is to reassure parents that the process is common and self-limited and provide them with some basic measures to try: (1) provide motion, as in a mechanical swing, rocker, or papoose, or a steady hum, as in a car or lying on top of a dryer; (2) provide snug bundling; (3) provide warmth such as laying the infant on his or her stomach on a heating pad set low; and (4) ensure that the infant burps well and frequently during and after feeding. Often the physician's most important roles are providing support over time and legitimizing the parents' sense of frustration, even anger, with the situation. The physician should also encourage parents to help each other to care for the infant and whenever possible to enlist the help of others so they have an opportunity to take a break. Parents should also be given permission, when all other measures have failed, to leave the infant alone in a secure location until the crying stops.[14]

The role of *allergy* or *intolerance to cows' milk protein* is controversial. There is evidence that switching infants on a cows' milk-based formula to a casein hydrolysate formula is beneficial in up to 70% of infants, especially if there is a family history or other signs of allergy. Similarly, some breast-fed infants are sensitive to the cows' milk protein in the diet of their mothers, and a trial of excluding all dairy products from the mother's diet for at least 1 week may be warranted. Infants who benefit from avoiding cows' milk protein often have only transient intolerance and should be challenged with cows' milk again 1 to 2 months later.

Infants who have more prolonged, severe bouts of crying, especially if these appear intermittently throughout the day, may have at least a partial organic cause. If such a child seems to pass a lot of gas with relief, try simethicone (Mylicon). *Constipation* is treated as in other infants (Table 4.2). Frequent vomiting, especially if accompanied by poor feeding and failure to thrive, may indicate *gastroesophageal reflux*. A trial of antacids is warranted and further workup suggested if the antacids are not effective. Although anticholinergic agents have been advocated in the past, their efficacy probably has more to do with their sedating effect than any specific effect on the gastrointestinal muscles. With their potential for severe side effects, their use is discouraged.

FAILURE TO THRIVE

Failure to thrive (FTT) can be defined as failure to grow at an appropriate rate, with weight crossing two major channels on the National

TABLE 4.2. Approaches to common problems of the infant

HEENT (head, ears, eyes, nose, throat)

THRUSH (pearly white pseudomembranes on the oral mucosa): *Causes:* transmission from vaginal mucosa during delivery; contaminated fomites (nipples, both breast and bottle; toys; teething rings). *Rx:* clean fomites (boil bottle nipples, toys); oral nystatin 200,000–500,000 units every 4–6h until clear for 48 hours.

NASOLACRIMAL DUCT OBSTRUCTION (incomplete canalization with tearing and accumulation of mucoid or mucopurulent discharge, 5% of newborns). Congenital but symptoms usually delayed until days to weeks after birth. *Rx:* Nasolacrimal massage, BID-TID, and cleansing of eyelids with warm water; topical antibiotics for secondary conjunctivitis; surgical duct dilatation if not resolved by the age of 9–12 months.

STRABISMUS (misalignment of eyes). Screen with corneal light reflex and cover test. *Rx:* ophthalmology referral for persistent deviation > several weeks or any deviation after 6 months of age.

HEARING LOSS. Screen those at risk: family history; congenital infection; craniofacial abnormalities; birth weight < 1500 g; hyperbilirubinemia requiring exchange transfusion; severe depression at birth; bacterial meningitis. *Screening:* auditory response cradle; auditory brain stem response.

TEETHING (painful gums secondary to eruption of teeth with irritability, drooling). Fever and other systemic effects are *not* caused by teething. *Rx:* chewing on soft cloth, teething ring, dry toast hastens eruption; topical and systemic analgesia.

Skin problems

CIRCUMCISION: Elective procedure performed only on healthy, stable infants. Contraindicated if any genital abnormalities. *Advantages:* decreased incidence of phimosis and male infant urinary tract infections. *Risks* (small): sepsis; amputation; urethral injury; removal of excessive foreskin.

UMBILICAL GRANULOMA (exuberant soft, vascular, red-pink granulation tissue after cord separation). *Rx:* cauterization with silver nitrate.

DIAPER DERMATITIS (erythematous, scaly eruptions that may advance to papulovesicular lesions or erosions; may be patchy or confluent; genitocrural folds often spared). Due to reaction to overhydration of skin, friction, or prolonged contact with urine, feces, chemicals such as in diapers, and soaps. *Rx:* frequent changing of diapers; exposure to air; bland, protective topical ointment (petrolatum, zinc oxide) after each diaper change; advanced cases may require 1% hydrocortisone ointment.

CANDIDAL SUPERINFECTION of the diaper area (pronounced erythema with sharp margins, satellite lesions, involvement of genitocrural folds). *Rx:* topical antifungal; treat associated thrush.

MILIA (superficial 1- to 2-mm inclusion cysts). Common on face and gingiva. *Rx:* none needed.

MILIARIA (clear or erythematous papulovesicles in response to heat or overdressing; especially in flexural areas). *Rx:* resolves with cooling.

SEBORRHEIC DERMATITIS (most commonly greasy, yellow scaling of scalp or dry, white scaling of inguinal regions; may be more extensive). *Rx:* generally clears spontaneously; may require 1% hydrocortisone cream; mild antiseborrheic shampoos for scalp lesions; mineral oil with gentle brushing after 10 minutes for thick scalp crusts.

TABLE 4.2. (*continued*)

ATOPIC DERMATITIS (intensely pruritic, dry, scaly, erythematous patches). Acute lesions may weep. Typically involves face, neck, hands, abdomen, and extensor surfaces of extremities. Genetic propensity with frequent subsequent development of allergic rhinitis and asthma. *Rx:* mainstay is avoidance of irritants (temperature and humidity extremes, foods, chemicals) and drying of the skin (frequent bathing, soaps) with frequent application of lubricants (apply to damp skin after bathing). Severe disease usually requires topical steroids; acute lesions may require 1:20 Burow's solution and antihistamines (diphenhydramine, hydroxyzine).

Cardiac murmur

INNOCENT OR FUNCTIONAL (typically diminished with decreased cardiac output, i.e., standing)

Newborn murmur. Onset within first few days of life that resolves by 2–3 weeks of age. Typically soft, short, vibratory, grade I–II/VI early systolic murmur located at lower left sternal border that subsides with mild abdominal pressure.

Still's murmur. Most common murmur of early childhood. May start during infancy. Typically loudest midway between apex and left sternal border. Musical or vibratory, grade I–III early systolic murmur.

Pulmonary outflow ejection murmur. May be heard throughout childhood. Typically soft, short, systolic ejection murmur, grade I–II and localized to upper left sternal border.

Hemic murmur. Heard with increased cardiac output (fever, anemia, stress). Typically grade I–II high-pitched systolic ejection murmur heard best in aortic/pulmonic areas.

PATHOLOGIC OR ORGANIC MURMURS. Any diastolic murmur. Consider when a systolic murmur has one or more of the following features: grade III or louder; persistent through much of systole; presence of a thrill, abnormal second heart sound, or a gallop. Other ominous signs: congestive heart failure, cyanosis, tachycardia. *Evaluation:* chest radiography, ECG; if persistent or any distress, cardiology consult.

Gastrointestinal disturbance

CONSTIPATION (intestinal dysfunction in which the bowels are difficult or painful to evacuate). Associated failure to thrive, vomiting, moderate to tense abdominal distension, or blood without anal fissures requires ruling out organic disease (Hirschsprung's, celiac disease, hypothyroidism, structural defects, lead toxicity). *Common causes:* anal fissures, undernutrition, dehydration, excessive milk intake, and lack of bulk. Less common with breast-feeding. Rarely caused by iron-fortified cereals. *Rx:* during early infancy increase amount of fluid or add sugars (Maltsupex); later add juices (prune, apple) and other fruits, cereals, and vegetables; may add artificial fiber (Citrocel). Severe disease may require brief use of milk of magnesia (1–2 tsp), docusate sodium, and glycerin suppositories; when persistent requires ruling out organic disease.

PYLORIC STENOSIS (nonbilious vomiting immediately after feeding, becoming progressively more projectile). Male/female preponderance by 4:1. Onset 1 week to 5 months after birth (typically 3 weeks). May be intermittent. *Diagnosis:* palpation of pyloric mass (typically 2 cm in length, olive-shaped) that may be easier to palpate after vomiting; ultrasonography preferred method to confirm difficult cases (90% sensitivity). *Rx:* surgery.

Anemia

Improved nutrition has reduced incidence, but infants remain at significant risk. *Additional risk factors:* low socioeconomic status, consumption of cows' milk prior to age 12 months, use of formula not iron-fortified, low birth weight, prematurity. *Effects:* fatigue, apathy, impairment of growth, and decreased resistance to infection. *Causes:* iron deficiency most common (usually sufficient birth stores to prevent occurrence prior to age 4 months), sickle cell disease, thalassemia, lead toxicity. *Screening:* hemoglobin or hematocrit between ages 6 and 9 months (some recommend only for infants with risk factors). *Rx:* if microcytic give trial of iron (elemental iron, Feosol, 3–6 mg/kg/day); if not microcytic or unresponsive to iron, consider other causes (family history, environment).

TABLE 4.2. (*continued*)

Sleep disturbances
Infant's sleeping pattern disrupts the parent's sleep. About 70% of infants can sleep through the night by age 3 months. Most 6-month-olds no longer require nighttime feeding. *Screening:* a sudden change in sleeping pattern should prompt a search for new stresses: physical (e.g., infection, esophageal reflux) or emotional (e.g., new surroundings or household members). *Rx:* establish realistic parental expectations (consider the natural sleeping patterns of the infant); allow infants awakening at night to learn how to fall asleep by themselves (keep bedtime rituals simple and put the infant to bed awake; do not respond to infant's first cry; keep interactions during the night short and simple; provide a security object for older infants); slowly change undesirable sleeping patterns (move bedtime hour up and awaken infant earlier in the morning; decrease daytime napping).

Center for Health Statistics (NCHS) growth curve or falling below the 5th percentile for age and sex after correcting for parents' stature, prematurity, or growth retardation at birth.[15,16] Because of a high prevalence of FTT in urban and rural areas (5–10%) and significant morbidity (developmental delay, permanent cognitive deficits, behavioral disorders, short stature, chronic physical problems, and medical illness), it is advisable to begin following any child whose weight declines across one NCHS channel or if a parent suspects a growth problem.[17]

Diagnosis. Although the consequences of malnutrition sometimes obscure the original causes, a thorough history and physical examination detect most organic, behavioral, family, and environmental problems that contribute to FTT. This initial assessment should include (1) prior records including growth charts and prenatal history (prematurity, growth retardation); (2) nutrition (diet, behavior); (3) development (cognitive, motor, behavioral, emotional); (4) social context (parental knowledge, family dysfunction, drug abuse, social support, isolation); and (5) environment (poverty, shelter, toxic exposures to lead or pesticides). Diagnostic studies can follow in a stepwise manner, based on severity and history.

Step 1: CBC, fasting chemistry panel, electrolytes, urinalysis
Step 2: thyroid, stool (culture, ova and parasites, fat), sweat chloride
Step 3: tuberculosis, HIV, skeletal survey, renal studies

Treatment. Hospitalization is indicated when there is (1) severe malnutrition; (2) suspected abuse or neglect; (3) an extreme problem with parent–child interaction; (4) family dysfunction (e.g., barriers to follow-up, disorganization, depression, chemical dependence, violence); or (5) failure of outpatient treatment. Outpatient treatment is often appropriate when FTT is moderate (infant's weight is more than 60% the average weight for age *and* more than 80% average weight for height). Weekly follow-up may be lengthened after sustained weight gain. Collaborative, interdisciplinary treatment involves the parents, physician, social worker, nutritionist, and psychologist. It implements one or more of the following strategies: (1) treating organic factors first; (2) implementing a written nutritional plan for meals and snacks with caloric intake 1.5 to 2.0 times normal; (3) beginning a vitamin supplement; (4) supporting parents with mealtime observation and coaching; (5) treating specific family problems that interfere with the family's ability to care for the infant (misunderstanding, depression, drug abuse); (5) enlisting social support (family, friends, church); (6) mobilizing community and economic resources for the family; (7) establishing continuity of care and access to the treatment team; (8) promoting parental competence.

Fever

For children under 3 years of age, if a source for fever cannot be determined or if otitis media is found, 3% to 11% have occult bacteremia. The risk is even higher in infants under age 3 months, who have an 8.6% risk of having a serious bacterial infection.[18,19] In an attempt to provide a framework for evaluating these children, a set of guidelines was published in *Pediatrics* in 1993; it presents a reasonable outline of how to approach this vexing problem.[19] The basic elements of the guidelines, with some variations proposed by others[18,20] are as follows.

TOXIC-APPEARING INFANTS

Children with signs of sepsis (e.g., lethargy, poor perfusion, hypoventilation, hyperventilation, cyanosis) should be hospitalized for a full septic workup with blood and urine cultures and lumbar puncture. Antibiotics are initiated pending culture results. In infants under 1 to 2 months of age, antibiotic choices should follow the recommendations made earlier in this chapter for neonates. Older children are most frequently treated with either cefotaxime (50 mg/kg IV q8h) or ceftriaxone (100 mg/kg IV q24h).

LOW-RISK INFANTS

The clinical criteria defining low risk infants are (1) previously healthy; (2) nontoxic appearance; (3) no focal bacterial infection (except otitis media); and (4) the ability to be closely monitored by caregivers. Laboratory criteria are a WBC count of 5,000 to 15,000/mm^3 (< 1500 bands/ mm^3); normal urinalysis, defined as < 5 WBCs per high power field (hpf); and when diarrhea is present fewer than 5 WBCs/hpf in the stool. Most experts recommend obtaining the urine sample by catheterization.

Age Less Than 28 Days. Most of the experts formulating the guidelines recommend admitting all low-risk neonates less than 28 days old with rectal temperatures over 38°C (100.4°F) for the septic workup described earlier in this chapter for neonates, with or without antibiotic coverage, pending culture results. However, one study indicated that many community pediatricians prefer to treat very low risk infants as outpatients, with or without antibiotics. If treated as outpatients, such infants must be monitored closely and reevaluated within 24 hours. If blood cultures are positive, they are then admitted for a sepsis evaluation and parenteral antibiotics.[20] If a urine culture is positive and there is persistent fever, the neonate is admitted for septic evaluation and parenteral antibiotics; however, outpatient treatment with oral antibiotics can be used if the patient is afebrile and well. Further studies are needed to better define the most appropriate course to follow in this group of infants.

Age 28 to 90 Days. The 28- to 90-day-old infants with a rectal temperature over 38°C, when at low risk, can be managed as outpatients. Some investigators recommend culturing both urine and blood, others only one of these, and some add a lumbar puncture and analysis. If there is any suspicion of bacteremia, most experts recommend getting at least a blood culture and giving a dose of parenteral antibiotics, most often ceftriaxone (50 mg/kg IM, maximum 1g). These infants are then reevaluated within 24 hours. Those with positive cultures can be treated similarly to the outpatients less than 28 days old; however, infants with blood cultures positive for *Streptococcus pneumoniae,* known to be sensitive to penicillin, can be treated with oral penicillin or amoxicillin. Otherwise treatment is based on the infant's clinical appearance at the time of reevaluation.

Age 3 to 36 Months. There is no need to screen for occult bacteremia in infants 3 to 36 months old with temperatures less than 39°C (102.2°F). Infants with persistent fever (>2–3 days), a worsening clinical appearance, or temperatures of 39°C or more without an apparent source for the fever other than otitis media constitute a higher-risk group. They should be evaluated with a WBC count. If the count is 15,000/mm^3 or higher, a blood culture is indicated, as well as injection of a parenteral antibiotic (most commonly ceftriaxone 50 mg/kg IM to a maximum of 1 g) while the culture is pending. In addition, a urine sample by catheter should be cultured from all male infants less than 6 months of age or female infants less than 2 years of age who are treated with antibiotics. This higher risk group is reevaluated and treated as described above for outpatient infants 28 to 90 days old.

Sudden Infant Death Syndrome

Sudden infant death syndrome (SIDS) is the leading cause of death for infants past the neonatal period, peaking at age 2 months. Characterized by being unexpected and without an apparent cause, despite thorough postmortem examination, it represents a collection of etiologies involving an abnormality of cardiorespiratory regulation. This divergence of etiologies has so far frustrated attempts to develop reliable screening and prevention methods. Many have recommended using electronic home monitoring for apnea and bradycardia for infants judged to be at high risk, including siblings of SIDS casualties, infants who had apparent life-threatening episodes, and those with the other risk factors cited below. However, such monitors have generally had little effect on reducing the incidence of SIDS, in part because of frequent poor parent compliance with their use. When employed, they can be discontinued if there are no episodes of true apnea for 16 consecutive weeks. The use of event recorders with the monitors has made identifying apneic episodes more objective and seems to allow shorter periods of monitoring.

At this time the greatest impact on reducing the incidence of SIDS has involved targeting the risk factors known to be associated with a two- to threefold increase in the risk of SIDS. These factors include maternal smoking or drug use, poor prenatal care, complications of delivery and prematurity, and prone (stomach) sleeping position. To address the last risk factor, infants who have no medical contraindications should be placed for sleep in the supine (back) or side position, although there are no controlled studies demonstrating efficacy.[21,22]

Other Common Problems of the Infant

Table 4.2 provides short summaries of other frequent problems of infancy and their management.

Family and Community Issues

Child Care

More than 50% of infants under 1 year of age have parents who work outside the home. The physician can encourage parents to use paid and unpaid leave to maximize time with their child during the first year of life and to select child care carefully. A quality child care setting supports normal infant development, but many settings fail to protect health and safety or provide adequate developmental stimulation. Parents can find quality programs in both private homes and child care centers; nonprofit centers generally provide higher quality care than for-profit centers.[23] Parents can compare several programs by making scheduled and unscheduled visits to observe the emotional atmosphere and sanitation. The optimal adult/child ratio before 1 year of age is 1:3 and should not exceed 1:4. Staff should (1) be trained in child development; (2) be paid sufficiently to minimize turnover; (3) enjoy their interactions with

TABLE 4.3. Assessing resources and risks for early family development

Concept	Interview questions
Social support	Do you have at least one friend or relative you can turn to for support and advice? Do you work, attend school, or participate in a religious community?
Housing	Do you have any concerns about housing?
Child care	Do you have any concerns about child care?
Transportation	Do you have any concerns about transportation?
Finances	Will you have any problems paying for food and clothing? Vitamins and medications? Health care?
Safety	During the past year, has anyone you know: Made you afraid for your safety? Pushed, kicked, slapped, hit, or otherwise hurt you? Forced sexual or physical contact? Tried to control your activities, your friends, or other parts of your life? Do you have any guns in your house? Do you have any concerns about safety or violence in your neighborhood? Do you use a seat belt when you ride in a car? Does each infant and toddler in your family always ride in a rear seat and use an infant or car seat? Do your children always ride in a rear seat and use a seat belt?
Personal health	In general, how healthy do you consider yourself? (Excellent; Good; Fair; Poor)
STD and HIV risk	Have you ever had herpes, gonorrhea, *Chlamydia, Trichomonas,* genital warts, or a pelvic infection? Have you had two or more sexual partners during the past year?
Emotions	During the last 30 days, how much of the time have you felt downhearted and blue? (Very little; Sometimes; Often; Most of the time).
Alcohol and drugs	Have your parents had any problems with alcohol or drugs? Does your partner have any problems with alcohol or drugs? Have you had any problems in the past with alcohol or drugs? During the past 30 days, on how many days did you have at least one drink of alcohol? During the past 30 days, on how many days did you have five or more drinks of alcohol in a row (i.e., within a couple of hours)?
Tobacco	Does anyone in your home smoke tobacco? Do you currently smoke or use tobacco?

STD = sexually transmitted diseases; HIV = human immunodeficiency virus.

children, respond positively to children's accomplishments, and attend quickly when a child is upset; and (4) wash their hands after diapering and before food preparation, use disposable tissue for wiping runny noses, and routinely wash changing tables. After enrollment, encourage parents to continue occasional unscheduled visits and to investigate sudden changes in their child's behavior such as withdrawal, anxiety, or agitation.

Families and Infants: Risks and Resources

Normal infant development is promoted by fostering a family's strengths and resources but is threatened by individual, family, and environmental risk factors (see Chapter 2). *Individual* infant risk factors include chronic illness, physical handicap, low birth weight, growth failure, and developmental delay. *Family* factors include physical or sexual abuse, family violence, neglect, parental depression, chemical dependence, and chronic illness. *Environmental* factors include poverty and environmental toxins such as lead. Table 4.3 outlines systematic approach for identifying some common resources and risks for early family development. When possible, screening for such risk factors should start prenatally.

Early intervention programs promote healthy development and prevent developmental delay even when infants and families face serious medical, psychosocial, and environmental obstacles. Effective early intervention has five elements.

1. *Crisis intervention.* Take quick action to treat immediate threats to safety (e.g., family violence, physical or sexual abuse, severe neglect).
2. *Family-centered care.* Collaborate with parents and avoid labeling a child or parent. Describe the challenge the family faces and the strengths and resources they have to assist them. Teach parents about the unique needs and abilities of their infant. Be optimistic and adapt your interventions to the family's culture.
3. *Social support.* Help families identify supportive family, friends, church, or mutual-help groups.
4. *Community resources.* Help parents mobilize community resources to treat specific needs of the infant and family (e.g., specialized day care, parenting classes).
5. *Ecologic model of intervention.* Assess the individual infant, family, and physical environment and customize your intervention to use the family's specific strengths. Continue to coordinate the involvement of multiple professionals and ensure that the overall plan remains suitable for the family. Serve as an advocate and catalyst to ensure the treatment team addresses unanswered questions.

Chaotic families disrupted by family violence, sexual abuse, or chemical dependence may be difficult to work with, as these same problems tend to disrupt the doctor–patient relationship. It is important that family-centered care be respectful, culturally sensitive, and nonstigmatizing. The physician can take a leadership role by helping the team and family focus on the developmental potential of the infant and family.

INFANTS OF SUBSTANCE-ABUSING MOTHERS

Drug abuse during pregnancy significantly increases the risk for low birth weight, growth retardation, microcephaly, and other anomalies. Fetal alcohol syndrome includes the well described triad of growth retardation before or after biSrth, nervous system abnormalities, and mid-facial hypoplasia. Cardiac and renal systems may also be affected. Infants are typically irritable, have difficulty feeding, and show disorganized sleep patterns. The full syndrome occurs with heavy drinking throughout pregnancy but lower levels of exposure also affect development. The specific effects of prenatal exposure to cocaine and other drugs of abuse are less well described. Exposure to one substance is often confounded by abuse of other drugs and social and environmental factors (e.g., diet and prenatal care) that correlate with chemical dependence and are known to affect infant outcome.[24]

Parents should be encouraged to seek treatment for chemical dependence at any point during pregnancy or after birth. When maternal drug abuse is suspected, infants should be evaluated and treated for acute withdrawal symptoms and then referred for developmental assessment and early intervention.

ADOLESCENT PARENTS

Adolescent parents are often *perceived* as high risk, when in fact, adolescent girls who have access to appropriate resources, including pre- and postnatal care, give birth to healthy infants and raise children who are well adjusted. True risk factors are poverty, lack of access to health care, family violence, and substance abuse. Adolescents who grow up in a family with violence, sexual abuse, or chemical dependence initiate sexual intercourse at an earlier age than the general population and experience a higher rate of pregnancy.

When working with adolescent parents: (1) expect a positive outcome while offering respect and dignity; (2) encourage family support, if appropriate, including support of the father and his family; (3) encourage use of community resources (child care, parenting classes, education, early intervention programs); (4) initiate family planning early during the pregnancy; and (5) encourage continued education and delay of the birth of another child (delay by as little as 6 months and completion of high school improves long-term social and economic outcome).

PUBLIC POLICY

Federal law (PL99-457) encourages states to develop programs that identify and provide services to children at risk from birth to age 3 years. By statute these early intervention programs are to be individualized, family-centered, and *involve the primary care physician.* Implementation varies from state to state, making it important for physicians to familiarize themselves with local programs and resources.

References

1. Bloom RS, Cropley C, AHA/AAP Neonatal Resuscitation Program Steering Committee. Textbook of neonatal resuscitation. Elk Grove Village, IL: American Academy of Pediatrics, American Heart Association, 1994.
2. Centers for Disease Control and Prevention. Prevention of perinatal group B streptococcal disease: a public health perspective. MMWR 1996;45(RR-7):1–24.
3. Cole FS. Bacterial infections of the newborn. In: Taeusch HW, Ballard RS, Avery MA, editors. Schaeffer and Avery's diseases of the newborn. 6th ed. Philadelphia: Saunders, 1991.
4. American Academy of Pediatrics, Provisional Committee for Quality Improvement and Subcommittee on Hyperbilirubinemia. Practice parameter: management of hyperbilirubinemia in the healthy term newborn. Pediatrics 1994; 94:558–65.
5. Centers for Disease Control and Prevention. Zidovudine for the prevention of HIV transmission from mother to infant. MMWR 1994;43:285–8.
6. Centers for Disease Control and Prevention. U.S. Public Health Service recommendations for human immunodeficiency virus counseling and voluntary testing for pregnant women. MMWR 1995;44(RR-7):3–11.
7. Landesman SH, Kalish LA, Burns DN, et al. Obstetrical factors and the transmission of human immunodeficiency virus type 1 from mother to child. N Engl J Med 1996; 334:1617–23.
8. Chadwick EG, Yogev R. Pediatric AIDS. Pediatr Clin North Am 1995; 42:969–92.
9. Luzuriaga K, Sullivan JL. DNA polymerase chain reaction for the diagnosis of vertical HIV infection. JAMA 1996;275: 1360–1.
10. Shearer WT, Quinn TC, La Russo P, et al. Viral load and disease progression in infants infected with human immunodeficiency virus type 1. N Engl J Med 1997;336:1337–1342.
11. Lawrence PR. Breast milk: best source of nutrition for term and preterm infants. Pediatr Clin North Am 1994;41:925–42.
12. Dewey KG, Heinig MJ, Nommsen-Rivers LA. Differences in morbidity between breast-fed and formula-fed infants. J Pediatr 1995;126:696–702.
13. Hardy SC, Kleinman RE. Fat and cholesterol in the diet of infants and young children: implications for growth, development, and long-term health. J Pediatr 1994;125:S69–75.

14. Treem WR. Infant colic: a pediatric gastroenterologist's perspective. Pediatr Clin North Am 1994;41:1121–38.
15. Drotar D. Failure to thrive (growth deficiency). In: Roberts MC, editor. Handbook of pediatric psychology. New York: Guilford, 1995:516–36.
16. Leung AKC, Robson WLM, Fagan JE. Assessment of the child with failure to thrive. Am Fam Physician 1993;48:1432–8.
17. Ambuel JP, Harris B. Failure to thrive: a study of failure to grow in height or weight. Ohio State Med J 1963;59:997–1001.
18. Grubb NS, Lyle S, Brodie JH, et al. Management of infants and children 0 to 36 months of age with fever without a source. J Am Board Fam Pract 1995;8:114–19.
19. Baraff LJ, Bass JW, Fleisher GR, et al. Practice guideline for the management of infants and children 0 to 36 months of age with fever without source. Pediatrics 1993;92:1–12.
20. Young PC. The management of febrile infants by primary-care pediatricians in Utah: comparison with published practice guidelines. Pediatrics 1995;95:623–7.
21. Freed GE, Steinshneider A, Glassman M, Winn K. Sudden infant death syndrome prevention and an understanding of selected clinical issues. Pediatr Clin North Am 1994;41:967–89.
22. AAP Task Force on Infant Positioning and SIDS. Positioning and SIDS. Pediatrics 1992;89:1120–6.
23. Phillips DA, Howes C, Whitebook M. The social policy context of child care: effects on quality. Am J Community Psychol 1992;20(1):25–52.
24. Singer L, Farkos K, Kliegman R. Childhood medical and behavioral consequences of maternal cocaine use. J Pediatr Psychol 1992;17:389–406.

CASE PRESENTATION

Subjective

PATIENT PROFILE

Allison Harris is a 1-year-old white female child, here today with her mother.

PRESENTING PROBLEM

"For checkup and shots."

PRESENT ILLNESS

Over the first year of life, you have treated Allison for three episodes of otitis media. She has otherwise been well. She knows three words, walks alone, eats some table food, and drinks almost 2 quarts of milk daily.

PAST MEDICAL HISTORY

No serious illnesses or hospitalization during her first year of life.

SOCIAL HISTORY

She is the second child of her father who is a truck driver and her mother who works as a secretary in a business office.

FAMILY HISTORY

Her parents are living and well. Her grandfather has diabetes and coronary artery disease with angina, and her uncle is HIV-positive.

- What other information regarding Allison's health status would you like to know? Why?
- What are the possible implications of both parents working, and how might you address this issue?
- What more would you like to know about Allison's ear infections and her ability to hear?
- What is the possible significance of her milk consumption, and what else would you ask about her current diet?

Objective

VITAL SIGNS

Height 28 in; weight 32 lb; pulse, 82; respirations, 22; temperature, 37.2°C.

EXAMINATION

The 1-year-old child is alert and cheerful and makes good eye contact. Her left tympanic membrane is slightly dull but moves freely. Her eyes, throat, and neck are normal. The chest, heart, abdomen, and genitalia are unremarkable. Her musculoskeletal examination, including gait, is normal for her age.

- What other information derived from the physical examination might be important, and why?
- Are the patient's weight and height appropriate for her age, and how is this calculation made?
- How might you further evaluate Allison's ability to hear?
- What—if any—laboratory tests would you perform today?

Assessment

- How would you describe Allison's health status to her parents?
- What is the developmental status of this patient?
- What are your concerns regarding Allison's diet, and how would you further assess the potential problem?
- Would you do anything special in view of the family history of diabetes mellitus and coronary artery disease? Explain.

Plan

- Describe your recommendation regarding vitamins, medication, and follow-up on her ear infections.
- What immunizations would generally be appropriate at this visit?
- What diet recommendations would be appropriate? How might a problem have developed?
- Describe your recommendations for follow-up care of Allison.

5

Common Problems of the Elderly

James P. Richardson and Aubrey L. Knight

Older patients are a challenging but satisfying part of most family physicians' practices. Optimal care of geriatric patients occurs when the precepts of continuity of care, the team approach to the management of illness, the importance of the family, and the biopsychosocial model are followed. Because of the prevalence of chronic disease in the elderly, cure may be elusive, but appropriate care always improves the quality of the older adult's life. Some common problems of the elderly are reviewed in this chapter. More complete discussions may be found in textbooks of geriatric medicine.[1,2]

Falls

Falls are common, alarming, and worrisome to patients, their families, and their physicians. Most falls by the elderly do not result in serious consequences, but some cause hip fractures, other injuries, and rarely death. Unintentional injury is the sixth leading cause of death among the elderly, and most of these deaths are the result of falls.[3] Frequent falls may lead to consideration of a change in living arrangements or a severe limitation in socialization. Studies have clarified both the evaluation and management of patients who fall.[4]

The cause of a fall that results from loss of consciousness, a stroke or seizure, or an accidental or intentional blow to the body usually is easily discerned and managed. In most cases, however, the cause of a fall is not readily apparent. Falls may be classified as extrinsic (caused by slips or trips), intrinsic (caused by poor gait or balance, impaired sensation or proprioception, or cognitive impairment), nonbipedal (e.g., a fall out of bed), or nonclassifiable. Risk factors for falls from prospective studies include older age, white race, cognitive impairment, medication use, chronic diseases such as arthritis and Parkinson disease, foot problems, dizziness, and impaired muscle strength, gait, and balance.[4] Frequent fallers are likely to have more than one risk factor, but a significant number of older patients who fall have no risk factors. Acute illnesses such as pneumonia, sepsis, and congestive heart failure also may present with a fall.

Most falls occur in the faller's home, and the home environment is usually a factor in these falls. Many falls occur on stairs, with injuries more likely to occur while descending rather than climbing stairs. Other hazards are electrical cords, uneven surfaces such as throw rugs or carpeting, or objects left on the floor. Poor lighting may contribute to these hazards.

Medication use is a potentially easily modifiable risk factor for falls. Long-acting benzodiazepines, barbiturates, tricyclic antidepressants, and neuroleptics are associated with an increased risk of falls. Diuretics and other antihypertensive medicines also may increase the risk of falls by producing postural hypotension (see below and Chapter 8).

Numerous trials have been completed that examine methods of fall reduction and injuries due to falls. Low level exercise appears to reduce the frequency of falls but may not reduce the number of falls resulting in medical treatment[5] or fractures.[6] The multisite FICSIT (Frailty and Injuries: Cooperative Studies of Intervention Techniques) trial has demonstrated a modest decline in frequency of falls for the groups that underwent a variety of exercise interventions.[7] One FICSIT site used a multidisciplinary program to identify and reduce risk factors for falls. The intervention group underwent environmental hazards assessment, review of medications, treatment of postural hypotension, and physical therapy to improve strength and treat any balance or gait impairments. The rate of falls during the following year was reduced by 31%.[8]

More information should be forthcoming on useful interventions to reduce the risk of falls in the elderly. Known risk factors can be used to target the elderly for interventions, but because some elderly without risk factors experience falls as well, probably all elderly should be screened. At this time, effective strategies for the practicing physician include (1) a home assessment to eliminate environmental hazards, such as throw rugs, unlit stairs, or poorly arranged furniture (by the physician during a housecall or a home care agency); (2) review of all medications, with elimination of problematic drugs when possible; (3) office evaluation of gait and balance (by the physician with a screening instrument[9] or a physical therapist); (4) detection and treatment of postural hypotension or other chronic diseases that may cause weakness with standing (e.g., congestive heart failure, chronic obstructive pulmonary disease); (5) detection and treatment of sensory losses, including poor vision and proprioception (e.g., vitamin B_{12} deficiency); and (6) physical, medical, or surgical therapy for arthritis or other musculoskeletal disorders, especially when the feet are involved (see Chapters 17, 18).

Postural Hypotension

Postural or orthostatic hypotension is defined as a drop in systolic blood pressure of at least 20 mm Hg 1 minute after a patient changes from a supine to a standing position. Prevalence in community-dwelling elderly ranges from 10% to 30%. Syncope or near-syncope may be presenting symptoms, but elderly persons with postural hypotension may complain of nonspecific symptoms such as weakness, fatigue, or difficulty concentrating.

The most common causes of postural hypotension in older people are deconditioning, with loss of compensating autonomic reflexes, and medications, especially diuretics, tricyclic antidepressants, neuroleptics, antihypertensives, and dopaminergic drugs (e.g., levodopa). Treatment is the same for these patients. Deconditioned patients should be encouraged to gradually increase their activity, under the supervision of a physical therapist if necessary. Salt intake can be liberalized for most patients without heart failure. Raising the head of the bed on blocks 4 to 6 inches high also helps improve postural hypotension by stimulating autonomic reflexes and fluid retention. Offending drugs should be eliminated whenever possible. Patients with hypertension can be switched from a diuretic to a calcium channel blocker, angiotensin-converting enzyme inhibitor, or a β-blocker, as these classes of antihypertensives have a low incidence of postural hypotension when used alone. Until the postural hypotension improves, patients should be reminded to change positions slowly to give compensating mechanisms some time to work. Patients also can be instructed to tighten their calf muscles while standing, thereby decreasing the pooling of blood in the legs.

Rarer causes of postural hypotension are autonomic nervous system disease, either central (e.g., Shy-Drager or Parkinson disease) or peripheral (e.g., diabetes, amyloidosis). These patients may need to be evaluated by a neurologist experienced in these conditions. In addition to the therapies mentioned above, treatment is aimed at the underlying disease. In severe cases salt tablets and fludrocortisone may be necessary.

Urinary Incontinence

Urinary incontinence (UI) is defined as an involuntary loss of urine sufficient to be a problem. UI is a common clinical entity affecting 15% to 30% of noninstitutionalized persons older than 60 years of age. The prevalence is twice as high in women as in men. Institutionalized, hospitalized, and homebound elders have higher prevalence rates. It translates into a huge cost burden in both economic and human terms. UI is more common in the elderly population, but there are other identifiable risk factors, including pregnancy, urinary tract infection, medications, dementia, immobility, diabetes mellitus, estrogen deficiency, pelvic muscle weakness, and smoking.

Types of Urinary Incontinence

Most cases of UI can be categorized as due to one of four basic causes: (1) involuntary loss of urine with a strong urinary urgency (urge incontinence); (2) urethral sphincter pressure insufficient to hold urine (stress incontinence); (3) too high urethral resistance or insufficient bladder contractions (overflow incontinence); and (4) chronic impairment of physical or cognitive function (functional incontinence) (Table 5.1).

Urge incontinence, also referred to as detrusor instability, occurs when the involuntary bladder contractions overcome the normal resistance of the urethra. This type of incontinence is likely the most common cause of problematic incontinence, affecting up to 70% of persons with incontinence. The three basic mechanisms of action for this type of incontinence are loss of brain inhibition, involuntary detrusor contractions, and

TABLE 5.1. Treatment of urinary incontinence

Type	Signs and symptoms	Treatment
Urge (detrusor instability)	Inability to get to toilet Large volume loss Normal postvoid residual (PVR)	Treat underlying condition Prompted voiding Bladder training Anticholinergic agents
Stress (sphincter insufficiency)	Urine loss with increased intraabdominal pressure Small volume loss Normal PVR	Pelvic muscle exercises Estrogen α-Adrenergic agents Surgical correction
Overflow (outlet obstruction or hypoactive bladder)	Constant urine loss Abdominal pain/distension High PVR	Treat underlying condition α-Adrenergic blockers Intermittent catheterization Surgical correction
Functional	Inability or unwillingness to be continent Large or small volume loss Normal PVR	Treat underlying condition Remove hindrances

loss of the normal voiding reflexes. It is characterized by a strong desire to void followed by a loss of urine, often on the way to the bathroom.

Stress incontinence, also referred to as sphincter insufficiency, is most frequently encountered in postmenopausal women and is the result of reduced intraurethral pressure and an associated increase in intraabdominal pressure. There is usually a small amount of urine loss during coughing, sneezing, laughing, or other activities that lead to an increase in intraabdominal pressure.

Overflow incontinence is the result of the bladder not emptying properly. It can be secondary to an atonic or hypotonic detrusor or an obstruction of the bladder outlet from an enlarged prostate, urethral stricture, or stone. Detrusor hypoactivity can result from diabetes mellitus, lower spinal cord injury, or drugs. Overflow incontinence is characterized by a variety of symptoms that may be confused with symptoms more frequently associated with urge or stress incontinence. The urinary stream is often weak, and there is the sensation of incomplete emptying of the bladder.

Functional incontinence occurs in persons who, despite normal urinary tract functioning, are incontinent. It results from physical, psychiatric, or cognitive dysfunction or environmental limitations. This type of incontinence is frequently seen in the hospital setting when restraints or bedrails are utilized.

Evaluation

The evaluation of UI has as its goal confirmation of the diagnosis, identification of any reversible causes, and identification of factors that require further diagnostic or therapeutic interventions. A history focused on the neurologic and urologic systems is required. In addition, complete review of the medications, both prescribed and over-the-counter, is necessary. This phase should be accompanied by detailed exploration of the UI symptoms, including duration, frequency, timing, precipitants, and amount of urine lost. Associated symptoms such as nocturia, dysuria, hesitancy, urgency, hematuria, straining, and frequency should be noted. Finally, it is important to know about any medical or surgical treatment of such conditions as diabetes mellitus, neurologic diseases, or urologic problems. At the conclusion of the initial visit, if the patient cannot characterize the incontinence, a bladder record should be kept for several days.[10]

The physical examination focuses on abdominal, neurologic, and genitourinary tract examinations. Specifically, during the abdominal examination the bladder is palpated. The neurologic examination focuses on an assessment of cognitive function and on nerve roots S2–3. In men a genital examination to detect abnormalities of the foreskin, glans penis, and perineal skin as well as a rectal examination to test for perineal sensation, sphincter tone, fecal impaction, and prostatic enlargement is performed. In women a pelvic examination is done to assess perineal skin condition, pelvic prolapse, pelvic mass, and muscle tone. Finally, one can perform the cough stress test to observe urine loss with a full bladder.

Additional tests performed to evaluate all patients with UI include urinalysis and assessment of postvoid residual (PVR). A PVR of more than 100 ml is strongly suggestive of incomplete emptying of the bladder. Selected patients have a urine culture or blood testing that might include blood urea nitrogen (BUN), creatinine, glucose, calcium, electrolytes, and urine cytology. Further testing, including intravenous pyelography, ultrasonography, and computed tomography (CT), or referral to a specialist should be pursued when indicated by the history, physical examination, and simple testing.

Management

The first step in management is to identify and treat any reversible factors, remembering that there may be more than one cause. Seemingly small improvements may make a big difference to patients, and in many patients cure is possible. Further treatment is dictated by the type of UI. Management can be behavioral, surgical, or pharmacologic. Many of the medications used to treat UI can, if used in the wrong circumstance, worsen the symptoms. Dosages listed below are average; both starting and maintenance doses must be individualized.

Nonpharmacologic Therapy

Clinical guidelines from the Agency for Health Care Policy and Research (AHCPR)[10] recommend behavioral therapy in the form of bladder training, prompted voiding, or pelvic muscle exercises for most forms of UI. Bladder training is most effective in the setting of urge incontinence but also may be helpful for other forms of UI. It involves behavioral education through the use of urge inhibition and scheduled voiding; and it requires a cognitively intact individual. Prompted voiding, the nonpharmacologic treatment of choice in the cognitively impaired incontinent individual, involves scheduled voiding and requires prompting by the caregiver. Pelvic muscle exercises, a regimen of planned, active exercises of the pelvic muscles to increase periurethral muscle strength, are particularly helpful in women with stress incontinence.

Other nonpharmacologic means of managing UI include intermittent catheterization, indwelling urethral or suprapubic catheters, external collection systems, and protective undergarments. Chronic indwelling catheters should not be viewed as a viable treatment option except when all else has failed or when there is accompanying local skin breakdown.

Pharmacologic Agents

Postmenopausal women with stress incontinence should use topical or oral estrogen in postmenopausal doses unless contraindicated. For those with an intact uterus, a progestin is added. α-Adrenergic agents such as phenylpropanolamine (25–100 mg PO bid) or pseudoephedrine (15–30 mg PO tid) are also helpful in the setting of stress incontinence.

Anticholinergic agents such as oxybutynin (2.5–5.0 mg PO tid or qid), propantheline (7.5–30.0 mg PO tid), dicyclomine (10–20 mg PO tid), and imipramine or desipramine (25–100 mg PO day) are effective in those with urge incontinence. Anticholinergic medications should be used with caution, especially in the elderly, because of their side effects (confusion, constipation, and dizziness).

In patients with overflow incontinence, bethanechol (10–50 mg PO tid) can help facilitate bladder emptying. Men with prostatic hypertrophy and overflow incontinence can likely benefit from the α-adrenergic blockers prazosin, terazosin, or doxazosin (titrated up to 1–5 mg PO per day).

Surgical Treatment

Surgical therapy is indicated in certain circumstances. Stress incontinence with urethrocele has an 80% to 95% one-year success rate with suspension of the bladder neck.[10] Obstructive overflow incontinence with prostatic enlargement is often best treated with prostate surgery. Patients with urge incontinence and detrusor instability refractory to medical therapy often benefit from augmentation cystoplasty.

Prescription Drug Use

Elderly patients consume a disproportionate number of drugs; consequently, they suffer a disproportionate number of adverse drug reactions. Inappropriate overprescribing, or polypharmacy, has been defined as taking too many drugs, using drugs for too long a time, or using drugs at too high a dose.[11] Careful attention to appropriate prescribing can avoid many of these problems.

Risk Factors

Several risk factors have been identified. Older adults with chronic medical problems often consult several physicians. Vague complaints may tempt physicians to prescribe, or patients or their families may pressure physicians to prescribe. Both hospitalization and nursing home placement usually result in more medicines being prescribed. Medication is often added to a patient's regimen to treat the side effects of another drug. Physiologic changes of aging, including decreased body water and increased proportion of fat, can change the volume of distribution of some drugs and other pharmocokinetic characteristics and make the older person more prone to adverse drug effects.

Problematic Drug Classes

Neuroleptics, long-acting benzodiazepines, and tricyclic antidepressants have been associated with hip fractures resulting from falls[12] (see Chapters 22, 23). Antihypertensive agents, especially diuretics, can also lead to falls. Benzodiazepines, especially those with long half-lives, are associated with cognitive impairment. Cardiovascular drugs and nonsteroidal antiinflammatory drugs (NSAIDs) have high rates of adverse effects. Drug–drug interactions are less frequent causes of adverse effects, but the potential for these problems obviously increases as the number of drugs taken increases.

Principles of Prescribing

Simple changes in a patient's drug regimen can result in substantial improvements in a patient's condition. The following principles, modified from those first espoused by Vestal,[13] are helpful when prescribing for the elderly.

1. *Evaluate the need for drug therapy.* Drug therapy is not always necessary or helpful.
2. *Make a diagnosis before prescribing.* The potential for adverse reactions is reduced when a specific drug is given for a specific, confirmed diagnosis.
3. *A careful drug history is essential.* Patients do not always immediately recall drugs prescribed by other physicians.
4. *Know the pharmacology of the drugs you prescribe, especially with respect to the influence of the changes of aging.* Patient reactions are more predictable when the prescriber uses few drugs in each drug class.
5. *Start with small doses and titrate slowly to the desired response.* Establish reasonable goals, stopping titration when the goals are achieved or side effects start to develop.
6. *Keep the regimen simple to encourage compliance.* Once- or twice-a-day dosing is ideal. Careful instruction should be given to both the patient and a relative or friend, if possible.
7. *Review all medicines regularly and discontinue those that are ineffective or no longer indicated.* Ask the patient to throw all the drugs in their medicine cabinet into a paper bag and bring them to the office for review twice a year.

8. *Remember that drugs cause illness.* A new symptom may not be the result of a chronic or new medical condition. Always eliminate drug causes first.

Pain Management

Pain, acute or chronic, is one of the most common complaints of older individuals. Evaluating and treating pain syndromes in the elderly can be difficult. Many elderly patients are stoic. Cognitive impairment, especially in residents of nursing homes, may cause physicians to question the reliability of complaints of pain. Painful syndromes such as acute myocardial infarction and intraabdominal emergencies often present atypically or even silently in the elderly population. As a result, elderly patients are at risk for both over- and undertreatment of pain syndromes. Other consequences of improperly treated pain include depression, malnutrition, polypharmacy, cognitive dysfunction, and immobility. Acute pain is defined by its distinct onset and duration of less than 6 weeks; chronic pain lasts longer. Guidelines to the management of acute pain[14,15] and pain due to cancer[15,16] have been reported.

WHO Analgesic Ladder

Drug therapy is the cornerstone of treatment of acute and chronic pain due to cancer. The World Health Organization (WHO) analgesic ladder organizes drug therapy into three steps: (1) nonopioid drugs; (2) low-dose opioids; and (3) higher-dose opioids.[15] Treatment is begun with nonopioids, and opioid drugs are added as necessary. It is important to realize that when opioid–acetaminophen combinations are used [e.g., acetaminophen with codeine (Tylenol No. 3), oxycodone with acetaminophen (Percocet)], patients should receive no more than 4000 mg of acetaminophen per day. Adjuvant therapy, such as tricyclic antidepressants, caffeine, or anticonvulsants, may be added at any step.

Acute Pain

In the older patient with acute pain, physicians should determine the etiology of the pain while simultaneously making the patient comfortable. Rest, ice, compression, and elevation constitute the mainstays of treatment for acute injuries. In the elderly population, however, the period of rest should not exceed 48 to 72 hours, and early mobilization is encouraged. Physicians should start with the safest analgesics, such as acetaminophen, and add or substitute stronger analgesics as necessary. With respect to drug therapy, special considerations apply to the elderly.

Older persons are more sensitive to the analgesic properties of opioids and to their side effects, such as sedation and respiratory depression. In addition, constipation and central nervous system (CNS) effects (e.g., delirium and depression) are more common in elderly patients treated with narcotics. NSAIDs should be used with care because of their gastrointestinal, renal, and hepatic effects, especially in the frail elderly. Some physicians believe that older patients have higher pain thresholds, but there is no experimental evidence to support this belief.[14]

Chronic Cancer Pain

As in the case of patients with acute pain, the WHO analgesic ladder is followed for those with chronic pain, beginning with nonopioids such as acetaminophen and NSAIDs, adding opioids as necessary. NSAIDs may be particularly effective in cancer patients with bony metastases. Tricyclic antidepressants and the anticonvulsants carbamazepine and valproic acid are usually helpful in patients with neuropathic pain, although side effects (orthostatic hypotension, constipation, dry mouth) may limit the use of tricyclics.

Several principles help the physician provide optimal relief of cancer pain. Wide variation exists in the response of elderly patients to analgesics. Titration must be done carefully, with frequent follow-up to ensure that the drug is effective. Patients who have pain most of the day should receive their drugs regularly, not as needed. Side effects are treated aggressively. For example, sedation due to opioids can be particularly bothersome but can be treated by adding a stimulant such as caffeine or dextroamphetamine. Long-acting morphine and fentanyl patches are helpful for patients with severe cancer pain, but care must be taken when calculating equianalgesic doses.[15] Other patients may require patient-controlled analgesia (PCA), continuous epidural morphine, or local radiation therapy. Lastly, nonpharmacologic adjunctive therapies including exercise, transcutaneous nerve stimulation, acupuncture, chiropractic manipulation, or prayer may aid in the treatment of pain (see Chapter 26).

Nutrition

There are few data regarding the nutritional requirements in the aged population. Similarly, the effect of nutrition on the aging process in humans is unclear. Poor nutritional status does, however, contribute to the morbidity of chronic illnesses and worsens the prognosis when an older person becomes ill. Protein–calorie malnutrition is the most common nutritional abnormality in the elderly. In one study, hospitalized elders had a 44% prevalence of protein–calorie malnutrition as defined by height/weight and serum albumin.[17]

Many factors increase the risk for malnutrition in the elderly. A decrease in the acuity of taste and smell with aging serves to lessen the enjoyment of eating. Poor dentition or poorly fitting dentures may lead to chewing difficulties. Swallowing disorders are more common in older persons, and gastrointestinal motility declines with age. Other risk factors for malnutrition include depression, poverty, social isolation, certain medications, and dementia. Such conditions as pressure ulcers, chronic infections, malabsorption, sepsis, malignancy, and alcoholism can increase the metabolic demands and result in malnutrition.

Nutritional Assessment

The key to the evaluation of malnutrition in the elderly is maintaining a high index of suspicion. The patient is asked about symptoms such as nausea, vomiting, anorexia, swallowing difficulties, and abdominal pain. They are also asked about any new medications, diagnoses, or social issues. A careful weight history is obtained and the weight loss expressed as a percentage of the patient's usual weight. Weight loss of more than 10% of the patient's usual weight usually represents severe malnutrition.

Physical signs of malnutrition may be difficult to recognize in the elderly. Anthropometric measures such as weight, height, and skinfold thickness can be helpful for the initial assessment. The total lymphocyte count, hemoglobin, serum albumin, and cholesterol levels are important tests in the biochemical assessment of nutritional status. The farther the results are below normal values, the greater is the degree of malnutrition present. The Nutrition Screening Initiative (NSI) focused on the need for primary care physicians to consider the nutritional aspects of medical care.[18] The NSI developed a screening tool useful for evaluating risk for malnutrition.

Treatment

Treatment of malnutrition begins while efforts are made to identify the sources of nutrient losses and conditions that increase the metabolic needs. In addition, nutritional support begins early in those individuals who are at increased risk for malnutrition. In the nonstressed elderly, approximately 22 to 25 kcal/kg body weight is required. This support increases to 30 kcal/kg in the severely stressed elderly.

Oral supplementation with food is optimal. The goal is to optimize the types of food and consistency of the diet to improve the nutritional status of the individual. The addition of liquid supplemental feedings can also improve nutritional status. When there is refusal or an inability to swallow, enteral tube feeding with a small-bore nasogastric tube or gastrostomy/jejunostomy tube is required. The decision on which of these methods to use depends on patient preference, suspected length of time the feedings will be necessary, and patient tolerance of each method. Feeding can occur in a continuous fashion or with intermittent bolus feeds. Each of these methods of feeding carries a risk of aspiration. Diarrhea is a frequent complication in the tube-fed patient.

Total parenteral nutrition (TPN) is indicated in the elderly patient when there is an inability to use the gut to meet nutrient needs. Complications are more likely to occur in the elderly population, but it should not preclude the use of TPN in the appropriate clinical setting in an elderly patient. As with younger individuals, the use of TPN necessitates careful monitoring of the electrolyte and glucose levels as well as renal function.

Health Promotion and Disease Prevention

Elderly patients are living longer and longer. Average life expectancy for a 65-year-old man is at least 15 years more, and women live even longer. Thus it is important that physicians consider health promotion activities for their elderly patients, just as they do for children and younger adults.[19] Among the interventions that are probably helpful in the elderly are (1) immunizations for influenza, pneumococcal disease, and tetanus-diphtheria; (2) counseling for injury prevention (car safety belts, smoke detectors); (3) counseling for smoking cessation; (4) cervical cancer screening for women who have not been previously screened; (5) guaiac stool testing or sigmoidoscopy to detect colorectal cancer; and (6) hormone replacement therapy and calcium supplementation for women at risk of osteoporosis. Currently, no evidence exists for the elderly to support the use of prostate-specific antigen screening, mammography screening for breast cancer in women older than 69 years, or cholesterol screening, although physicians may choose to screen some older individuals for these conditions (see Chapter 2).[20]

Evaluating and Managing Nursing Home Patients

Every physician who takes care of older patients has some interaction with a nursing home. For some family physicians, this interaction may be limited to referring their ambulatory patients for admission when they can no longer remain in the community. Increasingly, however, family physicians will be asked to assume larger roles in nursing homes. Only about 5% of the elderly reside in nursing homes, but the lifetime chance of an older person being admitted to a nursing home is about 40%.[21]

Evaluating Elderly Patients for Nursing Home Placement

Most nursing home residents are admitted to a long-term care facility from the hospital. Not uncommonly physicians are asked to certify that an elderly person living in the community needs nursing home care. Usually these patients and their families present at a time of crisis. The patient may have been found wandering in the neighborhood, or they may have suffered recurrent falls and are thought to be unsafe in their home. Loss of function, usually as a result of cognitive impairment, is the common denominator.[22]

Careful assessment is important because a less restrictive environment may be a better solution and because patients and families often are not aware of these possibilities. Patients should have a complete history and physical examination, focusing on the function of the patient: activities of daily living (ADLs), such as bathing, eating, dressing, and instrumental activities of daily living (IADLs), such as using the phone or buying groceries. A mental status examination is important, as patients may appear relatively intact on casual questioning but be severely impaired. Patients and family members should be questioned closely regarding the possibility of major depression, which has a high incidence among severely medically ill elderly and nursing home residents. Medicines are reviewed to see if any can be eliminated, especially those that may impair function (see above). The social history explores personal and financial resources that could support other care options, and advance directives are reviewed. For patients found to require the services of a nursing home, a complete assessment provides an opportunity to stabilize chronic illnesses or to complete any evaluations that might be necessary prior to admission.

Integrating Nursing Home Practice into Office Practice

Family physicians can provide continuity of care for their elderly patients who are admitted to nursing homes by continuing to follow them after their admission. To avoid disrupting an office practice, however, it is wise for the physician to limit privileges to just a few facilities. Ideally, these nursing homes are near the physician's office, home, or hospital, so visits can be incorporated into the usual work day. In this way physicians can avoid wasting time driving between several facilities to see only one or two residents in each nursing home. Another benefit is that the physician becomes more familiar with the nursing staff and capabilities of those nursing homes.

After building up a sizable census in a few facilities, it becomes practical to set aside a half-day every 1 or 2 weeks to make rounds. Routine nursing home rounds gives the physician a chance to consult with the resident's usual nurses and observe them during therapy or other activities. Fewer phone calls from the nursing staff usually result as well. To minimize disruptions in the office, some physicians ask nursing homes to call at previously agreed on times for routine problems.

Physicians with an interest in the organization and administration of nursing homes may wish to work as a medical director. Most medical directors approve policies and procedures, act as liaisons with the medical staff, supervise employee health issues, address quality improvement, and help keep the facility abreast of new regulations or medical treatments. New medical directors can find resources to help them through the American Medical Directors Association (10480 Little Patuxent Parkway, Suite 760, Columbia, MD 21044; phone 1-800-876-AMDA).

Pressure Sores

Pressure sores are defined as changes in the skin and underlying tissue that result from pressure over bony prominences. If not attended to, these forces cause ulceration. The best treatment for pressure sores is prevention; but even under the best conditions it is not always possible.

Epidemiology

The incidence of pressure sores is greatest among the elderly population, especially during long hospital or nursing home confinements.[23–25] In addition, patients with spinal cord injuries[26] or cerebrovascular disease[27] are at risk for the development of pressure sores. Factors that may contribute to the likelihood of developing pressure sores include nutritional deficiencies, volume depletion, increased or decreased body weight, anemia, fecal incontinence, renal failure, diabetes, malignancy, sedation, major surgery, numerous metabolic disorders, cigarette smoking, and being bed- or chairbound.[23–30] Finally, the aging skin itself, because of reduced epidermal thickness and elasticity, increases the risk for pressure changes.

Etiology

There are four primary mechanisms in the development of pressure sores: pressure, shearing forces, friction, and moisture.[31] More than 90 percent of pressure sores occur over the bony prominences of the lower part of the body. The amount of time and pressure necessary to cause tissue damage depends on the number of risk factors present. The second etiologic factor, shearing forces, is caused by the sliding of adjacent surfaces. This sliding results in compression of capillary flow in the subcutaneous layer. An example of shearing forces is elevation of the head of the bed, which causes the body to slide down, producing a shear in the sacral and coccygeal region. Friction is the force created when two surfaces move across each other, such as would occur when maneuvering a patient on the bed. The impact of friction damages the epidermis, which is already vulnerable in the elderly. This damage accelerates the onset of ulceration. Finally, moisture increases the risk of pressure ulceration. A high correlation exists between urinary or fecal incontinence and ulceration. Because of the increased risk of skin infection, the presence of a sacral pressure sore is an indication for a chronic indwelling urethral catheter in the incontinent patient.

Clinical Evaluation

The best method for evaluating a pressure sore is to classify the sore by its severity. There are several classification schemes for pressure sores. The National Pressure Ulcer Advisory Panel has proposed a staging system[32] that divides pressure sores into four grades, depending on the depth of tissue involvement.

Grade I pressure sore (Fig. 5.1A): Acute inflammatory response in all layers of the skin. The clinical presentation of a grade I pressure sore is a well defined area of nonblanchable erythema of the intact skin.

Grade II pressure sore (Fig. 5.1B): Presents as a break in the epidermis and dermis, with surrounding erythema, induration, or both. It is caused by an extension of the inflammatory response leading to a fibroblastic response.

Grade III pressure sore (Fig. 5.1C): Inflammatory response characterized by an irregular full-thickness ulcer extending into the subcutaneous tissue but not through underlying fascia. There is often a draining, foul-smelling, necrotic base.

Grade IV pressure sore (Fig. 5.1D): Penetrates the deep fascia, eliminating the last barrier to extensive spread. Clinically, it resembles a grade III sore except that bone, joint, or muscle can be identified.

The complications of pressure sores are associated with significant morbidity and mortality. Most of the complications occur with grade III and IV sores and include cellulitis, osteomyelitis, septic joints, pyarthrosis, and tetanus. Tetanus may complicate pressure sores, and for this reason immunoprophylaxis against tetanus is recommended in patients with pressure sores.[33]

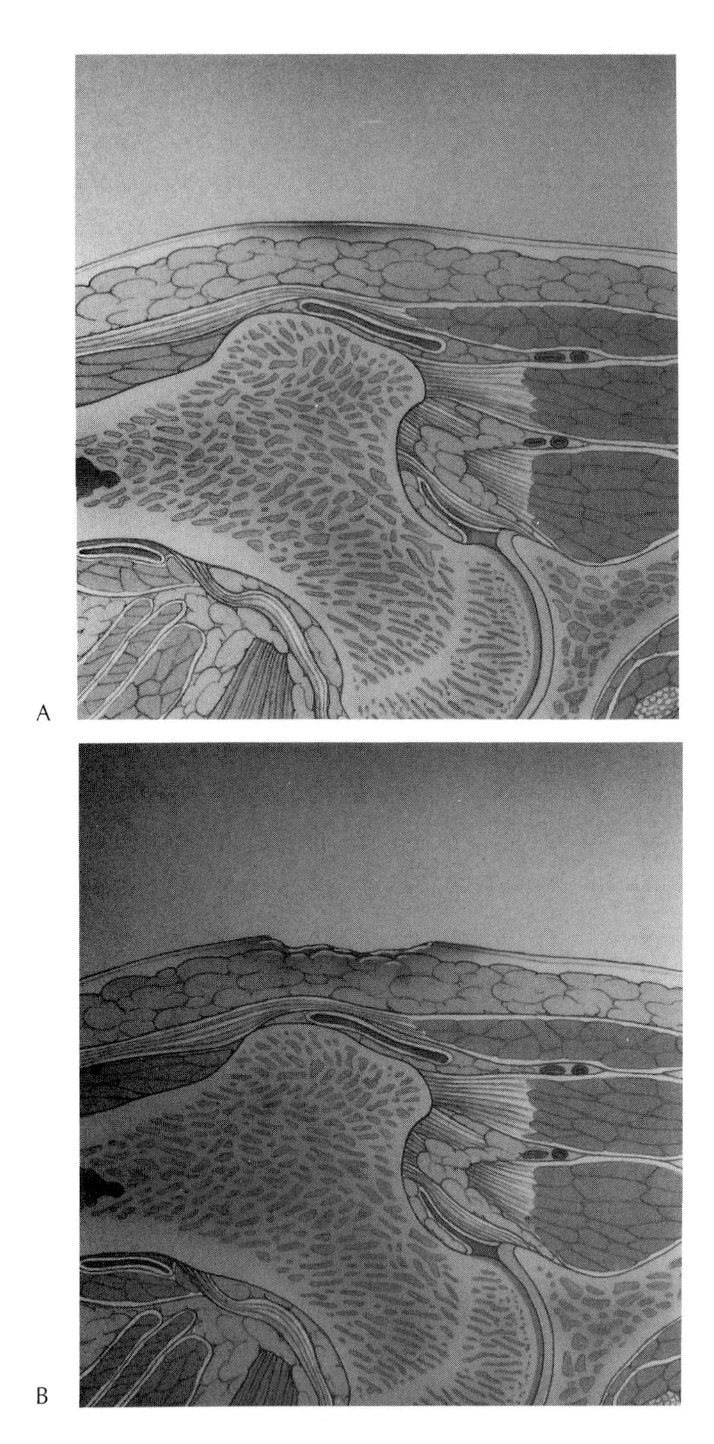

FIGURE. 5.1. National Pressure Ulcer Advisory Panel staging system. (A) Grade I pressure sore, characterized by inflammatory reaction of the epidermis and dermis. It presents clinically as nonblanchable erythema over an area of pressure. (B) Grade II pressure sore, characterized by epidermal and dermal skin breakdown with surrounding erythema.

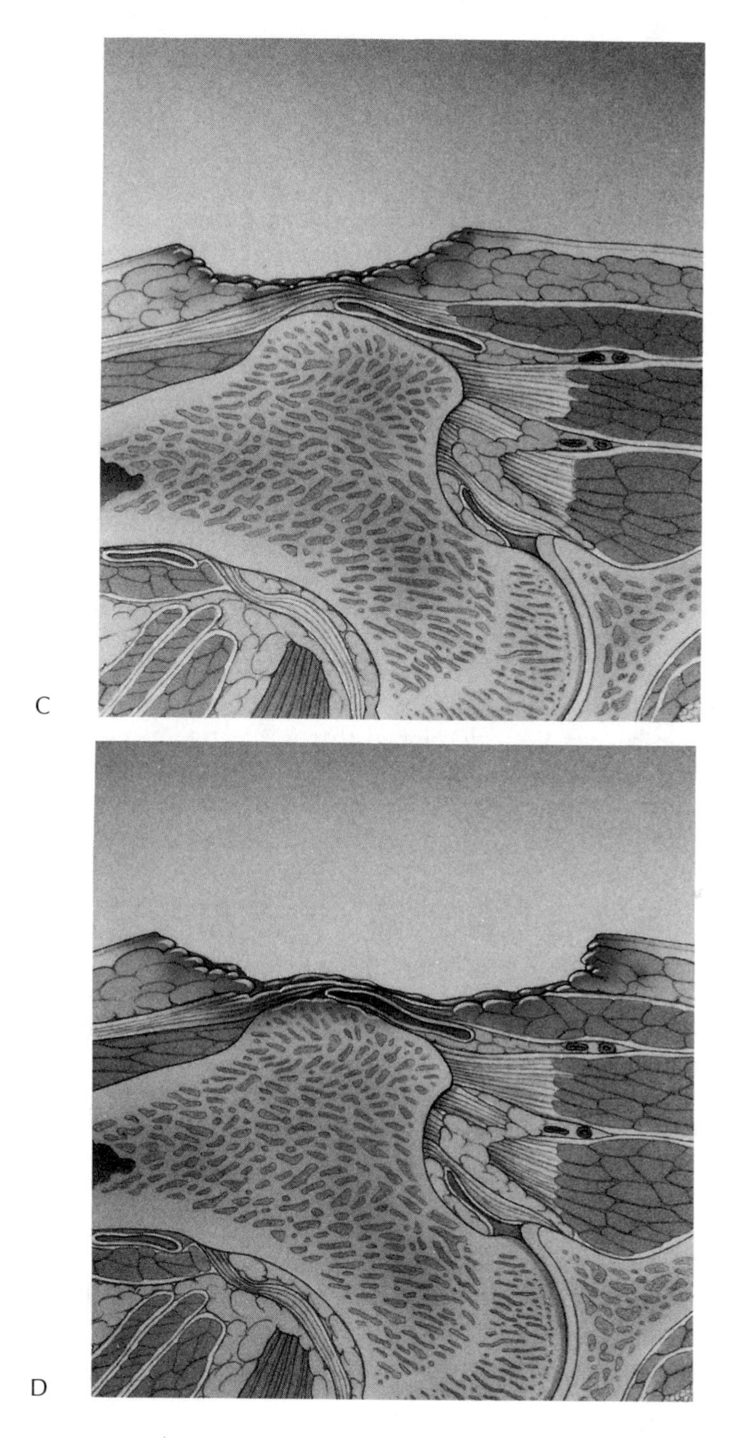

FIGURE. 5.1.(*continued*) (C) Grade III pressure sore characterized by an ulcer extending into the subcutaneous tissue, frequently with necrosis. (D) Grade IV pressure sore characterized by extension of the ulcer beyond the fascial layer and thus involving muscle, bone, or other structures. (Source: National Pressure Ulcer Advisory Panel.[32] With permission.)

Prevention

Because of the great morbidity and mortality associated with pressure sores and the financial burden incurred by treating this problem, their prevention is the primary goal of physicians and health care facilities taking care of patients at risk. Identifying persons at risk is the first step in employing intensive preventive measures.

Persons at risk should undergo frequent assessment and be placed in an environment that enhances soft-tissue viability, which can be achieved through use of proper positioning techniques and support surfaces. At the time of positioning, the patient's skin is examined for areas of redness that indicate early pressure changes. When repositioning, the patient is lifted, not dragged, from a bed or wheelchair to avoid friction and subsequent damage to the epidermis. Elevating the head of the bed to more than 30 degrees is avoided to minimize the shearing forces.

Special pads, beds, and mechanical devices are available and prevent pressure sores by altering the pressure over bony prominences. Devices such as gel pads, foam cushions, wheelchair cushions, and sheepskin pads are practical for preventing pressure sores at specific anatomic sites. No single device has yet been developed that is effective in preventing all pressure sores. Static flotation mattresses, low air loss mattresses, alternating air pressure mattresses, and air-fluidized beds help to prevent and treat pressure sores. These beds tend to relieve pressure by using air or buoyancy to keep the patient's weight evenly distributed. Such devices, however, cannot be relied on as a substitute for basic nursing care.

Preventive care of pressure sores also involves improvement of medical conditions that predispose the individual to the development of pressure changes. In particular, nutritional deficiencies, incontinence, and immobility should be minimized. Nutritional status is assessed on admission to the hospital or nursing home: Once a pressure sore has developed, nutritional status usually is already severely compromised and is difficult to correct.

Management

The first step in the management of pressure sores is assessing the extent of the sore and the patient's overall status, including his or her nutritional state. Regardless of the grade of the sore, adherence to the principles of prevention outlined above remain important.

WOUND CLEANSING AND DÉBRIDEMENT

The primary goal of therapy for pressure sores is to create an environment that promotes healthy granulation tissue. Wounds are cleansed as atraumatically as possible with normal saline-soaked gauze, wound irrigation, and whirlpool baths. Most antiseptics, such as hydrogen peroxide and povidone-iodine, are cytotoxic and should be avoided.

Necrotic tissue prevents healing and creates favorable conditions for bacterial contamination. The ideal method for débriding pressure sores is sharp dissection of the necrotic tissue. Enzymatic débridement using such agents as fibrinolysin, collagenase, and dextranomer should be used only during intervals between surgical débridement to help dissolve thin necrotic layers that are less accessible to excision.[34] The inability of these agents to penetrate eschar or to remove large amounts of tissue limits their usefulness. There is no proof that topical antibiotics are superior to careful cleansing and wet-to-dry dressings. In addition, topical antibiotics may sensitize the tissue, promote the appearance of resistant organisms, and have systemic toxicity.[25]

Dressings

Once the wound is clean with granulation tissue visible, the use of dressings that promote healing is advisable. The cardinal rule is to keep the ulcer moist and the surrounding skin dry.[35] Additional factors when selecting dressings include exudate control and caregiver time requirements. Dressing options include saline-soaked gauze and occlusive dressings. The appeal of the occlusive dressings is that they can usually remain on the pressure sore for several days, whereas gauze dressings should be changed several times daily. This convenience is particularly useful for outpatient management of pressure sores. These dressings should be avoided in the presence of clinical infection.

Managing Complications

The two most frequently encountered complications are nonhealing and infection. For clean wounds that fail to heal, reassessment of the patient's overall status and a 2-week trial of a broad-spectrum topical antibiotic are recommended.[35] In patients who are operative candidates, surgical repair of the nonhealing wound may be considered. Appropriate systemic antibiotics are employed when the condition is complicated by bacteremia, soft-tissue infection, or osteomyelitis.

References

1. Hazzard WR, Bierman EL, Blass JP, Ettinger WH, Halter JB, editors. Principles of geriatric medicine. 3rd ed. New York: McGraw-Hill, 1994.
2. Kane RL, Ouslander JG, Abrass IB. Essentials of clinical geriatrics. 3rd ed. New York: McGraw-Hill, 1994.
3. Tinetti ME. Falls. In: Hazzard WR, Bierman EL, Blass JP, Ettinger WH, Halter JB, editors. Principles of geriatric medicine. 3rd ed. New York: McGraw-Hill, 1994:1313–20.

4. King MB, Tinetti ME. Falls in community-dwelling older persons. J Am Geriatr Soc 1995;43:1146–54.
5. Hornbrook MC, Stevens VJ, Wingfield DJ, et al. Preventing falls among community-dwelling older persons: results from a randomized trial. Gerontologist 1994;34:16–23.
6. Vetter NJ, Lewis PA, Ford D. Can health visitors prevent fractures in elderly people? BMJ 1992;304:888–90.
7. Province MA, Hadley EC, Hornbrook MC, et al. The effects of exercise on falls in elderly patients: a pre-planned meta-analysis of the FICSIT trials. JAMA 1995;273:1341–7.
8. Tinetti ME, Baker DI, McAvay G, et al. A multifactorial intervention to reduce the risk of falling among elderly people living in the community. N Engl J Med 1994;331:821–7.
9. Tinetti ME. Performance-oriented assessment of mobility problems in elderly patients. J Am Geriatr Soc 1986;34:119–26.
10. US Department of Health and Human Services. Clinical practice guideline: urinary incontinence in adults. Rockville, MD: DHHS, 1992:38–65. AHCPR Publ. No. 92-0038.
11. Michocki RJ, Lamy PP, Hooper FJ, Richardson JP. Drug prescribing for the elderly. Arch Fam Med 1993;2:441–4.
12. Ray WA, Griffin MR, Schaffner W, et al. Psychotropic drug use and the risk of hip fracture. N Engl J Med 1987;316:363–9.
13. Vestal R. Clinical pharmacology. In: Hazzard WR, Andres R, Bierman EL, Blass JP, editors. Principles of geriatric medicine and gerontology. 2nd ed. New York: McGraw-Hill, 1990:201–11.
14. Acute Pain Management Guideline Panel. Acute pain management: operative or medical procedures and trauma; clinical practice guideline. Rockville, MD: Agency for Health Care Policy and Research, Public Health Service, US Department of Health and Human Services, 1992. AHCPR Publ. No. 92-0032.
15. American Pain Society. Principles of analgesic use in the management of acute pain and cancer pain. 3rd ed. Skokie, IL: American Pain Society, 1992.
16. World Health Organization. Cancer pain and palliative care: report of a WHO expert committee. Geneva: WHO, 1990:1–75. World Health Organization Technical Report Series 804.
17. Bistrian BR, Blackburn GL, Vitale J, et al. Prevalence of malnutrition in general medical patients. JAMA 1976;235:1567–70.
18. White JV, Dwyer JT, Posner BM, et al. Nutrition Screening Initiative; development and implementation of the public awareness checklist and screening tools. J Am Diet Assoc 1992;92:163–7.
19. Richardson JP. Health maintenance for the elderly. In: Taylor RB, editor. The manual of family practice. Boston: Little, Brown, 1997;24–7.
20. United States Preventive Services Task Force. Guide to clinical preventive services. 2nd ed. Baltimore: Williams & Wilkins, 1996.
21. Kemper P, Murtaugh CM. Lifetime use of nursing home care. N Engl J Med 1991;324:595–600.
22. Richardson JP. Outpatient evaluation for nursing home admission. In: Yoshikawa TT, Cobbs EL, Brummel-Smith K, editors. Ambulatory geriatric care. 2nd ed. St. Louis: Mosby-Year Book, in press.

23. Brandeis GH, Morris JN, Nash DJ, Lipsitz LA. The epidemiology and natural history of pressure ulcers in elderly nursing home residents. JAMA 1990;264:2905–9.
24. Reuler JB, Cooney TG. The pressure sore: pathophysiology and principles of management. Ann Intern Med 1981;94: 661–6.
25. Longe RL. Current concepts in clinical therapeutics: pressure sores. Clin Pharm 1986;5:669–81.
26. Sather MR, Weber CE Jr, George J. Pressure sores in the spinal cord injury patient. Drug Intell Clin Pharm 1977;11: 154–69.
27. Berlowitz DR, Wilking SVB. Risk factors for pressure sores: a comparison of cross-sectional and cohort-derived data. J Am Geriatr Soc 1989;37: 1043–50.
28. Allman RM, LaPrade CA, Noel LB, et al. Pressure sores among hospitalized patients. Ann Intern Med 1986;105:337–42.
29. Pinchcofsky-Devin GD, Kaminski MV Jr. Correlation of pressure sores and nutritional status. J Am Geriatr Soc 1986;34: 435–40.
30. Guralnik JM, Harris TB, White LR, Cornoni-Huntley JC. Occurrence and predictors of pressure sores in the National Health and Nutrition Examination Survey follow-up. J Am Geriatr Soc 1989;36:807–12.
31. Knight AL. Medical management of pressure sores. J Fam Pract 1988; 27:95–100.
32. National Pressure Ulcer Advisory Panel. Pressure ulcers prevalence, cost and risk assessment: consensus development conference statement. Decubitus 1989; 2(2):24–8.
33. Richardson JP, Knight AL. The prevention of tetanus in the elderly. Arch Intern Med 1991;151:1712–17.
34. Seiler WO, Stahelin HB. Decubitus ulcers: treatment through five therapeutic principles. Geriatrics 1985;40:30–44.
35. Pressure Ulcer Guideline Panel. Pressure ulcer treatment. Am Fam Physician 1995;51:1207–22.

CASE PRESENTATION

Subjective

PATIENT PROFILE

Harold Nelson is a 76-year-old married white male retired welder.

PRESENTING PROBLEM

"I can't control my urine."

PRESENT ILLNESS

There is a 2-day history of urinary incontinence, and on three occasions, the patient has lost control of his urine, wetting his clothing. This follows a several-month history of urinary hesitancy and difficulty initiating the stream. There has been no dysuria, but the patient has been out of bed several times to pass urine during each of the past few nights.

PAST MEDICAL HISTORY

Mr. Nelson has had type 2 diabetes mellitus for 24 years and is now taking glyburide. He has had osteoarthritis of multiple joints for 20 years and underwent a lumbar laminectomy at age 60.

SOCIAL HISTORY

Mr. Nelson lives with his wife, aged 71.

HABITS

He does not smoke. He takes "a few drinks" each evening and drinks 2 cups of coffee daily.

FAMILY HISTORY

Both parents died in their mid-80s of "old age."

REVIEW OF SYSTEMS

He has had a recent cold with nasal congestion and cough.

- What additional medical history might be useful, and why?
- What more might you ask about his alcohol intake? How would you address this issue?
- What might be pertinent about his "cold?"
- What might be significant about the family's reaction to his recent incontinence, and how would you inquire about this issue?

Objective

VITAL SIGNS

Height, 5 ft 7 in; weight, 156 lb; blood pressure, 150/84; pulse, 90; temperature, 37.4°C.

EXAMINATION

The abdomen has no mass or organ enlargement. There is mild suprapubic tenderness. No costovertebral angle tenderness is present. His genitalia are normal for age, and there is no hernia. The prostate is 3 plus enlarged, smooth, and symmetric.

LABORATORY

A urinalysis shows 4 to 6 white blood cells per high-powered field; no glucose is present.

- What more—if anything—would you include in the physical examination, and why?
- Are there any diagnostic maneuvers that may be helpful today?
- What—if any—additional laboratory tests might be helpful in evaluating today's problem?
- What—if any—diagnostic imaging studies should be obtained today?

Assessment

- What seems to be Mr. Nelson's problem, and how would you describe this to the patient and the family?

- What are likely causes of the problem?
- What might be the meaning of this illness to the patient and the family?
- What might be unspoken concerns of the patient regarding today's problem? How might these concerns relate to his age?

Plan

- What therapeutic recommendations would you make today?
- How would you advise the patient and his family regarding the possibility of future urinary problems?
- What is the appropriate locus of care for this patient's problem? Is a consultation with a urologist likely to be needed now or in the future?
- What follow-up would you recommend to Mr. Nelson?

6

Domestic Violence

VALERIE J. GILCHRIST AND ANN CARDEN

Although domestic violence may refer to all aspects of family violence this chapter focuses on violence within an intimate relationship. Ninety-five percent of such abuse involves a man abusing his female partner. Although several studies have shown an almost equal number of episodes of violence perpetrated by men and women, the context, intent, and outcome of these episodes result in injury and fear in the female partner.[1] There is little published information concerning the remaining 5% of incidents, most of which occur between homosexual partners (male or female) and are even more likely than heterosexual abuse to be unreported by victims and unrecognized by clinicians.

Background

In the United States today, violent crimes occur more frequently within families than among strangers. According to U.S. Federal Bureau of Investigation (FBI) statistics, 52% of female murder victims in 1990 were killed by a current or former partner, and men kill their female partners more than twice as often as women kill their male partners. Battery is the single greatest cause of injury to women.[1]

The goal of the abuse is power and control by the perpetrator. Figure 6.1, based on descriptive data from more than 200 battered women, depicts eight tactics employed by batterers. Ultimately, ongoing ego-battering erodes the victim's self-image. She comes to believe that she is somehow to blame for the violence she suffers and that she is worthless, helpless, and incapable of survival without her abuser.[2]

Prevalence

An intimate partner's physical, emotional, or sexual abuse affects up to one-half of women in the United States at some time in their lives.[3] This figure may be an underestimation, as surveys exclude individuals who are

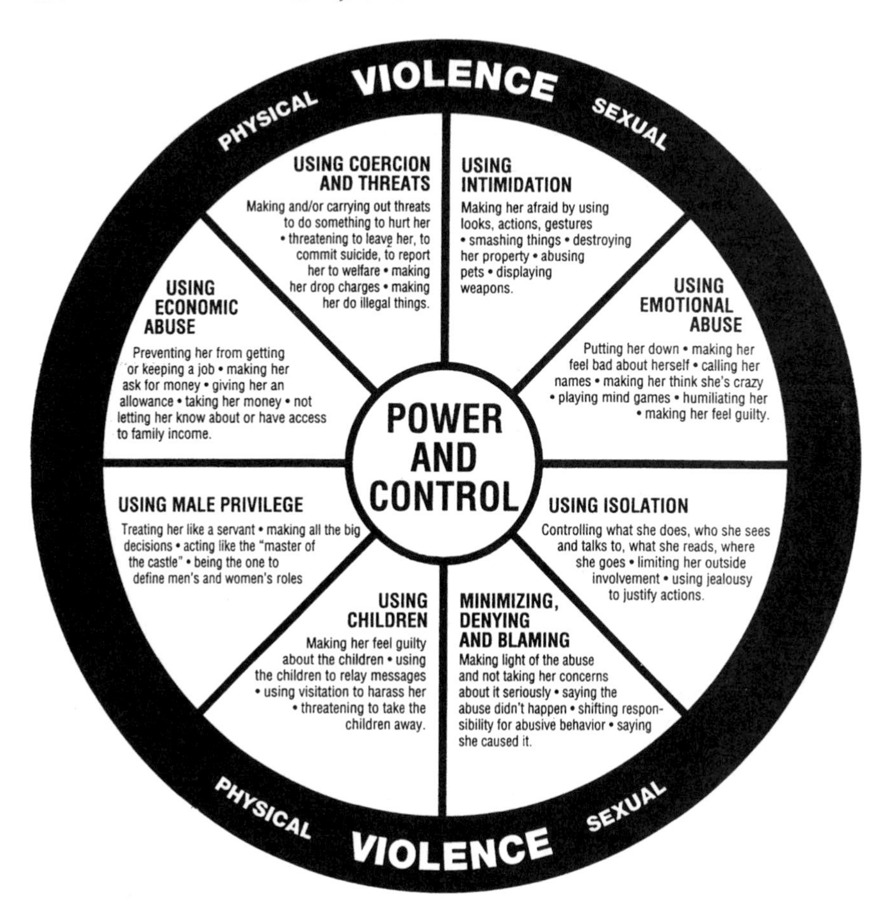

FIGURE. 6.1 "Power and control wheel" illustrates many components of domestic violence, all of which are ultimately enforced by the threat or actuality of physical and sexual violence. [Reprinted with permission by the Domestic Abuse Intervention Project, Minnesota Program Development, Inc., 206 West Fourth Street, Duluth, MN 55806-2720. Phone (218) 722-4134.]

hospitalized, homeless, institutionalized, incarcerated, or non-English-speaking. As many as 35% of women who visit emergency departments are battered, and studies in these settings reveal a lifetime prevalence of 11% to 54% depending on the definition of abuse and the survey method used.[3] Domestic violence may present as chronic with acute exacerbations. Two surveys in family practice settings revealed current abuse in 25% to 48% of women, with a lifetime prevalence of 38.8%.[4] One-third to one-half of women presenting to mental health centers have been battered.[1] As many as one in five women are battered during pregnancy, and this abuse may become more frequent during the postpartum period.[3,5] It is unclear when domestic violence ends as many, and in some studies the majority, of battered women have no current partner but fear or suffer abuse from past partners.

Cycle of Violence

On the basis of information obtained in a series of intensive interviews with battered women, Walker proposed the cycle theory of spousal violence.[6] After an abusive episode comes the *honeymoon phase*. The abuser is apologetic, often courting the victim with gifts and attention, promising that he will never hurt her again. This phase invariably shifts into the *tension-building phase* during which the woman lives in an atmosphere of extreme tension and fear as her partner threatens and isolates her. She is systematically stripped of the resources that would allow her to leave: her self-respect, pride, career, money, friends, and family. The tension-building phase ultimately culminates in the *violent phase* of battery and abuse. With repetition the cycle increases in frequency and severity.

Clinical Presentation

Battered women present with repeated, increasingly severe physical injuries, self-abuse, and psychosocial problems that include depression, drug or alcohol abuse, and suicide attempts. The battering injuries are often bilateral and only in areas covered by clothing. There may be contusions, lacerations, abrasions, pain without obvious tissue injury, evidence of injuries of different ages, and evidence of rape.

Eight percent to 39% of battered women report receiving medical care. Ten percent require hospital treatment, although most women present for routine, not emergency, medical care and most injuries do not require hospitalization.[1] Abused women have an increase in surgical procedures, pelvic pain, functional gastrointestinal problems, chronic headaches, and chronic pain problems in general.[1,2] Women who experienced serious assault averaged almost double the number of days in bed due to illness compared with other women. Fear of abuse has limited partner notification of human immunodeficiency virus (HIV) status.

Pregnancy may incite the initial episodes of abuse or cause ongoing abuse to increase. Abused women are twice as likely to delay seeking prenatal care, twice as likely to miscarry, and four times as likely to have a low-birth-weight infant; and these infants are 40% more likely to die during the first year of life.[5]

The diagnosis of borderline personality disorder and substance abuse are particularly common among abused women, although in a family practice center study depression was the strongest indicator of domestic violence.[4] Domestic violence is a cause of posttraumatic stress disorder, the intensity of which correlates directly with the intensity of the abuse. One in ten victims of abuse attempts suicide.

After battery, victims have demonstrated a 9-fold increased risk for drug abuse, and the use of alcohol increased 16-fold. There is concurrent use of alcohol and drugs during 25% to 80% of the battering episodes, and the presence of one factor should initiate questions about the other.[1]

Abused Women

Women who are divorced or separated, young, and of a low socioeconomic status report higher prevalence rates of abuse; but there is no characteristic premorbid personality profile of the abused woman.[2,3] Isolation, power imbalance, and alternating abusive and kind behaviors predispose victims to the formation of strong emotional attachments to their abusers, which explains why battered women must struggle to separate themselves emotionally from their abusers and often return after leaving.[7]

Abusing Men

Batterers do not lose control; rather, they take control.[8] Common characteristics among batterers include dependence on and jealousy of their partners, a belief in traditional gender roles, an extreme need for control, hostility, difficulty with trust, and refusal to accept responsibility for their violent behaviors. Ninety percent of men who batter have no criminal record.

Children

Parents often claim that the children are unaware of the violence, but 40% to 80% are present, the rest hear it from another room or witness the results and 30% to 40% experience physical abuse. Spousal abuse is, in and of itself, child abuse. In 45% to 60% of child abuse cases, there is concurrent domestic violence.[9]

The symptoms manifested by child witnesses of spousal abuse fall into three categories: internalizing behaviors (sadness, withdrawal, somatic complaints, fears, anxiety), externalizing behaviors (aggression, cruelty to animals, defiance of authority, destructiveness), and defects in social competence (poor school achievement, peer relations, participation in sports and other extracurricular activities). These children are predisposed to later enactment of abuse against, or victimization by, an intimate partner.[9]

Diagnosis

The single most important step medical professionals can take is to ask every woman if she is being or has been abused. Domestic violence cuts across all ages and socioeconomic, racial, ethnic, religious, and professional groups, although social and ethnic backgrounds may influence both the victim's and perpetrator's perception of domestic violence. Domestic violence occurs at a frequency comparable with that of breast cancer and is more common than other conditions for which screening is routine, such as colon cancer and thyroid dysfunction. Questioning communicates to the patient that the problem is not trivial, shameful, or irrelevant. It conveys to all women the physician's belief that it is important to talk about abuse.

While a single screening question may be appropriate for an emergency room setting, family practitioners should attempt to explore family violence with every patient. It is important to remain nonjudgmental and relaxed because abused women are extremely sensitive to nonverbal cues. Physicians should begin with general questions and then become more specific. Ask about the relationship (How are things going at home?) and then about conflict resolution (How do you and your partner resolve differences?). Next ask about nonviolent but psychologically abusive acts (Are you insulted, threatened, or fearful?). Inquire about the use of force, such as grabbing or restraining, pushing, throwing objects (be specific about the type of objects thrown). Finally, ask about more serious violence: forced sex, clubbing, beating, choking, and the use of weapons. Negative responses to more general questions do not preclude positive responses to more specific questions. Physicians must not only diagnose domestic violence but establish its severity and the risk to the patient.

Battered women may lack money for or transportation to medical facilities, or they may be prevented by their abuser from seeking medical care. Once with a clinician, victims may withhold information because they feel ashamed or humiliated; or they may think that the injuries are not serious or that they deserved it. Victims also may lie about the source of injuries in an effort to protect a partner or children or because they fear retribution for any disclosure or police involvement.

Domestic violence is a complex social problem that requires physicians to step beyond the basic medical paradigm to confront their own personal feelings and social beliefs.[10,11] Up to 38% of physicians report personal histories of violence. Among unselected patients, physicians identified only 1.5% to 8.5% of victims. Only 6 of 394 women surveyed in a family practice center had been asked about abuse, and only 3 of 139 women giving a history of abuse had the diagnosis of domestic violence or spouse abuse recorded.[4] Teenagers, elderly women, and never-married women are rarely identified. Physicians tend to believe that domestic violence is a problem but not among their patients.

Physicians believe they have not been trained to deal with domestic violence, and they sometimes avoid asking about it because they believe they are "opening a can of worms."[12] They cite lack of time or fear of offending patients, and believe themselves powerless to effect change. If incidents are discovered, abusers commonly accuse their partners of exaggeration and do not define their actions as violent, or dismiss the incident as an exception or justifiable.

Physicians may also inadvertently retraumatize the woman by blaming her.[10] They may diagnose anxiety, depression, or substance abuse without realizing they are a result of ongoing abuse. This practice labels the victim, delays appropriate intervention, and, if psychocoactive drugs are prescribed, increases the risk of suicide.

Management

There are several "do's and don'ts" for treating abused women (Table 6.1). The quality of medical care a battered woman receives often determines if she will follow through with referrals to legal, social service, and health care agencies. It is critical for the physician to breach the battered woman's isolation and validate her view of reality.

Once domestic violence has been recognized, the *immediate danger* must be assessed. The best way to ascertain the woman's risk is to ask: Are you safe tonight? Can you go home now? Are your children safe? Where

TABLE 6.1. Do's and don'ts of treating domestic violence

Do

Ask every woman patient about violence in the home.
Tell her spouse abuse is a crime. There is nothing she did to deserve the abuse. It is not her fault.
Tell the patient things can improve, and that her feelings of defeat are a result of the abuse.
At each visit assess safety, establish and review a "safe plan," review high risk factors, and remind her of the cycle of violence.
Give practical advice such as the local women's shelter or crisis number. Caution her that she may encounter prejudices. Direct patient to support groups.
Use neutral but precise and descriptive language in the medical record.

Do not

Assume domestic violence is not occurring in your neighborhood or among your patients.
Question the patient's sense of danger.
Rationalize, minimize, or excuse the abuser's violence.
Recommend family therapy. Separation from and treatment for the abuser must be accomplished first.
Insist that the patient terminate the relationship—she alone can make that decision.
Use judgmental statements and questions.
Underestimate her risk. Women are at even more risk when attempting to leave—most of the murders happen then.
Ask why she does not leave. (Ask, instead, why does he batter.)

is your batterer now? If she says she is in immediate danger, believe her and begin to explore safer options.[1,2,10] The physicians must review with the battered woman the *features associated with increasing risk:* (1) an increasing frequency of violence; (2) severe injuries; (3) the presence of weapons; (4) substance abuse; (5) threats and overt forced sexual acts; (6) threats of suicide or homicide; (7) surveillance; (8) abuse of children, pets, other family members, or the destruction of treasured objects; (9) increased isolation; (10) extreme jealousy and accusations of infidelity; (11) failure of multiple support systems; (12) a decrease or elimination of remorse expressed by the batterer.

The battered woman needs to develop a *safe plan* so she can escape quickly. It may save her life. A safe plan consists not only of consideration of where to flee but includes such things as a set of clothes packed for her and her children; an extra set of keys to home and car; evidence of abuse, such as names and addresses of witnesses, pictures of injuries, and medical reports; cash, checkbook, and other valuables; legal documents such as birth certificates, social security cards, driver's license, insurance policies, protection orders, prescriptions; something meaningful for each child (blanket, toy, book); a list of important telephone numbers and places to stay. If the children are old enough she should talk to them about safety: how to call for help and where to go to keep themselves safe.

Documentation

Once recognized, the abuse must be documented. The abused woman needs to know that her records are confidential unless she decides to use them. The physician's documentation provides the history and evidence of abuse. Notes should be nonjudgmental, precise, and document chronology. The chief complaint and a description of abusive events should use the patient's own words. Include a complete description of any injuries with body diagrams, describing the type, number, size, location, age, and the explanation offered of any injuries. Photographs are taken before medical treatment if possible and include a reference object and the face of the woman in at least one. All photographs are dated and kept with the consent form. The physician's record should also include the results of diagnostic procedures, referrals, and recommended follow-up and should record any contact with the abuser. The badge number of the investigating officer, if the police are notified, is important.[13]

Process of Leaving

Separation from an abusive partner is an ongoing process.[14,15] The abuser responds predictably when his partner leaves: He first tries to locate her, apologizing, then threatening, then promising religion or counseling, and often embarrassing her in public or harassing her. If she does not comply she is at risk for significant injury. Women are at the greatest risk of being brutally beaten or killed when they leave their abuser: 75% of calls to the police and 73% of emergency room visits occur after separation. Women are five times more likely to be murdered by their partner during the separation than before the separation or after divorce.[15]

Women report going through stages of "*reclaiming self*" as they separate from their abusive partners.[14] They progress from initial denial, shame, humiliation, guilt, shock, and fear, through staying in the relationship trying to minimize the abuse and hoping for improvement, to realizing the unavoidability of the abuse and the need to separate both emotionally and physically, to eventually establishing a safe and separate living situation, and finally to a new sense of themselves and their abuse history.

Continuing Care

Continued support, validation, risk assessment, and documentation comprise the physician's "treatment" of domestic violence. Scheduled follow-up visits provide the victim opportunities to acknowledge the validity of her experiences, the difficulties in her situation, and the chance to reassess her options. Physicians need to focus on the process of empowerment (Fig. 6.2) rather than the outcome of leaving. The battered woman must be reminded that she can take civil actions, which include requesting a protective order, injunction, or restraining order from the courts. She may also choose to file criminal charges including prosecution for assault and battery, aggravated assault or battery, harassment, intimidation, or attempted murder. However, the legal response to domestic violence is less than optimal, and the woman is likely to know whether the batterer will adhere to court orders. Physicians should refer batterers to an appropriate state certified batterer treatment program but also must realize that enrollment of the batterer in a program in no way guarantees a woman's safety.[8]

Prevention

Primary prevention of domestic violence is achieved only by challenging the roles of violence and patriarchy in society. Secondary prevention can be achieved by the interruption and elimination of intergenerational abuse of all kinds. Tertiary prevention can be achieved by identifying victims and their abusers and helping each one. When available, battered

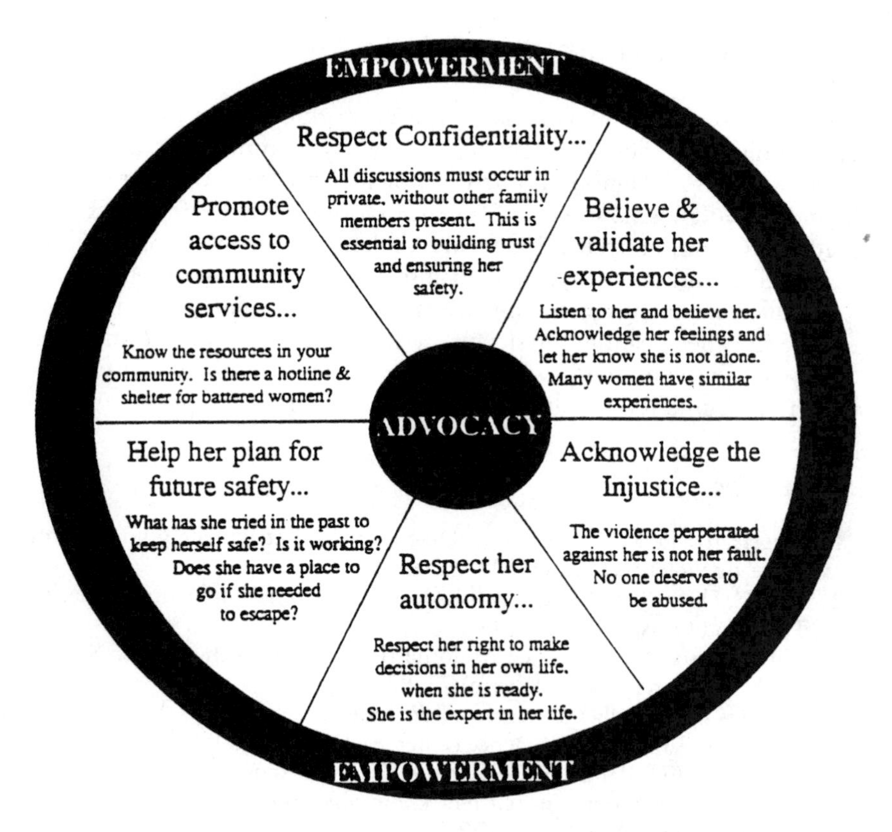

FIGURE. 6.2 "Empowerment wheel" describes the ways health care providers can help victims of domestic violence become empowered and change their lives. [Reprinted with permission by the Domestic Violence Project, Inc., 6308 8th Ave., Kenosha, WI 53143 Phone (414) 656-8502. Based on the "Power & Control and Equality Wheel" developed by the Domestic Abuse Intervention Project, 206 West 4th St., Duluth, MN 55806. Phone (218) 722-4134.

women's shelters are effective, although fewer than one-fourth of the women in need can access them. Court-ordered programs for male batterers have had some success in the reduction of battery. Most states require reporting of criminal assaults, and some states have mandatory reporting of domestic violence. Mandatory reporting, however, without the necessary support services places victims at risk, fearful of confiding in their physicians, and physicians are conflicted between their obligations to report and their concern for their patient's safety. The Joint Commission on Accreditation of Health Care Organizations requires policies for the identification and assessment of abuse victims and education of providers.

Family and Community Issues

Treatment of domestic violence requires working in partnership with community agencies (see Chapter 1). Many communities and states operate toll-free 24-hour domestic violence hotlines. Other resources include the National Domestic Violence Hotline (1-800-799-SAFE), the National Coalition against Domestic Violence (303-839-1852), and the National Coalition of Physicians against Violence (312-464-5000).

Families who engage in one form of family violence are likely to engage in others. Family physicians are in a unique position to interrupt the cycle of violence and to effect positive change in the lives of victims, abusers, and children involved in domestic violence.

References

1. American Medical Association. Diagnostic and treatment guidelines on domestic violence. Chicago: AMA, 1992.
2. Stark E, Flitcraft A. Women at risk: domestic violence and women's health. Thousand Oaks, CA: Sage, 1996.
3. Wilt S, Olson S. Prevalence of domestic violence in the United States. J Am Med Wom Assoc 1996;51(3):77–82.
4. Saunders DG, Hamberger K, Hovey M. Indicators of woman abuse based on a chart review at a family practice center. Arch Fam Med 1993;2:537–43.
5. Newberger EH, Barkan SE, Lieberman ES, et al. Abuse of pregnant women and adverse birth outcome: current knowledge and implication for practice [commentary]. JAMA 1992; 267:2370–2.
6. Walker LE. The battered woman syndrome. New York: Springer, 1984.
7. Barnett OW, Laviolette AD. It could happen to anyone: why battered women stay. Beverly Hills, CA: Sage, 1993.
8. Adams D. Guidelines for doctors on identifying and helping their patients who batter. J Am Med Wom Assoc 1996; 51(3):123–6.
9. Zuckerman B. Silent victims revisited: the special case of domestic violence. Pediatrics 1995;96:511–13.
10. Warshaw C. Domestic violence: changing theory, changing practice. J Am Med Wom Assoc 1996;51(3):87–91.
11. Gremillion D, Evins G. Why don't doctors identify and refer victims of domestic violence? NC Med J 1994;55:428–32.
12. Sugg NK, Inui T. Primary care physicians' response to domestic violence: opening Pandora's box. JAMA 1992;267:3157–60.
13. Hyman A. Domestic violence: legal issues for health care practitioners and institutions. J Am Med Wom Assoc 1996; 51(3):101–5.
14. Merritt-Gray M, Wuest J. Counteracting abuse and breaking free: the process of leaving revealed through women's voices. Health Care Wom Int 1995;16:399–412.
15. Campbell A. Epidemic of women battering. J Fla Med Assoc 1995;82:684–6.

Case Presentation

Subjective

Patient Profile

Ann Martino-Priestley is a 22-year-old married white female nursery school teacher found to be pregnant on her last visit 6 weeks ago.

Presenting Problem

"Routine prenatal visit."

Present Illness

The patient is now 13 weeks pregnant and no longer has nausea and urinary frequency. There is no vaginal spotting. She feels well and is "excited about this first pregnancy." Her appetite is good, and she is taking prenatal vitamins.

Past Medical History, Social History, Habits, and Family History

These are unchanged since her first prenatal visit (see Chapter 3).

Review of Systems

While taking the history, you noticed a bruise below her left eye, although this was not mentioned by the patient. When questioned, the patient reports that she walked into a partially opened bathroom door while going to the toilet at night.

- The husband insists on being present throughout the examination and the following consultation. How do you respond to this request?
- What additional information about the progress of the pregnancy would be important today?
- What might be the patient's goals for today's visit?
- What more would you like to know about the bruise below the left eye? How would you frame the question(s)?

Objective

VITAL SIGNS

Weight, 131 lb; blood pressure, 120/72; pulse, 74; temperature, 37.2°C.

EXAMINATION

There is no abdominal tenderness. The uterus is palpable at a 3-months' size. In addition to the fading ecchymosis below the left eye, there is a recent-appearing ecchymosis 2 to 4 cm in size of the left lower abdomen and another bruise 2 by 3 cm of the lateral right breast. The patient was apparently unaware of these bruises and reports that she does not know the cause.

LABORATORY

On laboratory examination, the urine is negative for protein and glucose.

- What additional information derived from the physical examination would be useful in regard to the pregnancy?
- What additional physical examination data might help clarify the cause of the bruising?
- What laboratory specimens—if any—should you obtain today?
- What diagnostic imaging—if any—would you obtain today?

Assessment

- What are the diagnostic possibilities, and how will you share these with the patient?
- What might be the significance of the pregnancy to the patient and her husband?
- What may be the patient's concerns, and how would you elicit these?
- What physical diseases could explain the bruising? What drugs might contribute to the bruising? How readily will you accept these possible explanations?

Plan

- What is your recommendation to the patient and her husband?
- What community agencies might become involved, and how should they be contacted?
- The patient expresses concern about the cost of prenatal care, hospital confinement, and delivery. How would you respond?
- As you are concluding the visit, the patient begins to cry and says, "I'm afraid." What would you do next?

7 Headache

Anne D. Walling

Headache is an almost universal experience, afflicting patients of any age or characteristic, although it is reported to be particularly frequent in young adults. Nearly 60% of men and 76% of women aged 12 to 29 years report at least one headache within any 4-week period.[1] The societal costs of headache are enormous but can be estimated only indirectly in terms of days lost from work or school, expenditures on medical services, and consumption of nonprescription medications. The total burden of suffering due to this symptom, including disruption of relationships and loss of normal activities, is incalculable. Although headache is given as the principal reason for more than 10 million physician office visits per year[2] and is consistently found to be one of the most frequent presenting complaints in family practice,[3] it is important to realize that most headache episodes are not brought to medical attention.

Headache is a symptom, not a diagnosis. Numerous conditions can produce cephalic pain (see Classification, below) as part of a localized or systemic process; thus headache may be a prominent symptom in the child with fever, the adult with sinusitis, or the elderly patient with temporal arteritis. The pathophysiology of "primary" headaches, such as migraine and cluster headaches, is a controversial, rapidly developing area with the principal developments focused on the role of neurotransmitters, endothelial cells, and whether neuronal tissue can itself generate pain.[4,5]

Whatever the etiology, each headache episode is interpreted by individual patients in terms of experience, culture, and belief systems. Thus a relatively minor degree of pain may prompt one patient to seek emergency care and comprehensive neurologic assessment, whereas a patient with extensive personal or family experience of recurrent headache may cope with several days of incapacitating symptoms without seeking medical assistance.

Both patients and physicians tend to be uncomfortable with the diagnosis and management of headache. Studies show that 75% of headache patients report some disappointment or dissatisfaction with their care,[6] and headache is frequently identified as a "heartsink" condition by physicians (i.e., the patient evokes "an overwhelming mixture of exasperation, defeat, and sometimes plain dislike"[7]). The reasons for this situation include the recurrent nature of most headache syndromes, the potential for secondary gain and iatrogenic complications (particularly overuse of narcotic analgesics), and fear of missing a potentially serious but rare intracranial lesion. The effective management of headaches requires the development of a "therapeutic alliance" between physician and patient based on objectivity and mutual respect.[8] Most chronic headaches are recurrent and cannot be completely cured. Physicians can, however, greatly help patients to understand their condition, develop effective strategies to reduce the number and severity of attacks, and follow healthy life styles not skewed by the presence or fear of headache.

Clinical Approach to the Headache Patient

With so many potential causes and complicating circumstances, a systematic approach to the headache patient is essential for objective, effective, efficient management. It can be achieved in four stages.

1. Clarification of the reasons for the consultation
2. Diagnosis (classification) of the headache
3. Negotiation of management
4. Follow-up

It is common to discover a significant headache history on systematic inquiry of a patient presenting for other reasons. The clinical approach to these patients may reverse the first question to identify why the patient avoided seeking medical help for headache symptoms.

Clarification of the Reasons for Consultation

Those headaches that lead to medical consultation have particular significance. It is important to have the patient articulate his or her beliefs about the symptoms and expectations of treatment.[8] Reasons for consultation range from fear of cancer to seeking validation that their current use of nonprescription medication is appropriate. Headache is frequently used as a "ticket of admission" symptom by the patient who wishes to discuss other medical or social problems. In practice, a change in the coping ability of the patient, family, or coworkers is as frequent a cause of consultation as any change in the severity or type of headache. Patients may also consult when they learn new information, particularly concerning situations in which a severe illness in a friend or relative presented as headache.

All headache patients should be asked directly what type of headache they think they have and what causes it. These issues must be addressed during the management even if they are inaccurate. Patients should also be asked about expectations of management. Successful management avoids dependence by emphasizing the patient's role in reducing the frequency and severity of headaches and increasing his or her ability to cope with a recurrent condition.

Background information from relatives and friends may give useful insights. Disruptive headaches lead to highly charged situations, and the physician must remain objective and avoid becoming triangulated between the patient and others. With good listening and a few directed questions, the background to the consultation can be clarified and the groundwork laid for accurate diagnosis and successful management. This short time is well invested. In headache patients presenting to family physicians, "listening" time makes a significantly greater contribution to the diagnosis and management than time spent on the physical examination or other investigation,[9] although all are appropriate.

Classification of Headaches

The 1988 International Classification of Headaches[10] established diagnostic criteria for 13 major types of headache with approximately 70 subtypes (Table 7.1). A useful grouping for family practice uses five categories.

1. Migraine (all types)
2. Cluster headaches
3. Tension/stress (or muscle contraction) headaches
4. Headaches secondary to other pathology
5. Specific headache syndromes (e.g., cough headache)

These categories are broad with considerable overlap. "Mixed headaches," where the clinical picture contains elements of more than one headache category, are common. Individual patients may also describe more than one type of headache; for example, migraineurs experience tension headaches on occasion.

Diagnosis

The diagnosis of headache syndromes (Table 7.2) requires systematic clinical reasoning based on the history augmented by physical examina-

TABLE 7.1. Headache types

Primary headaches	Secondary headaches
Migraine	*Associated with*
Without aura	Head trauma
With aura (several types)	Vascular disorders
Ophthalmoplegic	Intracranial disorders
Retinal	Substance use or withdrawal (including medication side effects)
Childhood syndromes	Systemic infections
Migraine complications	Metabolic disorders
Other	Structural disorder of head or neck
Tension type	Neuralgia syndromes
Episodic	
Chronic	
Other	**Unclassifiable headaches**
Cluster	
Episodic	
Chronic	
Chronic paroxysmal hemicrania	
Other	
Miscellaneous	
"Ice-pick"	
External compression	
Cold stimulus (including ice cream)	
Cough	
Exertional	
Coital	

tion and judicious use of investigations or consultation to establish the most probable etiology for the pain. A particular feature is the potential to use the diagnostic process to increase patient understanding and prepare him or her to take responsibility for long-term management in cooperation with the physician.

Tension headaches are by far the most prevalent type of cephalic pain encountered in family practice,[9,11] probably followed by headaches secondary to other causes. The medical literature, research efforts, and therapeutic innovations focus on migraine and other "interesting" syndromes, but all headache patients deserve a competent assessment and appropriate, individualized treatment for their symptoms.

History

Headache diagnoses depend on the medical history. An open-ended approach, such as "Tell me about your headaches," followed by specific questions to elucidate essential features usually indicates which of the diagnostic categories is most probable. The history should address the criteria shown in Table 7.2 and clarify the following:

TABLE 7.2. Diagnostic criteria for common primary headaches

Headache	Duration	Characteristics	Associated symptoms	Other
Migraine	4–72 hours	At least two: Unilateral Pulsating Moderate to severe Aggravated by activity	At least one: Nausea/vomiting Photophobia and phonophobia	No neurologic source for symptoms Multiple types (Table 7.1) At least 5 attacks for diagnosis
Cluster	Individual attacks: 15–180 minutes Cluster episodes: 1–8 attacks/day for 7 days to 1 year or longer	Unilateral orbital/temporal stabbing Severe to very severe	At least one: Conjunctival injection Lacrimation Nasal congestion Rhinorrhea Sweating Miosis Ptosis Eyelid edema	No neurologic source for symptoms At least 5 attacks for diagnosis
Tension/stress	Individual headaches: 30 minutes to 7 days Headaches < 15 days/month or < 180/year	At least two: Pressure/tightness Bilateral Mild to moderate Not aggravated by activity	No nausea Photophobia and phonophobia: absent or only one present, not both	No neurologic source for symptoms At least 10 episodes for diagnosis

1. *Characteristics:* nature of pain, location, radiation in head, intensity, exacerbating and relieving factors or techniques, associated symptoms and signs
2. *Pattern:* usual duration and frequency of episodes, precipitating factors, description of a "typical" episode, change in pattern over time, prodromes and precipitating factors, postheadache symptoms
3. *Personal history:* age at onset, medical history (including medication, alcohol, and substance use) with special emphasis on "secondary" causes of headache, such as depression or trauma; environmental and occupational exposure history
4. *Investigations and treatments:* previous diagnoses and supporting evidence, patient's degree of confidence in these diagnoses, patient's beliefs and concerns about diagnosis and potential treatments; previous treatments and degree of success; side effects of any investigations and treatments; patient preferences for treatment; current use of prescription and nonprescription medications
5. *Family history:* headache, other conditions, family attitudes to headache

The headache profile that emerges from the history has a high probability of correctly classifying the headache[8,9,12] without further investigation. It is important, however, to complete the usual review of systems to uncover additional data. Throughout the history-taking process, the physician forms a general impression of the patient. Although subjective, this should correlate with the headache profile and is particularly useful for assessing psychological components of the situation, including which management strategies are most likely to be successfully implemented and followed by the patient. By the end of the history taking the physician should have the answer to two questions: Which of the five headache groups best fits the story? and Is this diagnosis likely in this particular patient?

Physical Examination

The physical examination continues the dual processes of confirming a specific diagnosis and laying the groundwork for successful management. Unless the consultation coincides with an attack, many migraine, cluster, and other headache patients can be expected to have no abnormal findings on physical examination. Some authors recommend that only a targeted examination be performed, focusing on the most probable cause of the secondary headache elicited from the history,[9] whereas others emphasize the importance of complete physical and neurologic examination of every headache patient.[12] The time devoted to a complete examination may be a wise investment, as it documents both positive and negative physical findings, contributes to the "therapeutic alliance," and in many instances is therapeutic. Any physical examination targets the most probable diagnoses based on the symptoms presented by the patient and the physician's knowledge of conditions relevant to the individual.

Other Investigations

A logical test strategy is guided by the most probable diagnosis (or diagnoses) suggested by the history and physical examination. Targeted laboratory and radiologic investigations are most useful for confirming the underlying cause of secondary headaches. Tests are often performed to relieve either physician or patient distress and uncertainty. If the patient or family insists on tests the physician does not believe appropriate, the contributions and limitations of the test in question should be reviewed. Similarly, the physician experiencing the WHIMS (*w*hat *h*ave *I* *m*issed *s*yndrome) must review the data and attempt to make a rational decision as to the potential contribution of additional testing.

Most debate over the appropriate role of testing currently involves radiologic investigation, specifically computed tomography (CT) and magnetic resonance imaging (MRI). The role of these modalities is limited by the rarity of headaches caused by intracranial lesions in family practice. Serious intracranial pathology was the cause of only 0.4% of headaches presented to primary care physicians in two studies.[9,13] When deciding to refer a patient for advanced radiologic investigation, the family physician must seriously consider the potential benefits versus the potential radiation exposure (for CT), patient distress (MRI), and cost. As the investigations have different and often complementary abilities, one must also have a clear concept of what type of intracranial lesion is being sought and its likely location. CT is very sensitive to acute hemorrhage and certain enhancing solid lesions; MRI provides better resolution in the posterior fossa and superior detection of gliosis, infection, posttraumatic changes, and certain tumors.[14] Discussions with a neurologist or radiologist may be useful in this difficult area.

Family physicians should refer a patient for CT or MRI only when the history and physical examination indicate that an intracranial lesion is the probable diagnosis. This protocol is in general agreement with the National Institutes of Health (NIH) Consensus Development Panel, which recommended CT investigation of patients whose headaches were "severe, constant, unusual, or associated with neurological symptoms."[15] This recommendation can be problematic in practice, however, as more than half of the patients describe their headaches as severe.[9] The other elements of the NIH recommendations, particularly the presence of neurologic signs, are more useful; but the final decision to refer for CT or MRI remains a clinical judgment based on the characteristics of the patient and his or her symptom complex and risk factors for intracranial pathology.

Negotiation of Management

Migraine, cluster, tension/stress, and many secondary headaches are recurrent; hence the emphasis is on enabling the patient to successfully manage a lifestyle that includes headaches. The physician who sets a goal of abolishing headaches is being unrealistic in almost all cases.[8,9] More appropriate goals are effective treatment of individual headache episodes and minimizing the number and severity of these episodes. Most headache patients are open to the concept that they carry a vulnerability to headaches and are willing to learn how to manage this tendency. Patients who strongly resist this management approach are often highly dependent personalities who may have drug-seeking behavior or may change to another chronic pain symptom complex when offered aggressive treatment of headaches. The complete management plan includes patient education, treatment plans for both prophylaxis and acute management, and follow-up.

Patient education is essential for the patient and family to manage headaches. They must understand the type of headache and its treatment and natural history. In addition to providing information, the physician must address hidden concerns. Many myths and beliefs are associated with headaches, and patients are empowered to deal with their headaches once these beliefs are addressed. Patients may be embarrassed by their fears: For example, almost all migraine patients have feared cerebral hemorrhage during a severe attack.

Patient education and treatment overlap as the patient and family become responsible for identifying and managing situations that precipitate or exacerbate headache. These situations range from avoiding foods that trigger migraine attacks to practicing conflict resolution. Stress is implicated in almost all headaches; even the pain of secondary headaches is less easy to manage in stressful situations.

There are few "absolutes" in the pharmacologic treatment of headaches, and the large number of choices can be bewildering to both physicians and patients. In general, first-line analgesics and symptomatic treatment are effective, and narcotic use should be avoided. A common mistake is to appear tentative about therapy. The exasperated physician who uses phrases such as, "We'll try this," may convey the message that the medication is not expected to work. Conversely, implying to patients that one has selected a medication specific to their situation and based on an understanding of the headache literature, recruits the placebo effect and is much more likely to succeed. Patients gather information about headaches and their treatment from a wide variety of sources, including news media and the experience of friends. Patient knowledge and opinions of specific treatments should be established before issuing a prescription.

Nonpharmacologic advice is a powerful factor in building the placebo effect and therapeutic alliance. Physicians gather experiences from many patients and can pass on "tips" for headache management: such as Lamaze-type breathing exercises for tension headaches, cold washcloth over the eyes during a migraine attack, and vigorous exercise at the start of migraine, cluster, or tension headaches. Including such information in the overall treatment plan enhances the physician's credibility and reinforces the message that headache management is not solely dependent on medications.

Follow-up

With the exception of headaches secondary to acute self-limiting conditions, headaches tend to be a recurrent problem. Unless follow-up is well managed, the patient returns only at times of severe symptoms or exasperation at the failure of treatment. This pattern implies the risk of emergency visits at difficult times and consultation complicated by hostility or disappointment. In practice, patients manage well if given scheduled appointments, particularly if they are combined with the expectation that the patient will come to the consultation well prepared (i.e., with information on the number, pattern, response to treatment, and any other relevant information about headaches since the last visit). Some authors recommend a formal headache diary.[9]

Clinical Types of Headache

Migraine

Migraine-type headaches are estimated to affect more than 23 million Americans, approximately 17% of women and 6% of men.[16] Although all epidemiologic studies are complicated by differences in definitions and design, migraine is more common in women at all ages and has a peak prevalence during young adulthood. Up to 30% of women aged 21 to 34 report at least one migraine-type headache per year.[17]

Up to 90% of migraine patients have a first-degree relative, usually a parent, also affected by migraine.[17] Perhaps because of familiarity with the condition, significant numbers of migraine sufferers (up to 50%) do not seek medical assistance. Several classifications of migraine have been suggested. As shown in Table 7.2, the current international classification is based on clinical features, particularly the presence of aura. In practice, it is seldom useful to subclassify migraine.

Patients in the "classic" subgroup (approximately 20% of all migraineurs) experience a characteristic aura before the onset of migraine head pain. This aura may take several forms, but visual effects such as scotomas, zigzag lines, photopsia, or visual distortions are the most common. A much larger proportion of patients describe prodromal symptoms, which may be visceral, such as diarrhea or nausea, but are more commonly alterations in mood or behavior. Food cravings, mild euphoria (conversely, yawning), and heightened sensory perception, particularly of smell, are surprisingly common.

The headache of migraine is severe, usually unilateral, described as "throbbing" or "pulsating," and aggravated by movement. The pain usually takes 30 minutes to 3 hours to reach maximum intensity, and it may last several hours. The eye and temple are the most frequent centers of pain, but occipital involvement is common. Each patient describes a characteristic group of associated symptoms among which nausea predominates. Either nausea or photophobia and phonophobia are required for diagnosis along with the characteristic headache. During attacks, migraine patients avoid movement and sensory stimuli, especially light. They may use pressure and either heat or cold over the areas of maximal pain. The attack usually terminates with sleep. Vomiting appears to shorten attacks, and some patients admit to self-induced vomiting, although this phenomenon is not widely described in the literature. Many patients report "hangover" on waking after a migraine, but others report complete freedom from symptoms and a sense of euphoria. The cause of migraine remains unknown; research indicates that migraine begins in neurons as a biochemical process, and that vascular phenomena are secondary effects.[18,19]

The treatment of migraine typifies the approach of enabling patients to manage their own condition. A bewildering variety of therapies is available, and management should be individualized. The treatment plan has three aspects: avoidance of precipitants, aggressive treatment of attacks, and prophylactic therapy if indicated. Patients and their families can usually identify triggers of migraine attacks. The role of specific foods has probably been exaggerated,[20] although red wine and cheese continue to have a significant reputation as migraine triggers. Disturbance in daily routine, particularly missed meals, excessive sleeping, and relaxation after periods of stress, are notorious precipitants of migraine attacks. Certain women correlate migraines with the onset of menstruation each month, but the effect of oral contraception and postmenopausal hormone replacement are unpredictable. Migraines commonly disappear during pregnancy.

Patients should be encouraged to recognize their own aura or prodrome, as early treatment is most efficacious. Whatever treatment strategy is followed, early use of metoclopramide helps reduce nausea and counteract delayed gastric emptying. The multiple medications used for migraine may be regarded as falling into four groups.

1. Symptom control: principally analgesics, with or without adjunctive antiemetics or sedatives
2. Ergotamines: based on the theory that migraine pain is due to cerebral vasodilation
3. Serotonin (5-hydroxytryptamine, 5-HT) receptor agonists: new class of agents (prototype is sumatriptan) based on etiology
4. Prophylactic agents: large, diverse group of medications reported to reduce the frequency of attacks (Table 7.3).

A common problem in migraine treatment is subtherapeutic dosage of medication or failure to absorb medication because of vomiting and gastric stasis. Conversely, overzealous use of analgesics and ergotamines can trap paitents in chronic daily headache. This requires withdrawal over 1–2 weeks using regular analgesics with or without other medications. Hospitalization may be necessary.[21]

The choice of specific medications and route of delivery must be individualized. Factors contributing to the decision include the migraine characteristics (particularly the likelihood of vomiting), patient factors such as associated medical problems, and medication issues including efficacy, speed of onset, side effects, cost, and acceptability.[16] Patients frequently appreciate having more than one agent or combination of agents (e.g., ergotamine, analgesic, or sumatriptan) when they need to "keep going" and a combination analgesic and sedative for "backup" or situations when they can "crash." Many patients also report that a particular agent appears to work well for several months, but then they need to change it.

Narcotics have almost no place in migraine therapy. Even in the emergency room situation, controlled studies have shown that adequate analgesia, use of injections of antiemetics, or injectable ergotamines are superior to narcotics.[17] The migraine patient who demands narcotics or claims allergies to alternative treatments may be a drug abuser. Rarely, patients develop dehydration and "status migrainosus" when the attack lasts several days. These patients may require hospitalization and steroids in addition to fluids and aggressive therapy based on antiemetics plus sumatriptan or ergotamines.

The role of sumatriptan, zolmitriptan, naratriptan, and similar agents now in clinical trials is evolving.[22] Whereas many patients experience dramatic relief using the subcutaneous or oral forms of sumatriptan, others find its use limited by nausea, return of headache 3 to 6 hours after initial clearing, and an unpleasant autonomic reaction of flushing, nausea, hyperventilation, and "panic attack" as the medication is absorbed. A European study found comparable pain relief but fewer side effects when a combination of aspirin and antiemetic was compared to sumatriptan.[23] As with all migraine treatment, the importance of working with the patient to achieve optimal results from the many options cannot be overstressed. For some patients sumatriptan appears to be a "wonder drug" but for others an expensive disappointment. At least six "triptan" antimigraine drugs are available or in development. Each has specific advantages and disadvantages allowing therapy to be tailored to the specific patient experience.

If patients find normal life impossible because of the frequency and severity of migraine attacks, prophylactic treatment should be considered.[16] β-Blockers are the most widely studied agents. Those without intrinsic sympathomimetic activity (e.g., propranolol, nadolol, atenolol, metoprolol) are effective, but the dosage at which individual patients benefit must be established by clinical trial. Amitriptyline appears to prevent migraine at lower dosages than that used for treatment of depression. β-Blockers and amitriptyline are synergistic if used together. Many other drugs have been recommended, but the studies are often small and difficult to interpret because of the placebo effect and patient selection. Verapamil appears to have some prophylactic effect, but there is little evidence to support the use of other calcium channel blocking agents. Studies indicate that the anticonvulsant medication valproic acid can be prophylactic for migraine, and interest is growing in the use of fluoxetine and other selective serotonin-reuptake inhibitors for this indication.[16] The choice of any prophylactic agent must balance potential benefit against issues of compliance, side effects, and cost. Migraine patients can usually be assisted to find regimens that enable them to minimize attacks and deal effectively with those that do occur. They may be comforted by knowing that the condition tends to wane with age, has been associated with lower rates of cerebrovascular and ischemic heart disease than expected,[18] and has afflicted a galaxy of famous people.[17]

Cluster Headaches

The cluster headache, a rare but dramatic form, occurs predominantly in middle-aged men. The estimated prevalence is 69 per 100,000 adults with a 6:1 male preponderance.[17]

The headache is severe, unilateral, centered around the eye or temple, and accompanied by lacrimation, rhinorrhea, red eye, and other autonomic signs on the same side as the headache. Symptoms develop rapidly, reach a peak intensity within 10 to 15 minutes, and last up to 2 hours. During the attack the patient is frantic with pain and may be suspected of intoxication, drug-induced behavior, or hysteria.[8] This behavior, including talk of suicide because of the severity of the pain, is characteristic;

TABLE 7.3. Pharmacologic treatment of primary headaches

Headache type	Acute attack		Prophylactic therapy	
	Dose[a]	Comment	Dose	Comment
Migraine	Ergotamines Inhalation (0.5 mg/dose) Oral, sublingual (1–2 mg) Rectal IM or IV (0.2–2.0 mg)	Many formulations and combination drugs available Side effects: nausea, vasoconstriction	β-Blockers Propranolol (40–320 mg/day) Nadolol (40–240 mg/day) Timolol (10–60 mg/day) Atenolol (50–150 mg/day)	Dosage individualized; side effects include fatigue, GI upset; contraindicated with asthma, heart failure
	Analgesics Aspirin (650–1000 mg) Acetaminophen (<1000 mg) Ibuprofen (<600 mg) Naproxen (<550 mg)	Many analgesics and NSAIDs effective Dosage individualized Combination available with sedatives and antiemetics Side effects: mainly gastric upset	Amitriptyline (10–175 mg hs)	Sedation, weight gain, dry mouth; synergistic with β-blockers
	5-HT agonist: sumatriptan Subcutaneous (6 mg) Oral (25, 50, 100 mg) Nasal spray		Phenelzine (MAOI) (30–75 mg/day)	Insomnia, hypotension; interacts with tyramine in food
			Calcium channel blockers Flunarizine (10 mg hs) Verapamil (240–480 mg/day)	Pending FDA approval; dosage individualized

		Serotonin-receptor antagonists Pizotifen (0.5–4.5 mg/day) Methysergide (4–8 mg/day)	Pending FDA approval; sedation, weight gain, cramping, vasoconstriction, fibrosis
		Valproate (500–3000 mg/day)	Many potential side effects; other anticonvulsants may be effective
Cluster	Oxygen 100% 8–10 L/min for 10 minutes Ergotamine inhaler 0.5 mg/puff × 1–3 Lidocaine 4% 0.5–1.0 ml into nostril Methoxyflurane inhaled 10 drops	Prednisone (10–80 mg/day) Lithium (300–900 mg/day) Ergotamine (1–2 mg for attacks) Indomethacin (50–200 mg/day) Nifedipine (40–120 mg/day) Verapamil (240–480 mg/day)	
Tension-stress	Analgesics and NSAIDs (as for migraine but at lower dosages)	Amitriptyline (50–100 mg hs) Imipramine (25–75 mg)	

[a]Treatment must be of rapid onset. (1) All therapy should be started at first sign of attack. (2) Other symptomatic relief may be added, especially antiemetics and sedatives. (3) Encourage patients to find abortive therapy (e.g., caffeine, exercise, cold, ± pressure over the site of pain) to use in addition to above. (4) Narcotics are rarely necessary for migraine. (5) Available formulations may vary. Suppositories containing only ergotamine are currently difficult to obtain: parenteral formulation is D.H.E. 45.

but patients may be too embarrassed to volunteer this information. The diagnosis is based on the description of attacks, especially their severity, and is confirmed by the unique time pattern described by the patient. During a "cluster" period, which typically lasts 4 to 8 weeks, the patient experiences attacks at the same time or times of day with bizarre regularity. Approximately half of these attacks awaken the patient and are particularly frequent around 1 a.m. Most patients experience one or two cluster periods per year and are completely free from symptoms at other times. About 10% of patients develop chronic symptoms, with daily attacks over several years. During a cluster period, drinking alcohol almost inevitably precipitates an attack. It is speculated that the cluster headache is due to a disorder of serotonin metabolism or circadian rhythm (or both), but the cause remains unknown.[17]

Management strategies aim to provide relief from individual attacks and prophylactically to suppress cluster episodes (Table 7.3). Acute treatment must be of rapid onset and able to be administered by the patient or family. Conventional analgesics do not act quickly enough to provide relief, and all the current treatments of acute cluster headaches are difficult to administer to a patient who is restless and distracted with pain. Inhalation of oxygen is the traditional treatment, and inhalation or instillation of local anesthetics into the nostril on the affected side may also be effective. The only ergotamines likely to be effective during the acute attack are those delivered by inhaler or injection. European studies indicate that self-administered injections of sumatriptan are effective.[24]

The mainstay of cluster headache management is to suppress headaches during a cluster period. As shown in Table 7.3, several drugs are effective. Drugs may also be used in combination (e.g., verapamil 80 mg qid with ergotamine 2 mg HS).[25] Treatment should be initiated as soon as a cluster period begins and continued for a few days beyond the expected duration of the cluster. Only the previous experience of each patient can be used to judge duration of therapy. Each patient has a set length for his or her cluster period as well as a tendency to repeat the same time and symptom pattern of individual headaches. It is particularly important in the age group usually affected by cluster headaches to monitor prophylactic drugs such as lithium, prednisone, ergotamine, indomethacin, calcium channel blockers, and methysergide for side effects.

Tension-Stress (Muscle Contraction) Headaches

Tension-stress headaches are the most frequent of all headaches.[11,17] In one study of family practice consultations, they accounted for 70% of all new headache patients.[9] These patients represent a select sample of all tension headache patients, as most sufferers are believed to manage their symptoms using simple analgesics or other strategies.[24] Although physicians are familiar with the condition, it is difficult to define it because it presents in myriad forms and is known by several names. The formal definition (Table 7.2) contains both positive and negative criteria, but a common problem is to diagnose "tension headaches" only after searching for more "interesting" etiologies for the symptoms.

The etiology and pathophysiology of tension headaches are poorly understood. Stress, psychological abnormalities, muscle contraction, and abnormalities of neurotransmitters have been implicated. The clinical syndrome may represent more than one entry, and in many cases there is considerable overlap with migraine.[17]

As with migraine, more than 70% of tension headaches occur in women, and a substantial proportion of patients (40%) give a family history of similar symptoms. Tension headaches, however, tend to have their onset at an older age (70% after 20 years) and to produce symptoms daily or on several days per week, rather than occur as episodic attacks.

The clinical picture is characterized by long periods (up to several years) of almost daily headaches that vary in intensity throughout the day. Most patients "keep going" with daily activities, but going to bed early is characteristic. The pain is described in many ways, among which "pressure," "tight band," and "aching" predominate. Patients usually express exhaustion, and the patient's affect and body language convey weariness and frustration. Sleep disturbances are common.

Physical examination may be negative or may reveal tightness and tenderness of the muscles of the occipital area, posterior neck, and shoulders. Physical examination is important to rule out secondary headache and to assist in establishing the therapeutic relationship. Attempts to treat the headaches with analgesics before establishing patient confidence in the diagnosis risk failure despite escalating use of analgesics including narcotics.

The treatment of tension headaches is frequently unsatisfactory. Success depends on treatment of any underlying condition (particularly depression), patient education about the nature of the condition, and the control of symptoms without creating dependence or other adverse effects. Tension headache patients frequently take large quantities of analgesics, leading to gastrointestinal and other complications, or they use combination medicines containing sedatives. A wise investment during the history is to clarify all medication use, including nonprescription medication, and to explore previous encounters with physicians. Patients may have already been investigated extensively, and prior medical experiences color expectations and evaluation of management approaches.

Acute episodes of headache are best managed by first-line analgesics, such as acetaminophen, aspirin, or ibuprofen. Narcotics and combination drugs, especially those that contain barbiturates or caffeine, should be avoided. NSAIDs may be more effective than other analgesics,[11] especially if prescribed on a regular schedule for several days rather than on an as-needed basis. It is useful to teach the patient and family simple massage and relaxation techniques and to explore methods to resolve conflicts and enhance self-esteem. Not all patients require extensive counseling or biofeedback. The most significant predictor of symptom resolution after 1 year has been shown to be patient confidence that the problem had been fully discussed with a physician.[9] In addition to treating underlying depression, amitriptyline and other antidepressants raise pain thresholds and play a significant role in enabling patients to manage symptoms. The effective dosage may be lower than that required for depressive illnesses.

Secondary Headaches

Headache is part of the clinical picture of many conditions. Particularly in children, frontal headache is a common accompaniment of fever. In all age groups, almost any condition of the head and neck and several systemic conditions can present as headache. A careful history combined with physical examination and other investigations where appropriate can almost always differentiate secondary from primary headache.[3]

There is particular concern in family practice not to miss the rare but serious intracranial condition, especially brain tumor. The symptoms of an intracranial lesion depend on its size, location, and displacement effect on other tissues. No single characteristic headache picture can therefore be given. Suspicion should be raised about headaches of recent onset that appear to become steadily more severe, do not fit any of the primary classifications, and do not respond to first-line treatment. Close follow-up and repeated physical examinations may detect the earliest neurologic abnormalities; but if there is a high degree of suspicion, early radiologic investigation or specialist consultation should be obtained. With intracranial vascular lesions, the first symptom may be a catastrophic hemorrhage.

Specific Headache Syndromes

The literature describes several specific primary headache syndromes that are uncommon but may be encountered in practice (e.g., cough headache) (Table 7.1). These syndromes are more common in men and are characterized by the severity of the pain and the potential for confusion with serious intracranial conditions. Despite the dramatic history, the conditions are generally benign and many respond to indomethacin.[17] CT scans may be necessary to confirm the diagnosis. Explanation, reassurance, and symptom control are usually effective.

References

1. Diamond S, Feinberg DT. The classification, diagnosis and treatment of headaches. Med Times 1990;118:15–27.
2. National Ambulatory Medical Care Survey: 1991 Summary. Hyattsville, MD: Centers for Disease Control and Prevention/National Center for Health Statistics, 1994:21. DHSS Report No. (PHS)94-177.
3. Strayhorn G. Headache. In: Sloane PD, Slatt LM, Curtis P, editors. Essentials of family medicine. 2nd ed. Baltimore: Williams & Wilkins, 1993:185–93.
4. Olesen J. Understanding the biologic basis of migraine. N Engl J Med 1994;331:1713–4.
5. Appenzeller O. Pathogenesis of migraine. Med Clin North Am 1991;75:763–89.
6. Silberstein SD. Office management of benign headache. Postgrad Med 1996;93:223–40.
7. O'Dowd TC. Five years of heartsink patients in general practice. BMJ 1988;297:528–30.
8. Graham JR. Headaches. In: Noble J, editor. Textbook of primary care medicine. 2nd ed. St. Louis: Mosby, 1996:1283–319.
9. McWhinney IR. A textbook of family medicine. New York: Oxford University Press, 1989.
10. Headache Classification Committee of the International Headache Society. Classification and diagnostic criteria for all headache disorders, cranial neuralgias and facial pain. Cephalgia 1988;8(S7):1–96.
11. Clough C. Non-migrainous headaches [editorial] BMJ 1989; 299:70–2.
12. Diamond S, Dalessio DJ, editors. The practicing physician's approach to headache. 5th ed. Baltimore: Williams & Wilkins, 1992.
13. Becker L, Iverson DC, Reed FM, et al. Patients with new headache in primary care: a report from ASPN. J Fam Pract 1988;27:41–7.
14. Prager JM, Mikulis DJ. The radiology of headache. Med Clin North Am 1991;75:525–44.
15. NIH Consensus Development Panel. Computer tomographic scanning of the brain. In: Proceedings from NIH Consensus Development Conference, NIH, Bethesda. Washington DC: Government Printing Office, 1982:4:2.
16. Silberstein SD, Lipton RB. Overview of diagnosis and treatment of migraine. Neurology 1994;44 (Suppl 7):S6–16.
17. Raskin NH. Headache. 2nd ed. New York: Churchill Livingstone, 1988.
18. Blau J. Migraine: theories of pathogenesis. Lancet 1992;339: 1202–7.
19. Smith R. Chronic headaches in family practice. J Am Board Fam Pract 1992;5:589–99.
20. Lance JW. Treatment of migraine. Lancet 1992;393:1207–9.
21. Moore KL, Noble SL. Drug treatment of migraine: Part 1. Acute therapy and drug-rebound headache. Am Fam Physic 1997;56:2045–7.
22. Cady RK, Shealy CN. Recent advances in migraine management. J Fam Pract 1993;36:85–91.
23. Tfelt-Hansen P, Henry P, Mulder LJ, et al. The effectiveness of combined oral lysine acetylsalicylate and metoclopramide compared with oral sumatriptan for migraine. Lancet 1995;346:923–6.
24. Walling AD. Cluster headaches. Am Fam Physician 1993;47: 1457–63.
25. Kudrow L. Diagnosis and treatment of cluster headache. Med Clin North Am 1991;75:579–94.

CASE PRESENTATION

Subjective

PATIENT PROFILE

Lois Nelson Martino is a 44-year-old divorced white woman who works as a paralegal.

PRESENTING PROBLEM

Headaches.

PRESENT ILLNESS

For 6 months, Lois has had headaches that occur two or three times a month. The headaches are sometimes preceded by a sense of feeling a little "mentally fuzzy," and there may be slightly blurred vision. The headache pain, which begins about 20 to 30 minutes after the onset of the initial symptoms, is severe, throbbing, and generally right-sided, although it sometimes is on the left or spreads to involve the whole head. Lois reports that nausea often accompanies the pain but that she has never vomited during a headache. When the headache is present, she is especially sensitive to noise or bright lights, and she generally retreats to a dark room for the duration of the pain, which is usually some 3 to 6 hours. The patient has used aspirin and ibuprofen (Advil) for pain, but these afford little relief. She is concerned because the headaches sometimes occur during the day and are interfering with her work.

PAST MEDICAL HISTORY

She had an appendectomy at age 16 and is the mother of one child, aged 22.

SOCIAL HISTORY

Mrs. Martino has been employed with the same law firm for 8 years. She left her previous job at the time of her divorce 10 years ago; her ex-husband, Ralph Martino, is an attorney. She lives alone in an apartment not far from the home of her daughter Ann and son-in-law Luke Priestley.

HABITS

She has never smoked and uses alcohol only rarely. She takes no daily medications. Her meals are often at irregular times, and she drinks approximately six cans of diet cola each day.

FAMILY HISTORY

Her father, aged 76, has osteoarthritis and type 2 diabetes mellitus. Her mother, aged 71, has hypertension and sometimes takes medication for depression. She has three siblings.

REVIEW OF SYSTEMS

The patient believes that she sometimes feels excessively tired at the end of the day and sometimes awakes in the middle of the night and has trouble getting back to sleep.

- What more do you wish to know about the patient's headaches?
- How would you inquire to learn more about events in her personal life and at work?
- What else would you ask about the family history? Why?
- Are you listening carefully to what the patient is trying to tell you?

Objective

GENERAL

Mrs. Martino seems slightly anxious. She uses notes and a calendar while describing her symptoms.

VITAL SIGNS

Height, 5 ft 6 in; weight, 133 lb; blood pressure, 126/82; pulse, 74; temperature, 37.1°C.

EXAMINATION

The eyes, ears, nose, and throat are normal, including an unremarkable funduscopic examination. There are no abnormalities of the neck and thyroid. Cranial nerves II to XII are normal. The finger-to-nose test, deep tendon reflexes, and Romberg test are all normal.

LABORATORY

No office laboratory tests are performed at this visit.

- What more—if anything—would you include in the physical examination, and why?
- What additional neurologic tests might be useful?
- What laboratory tests—if any—might be helpful?
- What diagnostic imaging—if any—might be important and cost-effective?

Assessment

- What appears to be Mrs. Martino's problem, and how would you explain it to her?
- What do you think is the patient's chief concern about her headaches? Explain.
- How are her headaches likely to be affecting her life at home and at work?
- What is the possible significance of her tiredness and sleep disturbance?

Plan

- What medical therapy would you recommend today? Why did you choose this regimen?
- What diet and life-style changes would you advise?
- How might you help Mrs. Martino deal with the impact of the headaches on her work?
- If the headaches become more severe or more frequent over the next few months, what would you do then?

8

Hypertension

STEPHEN A. BRUNTON AND RITA K. EDWARDS

Despite widespread efforts to improve education and enhance public awareness, up to 33% of persons with hypertension remain undiagnosed, and only about 50% of those known to have hypertension are adequately controlled. The percentages of patients who are aware that they have hypertension, who are treated, and who are controlled have increased since the 1970s (Table 8.1). Most have stage 1 hypertension, and controversy still exists concerning the appropriate approach to these patients. Nonpharmacologic therapy is often the first choice, and this approach continues to evolve.[1] Of the 20 million to 30 million hypertensives who receive pharmacologic therapy, fewer than 50% adhere to their therapeutic regimen for more than 1 year, and 60% of these patients reduce the dosage of their drug owing to adverse effects. A negative impact on the patient's quality of life may occur as a result of just making the diagnosis. Effects such as increased absenteeism, sickness behavior, hypochondria, and decreased self-esteem have been noted in cohorts of previously well individuals who have been told they were hypertensive.[2] A 1987 survey of physicians revealed that they regarded quality of life changes to be the primary impediment to effective pharmacologic treatment of hypertension.

The challenge to the clinician is to provide patient education and develop a hypertensive regimen that effectively lowers blood pressure or reduces cardiac risk factors, minimizes changes in concomitant disease states, and maintains or improves quality of life. Putting the patient first necessitates integrating the individual patient's life style and current disease states with a thorough understanding of the effect of drug and nondrug therapy on quality of life. This chapter reviews nonpharmacologic and pharmacologic therapy, with special emphasis on individualizing patient regimens to improve adherence.

The assistance of Janet Pick, Pharm. D., with Table 8.1 is gratefully acknowledged.

TABLE 8.1. Hypertension[a] awareness, treatment, and control rates

Factor	1971–1972[b]	1974–1975[b]	1976–1980[c]	1988–1991[d]	1991–1994[e]
Aware: percent of hypertensives told by physician	51	64	(54) 73	(65) 84	(68.4%)
Treated: percent of hypertensives taking medication	36	34	(33) 56	(49) 73	(53.6%)
Controlled: percent of hypertensives with blood pressure < 160/95 mm Hg on one occasion and reported currently taking antihypertensive medication	16	20	(11) 34	(21) 55	(27.4%)

Source: National Institutes of Health.[1,3]
[a]Defined as 160/95 mm Hg or more on one occasion or reported currently taking antihypertensive medication. Numbers in parentheses are percents at 140/90 mm Hg or more.
[b]*Source:* National Health and Nutrition Examination Survey I.
[c]*Source:* National Health and Nutrition Examinaton Survey II.
[d]*Source:* National Health and Nutrition Examination Survey III (phase 1).
[e]*Source:* National Health and Nutrition Examination Survey III (phase 2).

Detection

The diagnosis of hypertension should not be based on any single measurement but should be established on the basis of at least three readings with an average systolic blood pressure of 140 mm Hg and a diastolic pressure of 90 mm Hg. Mechanisms should be established to standardize the measurement process: (1) The patient should be seated comfortably with the arm positioned at heart level. (2) Caffeine or nicotine should not have been ingested within 30 minutes before measurement. (3) The patient should be seated in a quiet environment for at least 5 minutes. (4) An appropriate sphygmomanometer cuff should be used (i.e., the rubber bladder should encircle at least two-thirds of the arm). (5) Measurement of the diastolic blood pressure should be based on the disappearance of sound (phase V Korotkoff sound). Table 8.2 describes the classification of blood pressure for adults.

Evaluation

Evaluation is directed toward establishing the etiology of hypertension, identifying other cardiovascular risk factors, and evaluating the possibility of target organ damage. Although most hypertension is considered "essential," primary, or idiopathic, it is necessary to eliminate secondary causes of hypertension, including renovascular disease, polycystic renal disease, aortic coarctation, Cushing syndrome, and pheochromocytoma. It is important to ensure that the patient is not on medications that may result in increased

TABLE 8.2. Classification of blood pressure for adults aged 18 years and older[a]

Category	Systolic (mm Hg)	Diastolic (mm Hg)
Optimal[b]	< 120	< 80
Normal[b]	< 130	< 85
High normal	130–139	85–89
Hypertension[c]		
Stage 1 (mild)	140–159	90–99
Stage 2 (moderate)	160–179	100–109
Stage 3 (severe)	≥ 180	≥ 110

Source: National Institutes of Health.[1]

Note: In addition to classifying stages of hypertension based on average blood pressure levels, the clinician should specify the presence or absence of target organ disease and additional risk factors. For example, a patient with diabetes, a blood pressure of 142/94 mm Hg, and left ventricular hypertrophy should be classified as "stage 1 hypertension with target organ disease (left ventricular hypertrophy) and with another major risk factor (diabetes)." This specificity is important for risk classification and management.

[a]Not taking antihypertensive drugs and not acutely ill. When systolic and diastolic pressures fall into different categories, the higher category should be selected to classify the individual's blood pressure status. For instance, 160/92 mm Hg should be classified as stage 2 and 180/120 mm Hg as stage 3. Isolated systolic hypertension is defined as systolic pressure of 140 mm Hg or more and diastolic pressure of less than 90 mm Hg and staged appropriately (e.g., 170/85 mm Hg is defined as stage 2 isolated systolic hypertension).

[b]Optimal blood pressure with respect to cardiovascular risk is systolic pressure < 120 mm Hg and diastolic pressure < 80 mm Hg. However, unusually low readings should be evaluated for clinical significance.

[c]Based on the average of two or more readings taken at each of two or more visits after an initial screening.

blood pressure, such as oral contraceptives, nasal decongestants, appetite suppressants, nonsteroidal antiinflammatory drugs (NSAIDs), steroids, and tricyclic antidepressants.

Medical History

The medical history should include a review of the family history for hypertension and cardiovascular disease, previous measurements of blood pressure, symptoms suggestive of secondary causes of hypertension, and other cardiovascular risk factors including smoking, hyperlipidemia, obesity, and diabetes. Environmental and psychosocial factors that may influence blood pressure control or the ability of the individual to comply with therapy should also be considered.

Physical Examination and Laboratory Tests

The physical examination should include more than one blood pressure measurement in both standing and seated positions with verification in the contralateral arm. (If a discrepancy exists, the higher value is used.) The rest of the physical examination includes (1) an evaluation of the optic fundi with gradation of hypertensive changes; (2) examination of the neck for bruits and thyromegaly; (3) a heart examination to evaluate for hypertrophy, arrhythmias, or additional sounds; (4) abdominal examination to search for evidence of aneurysms or kidney abnormalities; (5) examination of the extremities to check the pulses; and (6) a careful neurologic evaluation.

Some baseline laboratory tests may be helpful for the initial evaluation. They might include urinalysis and serum potassium, blood urea nitrogen, and creatinine levels. A lipid panel may help evaluate cardiovascular risk.

Treatment

The goal of therapy is not just to bring the blood pressure lower than 140 mm Hg systolic and 90 mm Hg diastolic but, rather, to prevent the morbidity and mortality associated with hypertension. As such, the decision to treat hypertension is based on documentation that blood pressure has remained elevated and assessment of the risk for that particular patient.

In general, individuals with diastolic blood pressure ranges considered borderline high (i.e., 85–89 mm Hg) should have their blood pressures rechecked within 1 year. Blood pressures in the mild range should be confirmed within 2 months by repeated measurements; however, certain life-style approaches are appropriate even at this level. Blood pressures that are markedly elevated (e.g., 115 mm Hg) or those associated with evidence of existing end-organ damage may require immediate pharmacologic intervention. In general, whether pharmacologic intervention is initiated, a nonpharmacologic approach is the foundation of any management strategy.[1]

Nonpharmacologic Therapeutic Approaches

Information concerning dietary modifications, exercise, weight reduction, the role of cations, and the possible role of relaxation and stress management techniques for reducing blood pressure have opened the door for greater acceptance of multiple nonpharmacologic approaches to the treatment of hypertension. The report of the Joint National Committee (JNC) on the Detection, Evaluation, and Treatment of High Blood Pressure recommended that "Nonpharmacological approaches be used both as definitive intervention and as an adjunct for pharmacological therapy and should be considered for all antihypertensive therapy."[1,3]

Several studies have shown positive correlation of increased blood pressure with alcohol consumption of more than 2 ounces/day.[4] Although smoking has not been shown to cause sustained hypertension, it is associated with increased cardiovascular, pulmonary, and hypertension risks and therefore should be eliminated.[5]

Weight reduction has a strong correlation with decreased blood pressure in obese individuals. Stamler et al. reported that a 10-pound weight loss maintained over a 4-year period allowed 50% of participants previously on pharmacologic management to remain normotensive and free of medication.[6]

Sodium restriction has been a mainstay of hypertension control, as a 100-mEq drop in daily intake can result in a 2 to 9 mm Hg decline in systolic blood pressure in salt-sensitive individuals. This goal is one of the easiest for a patient to accomplish, as moderate restriction can be accomplished by eliminating table salt for cooking, avoiding salty foods, and using a salt substitute.[7]

Regular aerobic exercise not only assists with weight reduction but also appears to lower diastolic blood pressure. Cade and associates reported a decline from 117 mm Hg to 97 mm Hg diastolic blood pressure after 3 months of daily walking or running for 2 miles. This effect appeared to be independent of weight loss, and some benefit persisted even if the patient became sedentary.[8]

Vegetarian diets high in polyunsaturated fats, potassium, and fiber result in lower blood pressures than diets high in saturated fats. Dietary fat control also contributes to the reduction of cholesterol and coronary artery disease risk.[9] The role of cations such as potassium, magnesium, and calcium in lowering blood pressure has now been investigated. High potassium intake (> 80 mEq/day) may result in a modest decline in blood pressure while offering a natriuretic and cardioprotective effect. These effects are more pronounced in hypokalemic individuals.[10] Magnesium and calcium supplementation of more than 300 mg/day and 800 mg/day, respectively, have been shown to lower the relative risk of developing hypertension in a large cohort of women. The impact of individual supplementation is less clear, and the role of these substances is still controversial.[11]

Stress management and relaxation techniques over a 4-year period have been shown to reduce systolic blood pressure 10 to 15 mm Hg and diastolic blood pressure 5 to 10 mm Hg. However, these results are variable and are largely dependent on the instructor–patient relationship.[12]

The effects of nonpharmacologic approaches can be additive and certainly are beneficial even if the patient requires drug therapy. Stamler and associates documented that reducing weight and lowering salt and alcohol intake allowed 39% of patients previously on therapy to remain normotensive without medication over a 4-year period. In the mildly hypertensive individual, these life-style modifications should be tried for at least 6 months before initiating pharmacologic therapy.[13]

Pharmacologic Therapy

Pharmacologic therapy is considered when the diastolic blood pressure remains higher than 90 to 94 mm Hg despite life-style modifications. The decision to initiate drug therapy requires consideration of individual patient characteristics, such as age, race, sex, family history, cardiovascular risk factors, concomitant disease states, compliance, and ability to purchase the prescribed therapeutic agent. Treatment of moderate to severe hypertension (diastolic pressure > 104 mm Hg) has reduced cardiovascular morbidity and mortality dramatically since the 1960s. Some controversy still exists regarding the appropriate treatment of stage 1 hypertension [diastolic blood pressure (DBP) 90–99 mm Hg] because of adverse drug reactions compromising quality of life, the cost of therapy, and little change in coronary heart disease morbidity and mortality. The incidence of stroke, congestive heart failure, and left ventricular hypertrophy has decreased among treated mild hypertensives, and therapy is recommended if the patient has one or more cardiovascular risk factors.

The ideal antihypertensive agent would improve quality of life, reduce coronary heart disease risk factors, maintain normal hemodynamic profiles, reduce left ventricular hypertrophy, have a positive impact on concomitant disease states, and reduce end-organ damage while effectively lowering blood pressure on a convenient dosing regimen at minimal cost to the patient. This "magic bullet" has yet to be synthesized, although several of the newer antihypertensive classes offer the possibility of many of these positive outcomes.

The selection of an appropriate antihypertensive agent may be based on the current recommendations of the Joint National Committee (JNC) on the Detection, Evaluation and Treatment of High Blood Pressure or individualized to the specific medical, social, psychological, and economic situation of each patient.[1,3] The previous stepped-care approach has been modified by the JNC into an algorithm that permits an individualized approach to the patient (Fig. 8.1). Many clinicians have moved away from the stepped-care philosophy toward a monotherapy approach, which maximizes the dose of one drug before substituting or adding another. Combination therapy with lower doses of several agents may also be utilized to minimize adverse effects. Therapeutic choices must be based on a sound understanding of the mechanism of action, pharmacokinetics, adverse effect profile, and cost of available agents.

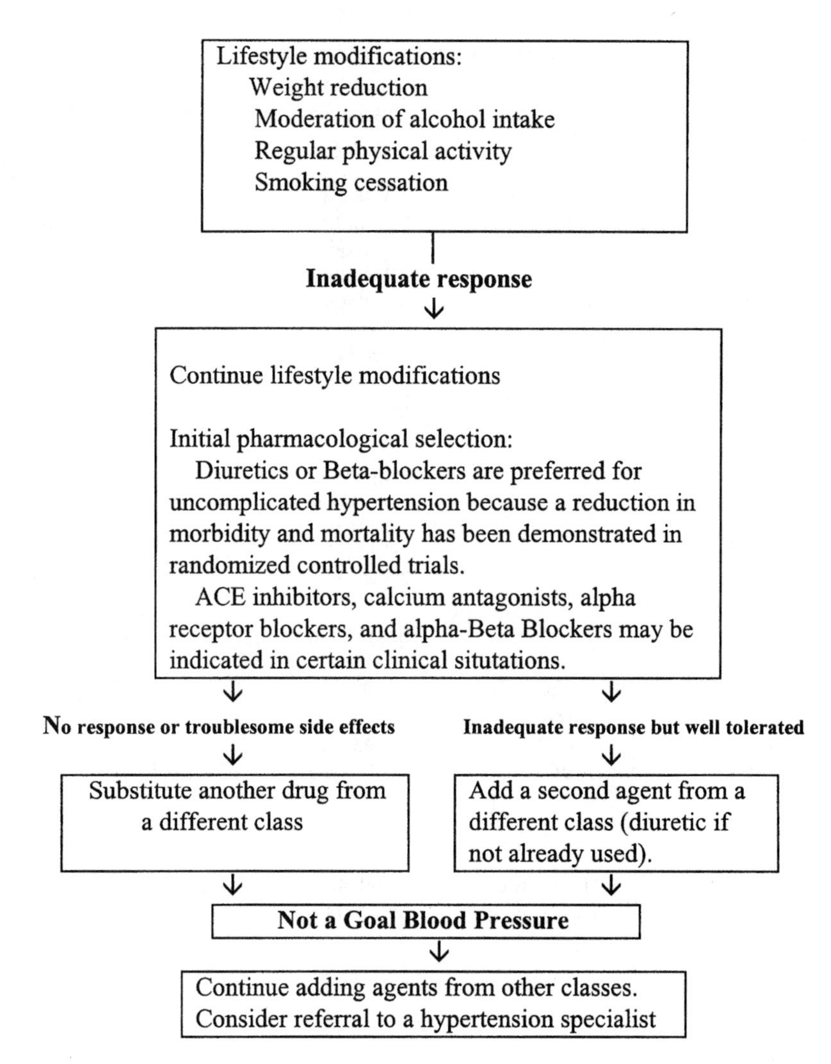

FIGURE 8.1. Treatment algorithm. (Adapted from National Institutes of Health.[1,3])

Major Antihypertensive Classes

ACE Inhibitors

Angiotensin-converting enzyme (ACE) inhibitors (Table 8.3) block the conversion of angiotensin I to angiotensin II, resulting in decreased aldosterone production with subsequent increased sodium and water excretion. Renin and potassium levels are usually increased as a result of

TABLE 8.3. Antihypertensive drugs

Drug class	Available doses (mg)	Usual dose/schedule (mg/day)	Half-life (hours)	Peak (hours)	Pregnancy class
ACE inhibitors					
Benazepril (Lotensin)	5, 10, 20, 40	10–40 qd	10	2–4	X
Captopril (Capoten)	12.5, 25, 50, 100	25–50 bid–tid	2	1–2	X
Enalapril (Vasotec)	2.5, 5, 10, 20	5–40 qd	11	4	X
Fosinopril (Monopril)	10, 20	10–40 qd	12	2–6	X
Lisinopril (Prinivil, Zestril)	2.5, 5, 10, 20, 40	10–40 qd	12	6	X
Moexipril (Univasc)	7.5, 15	7.5–30 qd	2–10	1.5	X
Quinapril (Accupril)	5, 10, 20, 40	10–80 qd	2	2–4	X
Rampril (Altace)	1.25, 2.5, 5, 10	2.5–20 qd	2	3–6	X
β-Blockers					
Atenolol (Tenormin)	25, 50, 100	50–100 qd	9	B_1	C
Acebutolol (Sectral)	200, 400	400–800 qd	4	B_1, ISA	B
Betaxolol (Kerlone)	10, 20	10–20 qd	22	B_1	C
Bisoprolol (Zebeta)	5, 10	5–20 qd	11	B_1	C
Carteolol (Cartrol)	2.5, 5	2.5–10 qd	6	B_1, B_2, ISA	C
Labetolol (Normodyne)	100, 200, 300	100–400 bid	6	B_1, B_2, α	C
Nadolol (Corgard)	20, 40, 80, 120, 160	40–80 qd	24	B_1, B_2	C
Metoprolol (Lopressor)	50, 100	100–450 qd	3	B_1	C
Penbutolol (Levatol)	20	20–80 qd	5	B_1, B_2, ISA	C
Pindolol (Visken)	5, 10	10–30 qd	4	B_1, B_2, ISA	B
Propranolol (Inderal)	SR 60, 80, 120, 160; 10, 20, 40, 60, 80, 90	80–160 SR qd	10	B_1, B_2	C
		20–120 bid	4	B_1, B_2	C
Timolol (Blocadren)	5, 10, 20	10–30 bid	4	B_1, B_2	C
Calcium entry antagonists					
Amlodipine (Norvasc)	2.5, 5, 10	2.5–10		6–12	C
Diltiazem (Cardizem)	SR 60, 90, 120	SR 60–120 bid		6–11	C
	CD 120, 180, 240, 300	CD 180–360 qd	6	12	
	30, 60, 90, 120	30–90 qid		2–3	
(Dilacor XR)	120, 180, 240	120–360 qd	4	4–6	C
Felodipine (Plendil)	SR 2.5, 5, 10	5–20 qd	16	2–5	C
Isradipine (Dynacirc)	2.5, 5	2.5–5 bid	8	1.5	C
Nicardipine (Cardene)	SR 30, 45, 60	SR 30–60 bid			
	20, 30	20–40 tid	4	0.5–2	C
Nifedipine (Procardia)	SR 10, 20, 30, 60, 90	30–120 qd	5	0.5–6	C
Nisoldipine (Sular)	10, 20, 30, 40	20–40 qd	10	6–12	C

TABLE 8.3. (*continued*)

Drug class	Available doses (mg)	Usual dose/schedule (mg/day)	Half-life (hours)	Peak (hours)	Pregnancy class
Verapamil (Calan, Isoptin)	SR 120, 180, 240 40, 80, 120	240–480 qd	7	1–2	C
Mibefradil (Posicor)	50, 100	50–100 qd,	17–25	1.2–1.7	C
α_1-Blockers					
Doxazosin (Cardura)	1, 2, 4, 8	1–16 mg qd	22	2–3	B
Prazosin (Minipress)	1, 2, 5	1–5 bid–tid	3	3	C
Terazosin (Hytrin)	1, 2, 5, 10	1–10 qd	12	1–2	C
Central α_2-agonists					
Clonidine (Catapres)	0.1, 0.2, 0.3 TTS 1, 2, 3	0.2–1.2 qd 1 patch weekly	16 19	3–5 2–3 days	C
Guanabenz (Wytensin)	4, 8	4–8 bid	6	2–4	C
Guanfacine (Tenex)	1, 2	1–3 qd	17	3	B
Methyldopa (Aldomet)	125, 250, 500	250–500 tid–qid	2	2–4	B
Vasodilators					
Hydralazine (Apresoline)	10, 25, 50, 100	10–50 qid	7	0.5–2	C
Minoxidil (Loniten)	2.5, 10	10–40 qd	4	2–3	C
αβ-Blockers					
Carvedilol (Coreg)	6.25, 12.5, 25	6.25–12.5 bid	7	3–4	C
Labetolol (Normodyne)	100, 200, 300	100 mg–400 bid	6	2–4	C
Selected thiazide diuretics					
Chlorothiazide (Diuril)	250–500	500–2000 qd	6–12	4	
Hydrochlorothiazide (Hydrodiuril)	25, 50, 100	25–50 qd	6–12	4–6	
Chlorthalidone (Hygroton)	25, 50, 100	25–100 qd	24–72	2–6	
Indapamide (Lozol)	1.25, 2.5	2.5–5 qd	36	2	B
Metolazone (Zaroxolyn)	0.5, 2.5, 5, 10	2.5–5 qd	12–24	2.6	B
Loop diuretics					
Bumetanide (Bumex)	0.5, 1, 2	0.5–2 qd	4–6	1–2	C
Furosemide (Lasix)	20, 40, 80	20–40 qd–bid	6–8	1–2	C
Potassium-sparing diuretics					
Amiloride (Midamor)	5	5–20 qd	24	6–10	B
Spironolactone (Aldactone)	25, 50, 100	25–100 qd	48–72	48–72	X
Triamterene (Dyrenium)	50, 100	100 bid	12–16	6–8	B

TABLE 8.3. (*continued*)

Drug class	Available doses (mg)	Usual dose/schedule (mg/day)	Half-life (hours)	Peak (hours)	Pregnancy class
Angiotensin receptor antagonists					
Losartan (Cozaar)	25, 50	25–100 qd	2–9	1–4	X
Valsartan (Diovan)	80, 160	80–320 qd	6	2–4	X
Irbesartan (Avapro)	75, 150, 300	75–300 qd	11–15	1.5–2	X

ISA = Intrinsic sympathomimetic activity. X = Fetal abnormalities may occur. Use contraindicated in pregnancy. C = Fetal risk documented in animals. B = Low fetal risk. SR = Slow release. CD = Controlled delivery.

this medication. The hemodynamic response includes decreased peripheral resistance, increased renal blood flow, and minimal changes in cardiac output and glomerular filtration rate. There is little change in insulin and glucose levels or in the lipid fractions. The adverse effects of ACE inhibitors include cough (1–30%), headache, dizziness, first-dose syncope in salt- or volume-depleted patients, acute renal failure in patients with renal artery stenosis, angioedema (0.1–0.2%), and teratogenic effects in the human fetus. Captopril (Capoten) has a higher incidence of rash, dysgeusia, neutropenia, and proteinuria than others due to a sulfhydryl group in the ring structure.[14]

The ACE inhibitors are good first-line agents for patients with diabetes, congestive heart failure, peripheral vascular disease, elevated lipids, and renal insufficiency. This class is effective in all races and ages, although black patients respond better with addition of a diuretic.[15,16]

Angiotensin Receptor Antagonists

Angiotensin receptor antagonists, a new class of antihypertensive agents, binds to the angiotensin II receptors, resulting in blockade of the vasoconstrictor and aldosterone-secreting effects of angiotensin II. In addition, bradykinin production is not stimulated. The first agent available in the United States was losartan (Cozaar). The physiologic effects of losartan include a rise in plasma renin and angiotensin II levels and a decrease in aldosterone production. There is no significant change in plasma potassium levels and no effect on glomerular filtration rate, renal plasma flow, heart rate, triglycerides, total cholesterol, high density lipoprotein (HDL) cholesterol, or glucose. Losartan use does produce a small uricosuric effect with lowering of plasma uric acid levels.

Losartan and valsartan (Diovan) are effective antihypertensives in adults and the elderly. Blood pressure-lowering effects are not as significant in black patients. Adverse effects include muscle pain, dizziness, cough, insomnia, and nasal congestion. As with ACE inhibitors, these drugs should not be used during pregnancy.

At this time the role of angiotensin receptor antagonists is not completely defined. Further study of the hemodynamic effects in large populations is needed to determine the role in cardiac patients. Losartan is an alternative antihypertensive agent for patients experiencing adverse effects from ACE inhibitors.[17]

Calcium Entry Antagonists

Calcium entry antagonists (CEAs) inhibit the movement of calcium across cell membranes in myocardial and smooth muscles. This action not only dilates coronary arteries but additional peripheral arteriole dilation reduces total peripheral resistance, resulting in decreased blood pressure. Although the mechanism of action for lowering blood pressure is similar for these agents, structural differences result in varying effects on cardiac conduction and adverse effect profiles. Verapamil (Calan, Isoptin) and diltiazem (Cardizem) slow atrioventricular (AV) node conduction and prolong the effective refractory period in the AV node. Cardiac output is increased by nifedipine (Procardia), nicardipine (Cardene), isradipine (Dynacirc), and felodipine (Plendil).

The calcium entry antagonists are contraindicated in patients with heart block, cardiogenic shock, or acute myocardial infarction. Common adverse effects include peripheral edema, dizziness, headache, asthenia, nausea, constipation, flushing, and tachycardia. Calcium entry antagonists have no significant impact on lipid profiles or glucose metabolism.[1]

These agents are effective at all ages and in all races. They are good choices for patients with diabetes, angina, migraine, chronic obstructive pulmonary disease (COPD)/asthma, peripheral vascular disease, renal insufficiency, and supraventricular arrhythmias.[15,16]

Diuretics

Thiazide, loop, and potassium-sparing diuretics have been the mainstay of antihypertensive therapy since the 1960s. They remain as first-line agents in the JNC V approach, although the ACE inhibitors and calcium entry antagonists are rapidly replacing diuretics as monotherapy for hypertension.

Thiazide diuretics increase renal excretion of sodium and chloride at the distal segment of the renal tubule, resulting in decreased plasma volume, cardiac output, and renal blood flow and increased renin activity. Potassium excretion is increased, and calcium and uric acid elimination is decreased.[14] Thiazides adversely affect lipid metabolism by increasing the total cholesterol level 6% to 10%, the low density lipoprotein (LDL) cholesterol 6% to 20%, and causing a possible 15% to 20% rise in triglycerides.[16] Plasma glucose levels increase secondary to a decrease in insulin secretion. Clinical adverse effects include nausea, vomiting, diarrhea, dizziness, headache, fatigue, muscle cramps, gout attacks, and impotence. Thiazides are inexpensive choices for initial therapy, but caution must be exercised in patients with preexisting cardiac dysfunction, lipid abnormalities, diabetes mellitus, and gout. The lowest effective dose is recommended to minimize these potential adverse effects. Suggested daily doses are hydrochlorothiazide (Hydrodiuril) 25 mg, chlorthalidone (Hygroton) 500 mg, and indapamide (Lozol) 2.5 mg daily. Indapamide is unique among thiazides in that it has minimal effects on glucose, lipids, and uric acid. Thiazides are good choices for volume/salt-dependent, low-renin hypertensives. Thiazides improve blood pressure control when added to ACE inhibitors, β-blockers, vasodilators, and α-blockers.

The loop diuretics—furosemide (Lasix), torsemide (Demadex), and bumetanide (Bumex)—inhibit sodium and chloride reabsorption in the proximal and distal tubules and the loop of Henle. These diuretics are effective in patients with decreased renal function. The primary adverse effects include ototoxicity with high doses in patients with severe renal disease and in combination with an aminoglycoside, photosensitivity, excess potassium loss, increased serum uric acid, decreased calcium levels, and impaired glucose metabolism. Patients may experience nausea, vomiting, diarrhea, headache, blurred vision, tinnitus, muscle cramps, fatigue, or weakness. Furosemide and bumetanide are utilized in patients with compromised renal function or congestive heart failure (CHF) and as adjuncts to volume-retaining agents such as hydralazine (Apresoline) and minoxidil (Loniten).

The potassium-sparing diuretics spironolactone (Aldactone), triamterene (Dyrenium), and amiloride (Midamor) are useful for preventing potassium wastage from thiazide and loop diuretics. Spironolactone competitively inhibits the uptake of aldosterone at the receptor site in the distal tubule, thereby reducing aldosterone effects. It is used for treatment of primary aldosteronism, CHF, cirrhosis with ascites, hypertension, and hirsutism. Triamterene is used in combination with hydrochlorothiazide as Dyazide or Maxzide and effectively prevents potassium loss. Amiloride inhibits potassium excretion at the collecting duct. Adverse reactions associated with spironolactone include gynecomastia, nausea, vomiting, diarrhea, muscle cramps, lethargy, and hyperkalemia. Triamterene and amiloride have adverse effects similar to those seen with the thiazide diuretics.[14–16]

Antiadrenergic Agents

β-BLOCKERS

β-Adrenergic blocking agents compete with β-agonists for B_1 receptors in cardiac muscles and B_2 receptors in the bronchial and vascular musculature, inhibiting the dilator, inotropic, and chronotropic effects of β-adrenergic stimulation. Clinical responses to β-adrenergic blockade include decreased heart rate, cardiac output, blood pressure, renin production, and bronchiolar constriction; there is also an initial increase in total peripheral resistance, which returns to normal with chronic use.

β-Blockers are contraindicated for sinus bradycardia, second or third degree heart block, cardiogenic shock, cardiac failure, and severe COPD/asthma. The adverse effect profile of β-blocking agents is partially dependent on their receptor selectivity (Table 8.3). Acebutolol (Sectral), penbutolol (Levatol), carteolol (Cartrol), and pindolol (Visken) have intrinsic sympathomimetic activity (ISA), resulting in less effect on cardiac output and lipid profiles. β-Blockers without ISA slow the heart rate, decrease cardiac output, increase peripheral vascular resistance, and cause bronchospasm. Common adverse effects include fatigue, impotence, depression, shortness of breath, cold extremities, cough, drowsiness, and dizziness. The more lipid-soluble agents, such as propranolol and metoprolol, have a higher incidence of central nervous system (CNS) effects. In diabetic patients β-blockers may mask the usual symptoms of hypoglycemia, such as tremor, tachycardia, and hunger.[14] Increased triglycerides (30%) and decreased HDL cholesterol (1–20%) occur with non-ISA agents.[16] β-Blockers are effective agents in the young and white populations. Black patients may not respond as well to monotherapy because of their lower renin levels. β-Blockers are good choices for patients with supraventricular tachycardia, high cardiac output, angina, recent myocardial infarction, migraine, and glaucoma. Caution should be exercised in those with diabetes, CHF, peripheral vascular disease, COPD/asthma, and an elevated lipid profile.[15]

Central Acting Drugs

Methyldopa (Aldomet), clonidine (Catapres), guanfacine (Tenex), and guanabenz (Wytensin) are central α_2-agonists. These agents decrease dopamine and norepinephrine production in the brain, resulting in a decrease in sympathetic nervous activity throughout the body. Blood pressure declines with the decrease in peripheral resistance. Methyldopa exhibits a unique adverse effect profile as it induces autoimmune disorders, such as those with positive Coombs and antinuclear antibody (ANA) tests, hemolytic anemia, and hepatic necrosis. The other agents produce sedation, dry mouth, and dizziness. Abrupt clonidine withdrawal may result in rebound hypertension. These drugs are good choices for patients with asthma, diabetes, high cholesterol, and peripheral vascular disease.

Peripheral Acting Drugs

Guanadrel (Hylorel), reserpine (Serpasil), and guanethidine (Ismelin) are peripheral antiadrenergic agents. Their mechanism of action is at the storage granule level of norepinephrine release. They are infrequently chosen because of their significant side effects, which include profound hypotension, sedation, depression, and impotence.

α_1-BLOCKERS

α_1-Receptor blockers have an affinity for the α_1-receptor on vascular smooth muscles, thereby blocking the uptake of catecholamines by smooth muscle cells. This action results in peripheral vasodilation. The currently available agents are prazosin (Minipress), terazosin (Hytrin), and doxazosin (Cardura). There is a marked reduction in blood pressure with the first dose of these drugs. It is recommended that they be started with 1 mg at bedtime and titrated slowly upward over 2 to 4 weeks. When adding a second antihypertensive, the α-blocker dose should be decreased and titrated upward again. Often a diuretic is added to α_1-blocker therapy to reduce sodium and water retention. The primary adverse effects of these three drugs are dizziness, sedation, nasal congestion, headache, and postural effects. They do not significantly affect lipids, glucose, electrolytes, or exercise tolerance. α_1-Blockers are good choices for young, active adults and patients with diabetes, renal insufficiency, CHF, peripheral vascular disease, COPD/ asthma, or elevated lipids.

Vasodilators

The two direct vasodilators, hydralazine (Apresoline) and minoxidil (Loniten), dilate peripheral arterioles, resulting in a significant fall in blood pressure. A sympathetic reflex increase in heart rate, renin and catecholamine release, and venous constriction occur. The renal response includes sodium and water retention. The patient often experiences tachycardia, flushing, and headache. Addition of a diuretic and a β-blocker relieves the major adverse effects of the vasodilators. Hydralazine may cause a lupus-like reaction with fever, rash, and joint pain. Chronic use of minoxidil often results in hirsutism, with increased facial and arm hair. These drugs are third or fourth line agents because of their adverse side effect profile.[14–16]

Quality of Life Issues

The need for life style changes and probable drug therapy increases the possibility that the patient's quality of life will be altered. The adverse physical, mental, and metabolic effects of antihypertensive therapy results in significant nonadherence to prescribed regimens. In 1982 Jachuck and associates investigated the effect of medications on their patients by asking the patient, their closest relatives, and their physicians a series of questions concerning their quality of life since starting the blood pressure medications. The physicians and patients thought there was either no change or improvement, whereas 99% of the relatives thought the patients were worse. They cited side effects such as memory loss, irritability, decreased libido, hypochondria, and decreased energy as major problems.[18] Other studies during the 1980s confirm that nonselective β-blockers, diuretics, and methyldopa compromised quality of life to a far greater extent than ACE inhibitors or calcium entry antagonists.[18–20] Further research in this area is necessary to assist the physician in determining the optimum strategy for blood pressure control to improve adherence and quality of life.

Antihypertensive Selection

It is important to consider the patient's life style, economic status, belief systems, and concerns about treatment when selecting an antihypertensive agent. Therapy should be initiated with one drug in small doses to minimize adverse effects. It is important to educate the patient about the long-term benefits of therapy, including the decreased incidence of stroke and renal and cardiac disease. Adequate follow-up visits are scheduled to assess adherence and adverse effects. During these visits the patient is asked to describe the mental, physical, and emotional changes that have occurred as a result of therapy. If adverse effects are bothersome, consider an alternative selection from a different drug class and attempt to maintain monotherapy. If a second drug is needed, agents can be combined that improve efficacy without significantly altering the adverse effect profile (e.g., adding a diuretic to an ACE inhibitor).

There are some special considerations when prescribing medications. Concomitant disease states must be considered and drugs selected that either improve or at least maintain the current clinical condition. Hypertension is a major risk factor for thrombotic and hemorrhagic strokes; smoking, CHF, diabetes, and coronary artery disease increase the risk. Patients with coronary artery disease may benefit from a calcium entry antagonist or β-blocker with ISA to decrease anginal pain while resulting in minimal changes in lipid profiles. CHF and hypertension respond well to ACE inhibitors and diuretic therapy. Diabetes may be adversely affected by thiazide diuretics and β-blockers. ACE inhibitors, calcium entry antagonists, and central α_2-agonists are appropriate choices.

Patients with severe renal disease are most effectively treated with loop diuretics, whereas ACE inhibitors and CEAs may decrease proteinuria and slow the progress of renal failure. As renal function declines, ACE inhibitors must be used with some caution as increased potassium and decreased renal perfusion may occur. A few agents such as methyldopa, clonidine, atenolol, nadolol, and captopril need dosage reduction in the presence of renal failure.

Asthma and COPD patients may be effectively treated with calcium entry antagonists, central α_2-agonists, and α_1-blockers. β-Blockers and possibly diuretics should be avoided because they might exacerbate bronchospasm.

The elderly are of special concern when selecting an antihypertensive. They have decreased receptor sensitivity, changing baroreceptor response, atherosclerosis, decreased myocardial function, declining total body water, decreased renal function, and memory loss. Blood pressure should be lowered cautiously using smaller than normal doses that are slowly titrated upward. Calcium entry antagonists, ACE inhibitors, and diuretics are possible choices for the elderly. β-Blockers are effective in the elderly especially in conjunction with diuretics. Larger doses may result in declining mental function, depression, fatigue, and impotence. α_1-Blockers and central α_2-agonists may be used with caution. First-dose syncope and sedation are the major concerns.

Black patients may not respond as well to ACE inhibitors or β-blockers as other races, perhaps due in part to low renin, salt/volume-dependent hypertension. Thiazide diuretics may adversely affect diabetes, gout, and lipids. Calcium entry antagonists, α_1-blockers, central α_2-agonists, and ACE inhibitors are possible choices.

Young women with hyperdynamic hypertension may respond best to a β-blocker to slow the heart rate and relieve symptoms of stress. An active young man would be better served with an ACE inhibitor, calcium entry antagonist, or α-blocker, as β-blockers and diuretics may cause impotence and exercise intolerance.[15]

Severe Hypertension and Emergencies

Patients with a DBP over 115 mm Hg must be treated upon diagnosis. The blood pressure should be lowered in 5 to 10 mm Hg increments with a goal of lowering it to less than 100 mm Hg after several weeks of therapy. Often more than one drug must be used initially to control the blood pressure. A hypertensive emergency exists if the DBP is over 130 mm Hg and evidence of end-organ damage exists, such as retinal hemorrhage, encephalopathy, pulmonary edema, myocardial infarction, or unstable angina. Drugs available for treatment in this situation include sodium nitroprusside, nitroglycerin, hydralazine, phentolamine, labetolol, and methyldopa. Patients must be hospitalized for appropriate monitoring. Hypertensive urgency exists when the DBP is over 115 mm Hg without evidence of end-organ damage. Oral agents such as nifedipine, clonidine, captopril, and minoxidil may be used to lower the DBP 10 to 15 mm Hg over several hours.[1] Nifedipine should be used with caution in patients with cardiac disease.[21]

Conclusion

Pharmacologic management of hypertension challenges the physician to understand the patient's social, psychological, and economic status in order to select an antihypertensive regimen that effectively lowers the blood pressure, alleviates concomitant disease states, and allows easy adherence to the regimen. Continual assessment of therapy is necessary to determine the effectiveness of the regimen, adverse side effects, and the patient's quality of life issues.

References

1. National Institutes of Health. Fifth Report of the Joint National Committee on Detection, Evaluation, and Treatment of High Blood Pressure. National High Blood Pressure Education. Bethesda: National Heart, Lung and Blood Institute, 1993. NIH Publication No. 93-1088.
2. Haynes RB, Sackett DL, Taylor DW, et al. Increased absenteeism from work after detection and labeling of hypertensive patients. N Engl J Med 1978; 297:741–4.
3. National Institutes of Health. Sixth Report of the Joint National Committee on Detection, Evaluation, and Treatment of High Blood Pressure. National High Blood Pressure Education. Bethesda: National Heart, Lung and Blood Institute, 1997. NIH Publication No. 98-4080.
4. Gordon T, Doyle JT. Alcohol consumption and its relationship to smoking, weight, blood pressure, and blood lipids. Arch Intern Med 1986;146:262–5.
5. Pooling Project Research Group. Relationship of blood pressure, serum cholesterol, smoking habit, relative weight and ECG abnormalities to incidence of major coronary events. J Chronic Dis 1978;31:201–6.
6. Stamler J, Farinaro E, Majonnier LM, et al. Prevention and control of hypertension by nutritional-hygienic means. JAMA 1980;243:1819–23.
7. Rose G, Stamler J. The Intersalt Study: background, methods and main results; Intersalt Cooperative Research Group. J Hum Hypertens 1989;3:283–8.
8. Cade R, Mars D, Wagemaker H, et al. Effect of aerobic exercise training on patients with systemic arterial hypertension. Am J Med 1984;77:785–90.
9. Margetts BM, Beilin LJ, Armstrong BK. A randomized control trial of a vegetarian diet in the treatment of mild hypertension. Clin Exp Pharmacol Physiol 1985;12:263–6.
10. Kaplan NM. Non-drug treatment of hypertension. Ann Intern Med 1985; 102:359–73.
11. Witteman JC, Willett WC, Stampfer MJ, et al. A prospective study of nutritional factors and hypertension among US women. Circulation 1989; 80:1320–7.

12. Patel C, Marmot MG. Stress management, blood pressure and quality of life. J Hypertens 1987;5 (Suppl 1):521–8.
13. Stamler R, Stamler J, Grimm R, et al. Nutritional therapy for high blood pressure. JAMA 1987;257:1484–91.
14. American Hospital Formulary Service Drug Information. Bethesda: American Society of Hospital Pharmacists, 1990.
15. Kaplan NM. Clinical hypertension. 5th ed. Baltimore: Williams & Wilkins, 1993.
16. Houston MC. New insights and new approaches for the treatment of essential hypertension: selection of therapy based on coronary heart disease, risk factor analysis, hemodynamic profiles, quality of life and subsets of hypertension. Am Heart J 1989;117:911–51.
17. Merck and Co. Cozaar monograph. Rahway, NJ: Merck, April 1995.
18. Jachuck SJ, Brierly H, Jachuck S, et al. The effect of hypotensive drugs on quality of life. J R Coll Gen Pract 1982;32:103–5.
19. Croog SH, Levine S, Testa MA, et al. The effects of antihypertensive therapy on the quality of life. N Engl J Med 1986;314:1657–64.
20. Steiner SS, Friedhoff AJ, Wilson BL, et al. Antihypertensive therapy and quality of life: a comparison of atenolol, captopril, enalapril and propranolol. J Hum Hypertens 1990;4:217–25.
21. Furberg CD, Psaty BM, Meyer JV. Nifedipine dose related increase in mortality in patients with coronary heart disease. Circulation 1995;92: 1326–31.

CASE PRESENTATION

Subjective

PATIENT PROFILE

Mary Nelson is a 71-year-old married white female retired teacher.

PRESENTING PROBLEM

High blood pressure.

PRESENT ILLNESS

Mrs. Nelson is here for continuing care of hypertension, which has been present since age 61. She currently takes 50 mg hydrochlorothiazide daily and feels well. Her last periodic health examination with laboratory tests and x-ray was 2 years ago.

PAST MEDICAL HISTORY

She had an abdominal hysterectomy for fibroids at age 50 and is currently taking no estrogen replacement. She has been treated for depression at times but is taking no medication now.

SOCIAL HISTORY

She retired as a middle school history teacher at age 62. She lives with her husband, Harold, aged 76, whom you recently treated for urinary incontinence (see Chapter 5), and son Samuel, aged 48.

HABITS

She does not use alcohol or tobacco. She drinks one cup of coffee daily.

FAMILY HISTORY

She is an orphan, adopted in infancy, and her biological parents are unknown. She and her husband, Harold, had four children. Three are living and have no serious illnesses; their son Samuel, aged 48, has COPD.

REVIEW OF SYSTEMS

She sleeps poorly and wakes early in the morning, unable to fall asleep again. She feels tired throughout the day and occasionally is inappropriately sad.

- What additional medical history might be helpful, and why?
- What questions might help elucidate target organ damage related to hypertension or problems with medication?
- What are possible reasons why the patient is not taking antidepressant medication, and how would you address this issue?
- Have you listened carefully to everything Mrs. Nelson would like to tell you today?

Objective

VITAL SIGNS

Height, 5 ft 3 in; weight, 122 lb; blood pressure, 162/84; pulse, 72.

EXAMINATION

The patient's affect seems somewhat dull and flat compared with previous visits. The head, eyes, ears, nose, and throat are normal. The neck and thyroid gland are normal. Her chest is clear to percussion and auscultation. The heart has a regular sinus rhythm with no murmurs.

- Is there any additional information regarding the physical examination that might be helpful, and why?
- What other areas of the body—if any—should be examined today?
- What—if any—laboratory tests should be obtained today?
- What—if any—diagnostic imaging should be obtained today?

Assessment

- What is the current status of Mrs. Nelson's hypertension? How would you explain this to the patient?

- Describe the pathophysiology of hypertension in the elderly patient. How might this influence your choice of therapy?
- What is the apparent status of her recurrent depression, and how would you explain this to the patient?
- What are some possible adaptations of this patient to her illnesses, and how might these be important in care?

Plan

- What would be your therapeutic recommendations today regarding diet and medication?
- What are possible interrelationships of Mrs. Nelson's problems and the medications that might be used to treat them?
- If Mrs. Nelson is your patient in a capitated plan for which you are a case manager, how might this influence your thinking and actions?
- What continuing care would you recommend for this patient?

9

Sinusitis and Pharyngitis

PAUL EVANS AND WILLIAM F. MISER

Sinusitis

Sinusitis is a common problem encountered in primary care, seen in 3% of patients with upper respiratory tract infections (URIs).[1] It is primarily caused by ostial obstruction of the anterior ethmoid and middle meatal complex due to retained secretions, edema, or polyps. Barotrauma, nasal cannulation, or ciliary transport defects can also precipitate infection.[1,2] The diagnosis is sometimes elusive, requiring skillful medical detective work and careful clinical evaluation to identify the problem.

Acute Sinusitis

CLINICAL PRESENTATION

Acute sinusitis usually presents with nasal congestion, purulent nasal discharge, headache, fever, facial pain, paranasal pressure, and dental pain. A change of head position or barometric pressure may also increase discomfort.[3] Frontal sinus involvement usually presents with lower forehead pain, whereas maxillary sinusitis is characterized by tenderness in the cheek with pain referred to the upper teeth. Ethmoidal sinusitis presents as retroorbital pain and tenderness over the lateral aspect of the nose. Sphenoid sinusitis frequently involves headache at the skull vertex.[4,5] Maxillary sinuses are most commonly infected, followed by ethmoidal, sphenoidal, and frontal sinuses.[3] Sneezing, watery rhinorrhea, and conjunctivitis may be seen in sinusitis associated with an allergy.

PHYSICAL FINDINGS

Examination may reveal nasal mucosal erythema and edema with purulent nasal discharge. Fever may or may not be present. Palpatory or percussive tenderness over the involved sinuses, particularly the frontal and maxillary sinuses, with dullness on sinus transillumination, is common.[6] Drainage from the maxillary and frontal sinuses may be seen at the middle meatus, or sinus ostial opening. The ethmoids drain from either the middle meatus (anterior ethmoid) or superior meatus (posterior ethmoid). The sphenoid drains into the superior meatus.

DIAGNOSIS

Definitive diagnosis is based on clinical presentation and the use of diagnostic imaging studies with laboratory corroboration. Plain sinus radiographs may show air-fluid levels, mucosal thickening, and possibly anatomic abnormalities that predispose to the condition, such as nasal polyps. Views specific to each sinus are the Caldwell (frontal), Waters (maxillary), lateral (sphenoid), and submentovertical (ethmoid).[5] Computed tomography (CT) is more sensitive and may better reveal pathology, with focused sinus CT now a cost-competitive alternative to the radiographic sinus series for both initial and follow-up studies.[7–10] Nasopharyngeal cultures and antral puncture by consultants may elucidate specific pathogens.

MICROBIOLOGY

Bacterial pathogens responsible for acute sinusitis commonly include *Streptococcus pneumoniae, Haemophilus influenzae,* group A streptococci, and *Moraxella catarrhalis.*[11] Less commonly *Staphylococcus aureus, Streptococcus pyogenes, Mycoplasma pneumoniae,* and *Chlamydia pneumoniae* are seen. Anaerobic organisms play a role, with *Peptostreptococcus, Corynebacterium, Bacteroides,* and *Veillonella* having been described.[12,13] Adenovirus, parainfluenza, rhinovirus, and influenza virus may cause or exacerbate sinusitis. *Aspergillus fumigatus* and *Mucormycosis* can cause sinusitis, especially in those who are immunocompromised.[5]

NONMICROBIOLOGIC CAUSES

Sinusitis may be a complication of allergic rhinitis, foreign bodies, deviated nasal septum, nasal packing, dental procedures, facial fractures, tumors, barotrauma, and nasal polyps. The cause appears to be stasis of normal physiologic sinus drainage.[4,12] Prolonged nasal intubation may also be associated with sinusitis (presumably by the same mechanism) with subsequent infection by *Staphylococcus aureus, Enterobacter, Pseudomonas aeruginosa, Bacteroides fragilis, Bacteroides melaninogenicus,* and *Candida* sp.[2]

TREATMENT

Initial treatment of acute sinusitis consists of antibiotics, decongestants, and nonpharmacologic measures to maintain adequate sinus drainage.

1. *Antibiotics* (Table 9.1): Amoxicillin-clavulanate, trimethoprim-sulfamethoxazole, clarithromycin, or a second or third generation cephalosporin

TABLE 9.1. Antibiotics for sinusitis

Antibiotic	Dosage		Dosing frequency
	Adults (mg)	Children (mg/kg/day)	
Oral administration			
3. Trimethoprim-sulfamethoxazole[a]	160/300	8/40	bid
1. Ampicillin-clavulanate[a]	875/125	45/6.4	bid
Cefaclor	500	40	tid
Clarithromycin	500	15	bid
Amoxicillin	500	40	tid
Ampicillin	500	100	tid
Erythromycin-sulfisoxazole	N/A	50/150	qid
2. Cefuroxime axetil a.	250	30	bid
Cefixime	400	8	qd
Cefpodoxime-proxetil	200	10	qd
Cefprozil	500	30	bid
Loracarbef	400	30	bid
Clarithromycin	500		bid
Parenteral administration			
Imipenem	500		q6h IV
Meropenem	1000		q8 IV

Source: adapted from Gilbert et al.[11]
N/A = not available.
[a]Suggested primary regimen.

(e.g., cefaclor, cefuroxime axetil, loracarbef) are primary antibiotics for acute bacterial sinusitis. Duration of treatment is 14 to 21 days. Ampicillin may be used if β-lactamase organisms are locally uncommon.[11]

2. *Decongestants:* Normal saline nose drops loosen secretions, and steam treatments may help increase sinus drainage. Oxymetazoline 0.05% topical nasal spray can be used for no more than 3 to 4 days. Guaifenesin preparations can maintain sinus drainage by thinning secretions and thus decrease stasis.[14]
3. *Nasal steroids:* With allergic sinusitis, nasal steroids shrink edematous mucosa and allow ostial openings to increase. A two or three times per day dosage is commonly used.[15]
4. *Nonpharmacologic:* Increasing oral fluids, local steam inhalation, and application of heat or cold have had some success in reducing discomfort.[9]

Complications

Mucocele and osteomyelitis are rare but potentially life-threatening complications of sinusitis. Mucoceles, treated surgically, may be identified by radiography or sinus CT. Osteomyelitis, a serious infection of the surrounding bone, requires prolonged parenteral antibiotics and débridement of necrotic osseous structures, often with later cosmetic reconstruction.[5] Meningitis, cavernous sinus thrombosis, brain abscess, or hematogenous spread may also occur. Orbital infections occur more commonly in children.[16]

Chronic Recurrent Sinusitis

More than 32 million cases of chronic sinusitis occur annually in the United States. The definition of "chronic" is symptom duration of 3 weeks to 3 months, with epithelial damage as the hypothetic endpoint.[17,18] This condition is characterized by malaise, facial headache, and a cough. Predisposing factors include anatomic abnormalities, polyps, allergic rhinitis, ciliary dysmotility, foreign bodies, chronic irritants, adenoidal hypertrophy, nasal decongestant spray abuse (rhinitis medicamentosa), smoking, swimming, and chronic viral URIs. Pathogens are those listed above with an increase in involvement by *Bacteroides* sp., *Peptostreptococcus,* and *Fusobacterium*. Treatment involves organism-specific antibiotics.[11]

Surgical Management

When medical management fails (lack of clinical response to antibiotics), surgical management is indicated. Antral lavage techniques (sinus puncture) allow drainage of purulent sinus material. Functional endonasal sinus surgery techniques allow direct observation of sinus pathology and can create improved sinus ventilation and ciliary clearance.[19] Nasal antral window procedures have also been used successfully.

Sinusitis in Children

Maxillary and ethmoidal sinuses are the primary sites of infection in infants (12 months and younger). The sphenoid sinus develops during the third to fifth year of life and the frontal sinus during the sixth to tenth year. If a URI is severe or persists beyond 10 days in a child, suspect sinusitis. Common symptoms include fever over 39°C, periorbital edema, facial pain, and daytime cough.[16,20] Periorbital cellulitis is seen in infants with ethmoidal disease.

A single Waters view is an acceptable initial study; limited CT scans may be a better alternative.[21] The radiographic diagnosis is based on air-fluid levels, mucosal thickening of 4 mm or more, or sinus opacification. Organisms in antral cultures include *Streptococcus pneumoniae, Moraxella catarrhalis,* and *Haemophilus influenzae.*[22,23]

Amoxicillin is the initial antibiotic of choice. Trimethoprim-sulfamethoxazole, erythromycin-sulfisoxazole, amoxicillin-clavulanate, cefaclor, and cefuroxime axetil are useful in penicillin-allergic individuals or if β-lactamase-producing organisms are suspected. All antibiotics are given for 14 to 21 days. Antihistamines may impair ciliary clearing mechanisms and thicken secretions. If oral antibiotics are unsuccessful, parenteral cefuroxime or oxacillin plus chloramphenicol have been recommended (Table 9.1).[16]

Pharyngitis

Sore throat is one of the most common complaints seen by primary care physicians. Nearly 40 million visits are made each year for this complaint in the United States.[24–28] Nearly every step in the management of pharyngitis is controversial; the challenge for family physicians is to determine, in a cost-effective manner, which patients need antibiotic therapy.[29]

Epidemiology

The infectious causes for a sore throat are found in Table 9.2. Although viruses are the most common infectious etiologic agents of pharyngitis and tonsillitis, group A β-hemolytic *Streptococcus* (GABHS) is most important because of its potential sequelae. GABHS can be isolated by throat culture in 30% to 40% of children and 5% to 10% of adults, with the highest prevalence found in children age 6 to 11 years.[25,30,32,33] Groups C and G streptococci, *Mycoplasma pneumoniae,* and *Chlamydia pneumoniae* tend to cause pharyngitis most commonly in adolescents and young adults and are usually not associated with serious sequelae.[30,33,34] No infectious pathogen is found in 20% to 65% of patients, and noninfectious causes should be considered (Table 9.3).

The GABHS type pharyngitis is most frequently seen during late winter and early spring, whereas other infectious agents occur year-round.[28,29,33] All are spread by close contact or droplets. A higher incidence of disease occurs in schools, day-care centers, dormitories, and military barracks.[35] Pharyngitis, peritonsillar abscess, and acute rheumatic fever occur infrequently during the first 2 years of life.[29,33,35]

GABHS Pharyngitis

The classic features of GABHS pharyngitis (found in only 33–50% of patients) include the sudden onset of sore throat and moderate fever (39.0°–40.5°C), headache, anorexia, nausea, vomiting, abdominal pain, malaise, tonsillopharyngeal erythema, patchy, discrete tonsillar or pharyngeal exudate, soft palate petechiae, tender cervical adenopathy, or scarlet fever.[28,29,32,33] Most patients have mild or asymptomatic disease, and there is much overlap with these "classic" features and those of viral pharyngitis. One of the most useful clinical findings, tender anterior cervical adenopathy, may also occur with viral infections. Scarlet fever produces a rash characterized by a fine, blanching appearance and sandpaper texture, circumoral pallor, and hyperpigmentation in the skin creases. It is highly suggestive of GABHS but also may be seen with pharyngitis caused by *Arcanobacterium haemolyticus.* Exudative pharyngitis/tonsillitis, anterior cervical adenopathy, fever, and lack of other URI symptoms such as cough and

TABLE 9.2. Infectious causes of pharyngitis[a]

Primary bacterial pathogens (30% in children age 5–11 years old, 15% in adolescents, 5% in adults)
Group A β-hemolytic streptococci (GABHS)
Group B, C, and G streptococci
Neisseria gonorrhoeae (uncommon)
Cornybacterium diphtheriae (rare)
Treponema pallidum (unusual)
Tuberculosis (unusual)
Possible bacterial pathogens (5–10%, primarily in young adults)
Arcanobacterium haemolyticus
Chlamydia pneumoniae
Chlamydia trachomatis
Mycoplasma pneumoniae
Probable bacterial copathogens (all age groups)
Staphylococcus aureus
Haemophilus influenzae
Klebsiella pneumoniae rhinoscleromatis
Moraxella (Branhamella) catarrhalis
Bacteroides melaninogenicus
Bacteroides oralis
Bacteroides fragilis
Fusobacterium species
Peptostreptococcus
Viruses (15–40% in children, 30–60% in adults)
Adenovirus types 1, 2, 3, 5 (most common)
Parainfluenza virus
Coronavirus (uncommon)
Coxsackie virus
Echovirus
Herpes simplex virus
Epstein-Barr virus
Cytomegalovirus
Influenza viruses
Myxovirus
Reovirus
Respiratory syncytial virus
Fungal (uncommon in immunocompetent patient)
Candida albicans

Source: Data are from Denny[29] and Pichichero.[30, 31]
[a]No pathogen is isolated in 20% to 65% (average 30%) of cases of sore throat.

rhinorrhea are most predictive of a positive GABHS culture, with a probability of occurrence of 56% when all four are present.[38]

LABORATORY DIAGNOSIS

Additional laboratory tests are usually needed because clinical findings are unreliable. The "gold standard" for diagnosing acute GABHS pharyngitis is a properly processed and interpreted throat culture on sheep blood agar.[32,39] For best throat culture results, use a Dacron swab

TABLE 9.3. Noninfectious causes of pharyngitis

Postnasal drip
Sinusitis
Malignant disease: leukemia, lymphoma, squamous cell carcinoma
Behçet syndrome
Reiter syndrome
Kawasaki syndrome
Pemphigus
Erythema multiforme
Trauma: accidents, burns, other thermal injuries, child abuse
Foreign bodies
Contact stomatitis
Irritant exposure: cigarette smoke, smog
Lack of ambient humidity in home or work environment
Other

Source: Data are from Denny,[29] Pichichero,[30,31,36] and Bonilla and Bluestone.[37]

and thoroughly swab the palatine tonsils and pharyngeal wall, avoiding the tongue. Plating even a dry swab may be delayed as long as 24 hours without affecting culture results.[32,40,41]

There are more than 25 streptococcal rapid antigen tests available commercially. Most are highly specific (90–96%) but not as sensitive (41–93%) as throat cultures.[30,42] If a rapid antigen test is positive, one can be almost certain that GABHS is in the pharynx. If the test is negative, most authors recommend obtaining a throat culture for those whom one suspects has GABHS infection.[25,41,42] A newer test, the optical immunoassay (OIA), has better reported sensitivity than and comparable specificity to the rapid antigen tests.[40,43]

COMPLICATIONS

Suppurative complications include peritonsillar abscess, retropharyngeal abscess, and suppurative cervical lymphadenitis.[32,44] Peritonsillar abscess (PTA) occurs in fewer than 1% of patients treated with appropriate antibiotics.[42] It is seen most frequently in teenagers and young adults and is rare in children under the age of 5 years. Symptoms of an abscess are a severe unilateral sore throat associated with dysphagia, referred otalgia, pain with lateral movement of the neck, rancid breath, trismus, drooling from a partially opened mouth, and a muffled "hot potato" voice. About 3% to 10% of cases of PTA are bilateral.[45] There is generalized erythema of the pharynx and tonsils, with a deeper dusky redness overlying the involved area, swelling of the anterior pillar and soft palate above the tonsil, and uvular deviation to the opposite side.[28,46] Some have advocated the use of diagnostic ultrasonography[47] or CT scans[45] of the neck and head to distinguish between peritonsillar cellulitis and abscess.

In addition to intravenous penicillin, treatment options include repeated needle aspiration, incision and drainage, abscess tonsillectomy, and delayed (2–4 weeks) tonsillectomy. Penicillin therapy and needle aspiration, which can be done easily and safely in the outpatient setting by family physicians, eradicates the infection in 80% to 90% of patients within 3 days.[46,48] If needle aspiration fails, the patient is referred for the conventional methods of incision and drainage or immediate tonsillectomy.[49] Tonsillectomy is also indicated in those with recurrent PTA.

The erythrogenic toxin elaborated by GABHS causes the rash of scarlet fever, which now occurs infrequently in the United States. There have been increasing reports of streptococcal toxic shock-like syndrome (STSLS), which usually occurs in previously healthy adults and is marked by hypotension and progressive multisystemic failure.[44,50] Although usually associated with a soft tissue focus of infection, 10% to 20% of the cases of STSLS have been associated with an apparent pharyngeal infection.[44] The syndrome appears to be toxin-mediated and related to GABHS isolates of serotypes M-1, M-3, M-28, and T-11, M-nontypable.

Once the leading cause of death in children and adolescents in the United States, acute rheumatic fever (ARF) now occurs infrequently (0.3–3.0%) in untreated patients with acute GABHS pharyngitis.[41,44] Symptoms begin 2 weeks after the onset of pharyngitis with a symmetric polyarthritis, followed by cardiac valvulitis. Prevention of ARF depends on control and antibiotic treatment of GABHS tonsillopharyngitis.[41] Acute glomerulonephritis may occur 10 days after GABHS pharyngitis and presents as anasarca, hypertension, hematuria, and proteinuria. It generally is a self-limited condition, it almost never has permanent sequelae, and antibiotics do not prevent its occurrence.[32,42,51]

TREATMENT

A small but highly significant portion of patients with acute GABHS tonsillopharyngitis develop complications, which has led to efforts to identify and treat these patients with an effective antibiotic regimen.[44] However, treating all patients with sore throat as if they had GABHS infection overtreats at least 70% of pediatric and 90% of adult patients, which can be costly and problematic.[30]

Treating GABHS pharyngitis accomplishes four goals: (1) patients clinically improve more quickly[31,52]; (2) they become noninfectious within 24 hours[53] thereby preventing transmission of infection; (3) suppurative complications such as PTA are avoided[43]; and (4) ARF is prevented.[41] Children who complete a full 24 hours of antibiotics can be considered noninfectious and if they feel better may return to school. Although patients respond clinically within 1 to 2 days of antibiotics, treatment for 10 days remains the optimal duration to prevent ARF. Shortening the course increases the rate of treatment failure.[54] Patient compliance issues should be addressed; up to 80% do not complete a 10-day course.[28,42] Counseling on the importance of completing the 10-day course despite resolution of symptoms greatly increases compliance rates, as does twice-daily dosing.

The choice of antibiotic for GABHS pharyngitis (Table 9.4) should include cost, side-effects profile, and patient compliance. Penicillin remains the drug of choice because it is effective in preventing ARF, inexpensive, and relatively safe.[35,41,42,55] No evidence of penicillin-resistant GABHS has been identified.[41,42,51,56] Even when started as long as 9 days after the onset of acute pharyngitis, penicillin effectively prevents primary attacks of ARF. Intramuscular benzathine penicillin is the definitive treatment for GABHS but is infrequently used because injections are painful. For those allergic to penicillin, erythromycin is the antibiotic of choice, as resistance is not yet an appreciable problem in the United States. Clarithromycin and azithromycin have

TABLE 9.4. Treatment options for group A β-hemolytic streptococcal pharyngitis

	Dosage[a]			
Antibiotic	Adults (mg)	Children (mg/kg/day)	Dosing frequency[b]	Cost[c]
First-line treatment				
Benzathine penicillin G				
≤ 60 pounds (27 kg)	600,000 units IM	Same	Once	$
> 60 pounds (27 kg)	1,200,000 units IM	Same	Once	$–$$
Benzathine/procaine penicillin	900,000/300,000 IM	Same	Once	$
Penicillin VK	500 mg total	250 mg total	bid	$
Penicillin-allergic				
Erythromycin estolate	250	20	bid	$
Erythromycin ethylsuccinate	400	40	tid	$–$$
Second-line treatment				
Amoxicillin	250	20	qd to tid	$
Cephalexin	250	30	tid	$–$$$$
Cefadroxil	1000	30	qd	$$$–$$$$$
Cefaclor	250	20–30	tid	$$$$
Cefuroxime axetil	125	15	bid	$$–$$$
Cefixime	200	8	qd	$$$–$$$$$
Amoxicillin-clavulanate	250	20	tid	$$$$
Clarithromycin	250	—	bid	$$$$$
Azithromycin	500 mg on day 1 250 mg on days 2–5	—	qd	$$$–$$$$

Source: Data are from Sanford et al.,[11] Vukmir,[28] Denny,[29] Klein,[35] Dajani et al.,[41] and Kline and Runge.[42]

[a]Unless otherwise indicated, antibiotic is given orally for 10 days.

[b]qd = once daily, bid = twice daily, tid = three times daily

[c]Cost for therapeutic course based on average wholesale price from *1996 Drugs Topics Red Book;* prices for generic drugs were used when available; $ = 0–15 dollars; $$ = 15–30 dollars; $$$ = 31–45 dollars; $$$$ = 45–60 dollars; $$$$$ = more than 60 dollars.

a susceptibility pattern similar to that of erythromycin but with less gastrointestinal distress and may be administered once or twice a day. Azithromycin is the first oral antibiotic approved by the U.S. Food and Drug Administration (FDA) for a 5-day treatment regimen for GABHS pharyngitis. However, cost and nonapproval for children under age 16 years make these antibiotics second-line choices.[41] Amoxicillin offers a low cost, better-tasting efficacy, similar to that of penicillin VK but has a higher incidence of side-effect rashes. Cephalosporins are more expensive, may hasten the development of resistant bacteria, have never been proved to prevent ARF, and should not be used in patients with a history of immediate (anaphylactic) hypersensitivity to penicillin.[30]

Other Infectious Causes of Pharyngitis

Groups C and G streptococci and *A. haemolyticus* can produce tonsillopharyngitis that is indistinguishable from GABHS but have minimal suppurative or nonsuppurative sequelae.[29] The tonsillopharyngitis of *M. pneumoniae* and *C. pneumoniae* is similar to GABHS infection but is usually (75%) accompanied by a cough associated with tracheobronchitis, pneumonia, or both.[30,34] Membranous pharyngitis with a gangrenous exudative appearance is usually found with Vincent's angina or diphtheria.[28] Herpangina (caused by the Coxsackie A virus) is characterized by a severe sore throat, fever, and 1- to 2-mm pharyngeal vesicles that subsequently ulcerate and resolve within 5 days. Hand-foot-mouth disease (caused by Coxsackie A16 virus) presents as a pharyngitis accompanied by vesicles on the palm and sole surfaces. Patients with aphthous stomatitis have a sore throat and round, painful oral lesions that typically resolve within 2 weeks. Herpes simplex virus causes fever, oral fetor, submaxillary adenopathy, and a gingivostomatitis. Symptoms of infectious mononucleosis (Epstein-Barr virus) include a sore throat, anterior and posterior adenopathy, gray pseudomembranous pharyngitis, and palatine petechiae.

TREATMENT OF NONSTREPTOCOCCAL INFECTIONS

The same antibiotic choices exist for groups C and G streptococci and *A. haemolyticus.*[29] However, routine use of erythromycin in adult patients with non-GABHS pharyngitis is not recommended because of little benefit and potential for drug resistance.[57] Both *M. pneumoniae* and *C. pneumoniae* are sensitive to tetracycline and erythromycin, and treatment with either has been shown to be effective in patients who have pneumonia.[29] Treatment for diphtheria includes antitoxin and erythromycin 20 to 25 mg/kg IV q12h for 7 to 14 days. Vincent's angina is treated with penicillin, tetracycline, and oral oxidizing agents such as peroxide, with better oral hygiene. Treatment of viral pharyngitis with antivirals is not indicated. An oral rinse consisting of corticosteroids (Kenalog suspension) and topical tetracycline (250 mg/50 ml water) may hasten recovery in patients with aphthous stomatitis. Therapy for infectious mononucleosis is usually supportive but may include penicillin for simultaneous GABHS infection and steroids for respiratory obstruction. Amoxicillin, which causes a characteristic rash, should not be used for diagnosed cases of infectious mononucleosis.

Analgesia

Aspirin should be avoided in children and teenagers because of the risk for Reye syndrome. In addition, the use of aspirin and acetaminophen may actually prolong the common cold.[58] Ibuprofen 400 mg every 6 hours is superior to acetaminophen for alleviating throat pain.[42] Available suspension analgesics include ibuprofen 100 mg/5 ml and naproxen 125 mg/5 ml.[42] Warm liquids are an effective adjuvant treatment in combination with analgesics. Patients with severe inflammatory symptoms may benefit from corticosteroids, given as a short course of oral prednisone or a single 10 mg injection of dexamethasone.[26,42]

Cost Benefit of Treatment Strategy

There is no consensus on the best cost-effective approach to treating patients with a sore throat. Physicians must develop a rational policy for their practice based on the incidence of GABHS in their patient population, cost containment, avoidance of adverse outcomes (from both the use antibiotics and occurrence of sequelae from untreated GABHS), reducing unnecessary use of antibiotics, and patient priorities. When the probability of GABHS is greater than 20%, treating all patients with pharyngitis without testing may be rational.[59–61] Testing and antibiotic use should be avoided when the risk of GABHS is less than 5%, as the costs of evaluation and treatment and potential adverse reactions to antibiotics outweigh the potential problems associated with missed infection.[30] In cases where rapid antigen tests are negative and a confirmatory throat culture is pending, presumptive antibiotic use is based on severity of illness, risk of transmission to others, need to return to school or work, and the patient's willingness to accept risks of unnecessary use of antibiotics should the culture be reported as negative. When one family member has proved GABHS pharyngitis, all symptomatic family members can be treated without further testing.

Treatment Failures and Chronic Carriers

Posttreatment throat cultures are indicated only in those who remain symptomatic after completion of antibiotics, who develop recurrent symptoms within 6 weeks, or who have had rheumatic fever and are at unusually high risk for recurrence.[41,55] Reasons for treatment failures include poor patient antibiotic compliance, inactivation of penicillin by β-lactamase-producing bacteria normally present in the pharynx, and recurrent exposure to a family member who harbors GABHS ("ping-pong" infections).[29–31,54] The family pet is an unlikely reservoir for GABHS.[62] A chronic GABHS carrier is an individual with a positive throat culture who is asymptomatic.[31,42] As many as 20% to 50% of school-age children are GABHS carriers, are rarely contagious, and are at little risk for developing GABHS complications.[41,42,63] Indications to eradicate GABHS from the chronic carrier include a personal or family history of ARF and "ping-pong" spread within a family.[63] The treatment for those who fail an adequate course of antibiotics or who are GABHS carriers is a single injection of benzathine penicillin (Table 9.4). If this measure fails, a combination of oral penicillin for 10 days and rifampin 20 mg/kg/day (not to exceed 600 mg/day) in one or two equal doses concurrently for the last 4 days is efficacious.[31,42] Clindamycin 20 mg/kg/day (up to 450 mg/day) may be also given in three divided doses for 10 days.[64]

Tonsillectomy

Tonsillectomy is indicated for those who have recurrent peritonsillar abscesses or respiratory obstruction.[28] The American Academy of Otolaryngology and Head and Neck Surgery considers four or more infections of the tonsils per year, despite adequate medical therapy, as sufficient indication for tonsillectomy, although the benefit of decreased frequency of GABHS tonsillitis may last only 2 years.[65–67]

References

1. Jeffers J, Boynton S. Harrison's principles of internal medicine. 13th ed. New York: McGraw-Hill, 1995:418–21.
2. Linden B, Aguilar E, Allen S. Sinusitis in the nasotracheally intubated patient. Arch Otolaryngol Head Neck Surg 1988; 114:860–1.
3. Way L. Current surgical diagnosis and treatment. 10th ed. East Norwalk, CT: Appleton & Lange, 1994:874–7.
4. Simon H. Approach to the patient with sinusitis. In: Goroll A, May L, Mulley A, editors. Primary care medicine. 3rd ed. Philadelphia: Lippincott, 1995:1004–7.

5. Tierney L, McPhee S, Papadakis M. Current medical diagnosis and treatment. 34th ed. East Norwalk, CT: Appleton & Lange, 1995:182–4.
6. Ferguson B. Acute and chronic sinusitis: how to ease symptoms and locate the cause. Postgrad Med 1995;97:45–57.
7. Burke T, Guertler A, Timmons J. Comparisons of sinus x-rays with CT scans in acute sinusitis. Acad Emerg Med 1994;1:235–9.
8. Yousem D. Imaging of sinonasal inflammatory disease. Radiology 1993; 188:303–14.
9. Hopp R, Cooperstock M. Evaluation and treatment of sinusitis: aspects for the managed care environment. J Am Osteopath Assoc 1996;96 Suppl 4:S6–10.
10. Guarderas J. Acute and chronic sinusitis. Mayo Clin Proc 1996;71:882–6.
11. Gilbert DN, Moellenig RC, Sande MA. The Sanford guide to antimicrobial therapy 1998. 28th ed. Vienna, VA: Antimicrobial Therapy, Inc. 1998:35.
12. Hilger P. Diseases of the paranasal sinuses. In: Adams G, Boies L, Hilger P, editors. Fundamentals of otolaryngology. Philadelphia: Saunders, 1989: 249–70.
13. Nord C. The role of anaerobic bacteria in recurrent episodes of sinusitis and tonsillitis. Clin Infect Dis 1995;20:1512–24.
14. Malm L. Pharmacological background to decongesting and anti-inflammatory treatment of rhinitis and sinusitis. Acta Otolaryngol Suppl (Stockh) 1994;515:53–5.
15. Naclerio R. Allergic rhinitis. N Engl J Med 1991;325:860–9.
16. Tom L, Kennedy D. Rhinitis and sinusitis. In: Burg F, Ingelfinger J, Wald E, Polin R, editors. Current pediatric therapy. 15th ed. Philadelphia: Saunders, 1996.
17. Mellen I. Chronic sinusitis: clinical and pathophysiological aspects. Acta Otolaryngol Suppl (Stockh) 1994;515:45–8.
18. Chester A. Chronic sinusitis. Am Fam Physician 1996;53: 877–87.
19. Lazar R, Younis R, Long T. Functional endonasal sinus surgery in adults and children. Laryngoscope 1993;103:1–5.
20. Willett L, Carson J. Williams J. Current diagnosis and management of sinusitis. J Gen Intern Med 1994;9:38–45.
21. Behrman R, Kliegman R. Nelson textbook of pediatrics. 14th ed. Philadelphia: Saunders, 1992:1059–61.
22. Garcia D, Merly SC, Joyce M. Radiographic imaging studies in pediatric chronic sinusitis. J Allergy Clin Immunol 1994; 94:523–30.
23. Diaz I, Bamberger D. Acute sinusitis. Semin Respir Infect 1995;10:14–20.
24. Mainous A, Hueston W, Clark J. Antibiotics and upper respiratory infection: do some folks think there is a cure for the common cold? J Fam Pract 1996;42:357–61.
25. Pichichero M. Culture and antigen detection tests for streptococcal tonsillopharyngitis. Am Fam Physician 1992;45: 199–205.
26. O'Brien J, Meade J, Falk J. Dexamethasone as adjuvant therapy for severe acute pharyngitis. Ann Emerg Med 1993; 22:212–15.
27. Miser W. The content of outpatient family practice care in an Army community hospital: one physician's three-year experience. Mil Med 1992; 157:593–7.

28. Vukmir R. Adult and pediatric pharyngitis: a review. J Emerg Med 1992;10:607–16.
29. Denny F. Tonsillopharyngitis 1994. Pediatr Rev 1994;15: 185–91.
30. Pichichero M. Group A streptococcal tonsillopharyngitis: cost-effective diagnosis and treatment. Ann Emerg Med 1995;25:390–403.
31. Pichichero M. Controversies in the treatment of streptococcal pharyngitis. Am Fam Physician 1990;42:1567–76.
32. Kiselica D. Group A beta-hemolytic streptococcal pharyngitis: current clinical concepts. Am Fam Physician 1994;49: 1147–54.
33. Glezen W, Clyde W, Senior R, et al. Group A streptococci, mycoplasmas, and viruses associated with acute pharyngitis. JAMA 1967;202:119–24.
34. Williams W, Williamson H, LeFevre M. The prevalence of Mycoplasma pneumoniae in ambulatory patients with nonstreptococcal sore throat. Fam Med 1991;23:117–21.
35. Klein J. Management of streptococcal pharyngitis. Pediatr Infect Dis J 1994;13:572–5.
36. Pichichero M. Explanations and therapies for penicillin failure in streptococcal pharyngitis. Clin Pediatr 1992;31:642–9.
37. Bonilla J, Bluestone C. Pharyngitis: when is aggressive treatment warranted? Postgrad Med 1995;97:61–2, 65–6, 68–9.
38. Centor R, Witherspoon J, Dalton H, et al. The diagnosis of strep throat in adults in the emergency room. Med Decis Making 1981;1:240–6.
39. Wegner D, Witte D, Schrantz R. Insensitivity of rapid antigen detection methods and single blood agar plate culture for diagnosing streptococcal pharyngitis. JAMA 1992;267: 695–7.
40. Roddey O, Clegg H, Martin E, et al. Comparison of an optical immunoassay technique with two culture methods for the detection of group A streptococci in a pediatric office. J Pediatr 1995;126:931–3.
41. Dajani A, Taubert K, Ferrieri P, et al. Treatment of acute streptococcal pharyngitis and prevention of rheumatic fever: a statement for health professionals. Pediatrics 1995;96:758–64.
42. Kline J, Runge J. Streptococcal pharyngitis: a review of pathophysiology, diagnosis, and management. J Emerg Med 1994;12:665–80.
43. Fries S. Diagnosis of group A streptococcal pharyngitis in a private clinic: comparative evaluation of an optical immunoassay method and culture. J Pediatr 1995;126:933–6.
44. Shulman S. Complications of streptococcal pharyngitis. Pediatr Infect Dis J 1994;13:S70–4.
45. Patel K, Ahmad S, O'Leary G, Michel M. The role of computed tomography in the management of peritonsillar abscess. Otolaryngol Head Neck Surg 1992;107:727–32.
46. Epperly T, Wood T. New trends in the management of peritonsillar abscess. Am Fam Physician 1990;42:102–12.
47. Ahmed K, Jones A, Shah K, Smethurst A. The role of ultrasound in the management of peritonsillar abscess. J Laryngol Otol 1994;108:610–12.
48. Savolainen S, Jousimies-Somer H, Makitie A, Ylikoski J. Peritonsillar abscess: clinical and microbiologic aspects and treatment regimens. Arch Otolaryngol Head Neck Surg 1993;119: 521–4.

49. Chowdhury C, Bricknell M. The management of quinsy: a prospective study. J Laryngol Otol 1992;106:986–8.
50. Working Group on Streptococcal Infections. Defining the group A streptococcal toxic shock syndrome. JAMA 1993; 269:390–1.
51. Markowitz M. Changing epidemiology of group A streptococcal infections. Pediatr Infect Dis J 1994;13:557–60.
52. Krober M, Bass J, Michels G. Streptococcal pharyngitis: placebo-controlled double-blind evaluation of clinical response to penicillin therapy. JAMA 1985;253:1271–4.
53. Snellman L, Stang H, Stang J, et al. Duration of positive throat cultures for group A streptococci after initiation of antibiotic therapy. Pediatrics 1993; 91:1166–70.
54. Holm S. Reasons for failures in penicillin treatment of streptococcal tonsillitis and possible alternatives. Pediatr Infect Dis J 1994;13:S66–9.
55. Paradise J. Etiology and management of pharyngitis and pharyngotonsillitis in children: a current review. Ann Otol Rhinol Laryngol 1992;101:51–7.
56. Coonan K, Kaplan E. In vitro susceptibility of recent North American group A streptococcal isolates to eleven oral antibiotics. Pediatr Infect Dis J 1994;13:630–5.
57. Petersen K, Phillips RS, Soukup J, et al. The effect of erythromycin on resolution of symptoms among adults with pharyngitis not caused by Group A Streptococcus. J Gen Intern Med 1997;12:95–101.
58. Lorber B. The common cold. J Gen Intern Med 1996;11:229–36.
59. Slawson D, Squillace S, Franko J. Throat culture to rule out GABHS. J Fam Pract 1994;39:428.
60. Dippel D, Touw-Otten F, Habbema D. Management of children with acute pharyngitis: a decision analysis. J Fam Pract 1992;34:149–59.
61. Green S. Acute pharyngitis: the case for empiric antimicrobial therapy. Ann Emerg Med 1995;25:404–6.
62. Wilson K, Maroney S, Gander R. The family pet as an unlikely source of group A beta-hemolytic streptococcal infection in humans. Pediatr Infect Dis J 1995;14:372–5.
63. Gerber M. Treatment failures and carriers: perception or problems? Pediatr Infect Dis J 1994;13:576–9.
64. Tanz R, Poncher J, Corydon K, et al. Clindamycin treatment of chronic pharyngeal carriage of group A streptococci. J Pediatr 1991;119:123–8.
65. Paradise J, Bluestone C, Bachman R, et al. Efficacy of tonsillectomy for recurrent throat infection in severely affected children. N Engl J Med 1984;310:674–83.
66. Pichichero M. Recurrent streptococcal pharyngitis: indications for tonsillectomy and penicillin prophylaxis. Pediatr Infect Dis J 1994;13:83–4.
67. Deutsch E, Isaacson G. Tonsils and adenoids: an update. Pediatr Rev 1995;16:17–21.

Case Presentation

Subjective

Patient Profile

Luke Priestley is a 22-year-old married white male graduate student.

Presenting Problem

Sore throat.

Present Illness

For 2 days, Mr. Priestley has had a sore throat and fever. There has been slight pain in both ears and a mild cough. He is taking aspirin for the symptoms and has continued to attend classes.

Past Medical History

He had a positive tuberculin skin test on entering college 5 years ago. This finding followed a year as an exchange student in Korea.

Social History

Mr. Priestley is in his first year as a graduate student in an MBA program. He and his wife, Ann, are expecting their first child in 5 months.

Habits

He uses no tobacco, alcohol, or recreational drugs.

Family History

His father died of heart failure at age 55. His mother is living and well at age 57. His sister, aged 26, has mitral valve prolapse.

- What more would you like to know about the history of the present illness, and why?

- What further information would you like to know about Mr. Priestley's school work? Why?
- What family history might be pertinent, and why?
- What additional information might be pertinent about his positive tuberculin skin test?

Objective

VITAL SIGNS

Blood pressure, 120/78; pulse, 88; respirations, 26; temperature, 38.8°C.

EXAMINATION

The patient's face appears flushed, and the pitch of his voice seems altered by throat swelling. The tympanic membranes are both mildly injected but not retracted. The throat and tonsils are swollen bilaterally and erythematous. There is bilateral, tender cervical adenopathy. The thyroid is not enlarged. The chest examination reveals a few rhonchi at the bases bilaterally, but no wheezes are heard. The heart has a regular sinus rhythm without murmurs.

LABORATORY

A rapid screening test for β-hemolytic streptococcus is positive.

- What more—if anything—would you include in the physical examination, and why?
- Are there other areas of the body that should be examined, and why?
- What might cause you to be concerned about airway obstruction, and how would you address this concern?
- What—if any—laboratory or diagnostic imaging studies would you obtain today? Why?

Assessment

- What is your diagnostic impression, and how would you explain this to Mr. Priestley?
- What might be the meaning of this illness to the patient? To his wife?

- Mr. Priestley asks if he might develop complications of this illness. How would you respond?
- What are the risks that Mr. Priestley's wife or classmates might develop streptococcal pharyngitis, and what—if anything—should be done regarding this risk?

Plan

- Describe your therapeutic recommendations for the patient.
- If the patient were worse in 48 hours, what would you suspect? What would you do?
- Mrs. Priestley asks if her husband's illness presents any risk to the pregnancy. How would you respond?
- What follow-up would you advise?

10

Viral Infections of the Respiratory Tract

GEORGE L. KIRKPATRICK

Viral infections of the respiratory tract are responsible for large amounts of time lost from the workplace and significant morbidity and mortality in the very young and the very old. The worldwide pandemic of influenza in 1918 was alone responsible for nearly 30 million deaths in excess of those expected for influenza. National Health Survey data for 1978 in the United States showed that acute respiratory illness accounted for 50% of all disabling conditions annually.[1] That rate has continued unchanged for nearly 20 years. The common cold accounts for 40% of the respiratory illness and translates to more than 100 million disabling colds per year.

Viruses Involved with Upper Respiratory Tract Infections

Three studies, compared in Table 10.1, reflect prevalence rates for the most common respiratory tract viruses. A 12-month epidemiologic study of viral respiratory infections in Croatia from September 1, 1986, until August 31, 1987, involved 527 patients.[2] An Indian hospital-based study conducted from 1986 to 1989 on 736 children under the age of 5 years proved viral respiratory infections in 22% of the cases using nasopharyngeal cultures.[3] Finally, in a setting of institutionalized elderly, Falsey and Treanor found 149 nursing home residents with upper respiratory tract illnesses during a 3-month period.[4]

Table 10.2 compares the relative frequency of each common respiratory virus in four studies. Dowling[5] used epidemiologic data from numerous studies conducted during the late 1950s to define respiratory syndromes according to the viruses found by culture or rising antibody titers. Denny[6] studied the relative role of various viral causes of acute respiratory infections in children enrolled in day-care. The 1987 data in North Carolina were similar to Dowling's pooled data from the 1950s. In South Africa from 1982 to 1991 McAnerney[7] collected 966 throat swab

Table 10.1. Prevalence of common upper respiratory tract viruses

Virus	Croatia study[2] Patients (no.)	Croatia study[2] Prevalence (%)	Indian Hospital study[3] Patients (no.)	Indian Hospital study[3] Prevalence (%)	Nursing home study[4] Patients (no.)	Nursing home study[4] Prevalence (%)
Respiratory syncytial virus	177	33.6	37	5.0	18	12.1
Rhinoviruses					14	9.4
Herpes simplex	8	1.5			6	4.0
Parainfluenza (types 1, 2, 3)	12	2.3	38	5.2	3	2.0
Influenza (types A and B)	3	0.6	45	6.1	0	0
Adenoviruses	40	7.6	22	3.0		
Enteroviruses	18	3.4				
Measles virus			23	3.1		
Mixed infections	9	1.7			2	1.3
Total patients studied	527	—	736	—	149	—

Table 10.2. Frequency of upper respiratory tract viruses

Virus	Patients	Frequency (%) Dowling[5]	Denny[6]	McAnernay[7]	Monto & Sullivan[8]
Adenovirus	335	44	22	11	9
Parainfluenza	76	11	24	13	15
Enterovirus	101	14	14		
Rhinovirus	64	9	10		37
Influenza	58	9	5	55	22
Respiratory syncytial	17	2	10	3	10
Coxsackie	58	9	0		
Corona	20	2	0		
Total	729	100	85	82	93

culture results from 16 viral watch centers. There were 4133 specimens received, with a positive culture result in 23.4% of cases. Monto and Sullivan[8] studied families in Tecumseh, a small town in southeast Michigan, from 1965 to 1976 to determine the frequency of viral respiratory illnesses. Their results are similar to the others.

Respiratory Syncytial Virus

Respiratory syncytial virus (RSV), a single-stranded RNA paramyxovirus, is the leading cause of pneumonia and bronchiolitis in infants and children. Two antigenically distinct groups of RSV (A and B) are recognized. Community outbreaks of RSV usually appear during the winter and spring in temperate climates. The diagnosis of RSV in the acute setting is usually obtained by viral culture of nasopharyngeal secretions. A rapid diagnostic test (Abbott test pack RSV; Directigen RSV by Becton Dickinson) employing antigen detection in nasal secretions is 95% sensitive and 99% specific. Results are available in an hour.

The spectrum of illness associated with RSV is broad, ranging from mild nasal congestion to high fever and respiratory distress. What seems to begin as a simple cold may suddenly become a life-threatening illness. RSV tends to peak during early January most years. Evidence suggests that in infants group A viruses are associated with more severe infections than group B viruses.[9] Modes of spread are primarily via large-droplet inoculation (requiring close contact) and self-inoculation via contaminated fomites or skin. RSV is recoverable from countertops for up to 6 hours from the time of contamination, from rubber gloves for up to 90 minutes, and from skin for up to 20 minutes. Viral shedding of RSV in infants is a prolonged process averaging 7 days.

Strategies for controlling spread of RSV should be aimed at interrupting hand carriage of the virus and self-inoculation of the eyes and nose. Masks commonly employed for respiratory viruses have not been shown to be an effective measure for curtailing RSV outbreaks on pediatric wards. Hand-washing is probably the single most important infection control measure for RSV.

Influenza Viruses

Influenza, often considered a benign disease today, has ravaged human populations recently enough that there are still those living who can recall the 1918 worldwide pandemic called the "Spanish flu." This particular influenza was described as beginning with what appeared to be an ordinary attack of influenza and rapidly developing into severe pneumonia. Two hours after admission the patients had mahogany-colored spots over the cheek bones, and within a few hours cyanosis began to spread over the face. Death shortly overcame them as they struggled for air and suffocated. Severe influenza pandemics occur about every 7 to 11 years. They are always associated with extensive morbidity and a marked increase in mortality.

During 1977–1978 the National Health Survey estimated that 101 million acute respiratory illnesses caused by all types of respiratory viruses were medically attended in the United States. As many as 20 million cases could have been prevented by effective influenza prophylaxis. In addition to the predominant influenza virus that invades an area each season, many types, subtypes, or variants are identified during each epidemic period. These antigenically distinct viruses produce "herald waves." For several successive years, a relatively small wave of infections with an antigenically distinct virus can occur during the second half of an epidemic and herald the epidemic virus for the following year. These "herald waves" are useful to epidemiologists for predicting the viral antigens that should be included in each season's vaccine.

During the early stage of an epidemic, a disproportionate number of cases involve school-age children, 10 to 19 years old. Later in the epidemic, more cases are diagnosed in younger children and adults. The age shift suggests that the early spread of influenza viruses in a community is concentrated among schoolchildren.

Another characteristic of influenza virus is the decreased rate of infection in children living in urban areas compared to that of children in rural areas. In 1974 the rate of influenza B was four times greater for children living in rural areas of Michigan than in the urban areas. Children of low-income families in urban areas tend to become infected earlier in life and have milder illnesses. When these children experience intensive exposure to influenza type B during their school years, they may have immunity that is relatively more protective than that of children in the rural areas, who had less prior exposure.[10]

Parainfluenza Viruses

Parainfluenza is a single-stranded RNA virus of which four serotypes and two subtypes are recognized (parainfluenza types 1, 2, 3, 4A, and 4B). Peak activity of parainfluenza illness tends to occur in the fall and spring. These viruses can cause acute bronchitis, pneumonia, and bronchiolitis in young children. Most persons have been infected with parainfluenza virus by age 5. Immunity to parainfluenza is incomplete, and as with RSV, reinfection occurs throughout life. Parainfluenza types 1 and 2 tend to peak during the autumn of the year, whereas parainfluenza type 3 shows an increased prevalence during late spring. Adult infection results in mild upper respiratory tract symptoms, although pneumonia occasionally occurs. Outbreaks of parainfluenza types 1 and 3 have been reported from long-term care facilities.[11] Illness is characterized by fever, sore throat, rhinorrhea, and cough. The rate of pneumonia is relatively high.

Most studies suggest direct person-to-person transmission. Parainfluenza is stable in small-particle aerosols at the low humidity found in hospitals. Outbreaks tend to proceed more slowly than influenza or other aerosol-spread infections.[12] Infection control policies should emphasize hand-washing and isolation of patients.

Rhinoviruses

Rhinovirus is the most frequent cause of upper respiratory tract infections in adults. More than 100 antigenic types have been identified, and reinfection occurs throughout life. In temperate climates, rhinovirus infection shows spring and fall peaks of activity.[13] Rhinovirus infection is diagnosed by viral culture of nasopharyngeal secretions. In the healthy adult rhinovirus infection is self-limited and characterized by nasal congestion, rhinorrhea, and a mild sore throat. Although cough is common, direct viral invasion below the nasopharynx is rare. Cough is caused by reflex pathways. Unlike other respiratory viruses (influenza, adenoviruses) rhinovirus infections produce relatively minor damage to the nasal epithelium and probably no damage to the tracheal mucosa. Because rhinovirus replication is reduced at elevated body temperatures, direct invasion of the lower respiratory tract is unusual at all ages.

In one study, rhinovirus infections produced the first seasonal peak of respiratory infections in a long-term care facility.[14] Seasonal peaks occur most frequently between September and November. Rhinoviruses are easily transmitted by contact with infected secretions. The most efficient modes of spread are hand-to-hand contact or direct contact with a contaminated surface followed by inoculation of the nose or conjunctiva. Rhinoviruses remain infectious for as long as 3 hours on nonporous surfaces. Transmission can be decreased by hand-washing and disinfection of environmental surfaces.

Coronaviruses

Coronaviruses are single-stranded RNA viruses that have been identified as a major cause of colds in the general population. Epidemics occur during the winter and early spring.[15] Infections in volunteers have produced an illness similar to rhinovirus infection. Low-grade fever was present in approximately 20% of the patients. Upper respiratory tract infection is the most common result of coronavirus invasion. Coronaviruses have also been associated with exacerbations of chronic pulmonary diseases.

Diagnosis is difficult because the organism is not easy to isolate, and serology is generally not available. In a study of 11 long-term care facilities by Nicholson and Baker,[16] patients with respiratory illnesses were analyzed for evidence of coronavirus infections. Antibodies to the two best-studied antigenic strains of coronavirus (229 E and OC43) were detected by enzyme-linked immunosorbent assay (ELISA). It was noted that illnesses were indistinguishable from RSV and influenza virus infections. Lower respiratory complications, such as pneumonia, occurred in one-fourth of the infected residents.

Adenoviruses

Adenoviruses are double-stranded DNA viruses, with 41 recognized serotypes that most commonly cause infections in children. Coryza, pharyngitis, pneumonia, pharyngoconjunctival fever, and epidemic keratoconjunctivitis are attributable to adenoviruses. Transmission can occur by aerosolized droplets, fomites, and hand carriage as well as the fecal-oral route. The virus can be isolated for prolonged periods from respiratory secretions, conjunctival secretions, and stools of infected patients. The identification of adenoviruses can be confirmed by viral cultures, but the genetic heterogeneity of adenoviruses makes the information of little value. Outbreaks are uncommon in long-term care facilities for children or elderly patients. Should an outbreak of adenovirus occur, strategies for control should take into account the various modes of transmission.

Other Viruses

Herpes simplex and measles viruses are occasionally cultured from nasopharyngeal secretions of patients with upper respiratory infection. In one study[3] measles virus was found in 3% of nasopharyngeal cultures. The study showed a case-fatality rate of 43% among patients with upper respiratory infection from whom the measles virus was cultured. Similarly, herpes simplex virus showed a prevalence of 1.3% in nasopharyngeal cultures. There was no speculation about its involvement as a causative agent in the upper respiratory symptomatology.

Coxsackie and echoviruses are small RNA picornaviruses of about 60 types and subtypes. Most are transmitted from human to human by the fecal-oral route or by large-droplet spread. They tend to cause outbreaks during warm summer months. Clusters of cases are found in day-care centers, summer camps, and military camps. Coxsackie viruses are divided into two types, A and B, with about 20 subtypes of each. A variety of dissimilar syndromes vary with the age of the patient (Table 10.3).

Disease Presentations

Common Cold

The common cold, a disease of antiquity, is characterized by objective signs and subjective symptoms that are usually self-limited. Symptoms that occur with common colds include sneezing, watering of the eyes, nasal stuffiness, nasal obstruction, postnasal discharge, sore throat, hoarseness, cough, and sputum production. The common cold is a clinical diagnosis and lacks specificity because other ailments such as allergies and early symptoms of more serious illnesses mimic common cold symptoms. In the United States colds account for 23 million lost days of work and 26 million lost school days per year.

TABLE 10.3. Syndromes caused by Coxsackie and ECHO viruses, by subtype

Syndromes	Subtypes
Coxsackie type A viruses	
Herpangina	1–6, 8, 10, 22
Common cold	21
Pneumonia	9
Hand-foot-mouth disease	5, 10, 16
Coxsackie type B viruses	
Summer febrile illness with respiratory symptoms	All
Pleurodynia	All
Epidemic cervical myalgia	1–5
ECHO viruses	
Summer febrile illness	All
Common cold	11, 20

DIAGNOSIS

Rhinoviruses, coronaviruses, and RSV are most likely to cause cold symptoms. At times, influenza viruses, parainfluenza viruses, and adenoviruses do not cause their typical symptom patterns and appear as a minor illness. Five factors to consider in the differential diagnosis of the illness and virus are (1) age; (2) epidemiology; (3) physical findings; (4) progression of symptoms; and (5) laboratory tests.

Age. Rhinoviruses are by far the most common cause of respiratory illnesses in individuals age 5 to 40 years. Most of these infections manifest as the common cold. RSV and the parainfluenza viruses are common in those less than 2 years, manifesting as cold symptoms but suddenly progressing to more severe illness.

Epidemiology. Knowing the time of year and paying attention to the patterns of illness spreading through the community are helpful for distinguishing colds from other masqueraders.

Physical Findings. Physical findings should be limited to rhinorrhea and nasal congestion with minor contributions of other mild symptoms. Severe pharyngitis or any abnormal lung findings exclude the common cold from the diagnostic possibilities.

Progression of Symptoms. On the first day or two of other illnesses the prodromal symptoms may mimic a cold. After a few days, other illnesses progress to new or more severe symptoms, whereas a cold retains its original pattern. Patients should report changing symptom patterns to their physician.

Laboratory Testing. Influenza A and RSV can now be identified within 1 hour by rapid antigen tests available commercially. Nasopharyngeal washings are more likely to give a positive result than a nasal swab, but both are sensitive and specific. The other viruses may be identified in tissue cultures or by time-resolved fluoroimmunoassays (TR-FIAs) that are less widely available.

MANAGEMENT

There are as many ways to manage the common cold as there are physicians and mothers. Antibiotics have no effect on the causative viruses. Antihistamines have been shown to be of little use because the kinin system rather than histamine is responsible for rhinorrhea and congestion.[17–19] Antihistamines cause a generalized drying of the respiratory tract that may be unpleasant. More than 800 cold preparations are available over the counter in the United States.[20] The decongestant component in some remedies may be helpful but is dangerous for hypertensive patients. Aspirin, acetaminophen, and nonsteroidal antiinflammatory drugs (NSAIDs) are associated with a mild reduction in symptoms but have been shown to suppress the serum neutralizing antibody response and cause a highly significant increase in the rate of viral shedding.[21,22] They should not be used routinely but, rather, targeted for reducing myalgias and malaise. Even fever reduction is not a sacred reason for use of acetaminophen and antiinflammatory agents. Elevated body temperature has been shown to protect puppies from fatal viral infection.[23] Numerous studies have shown symptomatic improvement after raising the temperature of the nasal mucosa by inhaling heated vapor.[24,25]

Folk remedies such as hot chicken soup and vitamin C in large doses have large followings but no support in research literature. Zinc gluconate lozenges have enjoyed some interest as a possible treatment of common colds. Some research has shown strongly positive results with zinc.[26] Doses large enough to give positive results usually cause unacceptable side effects. In the future, antirhinovirus drugs and interferon may reach development levels where alleviation of symptoms or prevention of infection exceeds side effects.

COMPLICATIONS AND SEQUELAE

When the diagnosis of the common cold is accurate, complications and sequelae are minimal. Rhinoviruses and coronaviruses almost never progress to more serious disease. RSV, influenza virus, and parainfluenza virus infections frequently begin innocently but progress suddenly to life-threatening disease. Adenoviruses and Coxsackie viruses may appear to cause a cold but frequently produce additional symptoms and follow a different course.

Control and Prevention

Hand-washing is the most important way to prevent transmission of these viruses. With rhinoviruses and RSV, direct contact with a contaminated surface followed by inoculation of the nose or conjunctiva can result in infection. Use of masks and gloves and isolation of infected persons is the most effective way to limit the spread of cold viruses. With minimal symptoms and multiple sources of infection in the community, however, these measures are not practical.

Influenza

Influenza has one of the more characteristic sets of clinical findings. The onset is usually sudden, with shivering, sweating, headache, aching in the orbits, and general malaise and misery. Cough is often found early in the course, aggravating headaches and causing generalized aching. The onset is generally explosive, with fever in adults ranging up to 102°F. In children the fever may be higher than 102°F, and sore throat may be an early sign. The most consistent signs are the presence of polymyalgias, weakness, and malaise.

Diagnosis

Not surprisingly, the diagnosis of influenza is more accurate during epidemics and less accurate during nonepidemic periods. Influenza in the United States usually occurs during December, January, and February. Successful presumptive diagnosis requires appropriate clinical symptomatology at the right time of the year and a knowledge of the pattern of influenzal illness around the world. Influenza affects all ages, but children under age 2 years and elderly patients may be more severely affected. The cluster of symptoms tends to remain unchanged from beginning to end except in babies and the elderly, in whom progression to lower respiratory involvement may herald life-threatening illness. When spread of an A type influenza virus is reported, the rapid flu A (Directigen; Becton Dickinson) test can confirm infection in less than an hour. This antigen-based test is 91% sensitive and 95% specific, requiring only a throat swab or nasopharyngeal washings for detection. Conventional viral cultures and complement fixation tests are used only for retrospective study because they take 4 to 8 weeks for results. No rapid test is yet available for B type influenza.

Management

Management of influenza is generally symptomatic. If the family physician has a strong suspicion that the virus in question is type A influenza, the patient may benefit greatly from the use of amantadine or rimantadine. Amantadine (Symmetrel) or rimantadine (Flumadine) in a dose of 200 mg/day has long been known to be excellent prophylaxis against type A influenza.[27] It is most effective if started early in the course of the disease, although it does reduce symptoms and shorten the course of illness even if started 3 to 5 days into the disease process. The therapeutic dose of amantadine or rimantadine is 100 mg three times a day except in patients who have compromised renal function, for whom dosage adjustment is necessary. Because of the severity of the myalgias and headache associated with influenza, aspirin, and NSAIDs may not suffice to relieve pain, and a narcotic-containing product is frequently indicated. With good instructions, the patient can receive double benefit from codeine or hydrocodone, which reduces not only the myalgias but the cough.

COMPLICATIONS AND SEQUELAE

Pneumonia is usually blamed for excess mortality, but twice as many deaths during an influenza epidemic are attributable to ischemic heart disease than to pneumonia.[28] From July 1, 1975, through June 30, 1976, Glezen[28] studied 3301 hospitalized patients with the admission diagnosis of acute respiratory disease. Influenza and other respiratory disease were the cause 21.4% of the time. Glezen also noted that the rate of hospitalization with acute respiratory disease during the influenza A/Victoria epidemic varied by age group. Infants under age 1 had a hospitalization rate of 160 per 10,000 patients. Patients between age 1 and 65 had low hospitalization rates, whereas those over age 65 had a rate of 167 per 10,000. The rates of hospitalization were low in the school-age group, which would have had the highest rates with other infections.

CONTROL AND PREVENTION

Influenza vaccine is produced annually on the recommendation of the U.S. Food and Drug Administration (FDA) Vaccines and Related Biologicals Advisory Committee. Antigenic choices are based on (1) the viruses that have been seen during the previous year, (2) the viruses that are being seen in other parts of the world during the current year, and (3) the estimated antibody response in persons previously infected or vaccinated to these viruses.

There are two basic strategies for the use of vaccines and chemotherapy. A current strategy is to immunize high-risk groups (the elderly and children with underlying conditions including heart, pulmonary, malignant, and some metabolic diseases).[29] Healthy persons who become infected spread their infection to nonimmunized high-risk children. Another approach to the control of influenza is to immunize all schoolchildren, children in day-care, college students, military personnel, and employees of large companies. These groups have the highest susceptibility and, because of the nature of their activities, are the principal vectors of influenza virus in the community.

Bronchitis

DIAGNOSIS

Bronchitis is an inflammation of the major and minor bronchial branches. It is characterized by a cough that is frequently productive of sputum, depending on the inflammatory cause. Bacterial causes of bronchitis generally produce purulent-looking sputum. Viral causes of bronchitis can cause purulent-appearing sputum but more commonly produce either clear sputum or a nonproductive cough. On physical examination a patient with bronchitis has a noticeable cough, but the lungs are usually normal to auscultation except for a few scattered rhonchi. Rales, dullness to percussion, egophony, and other lower respiratory findings are usually absent. Cigarette smoking, other air pollutants, and chemical exposures that cause bronchial irritation may prolong an episode of bronchitis. Systemic lupus erythematosus is a cause of persistent bronchitis in a small number of affected patients.[30]

SPECTRUM OF INFECTION

Studies indicate that viral causes of acute bronchitis tend to be more common with influenza (types A and B), parainfluenza of all four serotypes, and RSV. Coronavirus and adenoviruses cause bronchitis less commonly. RSV and parainfluenza viruses are found more commonly in the young population, and coronaviruses and adenoviruses occur in older patients. Influenza causes bronchitis at all ages. Rhinovirus is the most frequent cause of upper respiratory tract infection in adults and can be a cause of coughing without bronchitis.

Glezen,[28] in a study of hospitalized patients with acute respiratory diagnoses, found acute bronchitis in 18.9%. He also found that adult admissions for bronchitis showed an appreciable increase only during the influenza A/Victoria epidemic, and pediatric admissions for bronchitis increased during the autumn parainfluenza types 1 and 2 epidemic and the RSV outbreak in December. Falsey and Treanor[4] reported that in institutionalized elderly patients RSV was likely to cause bronchitis, whereas rhinovirus was more likely to cause rhinorrhea with cough as a secondary symptom. Sputum production was considerably less frequent with the rhinovirus infection than with RSV infection.

Spasmodic Croup and Laryngotracheobronchitis

Spasmodic croup and laryngotracheobronchitis (LTB), or nonrecurrent croup, are different diseases caused by the same organisms. The focal points of their illnesses are croupy cough and inspiratory stridor. Spasmodic croup bursts into a family's life with a scary suddenness when their under-3-year-old child exhibits a croupy cough and stridor and appears dyspneic. This child has not been ill and has no fever. After a few frantic hours the croup clears, and the child is well until the next episode.

In contrast, LTB begins as a cold. For 3 to 5 days the young child has low-grade fever, rhinorrhea, congestion, sore throat, malaise, and cough. Fever gradually rises to 104° to 105°F, and the seal-like cough worsens to the point of inspiratory stridor. This child may be hoarse and may be wheezing too. Rarely airway obstruction requires intubation or bronchoscopy.

Both croups are the result of infection by a group of viruses including RSV, parainfluenza, influenza, adenoviruses, and coronaviruses. Influenza and RSV are more common during the winter months. The others are found in a fall and spring pattern. These viruses are transmitted by hand-to-hand contact or large-droplet aerosols. Knowing that influenza type A or RSV is in the community may be useful, as specific treatments are available.

Patients with spasmodic croup usually respond to breathing cool air (or in some cases warm mist in a steamed bathroom) and require little additional therapy. Resistant cases of spasmodic croup and most LTB cases respond to racemic epinephrine (0.05 ml/kg of 2.25% solution diluted in 3 ml of saline per application) administered as an aerosol. More severe cases of LTB require hospitalization for hydration and oxygen administration. Occasionally airway obstruction requires intubation. A single dose of intravenous steroid may preclude the need for intubation.

Bronchiolitis

CLINICAL PICTURE

Bronchiolitis is an acute viral respiratory disease generally found in children less than 2 years old. The typical clinical presentation is an upper respiratory infection with cough that progresses to a more severe cough and tachypnea. Respirations become rapid and shallow with a prolonged expiratory phase. Because the infants are not able to breathe well, they are also unable to suck or drink and can become dehydrated.

DIAGNOSIS

Physical findings include intercostal retractions and nasal flaring, which suggest pneumonia. A chest roentgenogram shows only hyperinflation with no infiltrates. Tight respiratory sounds (not entirely typical of wheezes found with asthma) are usually present, as are some rhonchi. Rales and dullness to percussion suggest the coexistence of pneumonia.

Bronchiolitis is most commonly caused by RSV, occurring predominantly during the winter and spring. Parainfluenza viruses, particularly types 1 and 2, can cause bronchiolitis during early winter. The most severe cases of bronchiolitis are usually caused by influenza viruses, especially type A. The virus involved can be identified by culture of nasopharyngeal secretions or rapid antigen tests for RSV and influenza A.

MANAGEMENT

Management of bronchiolitis depends on the progression of signs and symptoms. Hospitalization may be necessary to correct hypoxemia or dehydration. If fever is significant, pneumonia must be ruled out. Cases that appear to be recurrent bronchiolitis may be asthma, even if the child is less than 1 year old.

Outpatient treatment is generally supportive, with careful attention to hydration. If hospitalization becomes necessary to correct hypoxemia or dehydration, treatment is focused on oxygenation, mist, and mechanically clearing the upper airway.

COMPLICATIONS AND SEQUELAE

The most serious complication of bronchiolitis is respiratory failure requiring ventilatory assistance. It is best managed with continuous positive airway pressure and oxygen. Steroids and antibiotics are of questionable benefit for treating even the most severe cases of bronchiolitis. Ribavirin (Virazole) is useful as a continuous aerosol when RSV causes bronchiolitis. Ribavirin (6 g in 300 ml of water) is aerosolized in a small croup tent 16 to 20 hours a day for a minimum of 3 days up to 6 days.

FAMILY ISSUES

Family support is particularly important when infants require hospitalization. Many children subsequently wheeze with other viral respiratory illnesses, which alarms the family. The family needs to know that the long-term prognosis is excellent, although some research suggests that pulmonary function remains impaired in these children, especially those who have serious underlying respiratory or cardiovascular disease.

Pharyngoconjunctival Fever

Pharyngoconjunctival fever is an upper respiratory illness that affects teenagers and adults. It manifests as pharyngitis, cough, fever, headache, myalgias, malaise, and particularly conjunctivitis. This syndrome is caused by adenovirus serotypes 3 and 7, which are frequently found in natural bodies of water, reservoirs, and nonchlorinated swimming pools.

Symptoms may be similar to those of influenza. Conjunctivitis is generally not present with influenza but is always found with pharyngoconjunctival fever and usually at an early stage. There is a spring and summer seasonal prevalence. It can be diagnosed by viral cultures of nasopharyngeal and throat swabs or paired complement fixation antibody studies for adenovirus.

Management of pharyngoconjunctival fever is symptomatic. There is no indication for systemic antibiotic treatment or ophthalmic antibiotics. There are no long-term complications or sequelae. Recovery is generally within 1 to 2 weeks.

Laryngitis

There are six distinct causes of laryngitis, the most common being viral infections of the upper respiratory tract. Vocal cord tumors, allergies, and strain of the vocal cords caused by long periods of loud talking produce laryngitis. A fairly frequent cause of laryngitis is hard coughing associated with an upper or lower respiratory tract infection. The least frequent cause is a bacterial infection of the throat.

Most of the causes of laryngitis are obvious.[30] Viral laryngitis is difficult to distinguish from the less frequent bacterial laryngitis, which might require antibiotic treatment.

Children over age 2 and adults rarely have significant swelling of the throat that would put them at risk of airway obstruction. Children under age 2 are more likely to develop airway obstruction. Viral causes of laryngitis include the parainfluenza viruses, rhinoviruses, adenoviruses, and influenza viruses.

Voice rest makes the greatest impact on recovery. Patients who are able to gargle with warm, weak saline solution find it soothing. Patients should be told that laryngitis is not a serious disease and that adequate time to recover is the only therapy in most cases.

Herpangina

Herpangina accounts for up to 5% of all pharyngitis during the spring and summer. Several Coxsackie A subtypes are responsible for this common ailment of children and teenagers (Table 10.3). It is characterized by small numbers of vesicles on red bases that ulcerate on the soft palate and tonsillar pillars. The severity of the pain is out of proportion to the number and appearance of the small ulcers. Fever and headache are common. The punched-out red-based ulcers are so diagnostic that no cultures or prophylactic antibiotics are indicated. Treatment is symptomatic. Recovery is complete within 5 to 7 days.

TABLE 10.4. Patterns of viral illness in children and elderly patients

Virus	Signs and symptoms		
	Young children	Adults	Elderly
Respiratory syncytial virus	Wheezing, bronchiolitis, pneumonia, bronchitis	Nasal congestion and cough	Nasal congestion, cough, fever, pneumonia, wheezing, bronchitis
Influenza	Sore throat, high fever, myalgias, bronchitis, croup, bronchiolitis, rhinorrhea, otitis media	Fever, headache, myalgias, malaise, cough, weakness, bronchitis, laryngitis	Bronchitis, low-grade fever, sore throat, pneumonia
Parainfluenza	Croup, bronchitis, pneumonia, sore throat, bronchiolitis	Common cold, laryngitis	Rhinorrhea, sore throat, cough, pneumonia, fever
Rhinoviruses	Sore throat, rhinorrhea	Rhinorrhea, sneezing, cough, sore throat, laryngitis	Rhinorrhea, cough, sneezing
Coronaviruses	Croup, sore throat	Common cold, malaise, headache, sore throat, low-grade fever	Exacerbation of chronic pulmonary disease, pneumonia, bronchitis
Adenoviruses	Croup, sore throat	Coryza, sore throat, pneumonia, pharyngo-conjunctival fever, keratoconjunctivitis, laryngitis	Bronchitis rarely

Viral Respiratory Tract Infections in Very Young and Very Old Patients

Although most respiratory infections in children initially appear innocent, enough cases become severe to make them the third leading cause of death for infants 28 days to 1 year of age. Respiratory infections are the second leading cause of death from age 1 to 4 years.

Parents using the emergency room for evaluation of their children's colds have reasonable concern for the health of the child; but of 60,000 children seen at Cook County Hospital's Pediatric Emergency Room, Mayefsky and El-Shinaway[31] found more than 50% of the parents needed only reassurance that their child was not seriously ill.

Respiratory syncytial, influenza, and parainfluenza viruses are responsible for severe disease with excess mortality in very young children and elderly patients, while producing mild to moderate disease in everyone else. See Table 10.4 for a comparison of the effects of each virus on the three age groups. Mullooly and Barker[32] found rates of hospitalization three to five times higher during influenza epidemics for children under 4 years of age.

Many elderly persons living in long-term care facilities develop respiratory illnesses mistakenly attributed to bacterial pneumonia. Those illnesses due to RSV, influenza, and parainfluenza viruses frequently become severe and are responsible for excess mortality. A significant number of deaths during these infections are of cardiovascular origin rather than respiratory.

References

1. Acute conditions, incidence, and associated disability, United States, 1977–78. Washington, DC: US Department of Health Education and Welfare, 1977: 3. PHS 79-1560.
2. Milinaric G. Epidemiological picture of respiratory viral infections in Croatia. Acta Med Iugosl 1991;45:203–11.
3. Jain A. An Indian hospital study of viral causes of acute respiratory infection in children. J Med Microbiol 1991;35: 219–23.
4. Falsey AR, Treanor JJ. Viral respiratory infections in the institutionalized elderly; clinical and epidemiology findings. J Am Geriatr Soc 1992;40:115–19.
5. Dowling HF. Clinical syndromes in adults caused by respiratory viruses. Am Rev Respir Dis 1963;88: 61–72.
6. Denny FW. Acute respiratory infections in children: etiology and epidemiology. Pediatr Rev 1987;9:5.
7. McAnerney JM. Surveillance of respiratory viruses. S Afr Med J 1994;84: 473–7.
8. Monto AS, Sullivan KM. Acute respiratory illness in the community, frequency of illness and the agents involved. Epidemiol Infect 1993;110: 145–60.
9. McConnochie KM, Hall CB. Variation in severity of respiratory syncytial viruses with subtype. J Pediatr 1990;117:52–8.
10. Glezen WP. Consideration of the risk of influenza in children and indications for prophylaxis. Rev Infect Dis 1980;2:408–20.
11. Public Health Laboratory Service Communicable Disease Surveillance Center. Parainfluenza infections in the elderly 1976–1982. BMJ 1983; 287:1619.
12. Graman PS, Hall CB. Epidemiology and control of nosocomial viral infections. Infect Dis Clin North Am 1989;3:815–41.
13. Gwaltney JM, Mandell GL, Douglas RG Jr. Principles and practices of infectious diseases. 3rd ed. New York: Churchill Livingstone, 1989:1399–1404.
14. Grose PA, Rodstein M. Epidemiology of acute respiratory illness during an influenza outbreak in a nursing home: a prospective study. Arch Intern Med 1988;148:559–61.

15. Larsen HE, Reed JE. Isolation of rhinoviruses and coronaviruses from 38 colds in adults. J Med Virol 1980;5:211–19.
16. Nicholson KG, Baker DJ. Acute upper respiratory tract illness and influenza immunizations in homes for the elderly. Epidemiol Infect 1990;105:609–18.
17. Berkowitz RB, Tinkelman DG. Evaluation of oral terfenadine for treatment of the common cold. Ann Allergy 1991; 67:593–7.
18. Gaffey JJ, Kaiser DL. Ineffectiveness of oral terfenadine in natural colds: evidence against histamine as a mediator of common cold symptoms. Pediatr Infect Dis J 1988;7: 215–42.
19. Hutton N, Wilson MH. Effectiveness of an antihistamine-decongestant-combination for young children with the common cold: a randomized, controlled clinical trial. J Pediatr 1991;118:125–30.
20. Smith MBH, Feldman W. Over-the-counter cold medications. JAMA 1993;269:2258–63.
21. Graham NMH, Burrell CJ. Adverse effects of aspirin, acetaminophen, and ibuprophen on immune function, viral shedding, and clinical status in rhinovirus-infected volunteers. J Infect Dis 1990;162:1277–82.
22. Stanley ED, Jackson GG. Increased virus shedding with aspirin treatment of rhinovirus infection. JAMA 1975;231: 1248–51.
23. Carmichael LE, Barnes FD. Temperature as a factor in resistance of young puppies to canine herpesvirus. J Infect Dis 1969;120:669–78.
24. Ophir D, Elad Y. Effects of steam inhalation on nasal patency and nasal symptoms in patients with the common cold. Am J Otolaryngol 1987; 8:149–53.
25. Tyrrell D, Barrow I. Local hyperthermia benefits natural and experimental common colds. BMJ 1989;298:1280–3.
26. Eby GA, Davis DR. Reduction in duration of common colds by zinc gluconate lozenges in a double-blind study. Antimicrob Agents Chemother 1984;25:20–4.
27. Kobayashi JM. Control of influenza A outbreaks in nursing homes: amantadine as an adjunct to vaccine—Washington, 1989–90. MMWR 1991; 40:841–4.
28. Glezen WP. Serious morbidity and mortality associated with influenza epidemics. Epidemiol Rev 1982;4:25–43.
29. Liou YS, Barbour SD, Bell LM. Children hospitalized with influenza B infection. Pediatr Infect Dis J 1987;6:541–3.
30. Raz E, Bursztyn M. Severe recurrent lupus laryngitis. Am J Med 1992;92: 109–10.
31. Mayefsky JH, El-Shinaway Y. Families who seek care for the common cold in a pediatric emergency department. J Pediatr 1991;119:933–4.
32. Mullooly JP, Barker WH. Impact of type A influenza on children: a retrospective study. Am J Public Health 1982;72: 1008–16.

CASE PRESENTATION

Subjective

PATIENT PROFILE

Kendra Nelson is a 16-year-old single white female high school sophomore.

PRESENTING PROBLEM

Fever and weakness.

PRESENT ILLNESS

For the past day-and-a-half, Kendra has felt weak and achy. She has had a temperature of 103°F at home. There is a generalized headache, a mild cough, and a decreased appetite. A few of her schoolmates have had similar symptoms.

PAST MEDICAL HISTORY

No prior hospitalization or serious injury.

SOCIAL HISTORY

Kendra lives with her parents. She is a "good student" and has had a steady boyfriend for the past year.

HABITS

She uses no tobacco, alcohol, or coffee.

FAMILY HISTORY

Her parents are living and well. She has one sibling, aged 19, who is away from home in the Army.

- What additional historical information might be useful, and why?
- What might be the meaning of this illness to the patient?
- Would further information regarding her classmates or boyfriend be helpful? Why?
- What are likely adaptations of this teenager to her illness? Why might this be pertinent?

Objective

VITAL SIGNS

Blood pressure, 104/60; pulse, 86; respirations, 22; temperature, 38.6°C.

EXAMINATION

The patient is alert and ambulatory but looks "ill." The tympanic membranes are normal. The pharynx is mildly injected. The neck is supple without adenopathy, and the thyroid gland is normal. Her chest is clear. The heart has a normal sinus rhythm with no murmurs present.

- What further information about the physical examination might be useful, and why?
- What other areas of the body—if any—should be examined? Why?
- What—if any—laboratory tests should be obtained today? Why?
- What—if any—diagnostic imaging studies should be obtained today?

Assessment

- What is the likely diagnosis, and how would you explain this to the patient and her parents?
- Kendra's mother asks if Kendra is likely to be even worse during the next few days and what to do if this occurs. How would you reply?
- If the patient also had a rash, what diagnoses would you consider?
- What are the family/community implications of this illness?

Plan

- What would be your therapeutic recommendation to Kendra regarding medication, diet, pain relief, and return to school?
- Kendra asks about the possibility of others catching her illness. How would you reply?
- Kendra's mother asks about preventing such an illness in the future. How would you respond?
- What continuing care would you recommend?

11

Otitis Media and Otitis Externa

Jo Ann Rosenfeld and Greg Clarity

Otitis media and otitis externa are routinely and frequently diagnosed in office practice and are generally treated with few poor outcomes. They are usually easily diagnosed, and the organisms that cause them are well known. Yet, astonishingly, there remain several basic controversies in the treatment and care of individuals with these entities. Several large meta-analysis studies and multidisciplinary and specialist task forces have attempted to create a consensus on the treatment of these common disorders.

There are three separate, although related, diagnostic and therapeutic entities: acute otitis media, serous otitis media, and otitis externa. Acute otitis media is a sudden purulent infection of the middle ear that occurs often in children and is usually easily cured, although it can be recurrent or persistent. Serous otitis media is inflammatory and chronic. Otitis externa is an infection of the external canal. Although usually easily diagnosed and treated, all three diseases are common causes for physician visits and can have serious outcomes.

Acute Otitis Media in Children

Most children have an episode of acute otitis media (AOM) by age 3, and many have more than one.[1] AOM remains the most common diagnosis in children in office practice.[2,3] It accounts for one-third of all the visits to physicians by children under age 1 in the United States—up to 30 million visits annually[4,5]—and more than 25% of all antibiotic prescriptions.[3]

Etiology

Eustachian Tube Dysfunction

The most probable cause of AOM in children is eustachian tube (ET) dysfunction. In infants and small children, because of the ET's increased flexibility or the swelling of lymphoid tissue underneath the lining, fluid accumulates in the middle ear. Children have short, small ETs; the same volume of nasopharyngeal secretions that may be cleared by the adult ET may accumulate in children. Finally, the ET of children is more horizontal. When lying supine, especially while sucking or drinking as taking a bottle in bed, a child is more likely to have a reflux of fluid from the nasopharynx. Until age 6 children are less able to clear secretions in the middle ear by swallowing. Even in otologically normal children the ET does not work as competently as it does in adults. ET function improves with age.[6]

True mechanical dysfunction of the ET can be caused by congenital physical abnormalities, such as in children with Down syndrome or cleft lip or palate. Children with cleft palate may have undeveloped ET muscles that are often inserted incorrectly and predispose the child to AOM and serous otitis media (SOM).[4] Possible differences in ET anatomy among ethnic groups and between genders may account for the differences in the incidence of AOM.[7]

OTHER CAUSES

Other factors can complicate already poor ET function. Viral infections, including upper respiratory tract infections (URIs), are linked with the development of AOM. About 50% to 75% of children with URIs develop abnormal ET function.[6] Respiratory syncytial virus, adenoviruses, and rhinoviruses have all been cultured from middle ear fluid.[8]

Respiratory allergy plays a part in the etiology. Some children lack the ability to produce an adequate allergic response to eradicate bacteria in the middle ear.[9] Some children who have frequent AOM have elevated immunoglobulin E (IgE) levels, decreased IgG levels against *Streptococcus pneumoniae,* allergic rhinitis, and other signs of allergy.

Acute otitis media can occur rarely from local extension of infection or hematogenous spread. Primary mucosal disease of the middle ear due to allergy may be another factor.

Certain groups of children are more likely to develop AOM. Infants (preterm and term) and children under age 2 are more likely to have AOM; the incidence of AOM decreases with age.[5] Bottle-fed infants and infants put to bed with a bottle, perhaps because of the increased likelihood of reflux into the ET, are more likely to develop AOM.[10] Children with cleft lip or palate and Down syndrome often develop recurrent AOM. Native American children have a greater incidence of AOM.

Acute otitis media occurs more often during winter and spring, paralleling the incidence of URIs. Children who are more likely to acquire URIs, such as those in day care, those who have several siblings, and those who live in a house with smokers have a greater incidence of

AOM.[5] The 3.4 million office visits for AOM yearly can be attributed to parental smoking.[11]

Clinical Symptoms and Signs

The symptoms of AOM are characteristic in older children and less specific in infants. Older children complain of otalgia, often with fever, headache, nausea, anorexia, accompanying URI symptoms, and occasionally discharge from one ear. Younger children may present nonspecifically with fussiness, irritability, lethargy, vomiting, diarrhea, anorexia, abdominal pain, fever, and possibly pulling on one ear.

Diagnosis

The diagnosis is clinical and is made by direct otoscopy and confirmed by pneumatic otoscopy. The canal can be normal and pink, or swollen and red, or have a discharge that is yellow, white, or less commonly green. The tympanic membrane, instead of being pearly gray and translucent, is dull and red, with loss of sight of the bony landmarks in the middle ear. There may occasionally be pus, fluid, or air bubbles behind the membrane. Occasionally the membrane has ruptured, and then a discharge is present in the canal.

Pneumatic otoscopy confirms the diagnosis. Instead of normal bidirectional movement of the tympanic membrane (TM), there is usually no movement or occasionally only movement inward because of negative middle ear pressure. Although not necessary for the diagnosis of AOM, tympanometry can confirm the presence of fluid in the middle ear.

The diagnosis may be more difficult in children with canal wax accumulation and in small, anxious children or infants. Restraining children, allowing them to stay on the mother's lap, or giving them a bottle while making sure to pull the pinna back may improve the ease of the examination. If possible, the ears are examined before the child starts to cry because crying may cause erythema of the membrane. The mobility of the TM in the infant is decreased. Pneumatic otoscopy and tympanometry may not be reliable in infants younger than 7 months.[12]

Causative Organisms

In most children the bacterial organisms that cause AOM are the same organisms that are present in the nasopharynx, varying with the age of the child. From age 6 weeks until 4 years, *Streptococcus pneumoniae* and *Haemophilus influenzae* are the most common organisms, as well as *Moraxella catarrhalis,* and β-hemolytic streptococci. Above age 4, *H. influenzae* is less likely to cause AOM.

In children under age 2 months, most (85%) AOM is caused by the normal bacteria of the nasopharynx. However, approximately 15% of AOM in this group is caused by gram-negative enterobacteria, specifically *Escherichia coli* and *Klebsiella*. These infections are usually due to hematogeneous spread, making sepsis and meningitis, although rare, more likely sequelae than in the older children.[4]

The sensitivities of the bacterial organisms to the β-lactamase antibiotics have changed, as have the relative incidences of infection by organism. Up to 40% of *H. influenzae* and 90% of *M. catarrhalis* strains are now β-lactamase producers (BLP).[13] *M. catarrhalis* has become a more frequent cause of otitis media, being responsible for up to 22% of AOM. AOM caused by *M. catarrhalis* is less likely to be associated with fever and earache.[14]

Treatment

TO TREAT OR NOT TO TREAT?

The paradox of AOM is that it may resolve without pharmacologic intervention. Although the standard care has been antibiotic therapy, it is now being questioned. In up to one-third of cases of AOM, culturing the middle ear fluid produces no organisms.[15] Eichenwald reported that spontaneous resolution of AOM occurs in up to 60% of cases within 10 days of illness.[4] In 1981 Van Buchem, studying 171 children, found that reduction of pain, temperature, duration of discharge, and otoscopic appearances were all unrelated to any of four therapeutic methods: no treatment, myringotomy, antibiotics, or myringotomy and antibiotics. Few studies other than these have had a no-treatment group, so prevalent is the conviction that antibiotics are necessary. Most recently, Rosenfeld in a meta-analysis of 33 clinical studies involving 5400 patients, showed that 81% of patients improve without antibiotics or tympanocentesis.[16] Six of every seven children with AOM may not need antibiotics. Unfortunately, there is no reliable way to sort out which one needs treatment. All seven children must be given antibiotics to treat the one who actually needs them. The primary benefit of treating AOM with antibiotics may not be the alleviation of symptoms or the sterilization of fluid in the middle ear but, instead, the decrease of suppurative complications. Another study showed a modest reduction in pain from AOM with use of antibiotics by day 2 to 7. Seventeen children must be treated with antibiotics to prevent pain in one child.[17]

Until further studies have a no-treatment group, and it can be determined which child will worsen without treatment, it is reasonable to treat all cases of AOM with antibiotics, although time may more often cure AOM rather than the choice of a particular antibiotic.

ANTIBIOTIC CHOICE

Given these analyses, the choice of a particular antibiotic over another may become less important. Rosenfeld reported no significant differences in the efficacy of several antimicrobial agents and found that using an antibiotic with activity against BLPs did not improve cure.[7] Factors to take into account when choosing antibiotics include community bacterial resistance patterns, known or suspected allergies of the child, cost of the drug to the patient, dosing interval and its effect on compliance, approval on certain formularies, taste and palatability, and the child's and family's history with the drug.

First Choice. The antibiotic of choice for AOM is amoxicillin (Table 11.1). Amoxicillin is active against many strains of *H. influenzae* and *S. pneumoniae,* is not affected by food intake, and is relatively inexpensive.[2,18] Amoxicillin had the highest levels of penetration into middle ear fluid in one study, making it the preferred treatment for AOM.[19]

Another good choice, especially if the child is allergic to penicillin, is a fixed combination of trimethoprim-sulfamethoxazole (TMX-sulfa).[20] TMX-sulfa combinations are fairly inexpensive, are given only twice a day, and are effective against many organisms. They are not effective against *Streptococcus pyogenes* and should not be used if there is coexistent streptococcal pharyngitis.[2] The liquid preparations of TMX-sulfa are well tolerated in grape, fruit-licorice, or strawberry flavors. It should not be used in children with glucose-6-phosphate dehydrogenase (G6PD) deficiency or those who are folate-deficient. There is a significant, if small, percentage of children who become allergic to sulfa medications; and serious allergic complications including Stevens-Johnson syndrome are not rare.

Second Choices. There are a wide variety of second choices. The one chosen depends on individual sensitivity, tolerances, community patterns of bacterial resistances, and formularies (Table 11.2). If amoxicillin has been used, another antibiotic should be chosen, perhaps one effective against BLP.

The erythromycin-sulfisoxazole combination (Pediazole) has a wide spectrum of activity. It is moderately expensive and has a strawberry-banana taste. It can cause nausea, epigastric distress, and hemolysis in persons with G6PD deficiency. It should be given with food four times a day.[2] Two macrolide antibiotics, azithromycin (Zithromax) and clarithromycin (Biaxin) have liquid preparations approved for treatment of AOM. They cover BLPs, but the palatability of liquid clarithromycin is a problem for some patients.

Cefaclor (Ceclor) or cefuroxime (Ceftin), second generation cephalosporins, or cefixime (Suprax), an oral third generation cephalosporin, are significantly more expensive than amoxicillin but can be used as alternatives. Cephalexin is less expensive than the other ceph-

TABLE 11.1. Some common antibiotics used for acute otitis media

Agent	Flavor/dosing	Spectrum of activity	Comments
First-line drugs			
Amoxicillin	20–40 mg/kg/day tid; strawberry, bubble-gum flavored suspension	Covers *H. influenzae, S. pneumoniae,* some staphylococci	Some diarrhea; may be taken with food; not in penicillin-allergic patients; Stevens-Johnson and allergic reactions possible
Other first-line drugs			
Trimethoprim-sulfa-methoxazole (Bactrim; Septra)	8 mg/kg/day TMX/40 mg/kg/ day sulfa bid; strawberry, grape, fruit, licorice	Effective against *S. pneumoniae* and *H. influenzae* including some β-lactamase producers (BLPs)	Contraindicated in infants < 2 months; not in sulfa-allergic patients; significant intolerances and allergies (can be given generic)
Second-line drugs			
Penicillins			
Amoxicillin/ clavulanate (Augmentin)	20–40 mg/kg/day tid; banana, orange	Similar to amoxicillin with activity against BLPs	Use with caution in penicillin-allergic patients; chewable tablets; may cause diarrhea
Cephalosporins			
Cefaclor (Ceclor)	40 mg/kg/day tid/bid; grape, cherry	Effective against staphylococci, group A streptococci, *H. influenzae* including some BLPs	Can cause serum sickness-like reaction
Cefuroxime axetil (Ceftin)	250 mg bid in adults	Efficacy like that of cefaclor	Available only as a tablet, which may be crushed but has a bitter taste
Cephalexin (Keflex)	125 mg tid–qid; bubble-gum flavored	Spectrum like that for cefuroxime	Can be generic
Cefixime (Suprax)	8 mg/kg up to 400 mg qd or bid; strawberry	Effective only against group A β-hemolytic streptococci, *S. pneumoniae,* and *H. influenzae* including some BLP strains	Once-daily dosing may help compliance
Ceftriaxone	one single IM dose (up to 50 mg/kg)		Once-dosing IM may be useful in certain situations.
Others			
Erythromycin ethylsuccinate/sulfi-soxazole (Pediazole)	50 mg/kg/day eryth. qid; strawberry, banana	Effective against staphylococci, group A β-hemolytic streptococci and *H. influenzae*	Contraindicated in infants < 2 months; often used in patients allergic to penicillin

Table 11.1. (*continued*)

Agent	Flavor/dosing	Spectrum of activity	Comments
Clarithromycin (Biaxin)	7.5 mg/kg bid; cherry	Covers *S. pneumoniae* and *H. influenzae* including BLPs	Palatability may be a problem
Azithromycin (Zithromax)	10 mg/kg/day (1st day) then 5 mg/kg/day; cherry	Covers *S. pneumoniae* and *H. influenzae* including BLPs	Once daily dosing for 5 days
Sulfisoxazole (Gantrisin)	250 mg qid; strawberry	Effective against many gram-positive and gram-negative organisms; not totally effective against staphylococci or *H. influenzae* alone	Used for prophylaxis; can be generic
Sulfamethoxazole (Gantanol)	125–500 bid; cherry	As for sulfisoxazole	Used for prophylaxis; can be generic

alosporins; it is prescribed four times a day and has a bubble-gum flavor.[21] Cefaclor is well absorbed, moderately expensive, reaches good levels in the middle ear, and has two well tolerated flavors, grape and cherry; food does not decrease its absorption. Serum sickness is a serious reaction.[22]

Cefuroxime, although effective, is not currently available in liquid form, limiting its use in children.[21] Cefixime and cefpodoxime proxetil (Vantin) are the only oral third generation cephalosporins. They are effective against BLPs and many gram-negative bacilli, but not *S. aureus*.

A fixed combination of amoxicillin with clavulanic acid (Augmentin), which inactivates β-lactamase production, can be used. Its side effects include diarrhea and abdominal pain. It is moderately expensive, is not affected by food intake, and is given three times a day.[21] One IM dose of ceftriaxone (50 mg/kg) is clinically comparable in cure to 10 days of TMP/sulfa[23]

Table 11.2. Efficacy of selected antimicrobial agents on common pathogens for acute otitis media

Antibiotic	Streptococci	*H. influenzae*	*B. catarrhalis*	*S. pyogenes*	*S. aureus*
Amoxicillin	+	+/–	+/–	+	+/–
Erythromycin-sulfisoxazole	+	+	+	+	+
Trimethoprim-sulfisoxazole	+	+	+	–	–
Cefaclor	+	+	+	+	+
Cefixime	+	+	+	+/–	–

Length of Treatment and Compliance

Usually treatment is prescribed for 10 days.[4] A randomized double-blind, controlled trial comparing 3- and 10-day courses of amoxicillin showed little difference in the speed of resolution of symptoms and signs.[24] All children should have their ears rechecked for cure within 3 weeks.

Compliance may be a problem. In one study, nearly 40% of patients did not complete the course of antibiotics.[21] Compliance can be improved by using an antibiotic with fewer daily doses, by giving the parent verbal and written instructions, and by dispensing medications with calibrated measuring devices.[25] Many early treatment failures are caused by lack of compliance to the regimen. Compliance is better if the family is seen by their own doctor, not by partners or emergency room doctors. Compliance is also improved, especially in children, by using liquid preparations that have more acceptable flavors.

Surgical Treatment

There is no place for surgical treatment of AOM that is not persistent or recurrent. Although myringotomy, incision of the tympanic membrane, may provide symptomatic relief, it provides no improvement over antibiotics in terms of resolution, response, or audiometric tests and may in fact be ineffective in curing AOM.[21]

Adjuvant Measures for Comfort

It has been common practice to prescribe antihistamines or decongestants for relief of pain and alleviation of discomfort. These agents do not alter the course or improve the cure rate of AOM.[21] For otalgia, analgesic otic drops may be of benefit.[21]

Care of Infants with AOM

In infants age 6 weeks or younger, primary therapy may be cefaclor or amoxicillin-clavulanate, rather than amoxicillin because 10% to 15% of AOM is caused by gram-negative enteric bacilli and *S. aureus,* which may be resistant to amoxicillin.[21] These infants may require hospitalization and parenteral antibiotics, as AOM can be a sign of systemic infection. Continuing fever despite antibiotic therapy, dehydration, vomiting, toxic appearance, lethargy, anorexia, or severe diarrhea are indicators of the need for hospitalization.

There are times when immediate referral or admission to the hospital is recommended. Hospitalization may be indicated for children with AOM who are toxic or seriously ill, who have cystic fibrosis, who have a continued severe febrile course despite antibiotics, in whom suppurative complications occur, who are less than 6 months old, or who are immunocompromised. When a child treated for AOM presents with persistent headache, lethargy, malaise, irritability, continued severe otalgia, facial pain, stiff neck, focal seizures, ataxia, blurred vision, papilledema, diplopia, hemiplegia, aphasia, dysdiadochokinesia, intention tremor, dysmetria, hemianopsia, or persistent unremitting fever, a suppurative intracranial complication should be suspected. Although rare, these entities can be dangerous if not treated early and adequately.

Persistent Infectious Otitis Media

After a course of antibiotics the child should be reexamined at 10 to 30 days. If the tympanic membrane still is affected, an alternate antibiotic active against BLPs should be prescribed for another 10-day course. Studies suggest that early recurrent AOM may be a result of relapse with the initial infecting organism or noncompliance.[26] Only a few organisms obtained by tympanocentesis have been found to be resistant to the antibiotic initially chosen.[27] The child should be reexamined to document cure after another 10 to 30 days. If no improvement or worsening occurs, referral to an otolaryngologist for surgical drainage for therapy and culture might be indicated.

Recurrent Otitis Media

Some children clear one episode of AOM, with a documented cure, only to experience another soon after. The flora of the ear fluid of children with recurrent AOM, when episodes are separated by a month or more, is similar to that found during the first episode.[28] Spontaneous recovery is often the case, making the use of prophylaxis or surgery questionable. Thus second episodes of AOM should be treated in the same manner as the first episode. In these children chronic antibiotic prophylaxis may prevent recurrences of AOM.[29] Young children and those in day-care may benefit more by prophylaxis.[30]

Daily prophylactic antibiotics should be considered if there are three to four episodes within 6 to 18 months. Sulfisoxazole has been proved effective for preventing recurrent symptomatic AOM and is safe for long-term use (Table 11.3).[31,32] In a crossover double-blind study of 35 children ages 6 months to 5 years with recurrent infectious otitis media, sulfisoxazole reduced the rate of AOM recurrences by 40%.[33] Amoxicillin, erythromycin, or trimethoprim-sulfisoxazole have also been suggested for use. Treatment should continue for up to 6 months.[21]

A search should also be made for respiratory allergies or a physical abnormality of the pharynx. In older children sinusitis should be ruled out by radiography and treated if present (see Chapter 9). In some children immunologic studies are warranted, especially if other infections are present. Children with recurrent AOM should be examined for evidence of chronic middle ear effusions.[1]

Table 11.3. Antibiotics used for chronic prophylaxis against recurrent AOM

Antibiotic	Age group	Dose
Sulfamethoxazole	Children > 2	250 mg bid
	2–5 years	500 mg bid or 75 mg/kg/day bid
Erythromycin	All ages	20 mg/kg/day bid
Amoxicillin	All ages	20 mg/kg/day bid
Trimethoprim-sulfamethoxazole	> 2 months old	TMX 8 mg/kg/day

Influenza vaccine may decrease risk of developing AOM during the flue season[34]

AOM in Adults

Acute otitis media in adults presents differently than in children. The initial symptoms are usually pain, sore throat, hearing loss, discharge, and otorrhea but not fever.[29,35] The hearing loss is primarily conductive and usually mild to moderate. The physical examination is usually similar to that in children and may reveal a red eardrum or a nonhealing perforation of the eardrum. There is usually intermittent or recurrent discharge that is usually mucopurulent but can also be green and fetid. URIs usually accompany AOM.

Streptococcus pneumoniae is slightly less likely to be the cause of AOM in adults. *H. influenzae* has been found in increased frequency in older children and adults during 10% to 33% of AOM episodes.[32,36] Adults treated with oral antibiotics are less likely to recover than those not treated.[36] Treatment should provide coverage for *S. pneumoniae, H. influenzae,* and other gram-positive organisms.

Amoxicillin is still the drug of choice. Tetracycline, doxycycline, or cephalexin can be used; erythromycin or penicillin alone are inadequate. If there are a high incidence of BLPs in the community or if patients are at high risk, diabetic, or immunocompromised, cefuroxime axetil, amoxicillin-clavulanic acid, or trimethoprim-sulfisoxazole may be a better first choice.

Serous Otitis Media

Diagnosis and Etiology

Chronic serous otitis media (SOM) is the persistent presence of fluid in the middle ear. It can be painful, cause decreased hearing, or be asymptomatic, detected only on a follow-up visit for AOM or by chance.

The diagnosis is suggested by pneumatic otoscopy. Air bubbles, an air-fluid level, or decreased motion of the tympanic membrane with insufflation are diagnostic.

Tympanometry is 85% specific for diagnosing SOM. Normal tympanograms have a peaked appearance. Flat tympanograms suggest fluid behind the membrane and SOM.[24]

The etiology of SOM is complex and not completely understood. Eustachian tube dysfunction, AOM, allergies, passive smoke inhalation, and URIs can contribute to chronic SOM (CSOM). Serous effusions are found in as many as 40% of children after AOM.[4] There is a higher incidence of CSOM in children with allergy, URIs, and in children who live in urban areas and who have parental smoking in the home.[37–39] In one study, up to 76% of children with SOM had prior URIs.[7]

Significance of SOM in Children

The belief that SOM produces hearing loss and learning disabilities has driven physicians to great lengths to eradicate the fluid from the middle ear. Many believe that rapid, adequate treatment, with hopefully normalization of hearing, is essential for normal growth and development. More surgery is performed on children to correct SOM than for any other reason, although the natural course of the effusions in many cases is spontaneous resolution.[1,29,36,40,41] In one study of private pediatric practices, 70% of children had middle ear effusions at the conclusion of antimicrobial therapy at 2 weeks; without treatment only 40% continued to have effusions at 1 month, 20% at 2 months, and 10% at 3 months.[1]

Long-term, persistent fluid in the middle ear can produce a chronic hearing loss, which is usually conductive.[7,42] It is the most common complication of middle ear disease. Sensorineuronal involvement can also occur. The determination of when and how long effusions in the middle ear can cause severe enough hearing loss to affect growth and development is disputed. Several studies show developmental abnormalities in children with SOM, but many of these studies were retrospective.[41,43,44] There were several studies in which the associations between SOM and later developmental impairment were not found.[15,44,45]

There may be a critical period during infancy when SOM is particularly disabling, especially if it is bilateral.[7,18] One such time may be within the first 6 months of life (see Chapter 4). Other experts suggest that acquisition of language is not limited to specific and fixed periods of brain development, and most children catch up with their peers once the effusion resolves and hearing is restored.[4]

Treatment

The American Academy of Pediatrics, the American Academy of Family Physicians, and the American Academy of Otolaryngology convened a consensus panel to develop guidelines for management of otitis media with effusion (CSOM) in young children.[44] They did not find rigorous, methodologically sound research to support the belief that untreated SOM results in speech and language delay or deficits; they did find that SOM usually resolves spontaneously within 3 months. Observation and antibiotic therapy are treatment options for children with SOM less than 4 to 6 months in duration and at any time in a child without a hearing deficit. Myringotomy with tube placement is indicated in a child with bilateral CSOM for 3 months with a bilateral hearing deficit of at least 20 dB threshold loss or worse, or a child with 4 to 6 months of bilateral SOM and hearing deficit. Earlier surgical treatment may be an option in children with neurologic or balance disturbances. Steroids, antihistamines, adenoidectomy, and tonsillectomy are not recommended.

SURGICAL TREATMENT

Myringotomy and tympanostomy with tube placement (MTTP) is currently the most common surgical procedure requiring general anesthesia in children. Each year tympanostomy tubes are placed in 1 million children, and 600,000 children undergo tonsillectomy.[1]

Although MTTP cures SOM immediately, the tubes extrude within 4 to 8 months, and there is continuing controversy as to whether there is any long-term improvement in hearing or a decrease in the recurrence or persistence of SOM. Recurrence of middle ear effusions after extrusion of PE tubes is likely in as many as 20% to 40%.[7] Tympanograms of children 3 to 5 years after placement of PE tubes were no different from those of children who were not treated by surgery.[46] Little difference in hearing has been found with children treated surgically or not with 3 to 6 months of follow-up.[29]

The consensus panel concluded that MTTP is indicated in a child with bilateral CSOM for 3 months with a bilateral hearing deficit of at least 20 dB threshold loss or worse, or a child with 4 to 6 months of bilateral CSOM and hearing deficit.

TREATMENT OF SOM IN ADULTS

There is no consensus about treatment of SOM in adults. Treatment should be medical, as for children, with antibiotics and antihistamines. Unless there is demonstrable conductive hearing loss, surgery is probably not indicated. MTTP has been used in adults with some short-term improvement of hearing; long-term studies have not been done.[47]

Acute Otitis Externa

Acute Otitis Externa in Children

In children a common cause of acute otitis externa (AOE) is foreign bodies, which must be removed on detection. All varieties of objects have been found in the ears of children, from toys, paper, and jewelry to dirt. Some potentially serious objects include watch batteries, which must be removed immediately. These objects can be removed by simple instruments, irrigation, or suction.[48] Children and adults with abnormal or congenitally defective ears are more likely to develop otitis media.

Traumatic injury can cause otitis. Human bites to the pinna are usually infected and often serious; the infection frequently extends into the canal. Treatment includes simple closure of wounds, if clean. More complex injuries must be meticulously débrided with conservation of tissue. Any hematomas are drained by needle or incision, repeatedly if fluid reaccumulates. Some kind of pressure bandage should be used: fluffed gauze, Ace wrap, or a tie-through suture.

Swimmer's Ear (Acute Inflammatory Otitis Externa)

Prolonged exposure to swimming has been correlated with the development of "swimmer's ear," or acute inflammatory otitis externa. The inflammation is often accompanied by infection, making treatment somewhat more complicated than just avoidance of swimming. Swimmers who developed otitis media were more likely to have swum longer, more frequently, and with more frequent submersion of their head than swimmers without otitis media, independent of the type of water. Otitis media was more likely associated with swimming in freshwater rather than in the ocean and a pool; it increased with a month of exposure, but only in those who swam frequently.[49] Swimmer's ear is more likely in hot, humid climates, and 10 to 20 times more likely during the summer.[50]

Clinically, the patient complains of pain and itch for 1 to 2 days after prolonged swimming. There can be a history of local trauma, scratching or rubbing the canal, or prolonged occlusion of the canal. Clinical symptoms include otorrhea (which can be white, green, or foul-smelling), otalgia, pinna pain, and even hearing loss. Examination reveals a swollen canal that is often red, with discharge. Pulling the pinna up and backward often elicits discomfort.

The repeated exposure to water removes the protective waxy coating of the external auditory canal, allowing it to become macerated and predisposed to infection by gram-negative bacteria. *Pseudomonas aeruginosa,* the universal inhabitant of moist environments, is the most likely bacterial cause of external otitis. Other pathogens include *E. coli, Aerobacter, S. aureus,* streptococci, and some *Proteus* species.

Once the canal is infected and swollen, treatment includes gentle cleaning if possible. A topical medication is then the treatment of choice. Topical medications include acid/alcohol drops, which reduce inflammation and are antifungal (Otic Domeboro aqueous or Vosol Otic with propylene glycol). A 1:1 mixture of vinegar and rubbing alcohol is less expensive and probably just as effective, although it can be painful and thus difficult to administer to children. An antibiotic-steroid liquid preparation can be used to reduce inflammation and infection. The antibiotic preparations used can be a combination of polymyxin B and neomycin or colistin sulfate (to provide gram-negative and gram-positive coverage) or gentamicin alone. Both preparations, gentamicin and colistin-neomycin-hydrocortisone, produce few side effects. However, gentamicin is more likely to eradicate organisms, whereas the others relieve inflammation in a shorter period. Gentamicin drops can produce systemic allergies. Hydrocortisone is added to decrease inflammation.[50]

Topical medication should be given three or four times a day. If the canal is too swollen to allow easy access for the drops, a wick of 0.25 inch gauze or cotton may be inserted into the swollen external canal for 24 to 36 hours. Medication can then be dropped onto the wick. Treatment should be continued 7 to 10 days and ear canal protected from water for 2 weeks. Systemic antibiotics are seldom needed.

Most episodes of swimmer's ear can be prevented. Children or adults who often develop otitis externa can avoid prolonged exposure to moisture, utilize preventive antiseptics, or use water-repellent skin coating. Eardrops, such as Vosol or Otic Domeboro, can be utilized after swimming. Treating predisposing skin conditions such as eczema can minimize the incidence of swimmer's ear.

Chronic Otitis Externa

Chronic otitis externa is inflammatory (caused by conditions that affect other skin surfaces) or infectious. Psoriasis, eczema, and seborrhea can all cause chronic otitis externa (COE). Some people have chronically itching ears with dry, scaly skin. It is usually associated with dry skin elsewhere on the body and with aging. If it occurs only in the patient's ears, it may be a self-inflicted problem of habitual cleaning or picking at the ears. Treatment is education and a change of habits. The patient must be told to keep everything out of the external auditory canal and to place two or three drops of baby oil in the external ear canal on a daily or weekly basis. This regimen provides excellent relief.[50]

Some adults have excessive accumulation of cerumen, which may lead to conductive hearing loss, impaction with or without secondary infection, and pain and frustration when it has to be removed. Such excessive cerumen is worsened by patients who use cotton-tipped applicators, which irritate the canal and push the cerumen farther back. Treatment includes prior installation of a wax softener, such as olive or mineral oil, or use of carbamide peroxide (which should be used cautiously because it can cause dermatitis itself). Irrigation can then be used if the tympanic membrane is intact. After removal of the wax, the hearing function should be evaluated. Often a steroid-containing otic solution is given for 7 to 10 days to reduce subsequent swelling. Acetic acid drops may prevent further accumulation.

Psoriasis can cause persistent external otitis (see Chapter 19). It presents with dry, itchy, flaky skin and is treated with steroid cream or lotion. Seborrhea can cause a scaly inflammation in the external auditory canal (EAC) and behind the external ears. Usually it is accompanied by seborrhea of the eyelids, forehead, and face. It can be controlled by antiseborrheic shampoos daily and topical steroids. Allergic reactions can occur in the EAC as well as anywhere. Allergy may be caused by nickel-plated earrings. Eczema and atopic disease can affect the external ear as well. Symptoms include chronically itching ears.

Treatment of most forms of chronic inflammatory otitis externa includes removal of debris and reduction of swelling. Steroid otic solutions may help reduce the swelling. A few drops of oil can be used to reduce pruritus. A wick can be placed daily with Domeboro Otic. The patient should be counseled to avoid using anything to scratch the EAC. Systemic antibiotics are almost never used unless there is evidence of otitis media. If the patient has diabetes mellitus or arteriosclerosis, close observation is necessary for other infectious complications.

Chronic infection may be caused by recurrent infection of congenital cysts or sinus tracts. Treatment may include antibiotic therapy and local treatment such as hot packs. Incision of cysts may be necessary. Fungal infections of the external ear can be persistent and difficult to cure. They are more likely in adults, diabetics, and immunocompromised hosts. The discharge can be green or white or have white and black amorphous debris caused by *Aspergillus niger.* Fungi are an unusual cause of chronic otitis externa in temperate climates, though they are common in the tropics. The fungi recovered are saprophytes; *Aspergillus, Penicillium, Rhizopus,* and *Alternaria* are the most common species. *Candida* and tinea dermatophytes can cause a low-grade infection and inflammation. Treatment must be thorough. The canal must be cleaned well, possibly with an operating microscope, removing all loose surface skin. Application of sulfanilamide powder may be used.

Malignant Otitis Externa

Malignant otitis externa (MOE) was first reported in 1968 as an infection caused by *Pseudomonas aeruginosa*. Rare but potentially lethal, it is a rapidly progressive, necrotizing, serious infection that begins in the EAC. Among 150 reported cases, nearly all were in elderly patients (average age 68); 90% were in diabetics. Eight cases were reported in children with Stevens-Johnson syndrome, leukopenia, malnutrition, chemotherapy, AIDS, or diabetes mellitus.[52] MOE spreads to soft tissue underneath the temporal bone and may lead to facial nerve palsy, mastoiditis, multiple cranial nerve palsies, meningitis, and occasionally death. Recognized early and treated appropriately, sometimes with surgical débridement, the consequences of MOE have decreased in severity. Before combined carbenicillin-gentamicin therapy was common, the overall mortality was 50% to 63%. The mortality was higher if the patient developed nerve palsies. Now, 95% are cured.

The symptoms include an intensely inflamed ear filled with granulation tissue and pus. Examination reveals erythema, swelling, and tenderness of auricular and preauricular tissue, sometimes with a unilateral facial palsy, which is almost always permanent. Standard therapy is aggressive parenteral aminoglycoside and carbenicillin plus surgical débridement. Long-term therapy with outpatient tobramycin, carbenicillin, or both decreases its severity.

References

1. Bluestone CD, Klein JO, Paradise JL, et al. Workshop on effects of otitis media on the child. Pediatrics 1983;71:639–52.
2. Bluestone CD. Management of otitis media in infants and children: current role of old and new antimicrobial agents. Pediatr Infect Dis 1988;7:S129–36.
3. Bluestone CD. Modern management of otitis media. Pediatr Clin North Am 1989;36:1371–87.
4. Eichenwald HE. Developments in diagnosing and treating otitis media. Am Fam Physician 1985;31:155–64.
5. Howie VM, Schwartz RH. Acute otitis media. Am J Dis Child 1983;137: 155–8.
6. Klein BS, Dollete FR, Yolken RH. The role of respiratory syncytial virus and other viral pathogens in acute otitis media. J Pediatr 1982;101:16–20.
7. Rosenfeld JA, Clarity G. Acute otitis media in children. Prim Care Clin North Am 1996;23:677–85.
8. Chonmaitree T, Howie VM, Truant AL. Presence of respiratory viruses in middle ear fluids and nasal wash specimens from children with acute otitis media. Pediatrics 1986;77: 698–702.
9. Bernstein JM. Recent advances in immunologic reactivity in otitis media with effusion. J Allergy Clin Immunol 1988;81: 1004–9.

10. Shaefer O. Otitis media and bottle feeding. Can J Public Health 1971;62: 478–83.
11. Aligne CA, Stoddard JJ. Tobacco and children. Arch Pediatr Adolesc Med 1997;151:648–653.
12. Marchant CD, Shurin PA, Turczyk VA, et al. Course and outcome of otitis media in early infancy: a prospective study. J Pediatr 1984;104:826–31.
13. Barnett ED, Klein JO. The problem of resistant bacteria for the management of acute otitis media. Pediatr Clin North Am 1995;42:509–17.
14. Marchant CD. Spectrum of disease due to *Branhamella catarrhalis* in children with particular reference to acute otitis media. Am J Med 1990; 88:15S–19S.
15. Hoffman-Lawless K, Keith RW, Cotton RT. Auditory processing abilities in children with previous middle ear effusions. Ann Otol Rhinol Laryngol 1981;90:543–5.
16. Rosenfeld RM. Clinical efficacy of antimicrobial drugs for acute otitis media: metaanalysis of 5400 children form thirty-three randomized trials. J Pediatr 1994;14:731–7.
17. Delmar C, Glaziou P, Hyem M. Are antibiotics indicated as initial treatment for children with acute OM? BMJ 1997;314:1526–9.
18. Zenk KE, Ma H. Pharmacological treatment of otitis media and sinusitis in pediatrics. J Pediatr Health Care 1990;4:297–303.
19. Krause PJ, Owen NJ, Nightingale CH, et al. Penetration of amoxicillin, cefaclor, erythromycin-sulfisoxazole, and trimethoprim-sulfamethoxazole into the middle ear fluid of patients with chronic serious otitis media. J Infect Dis 1982; 145:815–21.
20. Barnett ED, Klein JO. The problem of resistant bacteria for the management of acute otitis media. Pediatr Clin North Am 1995;42:509–17.
21. Lorentzen P, Haugsten P. Treatment of acute suppurative otitis media. J Laryngol Otol 1977;91:331–40.
22. Giebink GS, Batalden PB, Russ JN, Le CT. Cefaclor v. amoxicillin in treatment of acute otitis media. Am J Dis Child 1984;138:287–92.
23. Barnett ED, Teele DW, Klein JO, et al. Comparison of ceftroaxone and TMP-sulfa for AOM. Pediatrics 1997;99:23–28.
24. Chaput de Saintonge DM, Levine DF, Savage, IT, et al. Trial of three day and ten day courses of amoxicillin in otitis media. BMJ 1982;284:1078–81.
25. Reed BD, Lutz LJ, Zazove P, Ratcliffe SD. Compliance with acute otitis media treatment. J Fam Pract 1984;19:627–32.
26. Barenkamp SJ, Shurin PA, Marchant CD, et al. Do children with recurrent *Haemophilus influenzae* otitis media become infected with a new organism or reacquire the original strain? J Pediatr 1984;105:533–7.
27. Legler JD. An approach to difficult management problems in otitis media in children. J Am Board Fam Pract 1991;4:331–9.
28. Jahn AF, Abramson M. Medical management of chronic otitis media. Otolaryngol Clin North Am 1984;17:673–7.
29. Bartelds AIM, Bowers P, Bridges-Webb C, et al. Acute otitis media in adults: a report from the international primary care network. J Am Board Fam Pract 1993;6:333–9.

30. Principi N, Marchisio P, Massironi E, et al. Prophylaxis of recurrent otitis media and middle ear infections. Am J Dis Child 1989;143:1414–18.
31. Liston TE, Foshee WS, Pierson WD. Sulfisoxazole chemoprophylaxis for frequent otitis media. Pediatrics 1983;71:524–30.
32. Sugita R, Fujimaki Y, Deguchi K. Bacteriologic features and chemotherapy of adult acute purulent otitis media. J Laryngol Otol 1985;99:629–35.
33. Schwartz RH, Puglise J, Rodriguez WJ. Sulfamethoxazole prophylaxis in the otitis-prone child. Arch Dis Child 1982;57: 590–3.
34. Clements DA, Langdon L, Bland C, Walter E. Influenza A vaccine decreases the incidence of otitis media in 6 to 30 month old children in day care. Arch Pediatr Adolesc Med 1996;150:652–3.
35. Froom J, Mold J, Culpepper L, Boisseau V. The spectrum of otitis media in family practice. J Fam Pract 1980;10:599–605.
36. Celin SE, Bluestone CK, Stephenson J, et al. Bacteriology of acute otitis media in adults. JAMA 1991;266: 2249–53.
37. Fireman P. Otitis media and nasal disease: a role for allergy. J Clin Immunol 1988;82:917–26.
38. Schenker MB, Samet JM, Speizer FE. Risk factors for childhood respiratory disease: the effect of host factors and home environmental exposures. Am Rev Respir Dis 1983;128: 1038–43.
39. Ferris BG, Ware JH, Berkey CS, et al. Effects of passive smoking on health of children. Environ Health Perspect 1985;62: 289–95.
40. Tos M, Holm-Jensen S, Sorensen CH, Mogenson C. Spontaneous course and frequency of secretory otitis in 4 year old children. Arch Otolaryngol 1982;108:4–10.
41. Rapin I. Conductive hearing loss effects on children's language and scholastic skills: a review of the literature. Ann Otorhinollaryngol Suppl 1979; 88:3–12.
42. Callahan CW, Lazoritz S. Otitis media and language development. Am Fam Physician 1988;37:186–90.
43. Paradise JL. Secretory otitis media: what effects on children's development? Adv Otorhinollaryngol 1988;40: 89–98.
44. Paradise JL. Otitis media during early life; how hazardous to development? A critical review of the evidence. Pediatrics 1981;68:869–73.
44. U.S. Department of Health and Human Services. Managing otitis media with effusion in young children. Clin Pract Guidel 1994;QR1–QR12.
45. Roberts JE, Sanyal MA, Burchinal MR, et al. Otitis media in early childhood and its relationship to later verbal and academic performance. Pediatrics 1986;78:423–30.
46. Gates G, Wachtendorf C, Hearne E, Holt G. Treatment of chronic otitis media with effusion: results of tympanostomy tubes. Am J Otolaryngol 1985;6:249–53.
47. Brenman AK, Meltzer CR, Milner RM. Myringotomy and tube ventilation in adults. Am Fam Physician 1982;26:181–4.
48. Amundson LH. Disorders of the external ear. Prim Care 1990;17:213–31.

49. Springer GL, Shapiro ED. Fresh water swimming as a risk factor for otitis externa: a case controlled study. Arch Environ Health 1985;40:202–6.
50. Marcy SM. Infections of external ear. Pediatr Infect Dis 1985; 4:192–201.
51. Reich JJ. Ear infections. Emerg Med Clin N Amer 1987;5:227–42.
52. Keim RJ. How aging affects the ear. Geriatrics 1977;12:97–9.

CASE PRESENTATION

Subjective

PATIENT PROFILE

Jason Harris is a 4-year-old white male child.

PRESENTING PROBLEM

Earache.

PRESENT ILLNESS

For 2 days, Jason has complained of a left earache. There has been a low-grade fever, sore throat, and nasal congestion. Jason has had three prior episodes of earache over the past 6 months.

PAST MEDICAL HISTORY

No serious illness or hospitalization since birth.

SOCIAL HISTORY

Jason attends day care 5 mornings per week.

FAMILY HISTORY

His parents are both living and well. There is a 1-year-old sibling.

- What other historical information might be pertinent, and why?
- What might be the significance of having had three prior episodes of ear infection?
- What—if anything—might be pertinent about the child's day-care experience?
- What more might you like to know about the family history, and why?

Objective

Vital Signs

Pulse, 78; respirations, 22; temperature, 38.0°C.

Examination

Patient is alert but in pain with a left earache. The left tympanic membrane is injected but not retracted or bulging. There is mild injection of the pharynx without tonsillar swelling or exudate. There are few enlarged left cervical lymph nodes. The chest is clear, and the heart is normal.

- What more—if anything—would you include in the physical examination, and why?
- How might you evaluate the child's hearing?
- What—if any—laboratory tests might you order today?
- If there were thick purulent drainage from the ear, what would be its significance?

Assessment

- What is the probable diagnosis? Describe the likely etiologic agent(s).
- How would you explain this diagnosis to the family?
- The parents ask if Jason needs a referral to an ear, nose, and throat specialist. How would you respond?
- What are the family implications of this illness?

Plan

- What therapeutic recommendations would you make regarding medication for relief of pain?
- When can Jason return to day care? What might influence your decision?
- If Jason's mother calls tonight to report that there is purulent drainage from the left ear, what would you advise?
- What follow-up would you advise for this illness?

12

Ischemic Heart Disease

JIM NUOVO AND AMIR SWEHA

Cardiovascular disease remains the most significant cause of morbidity and mortality in the United States. In 1995 approximately 1.5 million Americans experienced a myocardial infarction (MI) and 700,000 of them died.[1] It is estimated that 6.1 million Americans are alive today with a history of MI, angina, or both. The financial impact of this disease is enormous. The cost estimate for cardiovascular disease in 1995 was $110 billion. It is important for all primary care providers to implement screening and preventive care programs to reduce the burden of cardiovascular disease. Because of the high morbidity and mortality it is also important to recognize the early manifestations of this disease.

Unfortunately, in up to 20% of patients the first manifestation of ischemic heart disease (IHD) is sudden cardiac arrest.[2] Most deaths from IHD occur outside the hospital and within 2 hours of the onset of symptoms.[3,4] Since the 1960s a great deal of effort has been directed toward the practice of cardiopulmonary resuscitation and emergency cardiac care. These efforts have been directed toward minimizing the number of cardiac deaths.[5] Furthermore, there has been an substantial undertaking to identify and treat individuals with significant cardiovascular risk factors with the goal of lowering morbidity and mortality (see Chapter 2). This effort has been successful as noted by the decline in death rates from myocardial ischemia and its complications. The purpose of this chapter is to discuss three issues relevant to the family physician regarding IHD: the evaluation of patients with chest pain, the diagnosis and management of angina pectoris, and the diagnosis and management of MI.

Chest Pain

Chest pain is one of the common reasons for patients visiting primary care physicians.[6] The major diagnostic considerations for chest pain are listed (Table 12.1). Of the diagnostic considerations, which are the most commonly seen by family physicians? A Family Practice Research Network investigated this issue. Over 1 year the Michigan Research Net-

TABLE 12.1. Common causes of chronic and recurrent chest pain

Cardiac causes
Hypertrophic cardiomyopathy
Ischemic heart disease
Mitral valve prolapse
Pericarditis
Chest wall problems
Costochondritis
Myofascial syndrome
Gastrointestinal causes
Esophageal motility disorders
Gastroesophageal reflux
Neurologic causes
Radiculopathy
Zoster (postherpetic neuralgia)
Psychiatric causes
Anxiety
Depression
Hyperventilation
Panic disorder

work (MIRNET) prospectively collected information on 399 patients with episodes of chest pain. The most common diagnostic findings were (1) musculoskeletal pain (20.4%); (2) reflux esophagitis (13.4%); (3) costochondritis (13.1%); and (4) angina pectoris (10.3%).[7] The highest priority is generally given to distinguishing cardiac from noncardiac chest pain. Of the many diseases listed, the most common differential diagnostic considerations are of esophageal and psychiatric etiologies.

Noncardiac Chest Pain

Noncardiac chest pain remains a complex diagnosis and management problem. Studies have demonstrated that 10% to 30% of patients with chest pain who undergo coronary arteriography have no arterial abnormalities.[8,9] Follow-up studies of these patients have shown that the risk of subsequent myocardial infarction is low.[10–17] Fifty to seventy-five percent of these patients have persistent complaints of chest pain and disability.[12,14] The most common noncardiac problems in the differential are esophageal disorders, hyperventilation, panic attacks, and anxiety disorders.

ESOPHAGEAL CHEST PAIN

Of the patients who have undergone coronary arteriography and have been found to have normal coronary arteries, as many as 50% have demonstrable esophageal abnormalities.[17–19] Richter et al.[20] critically reviewed 117 articles on recurring chest pain of esophageal origin to clarify issues related to this disease. They paid specific attention to the following controversial issues: potential mechanisms of esophageal pain, differentiation of cardiac and esophageal causes, evaluation of esophageal motility disorders, use of esophageal tests for evaluating noncardiac chest pain, usefulness of techniques for prolonged monitoring of intraesophageal pressure and pH, and the relation of psychological abnormalities to esophageal motility disorders. They concluded that: (1) Specific mechanisms that produce chest pain are not well understood. (2) Esophageal chest pain has usually been attributed to the stimulation of chemoreceptors (acid and bile) or mechanoreceptors (spasm and distension). (3) Studies done to confirm direct associations between these factors and pain have not been consistent in their findings.

It appears that the triggers for esophageal chest pain are multifactorial and often idiosyncratic to a particular patient. Differentiating cardiac from esophageal disease can be frustrating. As many as 50% of patients with coronary disease have esophageal disease.[21] There are many esophageal disorders that produce pain mimicking myocardial ischemia.[22] Areskog et al.[23] have shown that esophageal abnormalities are common in patients who are admitted to a coronary care unit and are later found to have no evidence of cardiac disease. The clinical history frequently does not differentiate between cardiac and esophageal chest pain, although features may be helpful in this process. Features suggesting esophageal origin include pain that continues for hours, pain that interrupts sleep or is meal-related, pain relieved by antacids, or the presence of other esophageal symptoms (heartburn, dysphagia, regurgitation).[24] Conversely, it is well documented that gastroesophageal reflux may be triggered by heavy exercise and may produce exertional chest pain mimicking angina even during treadmill testing.[22]

Tests that can be done to determine the presence of esophageal disease include esophageal motility testing, continuous ambulatory esophageal pH monitoring, and provocative testing (e.g., acid perfusion and balloon distension).[25] Although findings from these tests have produced a better understanding of the pathologic conditions leading to the development of chest pain with esophageal disorders, there is no consensus as to the usefulness of these tests for the specific patient with chest pain. As noted by Pope,[26] "What is needed is a simple and safe provocative esophageal maneuver to turn on chest pain that possesses a high degree of sensitivity."

There is clearly an interaction between psychological abnormalities and esophageal disorders. Patients with esophageal disorders have been shown to have significantly higher levels of anxiety, somatization, and depression.[27] It is not clear if there is a cause-and-effect relation. Given the aforementioned difficulties in the diagnosis of esophageal chest pain, the differentiation of this pain from cardiac disease, and the close relation between cardiac, esophageal, and psychiatric disease, it is wise to maintain a consistent approach to the evaluation of these patients. Richter et al.[20] developed a stepwise approach for patients with recurring chest pain. They recommended exclusion of cardiac disease, with the subsequent evaluation to rule out structural abnormalities of the upper gastrointestinal (GI) tract (barium swallow, upper GI series, and endoscopy). Also recommended is a trial of antireflux therapy for 1 to 2 months. In those patients who fail to respond, specialized testing may then be appropriate (esophageal motility, 24-hour pH monitoring, provocative testing, and psychological evaluation).[25]

PSYCHIATRIC ILLNESS

There has long been a connection between psychiatric disorders and noncardiac chest pain. Katon et al.[28] reported the results of an evaluation of 74 patients with chest pain and no history of organic heart disease. Each patient underwent a structured psychiatric interview immediately after coronary arteriography. Patients with chest pain and negative coronary arteriograms were significantly younger, more likely to be female, more apt to have a higher number of autonomic symptoms (tachycardia, dyspnea, dizziness, paresthesias) associated with chest pain, and more likely to describe atypical chest pain. These patients also had significantly higher scores on indices of anxiety and depression that met *Diagnostic and Statistical Manual of Mental Disorders, Third Edition (DSM-III)* criteria for panic disorder, major depression, and phobias.

Waxler et al.[29] concluded that 40% of women with chest pain who had normal coronary arteries had hypochondriacal or neurotic behavior. In another study 19 of 46 patients with normal coronary arteries continued to experience chest pain despite reassurance that the pain was noncardiac. The authors believed that these patients tended to be chronically neurotic and socially maladjusted.[30] Iatrogenic uncertainty may also contribute to persistent pain. Specific medical therapy directed at anxiety and depression may help some of these patients. Cannon et al.[31] reported a study on a group of patients with chest pain despite normal coronary angiograms. Imipramine was shown to improve their symptoms. Patients who were given 50 mg nightly had a statistically significant reduction (52%) in episodes of chest pain.

Cardiac Chest Pain: Angina Pectoris

Angina is not simply one type of pain; it is a constellation of symptoms related to cardiac ischemia. The description of angina may fit several patterns.

1. *Classic angina.* It presents as a ill-defined pressure, heaviness (feeling like a weight), or squeezing sensation brought on by exertion and relieved by rest. The pain is most often substernal and left-sided. It may radiate to the jaw, interscapular area, or down the arm. Angina usually begins gradually and lasts only a few minutes.
2. *Atypical angina.* Similar symptoms are experienced but with the absence of one or more of the criteria for classic angina. For example, the pain may not be consistently related to exertion or relieved by rest. Conversely, the pain may have an atypical character (sharp, stabbing), but the precipitating factors are clearly anginal.
3. *Anginal equivalent.* The sensation of dyspnea is the sole or major manifestation.
4. *Variant (Prinzmetal's) angina.* This angina occurs at rest and may manifest in stereotyped patterns, such as nocturnal symptoms or symptoms that appear only after exercise. It is thought to be caused by coronary artery spasm. Its symptoms often occur periodically, with characteristic pain-free intervals, and are associated with typical electrocardiographic (ECG) changes, most commonly ST segment elevation.[32]
5. *Syndrome X (microvascular angina).* Some patients with the clinical diagnosis of coronary artery disease have no evidence of obstructive atherosclerosis. Several reports investigating this population have found a subset with metabolic evidence for ischemia (myocardial lactate during induced myocardial stress as evidence for ischemia). Kemp et al. reported this group to have "syndrome X."[33,34] It has been suggested that some of these patients have microvascular angina.[35]

It is important for clinicians to recognize the factors that may confound the clinical diagnosis of angina pectoris. Some of these factors are as follows: (1) The severity of pain is not necessarily proportional to the seriousness of the underlying illness. (2) The physical examination is not generally helpful for differentiating cardiac from noncardiac disease. A normal examination cannot be counted on to rule out significant cardiac disease. (3) The ECG is normal in more than 50% of patients with IHD. A normal ECG cannot be used to rule out significant cardiac disease. (4) Denial is a significant component in the presentation of chest pain caused by MI. (5) Some of the diseases common in the differential diagnosis of chest pain may present concurrently. Major depressive disorder and panic disorder are known to be prevalent in patients with esophageal disorders.[21] Colgan et al.[36] reported that of 63 patients with chest pain and normal angiograms 32 (51%) had evidence of an esophageal disorder, and 19 of the 32 (59%) had a current psychiatric disorder (anxiety or depression). Patients with concurrent disorders are particularly challenging to the clinician sorting out the cause of the chest pain.

Clinical Tools Used to Distinguish Cardiac from Noncardiac Chest Pain

Despite the difficulties noted above, there are important clinical tools that can be used to distinguish cardiac from noncardiac chest pain.

HISTORY

Despite the mentioned difficulties the history is key to distinguishing cardiac from noncardiac etiologies of chest pain. Noncardiac chest pain is often fleeting, brief, sharp, or stabbing. The pain may be reproduced by palpating the chest wall. The duration of pain is also important. Symptoms that last many hours or days are not likely to be anginal. A great deal of work has been done to assess the probability of IHD in a given patient based on the clinical presentation. In 1979 Diamond and Forrester[37] presented such an approach. Using data from the clinical presentation correlated with autopsy and angiographic information, they presented a pretest likelihood of coronary artery disease in symptomatic patients according to age, sex, and type of chest pain (nonanginal, atypical angina, or typical angina). Several observations can be made from this chart (Table 12.2): Men have a substantially greater risk than women for any given type of chest pain and for any given age. A middle-aged man with atypical chest pain is at high risk for having significant coronary artery disease. Young women (ages 30–40 years) with classic angina have a relatively low risk of having significant coronary artery disease.

DIAGNOSTIC TESTING

After establishing a pretest probability of IHD, there are a variety of tests available to help establish an accurate diagnosis. Although many tests are now firmly established in clinical practice, none is particularly suited to wide-scale, cost-effective application because each has limitations concerning sensitivity and specificity.

Exercise Tolerance Testing. In 1986 the American College of Cardiology and the American Heart Association Task Force on Assessment of

TABLE 12.2. Pretest likelihood of significant ischemic heart disease based on symptoms

	Likelihood of IHD, M/F (%)		
Age (years)	Nonanginal	Atypical angina	Typical angina
30–39	5.0/0.8	22/4	69/26
40–49	14/3	46/13	87/55
50–59	21/8	59/32	92/79
60–69	28/18	67/54	94/90

Source: Diamond and Forrester.[37] With permission.

Cardiovascular Procedures set guidelines for exercise treadmill testing (ETT).[38] For patients with symptoms suggestive of coronary artery disease there are five basic indications for undertaking exercise stress testing: (1) As a diagnostic test for patients with suspected IHD; (2) to assist in identifying those patients with documented IHD who are potentially at high risk due to advanced coronary disease or left ventricular dysfunction; (3) to evaluate patients after coronary artery bypass surgery; (4) to quantify a patient's functional capacity or response to therapy; and (5) to follow the natural course of the disease at appropriate intervals. The purpose of ETT for the patient with chest pain is to help establish whether the pain is indeed due to IHD.

Although there are many exercise protocols available, the protocols proposed by Bruce in 1956 remain appropriate. A review of the ETT for family physicians has been published.[39,40] In the standard ETT (Bruce protocol) the patient is asked to exercise for 3-minute intervals on a motorized treadmill device while being monitored for the following: heart rate and blood pressure response to exercise, symptoms during the test, ECG response (specifically ST segment displacement), dysrhythmias, and exercise capacity. Contraindications to ETT include unstable angina, MI, rapid atrial or ventricular dysrhythmias, poorly controlled congestive heart failure (CHF), severe aortic stenosis, myocarditis, recent significant illness, and an uncooperative patient. A significant (positive) test includes an ST segment depression of 1.0 mm below the baseline. Many factors influence the results of an ETT and can lead to false-positive or false-negative findings. Factors leading to false-positive results include (1) the use of medications such as digoxin, estrogens, and diuretics; and (2) conditions such as mitral valve prolapse, cardiomyopathy, and hyperventilation. Factors leading to false-negative results include (1) the use of medications such as nitrates, β-blockers, calcium channel blockers; and (2) conditions such as a prior MI or a submaximal effort.[38,41] The sensitivity of the ETT has been estimated to range from 56% to 81% and the specificity from 72% to 96%.[42] The key point is that given the vagaries of the ETT for diagnosing IHD (generally low sensitivity and specificity) a patient with a high pretest likelihood of IHD (e.g., a 50-year-old man with typical angina) still has a high probability of developing significant disease even in the face of a normal (negative) test. Furthermore, a patient with a low probability of IHD (e.g., a 40-year-old woman with atypical chest pain) still has a low chance of significant disease even if the test is positive.[37] The optimal use of diagnostic testing is for those patients with moderate pretest probabilities (e.g., a 40- to 50-year-old man with atypical pain).

In addition to the diagnostic implications of an ETT, there are prognostic implications. The following are considered to be parameters associated with poor prognosis or increased disease severity: failure to complete stage 2 of a Bruce protocol, failure to achieve a heart rate over 120 bpm (off β-blockers), onset of ST segment depression at a heart rate of less than 120 bpm, ST segment depression over 2.0 mm, ST segment depression lasting more than 6 minutes into recovery, ST segment depression in multiple leads, poor systolic blood pressure response to exercise, ST segment elevation, angina with exercise, and exercise-induced ventricular tachycardia.[38]

Radionuclide Perfusion Imaging. There are patients in whom the standard ETT is not a useful diagnostic tool and in whom a radionuclide procedure would be more appropriate. Patients with baseline ECG abnormalities due to digitalis or left ventricular hypertrophy with strain or those with bundle branch block (especially left bundle branch block) cannot have proper evaluation of the ST segment for characteristic ischemic changes. In these patients a radionuclide stress test is appropriate. The principle behind radionuclide testing is as follows: Myocardial thallium 201 chloride uptake is proportional to the coronary blood flow. A myocardial segment supplied by a stenotic coronary artery receives less flow relative to normal tissue, causing a thallium perfusion defect. Thallium washout is also slower in stenotic areas. With perfusion imaging, both stress and rest images are compared for perfusion. As a general rule, a defect is visible on thallium imaging if there is 50% or more stenosis in a coronary artery. In the standard exercise thallium test, repeat imaging is performed 3 to 4 hours after completion of the ETT. Some investigators advocate 24-hour imaging in patients with perfusion defects to look for delayed reversibility.

For patients unable to exercise, thallium imaging can be performed using dipyridamole (Persantine) as a coronary vasodilator. Adenosine may also be used. Its advantages over dipyridamole include an ultrashort half-life (less than 10 seconds) and better coronary vasodilation. Two technetium radiopharmaceuticals [technetium sestamibi (Cardiolyte) and technetium teboroxime (Cardiotech)] have been approved for myocardial perfusion imaging. These agents may eventually replace thallium because of more favorable imaging characteristics.[43,44]

Compared to the standard ETT, the thallium 201 ETT has the advantage of increased sensitivity (80–87%) and specificity (85–90%).[40] Dipyridamole, adenosine, and technetium perfusion testing has a sensitivity ranging from 70% to 95% and specificity from 60% to 100%. Unfortunately, the cost of these procedures is almost four times as great as a standard ETT ($175–$250 versus $1000–$1400).[39]

Stress Echocardiography. Ischemic heart disease can be detected with stress echocardiography. During stress-induced myocardial ischemia, the affected ventricular walls become hypokinetic. Studies suggest that physical exercise and dobutamine may be the preferable means of provoking ischemia in patients undergoing stress echocardiography.[45,46] Preliminary data suggest a higher sensitivity and specificity than for the standard ETT and increased usefulness for predicting subsequent myocardial events; however, the primary utility of this test appears to be for detection of ischemia in patients who are unable to exercise adequately. Similar values for sensitivity and specificity between stress echocardiography and perfusion imaging have been reported. Stress echocardiography may be particularly valuable in patients who have a questionable defect on perfusion imaging.[45,46]

Response to Nitroglycerin. Another approach employs clinical information to determine the probability of coronary artery disease based on response to treatment. One such study involved the use of sublingual nitroglycerin to determine the likelihood of disease. Horwitz et al.[47] evaluated the usefulness of nitroglycerin as a diagnostic aid for IHD. They found a sensitivity of 76% and a specificity of 80% in 70 patients with chest pain of anginal type. It was concluded that 90% of patients with recurrent, angina-like chest pain who exhibit a prompt response to nitroglycerin (within 3 minutes) have IHD; however, a delayed or absent response paradoxically indicates either an absence of IHD or unusually severe disease. Therefore failure to respond to nitroglycerin should not be used to exclude the diagnosis of IHD.

Angina Pectoris

Once the diagnosis of angina is established there are several important management considerations for this disease. The first is related to disease prognosis, the second to drug therapy, and the third to further investigative tests and invasive therapeutic interventions.

Prognosis

Three major factors determine the prognosis of patients with angina pectoris: the amount of viable but jeopardized left ventricular myocardium, the percentage of irreversibly scarred myocardium, and the severity of underlying coronary atherosclerosis. A number of studies were reported before invasive therapies were available that assess the prognosis of patients with stable angina. Most of them appeared between 1952 and 1973 and reported an annual mortality of 4%.[48,49] Since cardiac catheterization has come into general use, the prognosis has been modified and is based on the number of diseased vessels. During the 1980s the annual mortality rates for patients with one-vessel disease, two-vessel disease, three-vessel disease, and left main coronary artery disease (CAD) were 1.5%, 3.5%, 6.0%, and 8.0% to 10.0%, respectively.[50]

Exercise tolerance testing has been used to establish the prognosis in patients with symptomatic IHD. The exercise test parameters associated with a poor outcome have been described above.[38] There are no randomized studies available to assess the impact of medical therapy on the prognosis of patients with stable angina. Of interest is the impact of percutaneous transluminal coronary angioplasty (PTCA). It is unclear at this point that PTCA significantly improves the prognosis in patients with stable angina. A study of Coronary Artery Surgery Study (CASS) registry patients who were potentially suitable for PTCA revealed a 4-year survival of 96%.[51] A similar study of medically treated patients suitable for PTCA revealed a 5-year survival of 97%.[52]

When does angina signal severe coronary disease? Pryor et al.[53] developed a nomogram based on a point scoring system to help answer this question. They based the nomogram on the following factors: type of chest pain (typical, atypical, nonanginal), sex, selective cardiovascular risk factors (hypertension, smoking, hyperlipidemia, diabetes mellitus), anginal duration (months), and the presence of carotid bruits. By applying the nomogram for the individual patient one can determine the probability of severe disease (i.e., 75% narrowing of the left main coronary artery or three-vessel disease).

Drug Therapy

In patients with stable exertional angina who do not have severe disease the prognosis is excellent, and there is no difference between medical and surgical treatment as far as long-term mortality is concerned.[54] The goal of therapy is to abolish or reduce anginal attacks and myocardial ischemia and to promote a normal life style. For the relief of angina, the treatment strategy is to lower myocardial oxygen demand and increase coronary blood flow to the ischemic regions.

Patients are screened for the presence of significant cardiovascular risk factors and are advised to modify any that are present. Three classes of antianginal drugs are commonly used: nitrates, β-blockers, and calcium channel blockers. Each reduces myocardial oxygen demand and may improve blood flow to the ischemic regions. The mechanisms by which these agents reduce myocardial oxygen demand or increase coronary blood flow to ischemic areas differ from one class of drug to another. No greater efficacy in relieving chest pain or decreasing exercise-induced ischemia has been shown for one or another group of drugs.

NITRATES

Nitrates are potent venous and arterial dilators. At low doses venous dilation predominates, and at higher doses arterial dilation occurs as well. Nitrates decrease myocardial oxygen demand in the following ways:

Decreased venous return reduces left ventricular end-diastolic volume and ventricular wall stress. Increased arterial compliance and cardiac output lowers systolic blood pressure and decreases peripheral resistance (afterload). It also enhances myocardial oxygen supply by preventing closure of stenotic coronary arteries during exercise, dilating epicardial coronary arteries, and decreasing left ventricular end-diastolic pressure, thereby enhancing subendocardial blood flow and inhibiting coronary artery spasm. Nitrates are inexpensive and have a well documented safety record. Both short- and long-acting nitrates are available. Short-acting preparations are used for relief of an established attack, whereas long-acting nitrates are used for prevention.[55] The most significant concern about the long-acting nitrates is tolerance. Most studies have shown that tolerance develops rapidly when long-acting nitrates are given for anginal prophylaxis.[56]

With nitroglycerin patches tolerance can develop within 24 hours, and further therapy can lead to complete loss of the antianginal effect.[57] Various dosing strategies with oral and transdermal formulations have been used to overcome the development of nitroglycerin tolerance. Patch-free intervals of 10 to 12 hours are commonly used to retain the antianginal effectiveness.[56] For oral administration, nitroglycerin isosorbide dinitrate three times daily at 7 a.m., noon, and 5 p.m. appears to prevent the development of tolerance.[55] Because of the concern for intervals during which patients remain unprotected it is common to add another antianginal agent to the nitroglycerin regimen. Other problems with nitroglycerin include the fact that 10% of patients do not respond and 10% have associated intolerable headaches that may necessitate discontinuation.[56]

β-BLOCKERS

The antianginal effect of β-blockers is well established.[58] These agents improve exercise tolerance and reduce myocardial ischemia. The effect produces a reduction in myocardial oxygen demand through a reduction in heart rate and contractility. Many β-blockers are available. They may be divided into those that are nonselective (β_1 and β_2) (i.e., propranolol, timolol, nadolol), those that are β_1 selective (i.e., atenolol, metroprolol, acebutolol), and those that are nonselective and produce vasodilatory effects through the ability to block α_1-receptors and dilate blood vessels directly (i.e., labetolol). All β-blockers, irrespective of their selective properties, are equally effective in patients with angina.[58]

Some 20% of patients do not respond to β-blockers. Those who do not respond are more likely to have severe IHD. Furthermore, some patients do not tolerate the adverse side effects, such as fatigue, depression, dyspnea, and cold extremities. Other concerns include a small but significant aggravation of hyperlipidemia and precipitation of CHF and bronchospasm in susceptible individuals. Generally, β-blockers are dose-adjusted to achieve a heart rate of 50 to 60 bpm. Patients should be cautioned to not stop β-blockers abruptly, thereby avoiding a rebound phenomenon.

Calcium Channel Blockers

Calcium channel blockers are a diverse group of compounds, all of which impede calcium ion influx into the myocardium and smooth muscle cells.[59] These agents relieve myocardial ischemia by reducing myocardial oxygen demand secondary to decreased afterload and myocardial contractility. In addition, these agents dilate coronary arteries. There are three classes of calcium channel blockers: papaverine derivatives (verapamil), dihydropyridines (nifedipine, nicardipine), and benzothiazepines (diltiazem). Each of the drugs in the three classes has different effects on the atrioventricular (AV) node, heart rate, coronary vasodilation, diastolic relaxation, cardiac contractility, systemic blood pressure, and afterload. All three classes are effective for the management of patients with stable angina.[60] Most studies have shown them to have effects equal to those of β-blockers. Calcium channel blockers may be preferred in patients with obstructive airway disease, hypertension, peripheral vascular disease, or supraventricular tachycardia. In general, they are well tolerated. The most troublesome side effects include constipation, edema, headache, and aggravation of congestive heart failure.

Concern has developed that short-acting calcium channel blockers may be associated with an increased risk of MI. There has been evidence of a 58% to 70% increase in risk of MI compared to that in patients on β-blockers or diuretics. The phenomenon has been noted to be dose-related. At present the National Heart, Lung, and Blood Institute has issued a statement recommending caution with the use of short-acting calcium channel blockers.[61]

Combination Therapy

It is important to maximize therapy with any one class of antianginal drug before considering it a failed trial. If monotherapy fails, it is appropriate to add another agent. Generally β-blockers and nitrates or calcium channel blockers and nitrates complement each other. Because nitrates and nifedipine may increase the heart rate it is advisable to use a combination of nitrates plus verapamil or diltiazem.[62] Calcium channel blockers and β-blockers can be used together. Combination therapy may be more effective than either agent alone.[63] It is important to be cautious, as some combinations produce deleterious effects. For example, verapamil and β-blockers may produce extreme bradycardia or heart block.

ASPIRIN

Aspirin is effective for primary and secondary prevention of myocardial infarction, presumably by inhibiting thrombosis.[64] There is no evidence to support the idea that aspirin is effective for primary prevention of angina.[65] Although there is controversy as to the ideal therapeutic dose, "low-dose" therapy (80–300 mg) is generally recommended.[64]

Invasive Testing

Cardiac catheterization is not routinely recommended for initial management of patients with stable angina. Patients who warrant such an evaluation are those who exhibit evidence of severe myocardial ischemia on noninvasive testing or who have symptoms refractory to antianginal medications. In patients who undergo catheterization the most important determinant of survival is left ventricular function followed by the number of diseased vessels. Patients with left main artery disease or three-vessel disease with diminished left ventricular function are candidates for a coronary artery bypass graft procedure. Others (those with one- or two-vessel disease) are managed medically or considered for PTCA.

Unstable Angina Pectoris

Unstable angina manifests clinically either as an abrupt onset of ischemic symptoms at rest or as an intensification or change in the pattern of ischemic symptoms in a patient with a history of IHD. This intensification may be manifested by an increase in the frequency, severity, and duration of symptoms as well as an increasing ease of provocation (symptoms at rest or with minimal effort). Recurrence of ischemic symptoms soon after an MI (usually within 4 weeks) is also considered a sign of unstable angina. Unstable angina is generally diagnosed on clinical grounds alone. Because of the episodic nature of ischemia in unstable angina, however, transient ECG abnormalities (ST segment depression or elevation or T wave abnormalities, i.e., inversion, flattening, or peaking) may not be documented in 50% to 70% of patients with the clinical diagnosis of unstable angina. In studies in which prolonged Holter monitoring was used during the in-hospital phase of unstable angina, transient ischemic ST segment deviations have been described in 60% to 70% of cases, more than 70% of them being clinically unsuspected or silent.[66–68]

Prognosis

The prognosis of patients with unstable angina is clearly not as good as those with chronic stable angina. During the precatheterization era the mortality rate was estimated to be 12% to 15% for 3 months.[50] The rate of nonfatal MI is about 8% to 10% during the first 2 weeks. Mortality is increased in those who fail to respond to initial therapy, who have severe left ventricular dysfunction, and who have multivessel coronary artery disease (CAD) (particularly left main artery disease).

Management Strategy

The most important development in the management of unstable angina has been the 1994 report of the Agency for Health Care Policy and Research.[69] This report includes clinical practice guidelines that are based on a consensus panel of experts. The guidelines allow physicians to consider outpatient management for a select subgroup of patients with this problem, specifically those who are thought to be at low risk for myocardial infarction. According to the report, in the initial management physicians should use the information in Table 12.3 to determine whether a particular patient has high, intermediate, or low likelihood of having significant coronary artery disease. For example, the patient with low likelihood might be nondiabetic, have atypical chest pain, be younger (< 60 for men, < 70 for women), and have a normal ECG. The next step is to determine the level of risk for MI. The information in Table 12.4 allows a similar stratification of risk. For example, a low risk-patient is

TABLE 12.3. Likelihood of significant CAD in patients with symptoms suggesting unstable angina

High likelihood (any of the listed features)	Intermediate likelihood (absence of high likelihood features and any of the listed features)	Low likelihood (absence of high or intermediate likelihood features but may have the listed features)
Known history of CAD	Definite angina: men < 60, women < 70	Chest pain, probably not angina
Definite angina: men ≥ 60, women ≥ 70	Probable angina: men > 60 or women > 70	One risk factor but not diabetes
Hemodynamic changes or ECG changes with pain	Probably not angina in diabetics or in nondiabetics with ≥ two other risk factors[a]	T wave flat or inverted < 1 mm in leads with dominant R waves
Variant angina	Extracardiac vascular disease	Normal ECG
ST increase or decrease ≥ 1 mm	ST depression 0.05 to 1.00 mm	
Marked symmetric T wave inversion in multiple precordial leads	T wave inversion ≥ 1 mm in leads with dominant R waves,	

Source: Braunwald et al.[69]
[a]CAD risk factors include diabetes, smoking, hypertension, and elevated cholesterol.

TABLE 12.4. Short-term risk of death or nonfatal myocardial infarction in patients with symptoms suggesting unstable angina

High risk (at least one of the listed features must be present)	Intermediate risk (no high risk feature but must have any of the listed features)	Low-risk (no high- or intermediate-risk feature but may have any of the listed features)
Prolonged ongoing (> 20 min) rest pain	Rest angina now resolved but not low likelihood of CAD	Increased angina frequency, severity, or duration
Pulmonary edema	Rest angina (> 20 min or relieved with rest or nitroglycerin)	Angina provoked at a lower threshold
Angina with new or worsening mitral regurgitation murmurs	Angina with dynamic T wave changes	New-onset angina within 2 weeks to 2 months
Rest angina with dynamic ST changes ≥ 1 mm	Nocturnal angina	Normal or unchanged ECG
Angina with S_3 or rales	New onset of CCSC III or IV angina during past 2 weeks but not low likelihood of CAD	
Angina with hypotension	Q waves or ST depression ≥ 1 mm in multiple leads	
	Age > 65 years	

Source: Braunwald et al.[69]

one with a history of angina that is now provoked at a lower threshold but not at rest; and the ECG is normal or unchanged. Low-risk patients may be treated with aspirin, nitroglycerin, β-blockers, or a combination. Follow-up should be no later than 72 hours. High- or moderate-risk patients should be admitted for intensive medical management. Intensive medical management includes consideration of aspirin, heparin, nitrates, β-blockers, calcium channel blockers (if the patient is already on adequate doses of nitrates and β blockers or unable to tolerate them), and morphine sulfate.

Once the patient is stable he or she should be considered for noninvasive exercise testing to further define the prognosis and direct the treatment plan. Low-risk patients can be managed medically. Those at intermediate risk should be considered for additional testing (either a cardiac catheterization, radionuclide stress test, or echocardiographic stress test). Those at high risk should be referred for cardiac catheterization.[69]

ANTIPLATELET THERAPY

Antiplatelet therapy is an important addition for patients with unstable angina. A number of studies have demonstrated that a common cause of crescendo angina is platelet aggregation and thrombus formation on the surface of an ulcerated plaque.[70] In the Veterans Administration Cooperative Study, men with unstable angina who received aspirin (325 mg/day) had a 50% reduction in subsequent death from MI.[71]

Percutaneous Transluminal Coronary Angioplasty

There has been a marked increase in the use of angioplasty, and in 1990 more than 300,000 such procedures were done.[72] The American College of Cardiology and the American Heart Association Task Force have published guidelines for the selection of patients for coronary angioplasty.[73] Among patients with unstable angina, PTCA is recommended for those who do not show an adequate response to medical treatment (continued chest pain or evidence of ongoing ischemia during ECG monitoring) or who are intolerant to medical therapy because of uncontrollable side effects.

The long-term outcome after successful angioplasty has been reported to be excellent even when compared with patients undergoing bypass surgery.[74] Further research is important in the areas of long-term outcome for multiple lesions, extensive disease, and avoidance of complications. Technologies such as stents, laser angioplasty, and atherectomy await clinical evaluation.

Coronary Artery Bypass Graft

Large randomized trials have shown that surgical revascularization is more effective than medical therapy for relieving angina and improving exercise tolerance for at least several years. Development of atherosclerosis in the coronary artery bypass graft resulting in angina generally occurs within 5 to 10 years. However, patients with internal mammary artery grafts have substantially fewer problems with graft occlusion (90% patency rate at 10 years). Improved survival with surgical versus medical therapy is seen only in the subset of patients with severe CAD or left ventricular dysfunction.[75]

Silent Ischemia

Many investigations have established that most ischemic episodes in patients with stable angina are not accompanied by chest pain (silent ischemia). It remains unclear the precise nature of events that accompany ischemic events that do or do not produce pain. Patients with predominantly silent ischemia may be hyposensitive to pain in general; denial may play a role, or they may experience pain but attribute the symptoms to a less significant event. It is well documented that personality-related, emotional, and social factors can modulate the perception of pain. It is not surprising that the symptoms among cardiac patients with the same degree of disease vary greatly.[76] Personality inventory studies have shown that patients with reproducible angina have higher scores on indices of nervousness and excitability than do those who are free of symptoms.[77] Patients with clinical depression are also more likely to experience angina than control subjects.[78] Many studies have shown that stress of various types can influence the frequency and duration of ischemic episodes in patients with angina.[79,80]

Silent ischemia is prevalent. Seventy percent of ischemic episodes in patients with IHD are estimated to be asymptomatic. Among patients with stable angina who undergo 24-hour Holter monitoring, 40% to 72% of the episodes are painless. Among patients with unstable angina more than half manifest painless ST segment depression.

In 1988 Cohn[81] proposed classifying silent ischemia into three clinical types to help clarify the prevalence, detection, prognosis, and management of this syndrome. Type 1 includes persons with ischemia who are asymptomatic, never having had any signs or symptoms of cardiovascular disease. Type 2 includes persons who are asymptomatic after an MI but still show painless ischemia. Type 3 includes patients with both angina and silent ischemia. From Cohn's data 2.5% to 10.0% of middle-aged men have type 1 silent ischemia. Among middle-aged men known to have coronary artery disease, 18% have type 2 and 40% have type 3.

Methods of Detection

Certain tests can be used to assess the presence of silent ischemia: ETT, ambulatory ECG for ST segment changes (Holter monitor), radionuclide tests including thallium scintigraphy and gated pooled (MUGA) scan, and stress echocardiography. Of these tests, the most commonly considered are ETT and Holter monitoring.[82]

For Holter monitoring, when ST segment changes that meet strict criteria are seen in a patient with known IHD, it is generally accepted that they represent episodes of myocardial ischemia. Ischemic criteria include at least 1.0 mm of horizontal or downsloping ST segment depression that lasts for at least 1 minute and is separated from other discrete episodes by at least 1 minute of a normal baseline. The methodology has limitations, including difficulty reading ST segment changes in patients with an abnormal baseline (left ventricular hypertrophy with strain) or in those with a left bundle branch block.

It is not thought at this time that any of the methods to detect silent ischemia are useful for screening for the presence of IHD in apparently healthy populations. Although this subject remains controversial, it may be wise to screen those patients at high risk (i.e., diabetics or patients with two or more cardiac risk factors).

Prognostic Implications

The presence of frequent, prolonged ischemic episodes despite medical therapy in patients with stable and unstable angina has been associated with a poor prognosis. Using Cohn's classification system, those patients with type 2 silent ischemia have the worst prognosis, especially those with left ventricular dysfunction and three-vessel disease. Exercise tests done 2 to 3 weeks after an MI have shown an adverse 1-year prognosis associated with silent ischemia.[83] It is unclear whether those with type 3 have a worse prognosis.

Management

Antiischemic medical and revascularization therapies have been shown to reduce asymptomatic ischemia. It is prudent to consider patients with persistent asymptomatic ischemia to be at higher risk for subsequent events and therefore to be deserving of more aggressive therapy. Patients with type 1 are advised to modify risk factors and avoid activities known to produce ischemia. Those with strongly positive tests can be considered for angiography. For patients with types 2 or 3, treatment with β-blockers for a cardioprotective effect should be considered. It remains unresolved whether asymptomatic ischemia has a causal relation with subsequent MI and cardiac death or is merely a marker of high risk.[84]

Myocardial Infarction

Clinical Presentation

The classic initial manifestations of an acute MI include prolonged substernal chest pain with dyspnea, diaphoresis, and nausea. The pain may be described as a crushing, pressing, constricting, vise-like, or heavy sensation. There may be radiation of the pain to one or both shoulders and arms or to the neck, jaw, or interscapular area. Only a few patients have this classic overall picture. Although 80% of patients with an acute MI have chest pain at the time of initial examination, only 20% describe it as crushing, constricting, or vise-like.[85,86] The pain may also be described atypically, such as sharp or stabbing; or it can involve atypical areas such as the epigastrium or the back of the neck. "Atypical" presentations are common in the elderly.

Pathy[87] found that the initial manifestations of an acute MI were more likely to include symptoms such as sudden dyspnea, acute confusion, cerebrovascular events (e.g., stroke or syncope), acute CHF, vomiting, and palpitations. There is strong evidence that a substantial proportion of MIs are asymptomatic. In an update of the Framingham Study, Kannel and Abbott[88] reported that 28% of infarcts were discovered only through the appearance of new ECG changes (Q waves or loss of R waves) observed on a routine biennial study. These infarctions had been previously unrecognized by both patient and physician.

Physical Examination

For the patient with an "uncomplicated MI" there are few physical examination findings. The main purpose of the examination is to assess the patient for evidence of complications from the MI and to establish a baseline for future comparisons. Signs of severe left ventricular dysfunction include hypotension, peripheral vasoconstriction, tachycardia, pulmonary rales, an S_3, and elevated jugular venous pressure. Preexisting murmurs should be verified. A new systolic murmur can result from a number of causes: papillary muscle dysfunction, mitral regurgitation as a result of ventricular dilatation, ventricular septal rupture, and acute severe mitral regurgitation due to papillary muscle rupture.[86]

Electrocardiography

The classic ECG changes of acute ischemia are peaked, hyperacute T waves, T wave flattening or inversion with or without ST segment depression, horizontal ST segment depression, and ST segment elevation. Changes associated with an infarction are (1) the fresh appearance of Q waves or the increased prominence of preexisting ones; (2) ST segment elevations; and (3) T wave inversions.[89] It is important to recognize that with acute MI the ECG may be entirely normal or contain only "soft" ECG evidence of infarction.

In the past infarcts were classified as transmural or subendocardial, depending of the presence of Q waves. This terminology has now been replaced by the terms "Q-wave" or "non-Q-wave" MI. This distinction has more clinical relevance, as several studies have indicated differences in etiology and outcome.[86] The key differences between these two groups are as follows: (1) Q-wave infarctions account for 60% to 70% of all infarcts and non-Q-wave infarctions for 30% to 40%. (2) ST segment elevation is present in 80% of Q-wave infarctions and 40% of non-Q-wave infarctions. (3) The peak creatine kinase tends to be higher in Q-wave infarctions. (4) Postinfarction ischemia and early reinfarction are more common with non-Q-wave infarctions. (5) In-hospital mortality is greater with Q-wave infarctions (20% versus 8% for non-Q-wave infarctions). In general, it is thought that the non-Q-wave infarction is a more unstable condition because of the higher risk of reinfarction and ischemia.[86]

Laboratory Findings

Elevation of the creatine kinase MB (CK-MB) isoenzyme is essential for the diagnosis of acute MI. In general, acute elevations of this enzyme are accounted for by myocardial necrosis. Detectable CK-MB from non-cardiac causes is rare except during trauma or surgery. The peak level appearance of CK-MB is expected within 12 to 24 hours after the onset of symptoms. Therefore patients should have a CK-MB level determined on admission and every 12 hours thereafter (repeated twice). Reliance on a single CK assay in an emergency room setting to rule out myocardial infarction is not sensitive and should be discouraged. Myosin chains and the troponins are new markers that do not differ significantly from creatine kinase.[90,91]

In the event that a patient presents for evaluation past the time for a peak CK-MB to be of value, serum lactate dehydrogenase (LDH) levels may be used. LDH is less specific for myocardial necrosis because elevations may be induced by other diseases as well, such as liver and skeletal muscle disorders and trauma. There are five LDH isoenzymes. An increase in LDH-1 or an increase in the LDH-1/LDH-2 ratio is characteristically found with an acute MI. Concentrations of LDH isoenzymes usually become abnormal within 14 hours of the onset of infarction and can remain diagnostic for as long as 2 weeks after the infarction. The most common definition of abnormal is an LDH-1/LDH-2 ratio over 1.0.[92]

Management Guidelines

The main priority for patients with an acute MI is relief of pain. The frequent clinical observation of rapid, complete relief of pain after early reperfusion with thrombolytic therapy has made it clear that the pain of an acute myocardial infarction is due to continuing ischemia of living jeopardized myocardium rather than to the effects of completed myocardial necrosis.

Effective analgesia is promptly administered at the time of diagnosis.[93] Analgesia can be achieved by the use of sublingual nitroglycerin or intravenous morphine (or both). Sublingual nitroglycerin is given immediately unless the systolic blood pressure is less than 90 mm Hg. If the systolic blood pressure is under 90 mm Hg, nitroglycerin may be used after intravenous access has been obtained. Long-acting oral nitrate preparations are avoided for management of early acute MI. Sublingual or transdermal nitroglycerin can be used, but intravenous infusion of nitroglycerin allows more precise control. The intravenous dose can be titrated by frequently measuring blood pressure and heart rate. Morphine sulfate is also highly effective for the relief of pain associated with an acute MI. In addition to its analgesic properties, morphine exerts favorable hemodynamic effects by increasing venous capacitance and reducing systemic vascular resistance. The result is to decrease myocardial oxygen demand. As with nitroglycerin, hypotension may occur. The hypotension may be treated with intravenous fluids or leg elevation.

OXYGEN

Supplemental oxygen is given to all patients with an acute MI. Hypoxemia in a patient with an uncomplicated infarction is usually caused by ventilation-perfusion abnormalities.[94] When oxygen is used it is administered by nasal cannula or mask at a rate of 4 to 10 L/min. In patients with chronic obstructive pulmonary disease it may be wise to use lower flow rates (see Chapter 13).

THROMBOLYTIC THERAPY

In addition to relieving pain and managing ischemia, thrombolytic therapy must be considered. Thrombosis has a major role in the development of an acute MI. Approximately 66% of patients with MIs have ST segment elevation, making it likely that the process is caused by an occlusive clot. The goal of thrombolytic therapy is reperfusion with a minimum of side effects. The most commonly used thrombolytic agents are streptokinase, anisoylated plasminogen streptokinase activator complex (APSAC), recombinant tissue-type plasminogen activator (rt-PA), urokinase, and pro-urokinase.

Early administration of thrombolytic therapy, within 6 hours from the onset of symptoms, has been associated with a reduction in mortality. There have been several large international studies comparing the results with various thrombolytic agents. The Second International Study of Infarct Survival (ISIS-2) reported baseline and outcome data for 17,187 patients with suspected MI. Streptokinase was compared to placebo. A 23% reduction in vascular deaths was noted for patients on streptokinase.[95] Similar results were found in the GISSI-1[96] trial (8% reduction with streptokinase compared with placebo). Subsequent studies comparing the effectiveness of the various agents [GISSI-2[97] (rt-PA versus streptokinase)] failed to show a significant difference between the agents. Streptokinase is by far the least expensive of the agents ($125 versus $2800 for rt-PA), but it has more severe side effects (allergic reactions with repeat dosing and hypotension). The thrombolytic effect of streptokinase is more time-dependent. It is best used early (within 2 hours) after an acute MI, whereas rt-PA should be strongly considered for those patients in whom 3 hours has elapsed after infarction. To enhance thrombolysis and inhibit new thrombus formation, heparin is administered immediately as a bolus of 5,000 to 10,000 units and then by infusion of

1000 units per hour to maintain an activated partial thromboplastin time at two to three times control for 3 to 5 days. Low-dose aspirin (80 mg/day) is started immediately.[98]

Complications (Mechanical)

The most common complications of an acute MI are mechanical and electrical. Mechanical complications include those that are quickly reversible and those that are clearly life-threatening. Reversible causes of hypotension include hypovolemia, vasovagal reaction, overzealous therapy with antianginal or antiarrhythmic drugs, and brady- and tachyarrhythmias. Other, more serious etiologies include primary left ventricular failure, cardiac tamponade, rupture of the ventricular septum, acute papillary muscle dysfunction, and mitral regurgitation.

Killip and Kimball[99] developed a classification of patients with acute MI.

Class 1: Patients with uncomplicated infarction without evidence of heart failure as judged by the absence of rales and an S_3

Class 2: Patients with mild to moderate heart failure as evidenced by pulmonary rales in the lower half of the lung fields and an S_3

Class 3: Patients with severe left ventricular failure and pulmonary edema

Class 4: Patients with cardiogenic shock, defined as systolic blood pressure less than 90 mm Hg with oliguria and other evidence of poor peripheral perfusion

Cardiogenic shock has emerged as the most common cause of in-hospital mortality of patients with an acute MI. Despite advances in medical therapy, cardiogenic shock has a dismal prognosis (80–90% mortality).[100] The management of patients with cardiogenic shock includes adequate oxygenation, reduction in myocardial oxygen demands, protection of ischemic myocardium, and circulatory support. The potential for myocardial salvage with emergency reperfusion should be considered in all cases.

Complications (Electrical)

The past 30 years have seen major developments in the recognition and treatment of arrhythmias. The most common include the brady- and tachyarrhythmias, AV conduction disturbances, and ventricular arrhythmias. Organized treatment protocols have been developed for each of these dysrhythmias.[101]

Post-MI Evaluation

Recommendations for pre- and postdischarge evaluations of patients with an acute MI have been outlined by the American College of Cardiologists, the American Heart Association, and the American College of Physicians.[102,103] They include recommendations for testing exercise tolerance and strategies to determine those who would benefit from medical or surgical intervention. These recommendations include a submaximal ETT at 6 to 10 days and at 3 weeks to determine functional capacity.

Rehabilitation

The goal of cardiac rehabilitation includes maintenance of a desirable level of physical, social, and psychological functioning after the onset of cardiovascular illness.[104] Specific goals of rehabilitation include risk stratification, limitation of adverse psychological and emotional consequences of cardiovascular disease, modification of risk factors, alleviation of symptoms, and improved function. Risk stratification is accomplished by exercise tolerance testing. In addition, high risk patients include those with CHF, silent ischemia, and ventricular dysrhythmias. All patients should undergo an evaluation to reduce risk factors (smoking, hyperlipidemia, and hypertension) (see Chapter 2). Risk modification of these factors has been associated with significant reduction in subsequent cardiac events. Enrollment in a cardiac rehabilitation program with particular emphasis on exercise has been shown to reduce cardiovascular mortality.[105]

References

1. Deedwania PC. Clinical perspectives on primary and secondary prevention of coronary atherosclerosis. Med Clin North Am 1995;79:973–8.
2. Eisenberg MS, Cummings RO, Litwin PE, Hallstrom AP. Out-of hospital cardiac arrest: significance of symptoms in patients collapsing before and after arrival of paramedics. Am J Emerg Med 1986;4:116–20.
3. Kuller L. Sudden death—definition and epidemiologic considerations. Prog Cardiovasc Dis 1980;23:1–12.
4. Gordon T, Kannel WB. Premature mortality from coronary heart disease: the Framingham study. JAMA 1971;215: 1617–25.
5. American Heart Association. Advanced cardiac life support in perspective. In: Textbook of advanced life support. Dallas: American Heart Association, 1987:1–10.
6. Fulp SR, Richter JE. Esophageal chest pain. Am Fam Physician 1989;40: 101–16.
7. Klinkman MS, Stevens D, Gorenflo DW. Episodes of care for chest pain: a preliminary report from MIRNET. J Fam Pract 1994;38:345–52.
8. Kemp HG, Vokonas PS, Cohn PF, Gorlin R. The anginal syndrome associated with normal coronary arteriograms: report of a six-year experience. Am J Med 1973;54:735–42.

9. Marchandise B, Bourrassa MG, Chairman BR, Lesperance J. Angiographic evaluation of the natural history of normal coronary arteries and mild coronary atherosclerosis. Am J Cardiol 1978;41:216–20.
10. Proudfit WL, Bruschke AVG, Sones FM. Clinical course of patients with normal or slightly or moderately abnormal coronary arteriograms: 10-year follow-up of 521 patients. Circulation 1980;62:712–17.
11. Day LJ, Sowton E. Clinical features and follow-up of patients with angina and normal coronary arteries. Lancet 1979;2:334–7.
12. Ockene IS, Shay MJ, Alpert JS, et al. Unexplained chest pain in patients with normal coronary arteriograms: a follow-up study of functional status. N Engl J Med 1980;303:1249–52.
13. Waxler EB, Kimbiris D, Dreifus LS. The fate of women with normal coronary arteriograms and chest pain resembling angina pectoris. Am J Cardiol 1971;28:25–32.
14. Lavey EB, Winkle RA. Continuing disability of patients with chest pain and normal coronary arteriograms. J Chronic Dis 1979;32:191–6.
15. Isner JM, Salem DN, Banas JS, Levire HS. Long-term clinical course of patients with normal coronary arteriography: follow-up study of 121 patients with normal or nearly normal coronary arteriograms. Am Heart J 1981;102:645–53.
16. Kemp HG, Kronmal RA, Vlietstra RE, Frye RL. Seven year survival of patients with normal or near normal coronary arteriograms: a CASS registry study. J Am Coll Cardiol 1986;7:479–83.
17. DeMeester TR, O'Sullivan GC, Bermudez G, et al. Esophageal function in patient with angina-type chest pain and normal coronary angiograms. Ann Surg 1982;196:488–98.
18. Kline M, Chesne R, Studevant RL, McCallum RW. Esophageal disease in patients with angina-like chest pain. Am J Gastroenterol 1981;75:116–23.
19. Davies HA, Jones DB, Rhodes J. Esophageal angina as the cause of chest pain. JAMA 1982;248:2274–8.
20. Richter JE, Bradley LA, Castell DO. Esophageal chest pain current controversies in pathogenesis, diagnosis and therapy. Ann Intern Med 1989; 110:66–78.
21. Svensson O, Stenport G, Tibbling L, Wranne B. Oesophageal function and coronary angiogram in patients with disabling chest pain. Acta Med Scand 978;204:173–8.
22. Schofield PM, Bennett DH, Whorwell PJ, et al. Exertional gastro-oesophageal reflux: a mechanism for symptoms in patient with angina pectoris and normal coronary angiograms. BMJ 1987;294:1459–61.
23. Areskog M, Tibbling L, Wranne B. Noninfarction in coronary care unit patients. Acta Med Scand 1981;209:51–7.
24. Davies HA, Jones DB, Rhodes J, Newcombe RJ. Angina-like esophageal pain: differentiation from cardiac pain by history. Clin Gastroenterol 1985;7:477–81.
25. Glade MJ. Continuous ambulatory esophageal pH monitoring in the evaluation of patients with gastrointestinal reflux: diagnostic and therapeutic technology assessment (DATTA) JAMA 1995;274:662–8.

26. Pope CE. Chest pain: heart? gullet? both? neither? [editorial]. JAMA 1992;248:2315.
27. Clouse RE, Lustman PJ. Psychiatric illness and contraction abnormalities of the esophagus. N Engl J Med 1983;309: 1337–42.
28. Katon W, Hall ML, Russo J, et al. Chest pain: relationship of psychiatric illness to coronary arteriographic results. Am J Med 1988;84:1–9.
29. Waxler EB, Kimbiris D, Dreifus LS. The fate of women with normal coronary arteries and chest pain resembling stable angina pectoris. Am J Cardiol 1971;28:25–32.
30. Bass C, Wade C, Hand D, et al. Patients with angina with normal and near normal coronary arteries: clinical and psychosocial statistics 12 months after angiography. BMJ 1983; 287:1505–8.
31. Cannon RO, Quyyumi AA, Mincemoyer R, et al. Imipramine in patients with chest pain despite normal coronary angiograms. N Engl J Med 1994;330:1411–17.
32. Shub C. Stable angina pectoris. 1. Clinical patterns. Mayo Clin Proc 1990;65:233–42.
33. Kemp HG. Left ventricular function in patients with the angina syndrome and normal coronary arteriograms [editorial]. Am J Cardiol 1973;32:375–6.
34. Kemp HG, Elliott WC, Gorlin R. The anginal syndrome with normal coronary arteriography. Trans Assoc Am Physicians 1967;80:59–70.
35. Cannon RO. Angina pectoris with normal coronary angiograms. Cardiol Clin 1991;9:157–66.
36. Colgan SM, Schofield PJ, Whorwell DH, et al. Angina-like chest pain: a joint medical and psychiatric investigation. Postgrad Med J 1988;64: 743–6.
37. Diamond GA, Forrester JS. Analysis of probability as an aid in the clinical diagnosis of coronary-artery disease. N Engl J Med 1979;300:1350–8.
38. Guidelines for exercise testing: a report of the American College of Cardiology/American Heart Association Task Force on Assessment of Cardiovascular Procedures (Subcommittee on Exercise Testing). J Am Coll Cardiol 1986; 8:725–38.
39. Evans CH, Karunaratne HB. Exercise stress testing for the family physician. Part 1. Performing the test. Am Fam Physician 1992;45:121–32.
40. Evans CH, Karunaratne HB. Exercise stress testing for the family physician. Part 2. Am Fam Physician 1992;45:679–88.
41. Ellestad MH. Stress testing: principles and practice. 4d ed. Philadelphia: Davis, 1995.
42. Chaitman B. The changing role of the exercise electrocardiogram as a diagnostic and prognostic test for chronic ischemic heart disease. J Am Coll Cardiol 1986;8:1195–1210.
43. Rivitz SM, Deluca SA. Perfusion imaging in ischemic heart disease. Am Fam Physician 1993;48:1071–8.
44. Botvinick EH. Stress imaging: current clinical options for the diagnosis, localization, and evaluation of coronary artery disease. Med Clin North Am 1995;79:1025–61.

45. Afridi I, Quinones MA, Zoghbi WA, Cheirif J. Dobutamine stress echocardiography: sensitivity, specificity, and predictive value for future cardiac events. Am Heart J 1994;127: 1510–15.
46. Beleslin BD, Ostojic M, Stepanovic J, et al. Stress echocardiography in the detection of myocardial ischemia: head-to-head comparison of exercise, dobutamine, and dipyridamole tests. Circulation 1994;90:1168–76.
47. Horwitz LD, Herman MV, Gorlin R. Clinical response to nitroglycerin as a diagnostic test for coronary artery disease. Am J Cardiol 1972;29:149–53.
48. Frank CW, Weinblatt E, Shapiro S. Angina pectoris in men: prognostic significance of selected medical factors. Circulation 1973;47:509–17.
49. Kannel WB, Feinleib M. Natural history of angina pectoris in the Framingham study: prognosis and survival. Am J Cardiol 1972;29:154–63.
50. Hilton TC, Chaitman BR. The prognosis in stable and unstable angina. Cardiol Clin 1991;9:27–39.
51. Holmes DR, Vliestra RE, Fisher LD, et al. Follow-up of patient from the Coronary Artery Surgery Study (CASS) potentially suitable for percutaneous transluminal coronary angioplasty. Am Heart J 1983;106: 981–8.
52. Hlatky MA, Califf RM, Kong Y. Natural history of patients with single-vessel disease suitable for percutaneous transluminal coronary angioplasty. Am J Cardiol 1983;52:225–9.
53. Pryor DB, Shaw L, Harrell FE, et al. Estimating the likelihood of severe coronary artery disease. Am J Med 1991;90: 553–62.
54. Mock MB, Rinquist I, Fisher LD, et al. Survival of medically treated patients in the Coronary Artery Surgery Study (CASS registry). Circulation 1982;66:562–8.
55. Goodman LS, Gilman A. The pharmacologic basis of therapeutics. 8th ed. New York: Macmillan, 1990:727–43.
56. Bomber JW, Detullio PL. Oral nitrate preparations: an update. Am Fam Physician 1995;52:2331–6.
57. Thadani U, Whitsett T, Hamilton SE. Nitrate therapy for myocardial ischemic syndromes: current perspectives including tolerance. Curr Probl Cardiol 1988;13:725–84.
58. Thadani U, Davidson C, Singleton W, et al. Comparison of the immediate effects of five beta-adrenoceptor blocking drugs with different ancillary properties in angina pectoris. N Engl J Med 1979;300:750–5.
59. Braunwald E. Mechanism of action of calcium channel blocking agents. N Engl J Med 1982;307:1618–26.
60. Opie LH. Calcium channel antagonists. Part II. Use and comparative properties of prototypical calcium antagonists in ischemic heart disease, including recommendations based on analysis of 45 trials. Rev Cardiovasc Drug Ther 1987;1: 4461–75.
61. Psaty BM, Heckbert ER, Koepsell TD, et al. The risk of myocardial infarction associated with antihypertensive drug therapies. JAMA 1995;274: 670–5.
62. Thadani U. Medical therapy of stable angina pectoris. Cardiol Clin 1991;9:73–87.

63. Packer M. Drug therapy: combined beta-adrenergic and calcium entry blockade in angina pectoris. N Engl J Med 1989;320:709–18.
64. Hennekens CH, Buring JE. Aspirin in the primary prevention of cardiovascular disease. Cardiol Clin 1994;12:443–50.
65. Manson JE, Grobbee DE, Stampfer MJ, et al. Aspirin in the primary prevention of angina pectoris in a randomized trial of United States physicians. Am J Med 1990;89:772–6.
66. Shah PK. Pathophysiology of unstable angina. Cardiol Clin 1991;9:11–26.
67. Gottlieb SO, Weisfeldt ML, Ouyang P, et al. Silent ischemia as a marker for early unfavorable outcomes in patients with unstable angina. N Engl J Med 1986;314:1214–19.
68. Nademanee K, Intarachot V, Josephson MA, et al. Prognostic significance of silent myocardial ischemia in patients with unstable angina. J Am Coll Cardiol 1987;10:1–9.
69. Braunwald E, Mark DB, Jones RH, et al. Diagnosing and managing unstable angina: quick reference guide for clinicians, Number 10. Rockville, MD: US Department of Health and Human Services, Public Health Service, Agency for Health Care Policy and Research and National Heart, Lung, and Blood Institute, 1994. AHCPR Publication No. 94-0603.
70. Davies MJ, Thomas AC, Knapman PA, Hangartner JR. Intramyocardial platelet aggregation in patients with unstable angina suffering sudden ischemic cardiac death. Circulation 1986;73:418–27.
71. Lewis HD, Davis JW, Archibald DG, et al. Protective effects of aspirin against acute myocardial infarction and death in men with unstable angina: results of a Veterans Administration Cooperative Study. N Engl J Med 1983;309:396–403.
72. National Center for Health Statistics. 1986 Summary: National Hospital Discharge Survey. Hyattsville, MD: NCHS, 1987. DHHS Publ. No. (PHS) 87-1250.
73. Ryan TJ, Faxon DP, Gunnar RM, et al. Guidelines for percutaneous transluminal coronary angioplasty: a report of the American College of Cardiology/American Heart Association task force on assessment of diagnostic and therapeutic cardiovascular procedures (subcommittee on percutaneous transluminal angioplasty). Circulation 1988;78:486–502.
74. Faxon DP. Percutaneous coronary angioplasty in stable and unstable angina. Cardiol Clin 1991;9:99–113.
75. Sherman DL, Ryan TJ. Coronary angioplasty versus bypass grafting: cost-benefit considerations. Med Clin North Am 1995;79:1085–95.
76. Barsky AJ, Hochstrasser B, Coles A, et al. Silent myocardial ischemia: is the person or the event silent? JAMA 1990; 264:1132–5.
77. Droste C, Roskamm H. Experimental pain measurement in patients with asymptomatic myocardial ischemia. J Am Coll Cardiol 1983;1:940–5.
78. Sheps DS, Light KC, Bragdon EE, et al. Relationship between chest pain, exercise endorphine response and depression. Circulation 1989;80 Suppl II:591–4.
79. Freeman LS, Nixon PGF, Sallabank P, et al. Psychologic stress and silent myocardial ischemia. Am Heart J 1987;114: 477–82.

80. Rozanski A, Bairey CN, Krantz DS, et al. Mental stress and the induction of silent myocardial ischemia in patients with coronary artery disease. N Engl J Med 1988;318:1005–12.
81. Cohn PF. Silent myocardial ischemia. Ann Intern Med 1988; 109:312–17.
82. Mody FV, Nademanee K, Intarachot V, et al. Severity of silent myocardial ischemia on ambulatory electrocardiographic monitoring in patients with stable angina pectoris: relation to prognostic determinants during exercise stress testing and coronary angiography. J Am Coll Cardiol 1988; 12:1169–96.
83. Theroux P, Waters DD, Halphen C, et al. Prognostic value of exercise testing soon after myocardial infarction. N Engl J Med 1979;301:341–5.
84. Gottlieb SO. Asymptomatic or silent myocardial ischemia in angina pectoris: pathophysiology and clinical implications. Cardiol Clin 1991; 9:49–61.
85. Kinlen LJ. Incidence and presentation of myocardial infarction in an English community. Br Heart J 1973;35:616–22.
86. Lavie CJ, Gersh BJ. Acute myocardial infarction: initial manifestations, management, and prognosis. Mayo Clin Proc 1990;65:531–48.
87. Pathy MS. Clinical presentation of myocardial infarction in the elderly. Br Heart J 1967;29:190–9.
88. Kannel WB, Abbott RD. Incidence and prognosis of unrecognized myocardial infarction: an update on the Framingham study. N Engl J Med 1984;311:1144–7.
89. Marriott HJL. Practical electrocardiography. 6th ed. Baltimore: Williams & Wilkins, 1977:232–73.
90. Lee TH, Goldman L. Serum enzyme assays in the diagnosis of acute myocardial infarction: recommendations based on a quantitative analysis. Ann Intern Med 1986;105:221–33.
91. Guest TM, Jaffe AS. Rapid diagnosis of acute myocardial infarction. Cardiol Clin 1995;13:283–94.
92. Vasudevan G, Mercer DW, Varat MA. Lactic dehydrogenase isoenzyme determination in the diagnosis of acute myocardial infarction. Circulation 1978;57:1055–7.
93. Gunnar RM, Lambrew CT, Abrams W, et al. Task force IV: pharmacologic interventions. Am J Cardiol 1982;50:393–408.
94. Fillmore SJ, Shapiro M, Killip T. Arterial oxygen tension in acute myocardial infarction: serial analysis of clinical state and blood gas changes. Am Heart J 1970;79:620–9.
95. ISIS-2 (Second International Study of Infarct Survival) Collaborative Group. Randomized trial of intravenous streptokinase, oral aspirin, both, or neither among 17,187 cases of suspected acute myocardial infarction: ISIS-2. Lancet 1988; 2:349–60.
96. Gruppo Italiano per lo Studio della Streptochinasi nell'Infarto Miocardico (GISSI). Effectiveness of intravenous thrombolytic treatment in acute myocardial infarction. Lancet 1986; 1:397–401.
97. GISSI-2 Investigators. GISSI-2: a factorial randomized trial of alteplase vs streptokinase and heparin vs no heparin among 12,490 patients with acute myocardial infarction. Lancet 1990;336:65–71.

98. Lavie CJ, Gersh BJ, Chesebro JH. Reperfusion in acute myocardial infarction. Mayo Clin Proc 1990;65:549–64.
99. Killip T, Kimball JT. Treatment of myocardial infarction in a coronary care unit: a two-year experience with 250 patients. Am J Cardiol 1967;20:457–61.
100. Forrester JS, Diamond G, Chatterjee K, et al. Medical therapy of acute myocardial infarction by application of hemodynamic subsets. N Engl J Med 1976;295:1356–62.
101. American Heart Association. Putting it all together. In: Textbook of advanced cardiac life support. Dallas: American Heart Association, 1987: 235–48.
102. ACC/AHA Guidelines for the early management of patients with acute myocardial infarction: a report of the American College of Cardiology/American Heart Association Task Force on Assessment of Diagnostic and Therapeutic Cardiovascular Procedures (Subcommittee to Develop Guidelines for the Early Management of Patients with Acute Myocardial Infarction). Circulation 1990; 82:664–707.
103. American College of Physicians. Evaluation of patients after recent acute myocardial infarction [position paper]. Ann Intern Med 1989;110: 485–8.
104. Squires RW, Gau GT, Miller TD, et al. Cardiovascular rehabilitation: status 1990. Mayo Clin Proc 1990; 65:731–55.
105. O'Connor GT, Buring JE, Yusuf S, et al. An overview of randomized trials of rehabilitation with exercise after myocardial infarction. Circulation 1989;80:234–44.

Case Presentation

Subjective

Patient Profile

John McCarthy is a 54-year-old married white male restaurant operator.

Presenting Problem

"Chest pain, getting worse."

Present Illness

This is the second visit to the office for Mr. McCarthy, who is a well-controlled type 2 diabetic with angina pectoris for 1 year. His coronary artery disease has been stable, and he used three to four nitroglycerin tablets per month—especially after exertion and cold exposure—until the past week. He is now using three to five nitroglycerin tablets per day and has angina with mild exertion or when bending over. His pain radiates to the chin and to the left arm, which it seldom did before.

Past Medical History

No change since the past medical history recorded on his initial "get acquainted" office visit 6 months ago (see Chapter 1).

Social History

His restaurant business has been struggling recently; otherwise, no change since his last visit.

Habits

No change since his prior visit.

Family History

He is especially concerned about his son Mark, aged 28, who has been found to be HIV-positive.

REVIEW OF SYMPTOMS

No other pertinent symptoms noted.

- What further information regarding Mr. McCarthy's chest pain would you like to know? Why?
- What more would you like to know about the current status of his diabetes mellitus?
- What might have caused his chest pain to become worse, and how would you inquire about these possibilities?
- What might this change in symptoms mean to the patient, and how would you ask about this?

Objective

GENERAL

The patient appears apprehensive and describes his pain by holding his clenched fist to the midchest.

VITAL SIGNS

Height, 6 ft; weight, 194 lb; blood pressure, 152/100; pulse, 82; respirations, 22; temperature, 37.2°C.

EXAMINATION

The eyes, ears, nose, and throat are normal. The neck and thyroid gland are unremarkable, and there is no cervical bruit. The chest is clear to percussion and auscultation. The heart has a regular sinus rhythm of 82. There is no cardiac enlargement, rub, or murmur.

LABORATORY

An ECG performed in the office today is normal for age.

- What additional data from the physical examination are likely to be pertinent? Explain.
- What—if any—findings on physical examination might increase or ease your concerns regarding the patient's history today?
- What—if any—laboratory tests would you obtain today? Why?
- What other tests—diagnostic imaging, treadmill ECG, or radionuclide scan—might be important in making a diagnosis today? Explain.

Assessment

- Based on the data available and pending further tests, what is your tentative diagnosis? How would you explain this to Mr. McCarthy and his family?
- What are the implications of this diagnosis for the patient?
- The family asks about the long-term prognosis. How would you respond?
- What symptoms or physical findings—if present—would you consider especially worrisome in this clinical setting? Explain.

Plan

- What are your therapeutic recommendations, and how would you explain them to the patient?
- Is a subspecialist consultation needed? Explain your reasoning.
- The patient wishes to know how soon he can return to work. How would you respond?
- If you decide to admit the patient to the hospital, what is your role in hospital care?

13

Obstructive Airway Disease

HOWARD N. WEINBERG

Obstructive airways disease includes two entities that share many common characteristics, asthma and chronic obstructive pulmonary disease (COPD). Chronic cough, a prominent symptom of both ailments, is also discussed.

Background

Asthma

Asthma is a disorder of the pulmonary airways characterized by reversible obstruction, inflammation, and hyperresponsiveness.[1] Approximately 9 million to 12 million Americans are affected by this disease and experience an annual mortality of approximately 4000 to 5000.[2] Initial onset can be at any age, in either sex, and in every race. The severity of this illness is difficult to predict; some victims suffer a rapidly worsening course, whereas others appear to "outgrow" the disease.

The bronchospasm and inflammation may be triggered by allergens, infection, and psychophysiologic stressors. Allergens include inhaled substances such as molds, pollens, dust, animal danders, cockroaches, industrial pollutants, tobacco smoke (including side-stream), smoke from wood stoves, and cosmetics. Oral inducers may be food additives such as tartrazine coloring and preservatives containing sulfiting agents; and medications, especially aspirin and β-adrenergic antagonists (including selective agents and topical preparations), can be triggers.

Respiratory infections, particularly viral, are also major stimulators.[3] Occasionally a virus, such as the respiratory syncytial virus, induces bronchospasm in nearly all patients. Some patients have attacks only with infections.

Psychological factors certainly play a role in inducing asthma episodes. These triggers may be difficult to recognize and may manifest as part of a panic attack, as fear of the disease itself, or as a symptom of abuse. Panic attacks can also be confused with and misdiagnosed as asthma.

COPD

Chronic obstructive pulmonary disease is defined as an ailment characterized by abnormal expiratory flow that does not change significantly over time. This delineation was intended to exclude asthma as well as specific upper airway diseases such as cancers and conditions affecting the lower airways such as bronchiectasis, sarcoidosis, and cystic fibrosis.[4] Traditionally included in this category have been chronic bronchitis and emphysema. In some patients, however, the overlap with asthma is so strong that a significant distinction cannot be made. Indeed, the term COPD was developed in recognition of the tremendous overlap between asthma, chronic bronchitis, and emphysema.

Chronic bronchitis is defined as a cough that occurs at least 3 months a year for 2 consecutive years and involves excess mucous secretion in the large airways. A malady of adults, chronic bronchitis affects about 20% of men and is primarily caused by smoking. Unfortunately, the incidence in women is increasing as the percentage of women smokers increases. Other contributing factors include air pollution, occupational exposures, and infection.[5]

Emphysema has been defined as a permanent enlargement of distal airspaces with destruction of the acinar walls without fibrosis. This entity can be further subdivided into centriacinar, panacinar, and distal acinar types.[6] Like chronic bronchitis, this illness is found primarily in smokers. There is, however, a rare type of congenital emphysema and also a genetic syndrome associated with the lack of α_1-antitrypsin.

Chronic Cough

Although cough is an essential component of the presentation of both COPD and asthma, there are many other entities that can cause chronic coughing. The four most common causes are postnasal drip syndrome, COPD, asthma, and gastroesophageal reflux.[7] Other causes include acute and chronic infection, other lung diseases (embolism, cancer), aspiration, psychogenic factors, and cardiac failure. Cough can also result from medications, most prominent of which are probably angiotensin-converting enzyme (ACE) inhibitors. Also, a significant number of patients have two or more causes for cough.

Clinical Presentation

Asthma

The classic symptoms of asthma are cough, dyspnea, and wheezing. The wheezing may be audible or require auscultation. Infrequently, a patient may be so "tight" that wheezing is detected only after initial therapy. The patient might be resting comfortably or be in extreme respiratory distress. At such times there may be accessory muscle movement (subcostal, intercostal, or supraclavicular), nasal flaring (particularly in children), cyanosis, or altered mental status. Auscultation often reveals rhonchi, wheezing, and a reversal of the normal 2:1 inspiratory/expiratory ratio. An increase in respiratory rate, independent of fever, is also a cardinal sign.

Sometimes, especially in children, the only presentation of asthma is a chronic night cough. Another symptom complex includes wheezing and shortness of breath that occurs following exercise. This entity is known as exercise-induced asthma (EIA) or bronchospasm (EIB). Many Olympic-caliber athletes have EIB.

COPD

The typical picture of COPD is prominent cough, dyspnea, and often wheezing. In severe situations tachypnea, accessory muscle movement, breathing through pursed lips, cyanosis, and agitation are present. Long-standing disease may be indicated by a pronounced barrel chest (i.e., an increase in the anterior-to-posterior dimension). Copious sputum production may also be noted. Chest auscultation may reveal wheezes, rales, or rhonchi in varying intensity, or it can be normal. Heart sounds might be distant, or a gallop indicative of secondary heart disease may be detected. Examination of the extremities might reveal cyanosis of the nailbeds or clubbing of the fingers.

Chronic Cough

Clinical presentation of cough is self-explanatory: The patient is coughing. It is important to note whether the cough is dry or productive of sputum (thick, thin, purulent, bloody). The time of day or night often provides a clue to the extensive differential diagnosis as can evidence of allergy such as rhinitis, allergic shiners, or a transverse nose crease (the allergic salute). Of particular note are symptoms related to gastroesophageal reflux (i.e., heartburn, water brash, or increased belching). Finally, these patients may present with the signs and symptoms of a multitude of underlying diseases.

Diagnosis

Asthma and COPD

The diagnosis of asthma or COPD should be fairly evident after the history and physical examinations are completed. Laboratory and radiographic data usually cannot by themselves establish the diagnosis of either disorder but may provide confirmatory information and assist in the assessment of severity.

PULMONARY FUNCTION TESTS

Although extensive pulmonary testing may be indicated in the occasional patient, the most useful information is obtained from evaluating the forced expiratory volume in 1 second (FEV_1), the forced vital capacity (FVC), the FEV_1/FVC ratio, and the peak expiratory flow rate (PEFR). Obstructive disease is indicated by a reduced FEV_1 in the presence of a normal FVC, which also causes a reduction in the FEV_1/FVC ratio. Restrictive diseases (pure emphysema), on the other hand, shows a normal FEV_1, a decreased FVC, and an increased FEV_1/FVC ratio.

With asthma a useful test is to observe the change in FEV_1 following treatment with a bronchodilator. An increase of 15% is indicative of reversible airway disease.[4] Three stimulators—exercise, histamine, methacholine—may be used for provocative testing. A decrease in FEV_1 of 20% is considered positive. The PEFR may be obtained using a peak flowmeter and can easily be measured in the office or at home. It provides a quick, objective indication of the severity of an episode and can serve as a signal to start certain treatments. It is also a measure of the response to therapeutic intervention. It is highly recommended that patients be educated and provided with peak flowmeters. These devices must be demonstrated and practiced. Many patients have trouble mastering the technique. For the device to be fully effective, individuals must use it when they are feeling well in order to define a personal "best" for later comparison.

With COPD the spirometric abnormalities may be a mixture of obstructive and restrictive diseases. In asymptomatic patients, especially smokers, abnormal results can serve as an indicator of early illness and hopefully as a stimulus to quit smoking. In symptomatic patients, these measurements can serve as a sign of progression. Finally, the FEV_1 or PEFR may be used to evaluate the asthmatic component in the COPD patient.

ARTERIAL BLOOD GASES

Evaluation of the severity of disease may be assisted by the measurement of arterial blood gases (ABGs). Severe hypoxemia in the asthmatic or hypercapnia in the chronic lung patient might serve as an important factor in the decision to hospitalize a patient. Most outpatients do not need ABG measurements.

OTHER LABORATORY TESTS

Useful tests in ill patients include measurement of blood leukocytes as a sign of acute infection or hematocrit as indicative of an additional reason for hypoxemia if low or as a sign of long-standing hypoxemia if polycythemia is noted. Sputum evaluation is useful for identifying the pathogen in an acute infection.

CHEST RADIOGRAPHY

It is not necessary to obtain a chest radiograph on every patient with asthma or COPD. A radiograph may be useful in the undiagnosed patient with chronic cough and may help to identify complications in patients with obstructive disease. These problems might include pneumonia, pneumothorax, pneumomediastinum, or subcutaneous emphysema. In the newly discovered asthmatic (especially children) radiography should be done if foreign body aspiration is suspected. The chest radiograph of the COPD patient may be normal, show a mild increase in lung markings, demonstrate the hyperlucency, overinflation, and bullae often seen with emphysema, or show an enlarged heart or pulmonary congestion seen with heart failure. On occasion, a chest film holds the key to differentiating congestive heart failure with wheezing (cardiac asthma) from asthma. Other radiologic procedures, such as lung scans, computed tomography (CT) scans, and angiography have a role only in the management of complications.

Chronic Cough

The diagnosis and workup of chronic cough is often difficult, time-consuming, and expensive. Irwin and associates[7] presented a schema for evaluating previously undiagnosed patients. Their suggestions, in decreasing order of usefulness, include the history, physical examination, pulmonary function tests, methacholine challenge, upper gastrointestinal radiology, measurement of esophageal pH, sinus and chest radiography, and bronchoscopy. Following this design a diagnosis is possible in 99% of patients.

Management

The management of asthma and COPD is best viewed from a standpoint of both disease complexes. It includes avoidance, immunotherapy, exercise, drug treatment, and psychosocial support (Fig. 13.1).

Avoidance

The life style of any patient with pulmonary problems may be drastically affected by environmental factors: climate, outdoor air pollution, and indoor air pollution.

Asthma Maintenance

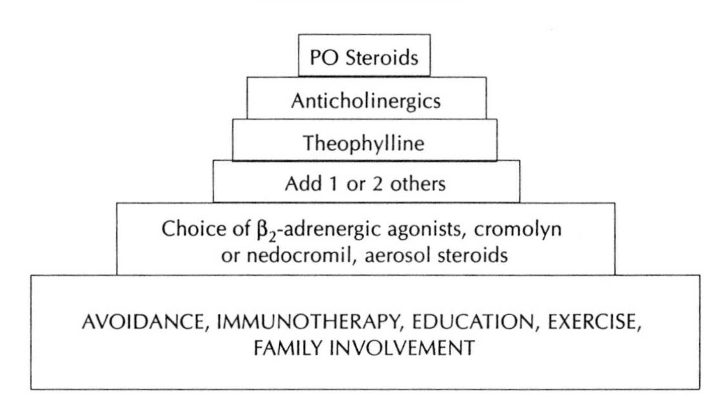

Acute Asthma

Admission

Corticosteroids

β_2-adrenergic agonists, Oxygen, Fluids

TREAT ASAP AND AGGRESSIVELY

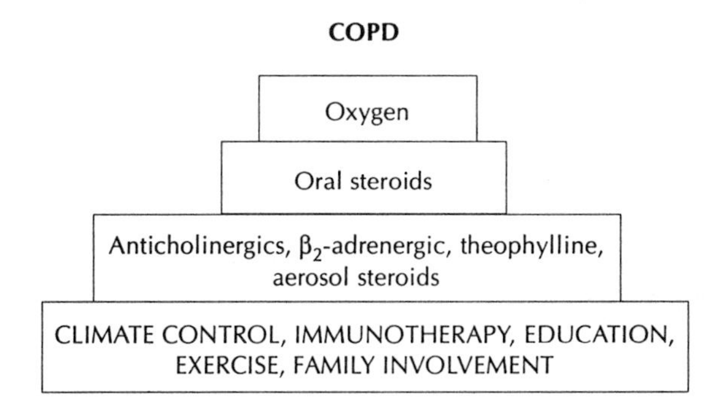

FIGURE 13.1. Recommended step treatment plan for asthma and COPD. ASAP = as soon as possible.

CLIMATE

Both asthmatic and COPD sufferers may be affected by changes in wind velocity, humidity, and temperature. Low wind velocity allows accumulation of allergens; high humidity leads to an increase in pollen-producing plants and molds; and sudden temperature drops cause a fall in airway conduction.[8] Barometric pressure changes are also associated with exacerbations of asthma and COPD. Extremes in climatic events, such as prolonged heat waves or air inversions, often result in increased mortality among COPD patients. Although patients cannot avoid climatic changes, they can stay inside on particularly bad days and can minimize the effects by using filtered air-conditioning and heating systems maintained at fairly constant temperature year round.

OUTDOOR AIR POLLUTION

Potential allergens are man-made (e.g., smoke and chemical fumes) and natural substances (e.g., pollens, dusts, and molds). Although difficult to avoid, some factors can be minimized by controlling the type of grass, ornamental shrubs, and flowering vegetation around the home.

INDOOR AIR POLLUTION

Fortunately, indoor allergens are much more readily controlled. It is of paramount importance to eliminate tobacco smoke. Other potential irritants include building materials, cleaning agents, air fresheners, pest control chemicals, decorative plants, dried flowers, and cosmetics. The bedroom is a critical room to allergy-proof. Attention is directed to pillows, mattresses, carpets, drapes, blankets, shelf ornaments, and stuffed animals (especially in the bed). Wood stoves and kerosene heaters have been shown to aggravate respiratory problems. Sometimes families must make sacrifices concerning pets. This entire aspect of avoidance must be stressed to all patients and may obviate the need for further treatment.

Education of patients is essential regarding all aspects of management. Excellent material is available through the National Asthma Education Program.[9]

Immunotherapy

DESENSITIZATION

If avoidance fails, allergic patients should be tried on antihistamines and nasal sprays and considered for allergy desensitization.[10]

IMMUNIZATION

Influenza and pneumococcal vaccines should be given to all patients with significant respiratory illness. Influenza vaccine is administered yearly about 2 to 3 months prior to anticipated outbreaks. October and November are the prime times to immunize in the United States. If a patient misses the vaccine, consideration should be given to prophylaxis with amantadine. Pneumococcal vaccine must be given only once.

Exercise

Aerobic exercise is important for both asthmatics and COPD patients. Proper and consistent exercise at least three times a week can lead to improved tolerance and endurance and an increase in the feeling of wellness.[11] Consider ordering pulmonary rehabilitation.

Drug Treatment

The choice of medication for these illnesses has greatly expanded since the 1980s and is currently continuing to undergo rapid changes in philosophy. It is especially true for asthma, where emphasis has shifted from treating just bronchospasm to treating inflammation as well.[1] Unfortunately, those who suffer with COPD have not experienced as great a revolution in drug treatment.

β_2-ADRENERGIC AGONISTS

The β_2-adrenergic agonist class of medication (Beta2s) is now the first step for treating bronchospasm. Available as liquids, short- and long-acting tablets, metered-dose inhalers (MDI), dry powder inhalers, nebulizable solutions, and injectables, these agents have many potential uses. Available in the United States are albuterol (Proventil, Ventolin), biltolteral (Tornalate), metaproterenol (Alupent, Metaprel), pirbuterol (Maxair), terbutaline (Brethaire, Brethine), and salmeterol (Serevent) (Table 13.1).

The choice of preparation depends on the patient's age and the acuteness of the situation. MDIs and nebulizers have an almost instantaneous onset of action, and sustained-released tablets offer assistance with nocturnal symptoms. Oral forms have their greatest use in young children. It is rarely necessary to use both the oral and inhalation route at the same time, a situation that leads to increased toxicity with little gain in benefit.

Beta2s are the treatment of choice for episodic or mild asthmatics and for EIB. Once the need is established for continual usage, as for moderate and severe asthmatics, some authorities use these agents as first-line treatment whereas others reserve their use for rescue efforts, preferring to

TABLE 13.1. Recommended dosages for theophylline, β_2-adrenergic agonists, and corticosteroids

Medication	Age group (years)	Route	Usual dosage
Theophylline	< 1	PO	Varies
	1–9	PO	24 mg/kg/day
	9–12	PO	20 mg/kg/day
	12–16	PO	18 mg/kg/day
	> 16, smoker	PO	18 mg/kg/day
	> 16, nonsmoker	PO	13 mg/kg/day
Albuterol	> 2	PO	0.1 mg/kg/ tid–qid, max 2 mg tid
	> 2	MDI	1–2 inhal q4h
	> 12	Nebulizer	2.5 mg q4h
Bitolterol	> 12	MDI	2 inhal q4h or 3 inhal q6h
Metaproterenol	< 6	PO	1.3–2.6 mg/kg/day tid–qid
	> 6	PO	10–20 mg tid/qid
	> 2	MDI	1–2 inhal q4h
	> 12	Nebulizer	0.2–0.3 ml q4h
Pirbuterol	> 12	MDI	1–2 inhal q4h
Salmeterol	> 12	MDI	2 inhal q12h
Terbutaline	> 12	PO	1.25–5.00 mg tid
	> 12	MDI	2 inhal q4h
Beclomethasone	> 6	MDI	2–4 inhal bid/qid, max 20/day
Flunisolide	> 6	MDI	2 inhal bid, max 8/day
Fluticasone	>6	MDI	3 different strengths
Triamcinolone	> 6	MDI	1–2 inhal tid/qid, max 16/day
Prednisone	1–12	PO	1–2 mg/kg/day, taper 5–10 days
	> 12	PO	40–80 mg/day, taper 5–10 days

Source: Data are from the *PDR.*[17]
MDI = Multiple-dose inhaler; inhal = inhalations

use antiinflammatory drugs first. Certainly, every patient with significant obstructive disease should always have this medication on hand.

The newest member of this class, salmeterol, is unique in its 12-hour action. It is indicated for maintenance and nocturnal symptoms. Shorter-acting agents may still be used between doses if rescue is needed, although tolerance may become a problem.[12]

In the near future, dry powder forms of MDIs should be available. This advance will hopefully reduce the problems associated with propellant gases and also be more compatible with the environment.

For the treatment of acute situations, Beta2s are the agents of choice. They can be administered by nebulizer (and repeated at 60- to 90-minute intervals if needed[13]) or by MDI using an InspirEase at the rate of one inhalation per minute for 5 minutes. The use of these agents has supplanted the need for older agents such as ephedrine, isoproterenol, and epinephrine. Even in the emergency situation, Beta2s have been found to be equally effective with significantly less toxicity when compared to subcutaneous epinephrine.[14]

Some patients experience great trouble utilizing an MDI. Proper technique must be taught and observed. For those too young or who cannot master the MDI, the following spacer devices are available: InspirEase, Inhal-aid, Paper tube, and Aerochamber.[15] Home-made alternatives are the inside of a paper towel roll or a small paper lunch bag. Any of these devices should work with all inhalers.

In the COPD patient these drugs have less application but are still valuable when bronchospasm is present. Pulse and blood pressure should be monitored, and inhalation is the route of choice.

CORTICOSTEROIDS

The use of steroids for asthma has received considerable impetus in recent years. Traditionally thought to be too strong for chronic use, the advent of MDI preparations has minimized side effects and pushed corticosteroids to the forefront. In addition, recognition of the importance of inflammation in the pathophysiology of asthma has made many authorities advocate corticosteroids as first-line treatment.[16] Unfortunately, the probably unfounded fear of the effect of steroids on growth and adrenal function has caused a reluctance to utilize this medication. For the moderate to severe asthmatic, for the unstable patient, and during an acute crisis, however, there should be no hesitancy to use steroids.

Aerosol preparations include beclomethasone (Beclovent, Vanceril), flunisolide (AeroBid), fluticasone (Flovent), and triamcinolone (Azmacort). The effect of these medications may not be fully seen for up to 4 to 8 weeks and are therefore not effective for the acute attack. They also do not protect against adrenal insufficiency. Oral medication must be tapered when switching to an aerosol (Table 13.1).

Oral steroids, usually in the form of prednisone, are essential for use during the acute exacerbation or for the severe, chronic patient with asthma or COPD. When used early during an episode, steroids may prevent a relapse[18] or the need for hospitalization. Some physicians prescribe oral steroids to any patient needing treatment in an emergency setting. Patients with long-standing disease often develop recognizable patterns of deterioration, such as with acute upper respiratory infections. These patients can be instructed to use steroids early to prevent exacerbations. Dosage varies with age and weight. For chronic treatment, every-other-day administration is preferred, whereas multiple daily dosing may be most effective in the acute situation.

Corticosteroids are also available for intravenous use, which is indicated whenever hospitalization is being considered. Unfortunately, there is no definitive proof as to the effectiveness of intravenous steroids for preventing hospitalization. If attempted, allow at least 4 hours for action.

CROMOLYN AND NEDOCROMIL

Primarily used as prophylactic agents for asthma, cromolyn and nedocromil are antiinflammatory and, due to their almost complete lack of side effects, represent a significant therapeutic advantage. Unfortunately, not all patients respond to them.

Cromolyn (Intal) is available for MDI or nebulizer. Its onset of action can be as long as 1 to 2 months. Dosage is two inhalations qid; tapering to less frequent dosage can be attempted. Once in usage this medication should be used throughout an acute episode so as not to lose the prophylaxis. Along with Beta2s and inhaled steroids, cromolyn is useful for EIB.

Nedocromil (Tilade) is the newer of the two agents, and its safety is comparable to that of cromolyn. Dosage recommendations are also similar. In addition, nedocromil may be effective in preventing the cough caused by ACE inhibitors.

LEUKOTRIENE ANTAGONISTS

This is a new and exciting class of medications that has just been released. There are currently three available: Zafirlukast (Accolate), Zileuton (Zyflo), and Montelukast (Singulair). Optimum dosing is still being worked out and comparative studies are lacking, but initial studies show great promise.

THEOPHYLLINE

Long the cornerstone of asthma treatment, theophylline is no longer the initial drug of choice. A bronchodilator, theophylline is best utilized for patients needing more than one maintenance drug and for those with pronounced nocturnal symptoms.[19] It is also worth a trial in COPD patients.

There are various formulations of theophylline: liquid, capsule, tablet, slow-release products, and the intravenous form. Most patients require several days of continuous usage to reach maximal effectiveness. Once a steady state is reached, it is best to maintain the same brand, as bioavailability may vary from product to product. Smokers and children tend to need higher doses due to rapid metabolism. Significant interactions are possible with erythromycins, fluoroquinolones, cimetidine, phenytoin, and oral contraceptives. Also, dosages need to be closely monitored in patients with liver failure or congestive heart failure. Serum theophylline levels are recommended for all the above situations and in difficult patients where fine tuning is needed. The serum therapeutic level has been changed from 10 to 20 mg/L to 8 to 15 mg/L.[20]

Older preparations that contain subtherapeutic doses of theophylline, Marax and Tedral, are no longer considered appropriate therapy (Table 13.1).

Children represent a special group who require close monitoring. With growth, dosage requires constant readjustment. For small children, slow-release capsules (SloBid, Theodur Sprinkles) are particularly useful when sprinkled onto food, thereby avoiding the nausea often associated with liquid preparations. Theophylline has come under scrutiny with regard to potential interference with school performance. To date no significant relationship has been established.

In the acute situation (office or emergency room) theophylline (as aminophylline) is no longer considered appropriate for intravenous usage as it does not represent a therapeutic advantage but does significantly increase toxicity.[21] It may be useful, however, once the patient has been hospitalized.

ANTICHOLINERGICS

The current choice of anticholinergic drug is ipratropium (Atrovent) for MDI or nebulizer. For COPD, because of fewer side effects, ipratropium may well be the preferred bronchodilator. The usual dosage is two inhalations qid, but this dosage can be exceeded in COPD patients.[20] For asthma use ipratropium if other treatment is not effective.

CALCIUM CHANNEL BLOCKERS

Calcium channel blockers have been suggested to have a mild bronchodilatory effect, but it has not been clinically demonstrated.[22] They are, however, effective for the treatment of hypertension in obstructive disease, especially compared to β-blockers and ACE inhibitors.

ANTIBIOTICS

For acute bacterial infections in patients with asthma and COPD, antibiotics are essential. There has been debate concerning when to treat the COPD-afflicted patient. The use of broad-spectrum antibiotics appears to be indicated when COPD sufferers have at least two of the following three symptoms: an increase in dyspnea, an increase in sputum production, or an increase in sputum purulence.[23]

MUCOLYTICS AND EXPECTORANTS

The value of mucolytics and expectorants has not been demonstrated in objective studies.[24]

OXYGEN

Except in the acute situation, oxygen should be reserved for chronic patients who are in distress when breathing room air. With COPD patients who retain high levels of carbon dioxide, the only functioning respiratory drive may be related to hypoxia. It is therefore critical to adjust the oxygen to a level where the hypoxic drive is not lost.

PREGNANCY AND BREAST-FEEDING

Pregnancy is complicated by asthma about 1% of the time, with a potentially large risk to the fetus if hypoxia develops. The use of theophylline, Beta2s, cromolyn, and steroids is generally considered safe. Some antibiotics and decongestants, live virus vaccines, and iodides must be avoided.

For lactating mothers the same medications considered safe during pregnancy are acceptable. Breast-feeding should be strongly encouraged, as studies suggest a delay in the onset of allergies and asthma in the infant.[1,19]

PSYCHOSOCIAL SUPPORT

Psychosocial support is a critical component in any management plan and is addressed later in the chapter.

Prevention

Asthma and COPD are at opposite extremes when it comes to treatment and prevention. Whereas there are several fine alternatives for asthma treatment, management of COPD is at best symptomatic. On the other hand, asthma is essentially unpreventable, whereas COPD should not exist.

Smoking cessation is the key to relegating COPD to medical history. Except for a rare genetic or occupational case (which should also be preventable with good industrial hygiene), most COPD is directly related to smoking. As a nation we are moving toward an atmosphere of nonsmokers' rights, but unfortunately children still have ready access to tobacco products and are starting to smoke in large numbers. Physicians therefore must remind each and every patient at every encounter to begin the process of cessation.

Control of smoking is also key to decreasing the morbidity of asthma. Even side-stream smoke has been shown to result in more attacks, more complications, and more frequent need for emergency services. It is critical that the parents of asthmatic children never smoke in the house or car their child rides in.

Prevention of death has always been a priority within the medical profession. It is certainly appropriate for asthma and COPD.

Asthma is usually viewed as a nonfatal disease, but it does carry the potential for death. Most studies show that preventable deaths and hospitalizations have been the result of delayed treatment due primarily to two factors: the patient's or family's inability to recognize the severity of an attack or the physician's poor assessment of the severity of an attack.[25,26] Suggestions for prevention include frequent use of peak flow meters as an objective guide to severity, establishing effective maintenance therapy, and emphasizing patient and family education. Education is aimed at recognizing an attack, knowing what measures to take at home, and learning to call for help early. The material provided in the national education program is superb and should be made available to all patients.[9]

On the other hand, COPD is a highly fatal disease, the fifth leading cause of mortality in the United States, with more than 75,000 deaths per annum.[27] Although little can be done to reverse this disease, good management of the environment, appropriate medication, and smoking cessation aid in improving the quality of life for the affected individual.

Family and Community Issues

Family support is an essential factor in the successful treatment of chronic lung disease. This point is especially true for children and the debilitated, who might be unable to care for themselves.

Asthma

Patient and family attitudes are critical in the patient's acceptance of this disease. Several factors have been identified with regard to poor patient attitude: the unpredictable nature of asthma leading to a feeling of "beyond my control"; a feeling of stigmatization; a false perception that asthma is psychogenic and therefore "in my head"; a tendency to deny the disease; and the fear elicited by an experience of being unable to breathe.[28] These attitudes may handicap all attempts at treatment and should be addressed via thorough patient and family education.

Also important is the tendency for families to label their asthmatics as ill. It is best to view the patient as a person with asthma and not as an asthmatic person. All activities should be continued, especially sports and physical education. It is far better to use an MDI and run than to sit on the sidelines and watch.

COPD

Emotional difficulties are common in COPD sufferers. The dyspnea and fatigue of this disease often leads to depression and fear. Quality of life may be reduced in all areas, including social, sexual, vocational, and recreational activities, leading to further loss of self-esteem and isolation.[29] Patients should be encouraged to do as much as possible for themselves and must be given every opportunity to participate in the usual family and community events, even if a wheelchair and oxygen are needed. When the illness becomes terminal, patients should be counseled to keep control of their own lives by participating in the decisions of how and where to die. They can be encouraged to make living wills or execute powers of attorney. If appropriate, patients should be allowed to die at home, and physicians should be willing to make house calls. This measure improves the final quality of life by affording the patient the comfort of dying in a familiar setting, surrounded by family and friends.

References

1. Guidelines for the diagnosis and management of asthma. National asthma education program, expert panel report. Bethesda: National Heart, Lung and Blood Institute, April 1997. NIH Publ. No. 97-4051.
2. Shuttari MF. Asthma: diagnosis and management. Am Fam Physician 1995; 52:2225–35.
3. Johnston SL, Pattemore PK, Sanderson G, et al. Community study of role of viral infections in exacerbations of asthma in 9–11 year old children. BMJ 1995;310:1225–9.
4. American Thoracic Society. Standards for the diagnosis and care of patients with chronic obstructive pulmonary disease (COPD) and asthma. Am Rev Respir Dis 1987;136:225–44.
5. Ingram RH. Chronic bronchitis, emphysema, and airway obstruction. In: Harrison's principles of internal medicine. New York: McGraw-Hill, 1994: 1197–1206.
6. Snider GL, Kleinerman J, Thurlbeck WM, Bengali ZH. The definition of emphysema: report of a National Heart, Lung and Blood Institute, Division of Lung Diseases workshop. Am Rev Respir Dis 1985;132:182–5.
7. Irwin RS, Curley FJ, French CL. Chronic cough, the spectrum and frequency of causes, key components of the diagnostic evaluation, and outcome of specific therapy. Am Rev Respir Dis 1990;141:640–7.
8. Kemp JP, Metzer EO. Getting control of the allergic child's environment. Pediatr Ann 1989;18:801–8.
9. Teach your patients about asthma: a clinician's guide. Washington, DC: National Institutes of Health, 1992. NIH Publ. No. 92-2737.
10. Abramson MJ, Puy RM, Weiner JM. Is allergen immunotherapy effective in asthma? A meta-analysis of randomized controlled trials. Am J Respir Crit Care Med 1995;151:969–74.
11. Gross NJ. COPD management: setting therapeutic goals. J Respir Dis 1996;17:92–100.
12. Anderson CJ, Bardana EJ. Asthma in the elderly: interactions to be wary of. J Respir Dis 1995;16:965–76.
13. Fanta CH, Israel E, Sheffer AL. Managing—and preventing—severe asthma attacks. J Respir Dis 1992;13:94–108.

14. Becker AB, Nelson NA, Simons FER. Inhaled salbutamol (albuterol) vs. injected epinephrine in the treatment of acute asthma in children. J Pediatr 1983;102:465–9.
15. Plaut TF. Holding chambers for aerosol drugs. Pediatr Ann 1989;18:824–6.
16. Szefler SJ. A comparison of aerosol glucocorticoids in the treatment of chronic bronchial asthma. Pediatr Asthma Allergy Immunol 1991;5:227–35.
17. Physician's desk reference. 50th ed. Oradell, NJ: Medical Economics, 1996.
18. Chapman KR, Verbeck PR, White JG, Rebeeck AS. Effect of a short course of prednisone in the prevalence of early relapse after the emergency room treatment of acute asthma. N Engl J Med 1991;324:788–94.
19. Weinberg H. Asthma in primary care patients, challenges and controversies. Postgrad Med 1990;88:107–14.
20. Gross NJ. COPD management: achieving bronchodilatation. J Respir Dis 1996;17:183–95.
21. Seigel D, Sheppard D, Gelb A, Weinberg PF. Aminophylline increases the toxicity but not the efficacy of an inhaled beta-adrenergic agonist in the treatment of acute exacerbations of asthma. Am Rev Respir Dis 1985;132: 283–6.
22. Olivier KN, Yankaskas JR. What role for calcium channel blockers in asthma? J Respir Dis 1991;12:703–7.
23. Anthonisen NR, Manfreda J, Warren CPW, et al. Antibiotic therapy in exacerbation of COPD. Ann Intern Med 1987;106:196–204.
24. Brain J. Aerosol and humidity therapy. Am Rev Respir Dis 1980;122 (Suppl):17–21.
25. Morray B, Redding G. Factors associated with prolonged hospitalization of children with asthma. Arch Pediatr Adolesc Med 1995;149:276–9.
26. Strunk RC. Death caused by asthma: minimizing the risks. J Respir Dis 1989;10:21–36.
27. Rosen MJ. Treatment of exacerbations of COPD. Am Fam Physician 1992;45:693–7.
28. Dirks JF. Patient attitude as a factor in asthma management. Pract Cardiol 1986;12(1):84–98.
29. Dowell AR. Quality of life: how important is managing COPD? J Respir Dis 1991;12:1057–72.

CASE PRESENTATION

Subjective

PATIENT PROFILE

Samuel Nelson is a 48-year-old single white male farm worker.

PRESENTING PROBLEM

"My breathing is worse."

PRESENT ILLNESS

For the past 5 years, Mr. Nelson has had gradually progressive cough, shortness of breath on exertion, and occasional wheezing. He has continued to smoke and does not take his medication regularly. When worse, he returns to the physician to refill his β-agonist inhaler for use as needed.

PAST MEDICAL HISTORY

He had pneumonia 3 years ago that did not require hospitalization.

SOCIAL HISTORY

Samuel was a high school dropout at age 16. He has never married and lives with his parents. He has no close friends.

HABITS

He has smoked two packs of cigarettes daily since age 15. He uses no alcohol or recreational drugs.

FAMILY HISTORY

His father, aged 76, has diabetes mellitus and osteoarthritis. His mother, aged 71, has high blood pressure. Three siblings are living and well.

- What additional information would you like about the history of present illness?

- What might be Mr. Nelson's reasons for the visit today? How would you inquire about this?
- What information about Mr. Nelson's work might be useful, and how would you ask about this?
- What more would you like to know about the patient's adaptation to his illness? Why might this be important?

Objective

VITAL SIGNS

Height, 5 ft, 10 in; weight 180 lb; blood pressure, 140/80; pulse, 76; respirations, 22; temperature, 37.2°C.

EXAMINATION

The patient is not in acute distress but has an occasional cough while talking. The head, eyes, ears, nose, and throat are normal. The neck and thyroid gland are normal. The chest has an increased anteroposterior diameter, and there are distant breath sounds throughout. No rales are present, but there are occasional faint wheezes on forced expiration. The heart has a regular sinus rhythm, and no murmurs are present.

- What more—if anything—might be included in the physical examination? Why?
- What—if any—laboratory tests would you order today? Why?
- What—if any—diagnostic imaging would you order today? Why?
- If, in addition to the symptoms described above, Mr. Nelson had lost 12 lb since a previous visit 6 months ago, what might you do differently? Explain.

Assessment

- What is your diagnostic impression today, and how would you explain this to the patient?
- How would you assess the meaning of the illness to Mr. Nelson?
- What is the apparent contribution of smoking to the patient's disease, and how would you describe this to him?
- The patient's employer calls to ask you about how Mr. Nelson is doing? How would you respond?

Plan

- What would be your therapeutic recommendations to the patient regarding medication, activity, and life style? How would you explain this to the patient?
- How might you persuade Mr. Nelson to stop smoking?
- What are the implications of this illness for the family and community?
- What continuing care would you advise? Explain.

14

Gastritis, Esophagitis, and Peptic Ulcer Disease

Alan M. Adelman and James P. Richardson

Dyspepsia/Epigastric Pain

Gastritis, esophagitis, and peptic ulcer disease present commonly with epigastric pain, or dyspepsia. Dyspepsia refers to upper abdominal pain or discomfort and is often associated with fullness, belching, bloating, heartburn, food intolerance, nausea, or vomiting. Dyspepsia is a common problem. Despite discoveries about the cause and treatment of peptic ulcer disease, dyspepsia remains a challenging problem to evaluate and treat.

Epidemiology

Dyspepsia is a common problem, with a annual incidence of 1% to 2% in the general population and a prevalence that may reach 20% to 40%. The four major causes of dyspepsia are nonulcer dyspepsia (NUD), peptic ulcer disease (PUD), gastroesophageal reflux disease (GERD), and gastritis. NUD, PUD, GERD, and gastritis account for more than 90% of all causes of dyspepsia. Other, less common causes of dyspepsia are cholelithiasis, irritable bowel disease, esophageal or gastric cancer, pancreatitis, pancreatic cancer, Zollinger-Ellison syndrome, and abdominal angina. Patients who seek medical attention for dyspepsia are more likely to be concerned about the seriousness of the symptom, worried about cancer or heart disease, and experiencing more stress than individuals who do not seek medical attention for dyspepsia.[1]

Presentation

No single symptom is helpful for distinguishing among the causes of dyspepsia, but some patient characteristics are predictive of serious disease. For example, as single symptoms, nocturnal pain, relief of pain by antacids, worsening of pain by food, anorexia, nausea, and food intolerance are not helpful for distinguishing the causes of dyspepsia. Age greater than 50 years, male gender, a history of smoking, and a history of peptic ulcer disease or hiatal hernia are likely to be associated with gastric carcinoma, ulcers, and esophageal strictures. There is tremendous overlap of symptoms described by patients with and without endoscopic confirmed diagnoses.[2] With the possible exceptions of peptic ulcer disease and duodenitis, there was no association of clinical value between endoscopic findings and dyspeptic symptoms. It is important to inquire about the use of nonsteroidal antiinflammatory drugs (NSAIDs), as their use is a frequent cause of peptic ulcer disease. It is also important to ask about symptoms related to serious complications of peptic ulcer disease, such as obstructive symptoms, hematemesis, melena, hematochezia, and weight loss. To summarize, symptoms are not useful for differentiating the causes of dyspepsia.

General Approach

Individuals with evidence of complications of PUD (e.g., gastric outlet obstruction or bleeding) or systemic disease (e.g., weight loss, anemia) should be thoroughly evaluated and promptly managed. This situation occurs uncommonly. Because age is the strongest predictor of finding "organic" disease on endoscopy, individuals over the age of 50 years should be thoroughly evaluated. For the remaining patients there are several possible strategies for the management of dyspeptic symptoms: 1) empiric anti-secretory therapy, 2) empiric anti-*H. pylori* therapy, 3) non-invasive testing for *H. pylori* and if positive, empiric therapy for *H. pylori,* 4) non-invasive testing for *H. pylori* and if positive, endoscopy, and 5) immediate endoscopy to determine a specific cause of the dyspeptic symptoms. The specific rationale for empiric anti-*H. pylori* therapy and non-invasive testing for *H. pylori* are discussed in the section on Peptic Ulcer Disease.

Empiric treatment for dyspepsia consists of standard antiacid therapy (Table 14.1). If antacids are tried initially and fail to relieve symptoms, a histamine$_2$ receptor antagonist (H_2RA), sucralfate, or a proton pump inhibitor (PPI) should be tried before further workup is undertaken.

The rationale for empiric treatment is based on four underlying principles. First, most patients have NUD, PUD, or GERD. Most of these individuals improve with standard antiacid therapies. Approximately 70% of patients with PUD are symptom-free within several weeks regardless of the therapy. Second, the risk of cancer, such as gastric or esophageal is small, especially in patients less than 50 years of age. Prompt, unrestricted use of endoscopy has not increased the early detection of gastric cancer. Even if a gastric carcinoma is initially treated empirically, a delay in definitive treatment for 4 to 8 weeks has no effect on the outcome. Third, the natural history of PUD (during the pre-*Helicobacter pylori* era), NUD, and GERD is marked by periodicity and recurrence. If

TABLE 14.1. Usual daily dosage of antiacid medications

Generic and brand names	Usual daily dosage
Antacids (Maalox, Mylanta)	15–30 ml 0.5 hour and 2 hours after meals and at bedtime
Histamine-2 receptor antagonists	
Cimetidine (Tagamet)	800 mg hs
Famotidine (Pepcid)	20 mg bid
Nizatidine (Axid)	150 mg bid
Ranitidine (Zantac)	150 mg bid
Sucralfate	1 g qid
Proton pump inhibitors,	
Omeprazole (Prilosec)	20 mg qd
Lansoprazole (Prevacid)	15 mg qd

symptoms recur, the patient should have a thorough evaluation. This approach potentially saves money, as only individuals with recurrent symptoms are evaluated with expensive procedures such as endoscopy.

When available, upper endoscopy is the procedure of choice for thorough investigation of dyspeptic symptoms. Although an upper gastrointestinal (UGI) series is less expensive and may be more readily available, it has a false-negative rate that exceeds 18% in some studies and a false-positive rate of 13% to 35%. In addition, the UGI series is poor for diagnosing GERD and gastritis, two of the most common causes of dyspepsia. A negative UGI does not rule out disease, and if indicated, further evaluation with upper endoscopy should be pursued. Upper endoscopy has lower false-positive and false-negative rates, and biopsy can be undertaken, although it is more costly, and its availability depends on the presence of a gastroenterologist. The indications for upper endoscopy recommended by the American College of Physicians are (1) persistence of symptoms after 6 to 8 weeks of therapy; (2) no response to therapy after 7 to 10 days; (3) signs of complications of peptic disease; (4) signs of systemic illness; and (5) symptom recurrence.[3]

Which approach is best is still unclear. Two decision analyses produced similar results. Ebell et al.[4] favored empiric *H. pylori* eradication or the use of serum *H. pylori* serology to identify patients for *H. pylori* eradication. Ofman et al.[5] Favored anti-*H. pylori* therapy as the most cost-effective approach. In the only randomized trial to test empiric treatment versus thorough evaluation, Bytzer et al.[6] reported that empiric treatment led to higher costs than prompt endoscopy. These higher costs were due to a greater number of sick days and greater use of antiulcer medications in the empiric treatment group. Several authors[7,8] have suggested that only those dyspeptic patients with a positive serology for *H. pylori* should be referred for upper endoscopy. Fraser et al.[7] reported that in the absence of NSAID use and a negative serology for *H. pylori,* peptic ulcer disease was unlikely.

Gastroesophageal Reflux Disease

Gastroesophageal reflux disease (GERD) is a common problem. About 10% of the general population report heartburn daily and 15% to 40% experience it monthly. GERD results from exposure of the lower esophagus to gastric acid, pepsin, or bile acids. Several factors may lead to GERD including hiatal hernia, incompetence of the lower esophageal sphincter (LES), inappropriate LES relaxation, impaired esophageal peristalsis and acid clearance, impaired gastric emptying, and repeated vomiting.[9] Exposure to excessive acid or pepsin can lead to damage of the esophageal mucosa, resulting in inflammation and ultimately scarring and stricture formation.

Presentation

The most reliable symptom of GERD is heartburn, a retrosternal burning sensation that may radiate from the epigastrium to the throat. Patients may also complain of pyrosis or water brash, the regurgitation of bitter-tasting material into the mouth. GERD can cause respiratory problems including laryngitis, chronic cough, aspiration pneumonia, and wheezing. Atypical chest pain can also be caused by GERD. Finally, patients may complain of odynophagia (pain with swallowing) or dysphagia.

Diagnosis

A young patient with no evidence of systemic illness requires no further workup and can be treated empirically. Older patients, particularly those with the complaint of odynophagia or dysphagia, require evaluation to rule out tumor or stricture. Upper endoscopy is the evaluation of choice. Ambulatory 24-hour pH monitoring is the most sensitive test for demonstrating reflux if endoscopy is negative. A barium swallow study or esophageal manometry may be necessary if a motility disorder is suspected, as endoscopy is often normal in patients with this problem.

The presence of hiatal hernia does not equate with a diagnosis of GERD. All patients with hiatal hernia do not have reflux, and all patients with GERD do not have a hiatal hernia. Approximately 50% of the population have a hiatal hernia, but most have no reflux symptoms.

Management

Gastroesophageal reflux disease is treated by nonpharmacologic and pharmacologic means. It is important to note that whereas patients with mild disease may respond to nonpharmacologic treatment, patients with moderate to severe symptoms or recurrent disease must continue to observe life style changes while drug therapy is added or intensified.

All patients with GERD should be advised to reduce weight (if over their ideal body weight), avoid large meals (especially several hours before going to sleep), refrain from lying down after meals, refrain from wearing tight clothing around the waist, and avoid exercise before sleep. Patients who experience nocturnal symptoms often find relief by putting the head of the bed on blocks 4 to 6 inches in height. Sleeping on more pillows or on a wedge may be less effective because of nocturnal movements. Because nicotine lowers LES pressure, smoking cessation is recommended. Medications that can lower LES pressure and should be avoided include alcohol, theophylline, calcium channel blockers, β-adrenergic agonists, and α-adrenergic antagonists.

Patients who do not respond to life style and medication changes alone are treated with pharmacologic agents. Antacids or over-the-counter H_2-blockers (cimetidine, famotidine, ranitidine) can be used for mild, intermittent heartburn. If symptoms are persistent or severe, a prokinetic agent or an H_2RA is substituted for or added.

Prokinetic agents are appealing from the theoretic standpoint that these drugs can increase esophageal contraction amplitude, increase LES pressure, and accelerate gastric emptying, three of the most significant motility problems in the pathogenesis of GERD.[10] Prokinetic drugs include metoclopramide, bethanechol, and cisapride. Metoclopramide is a dopamine antagonist that can cause extrapyramidal symptoms and, rarely, tardive dyskinesia; hence it is clearly a second-line agent for GERD. Bethanechol, a cholinergic agonist, is effective for GERD but can cause abdominal cramping, headache, reflex tachycardia, and flushing. Bethanechol should not be used alone for GERD because it may stimulate acid secretion through cholinergic mechanisms. Bethanechol has not been approved by the U.S. Food and Drug Administration (FDA) for treatment of GERD.

Cisapride works through serotonin receptors to increase the release of acetylcholine from the myenteric plexus.[11] Symptomatic relief has been documented, but healing of erosive esophagitis has not been demonstrated in trials in the United States.[12] Side effects are uncommon but include headache, nausea, and diarrhea. The starting dose of cisapride is 10 mg, taken at least 15 minutes before each meal and at bedtime. The maximum dose is 20 mg four times a day.

H_2RAs have been available for 20 years. Cimetidine, ranitidine, famotidine, and nizatidine suppress acid secretion by competing with histamine, thereby blocking its effect on parietal cells of the stomach. H_2RAs are effective when used for 6 to 12 weeks. Daytime and nocturnal acid production must be inhibited; therefore, twice-daily dosing is recommended rather than just nocturnal dosing. Sucralfate has also been shown to be efficacious for mild to moderate GERD. Sucralfate is a sulfated disaccharide that does not neutralize acid but appears to protect against acid by local effects on the mucosa.

For severe or refractory GERD, doubling the standard dose of H_2RAs may be effective. Combining H_2RAs with prokinetic agents may be better than using either agent alone. A PPI, such as omeprazole, decreases gastric acid secretion and is more potent than cimetidine or ranitidine for suppressing both basal and stimulated acid production. Omeprazole has been shown to be effective therapy when H_2RAs have failed. There has been concern about the long-term safety of omeprazole because of the increase incidence of gastric carcinoid tumors in rats on long-term therapy. Experience with omeprazole now totals more than 5 years in some patients; an increase in gastric carcinoid tumors has not been noted, and the FDA allows omeprazole for long-term therapy. A new PPI, lansoprazole, appears to be as effective as omeprazole for treatment of erosive esophagitis. Like omeprazole, lansoprazole is well tolerated, but long-term experience with it is lacking. For severe or refractory GERD, doubling the standard dose of the PPI may be needed.

With the advent of PPIs, few patients should require surgery for GERD. Possible indications for surgery are young age, nonadherence to medical therapy, disease refractory to high-dose PPI therapy, or complications of GERD, such as recurrent esophageal strictures or bleeding.[13] New laparoscopic procedures promise effective treatment without the morbidity of open procedures, but the experience of the surgeon is paramount for obtaining satisfactory results. Indications for antireflux surgery include recurrent esophageal strictures; aspiration resulting in recurrent pneumonia, asthma, or laryngitis; bleeding from Barrett's ulcers or gastric erosions in a hiatal hernia; intolerable or difficult-to-treat symptoms.[14] Spechler et al. showed that antireflux surgery was more effective than medical therapy in selected patients,[15] although the study was performed before omeprazole was available.

Peptic Ulcer Disease

The association of *H. pylori* with peptic ulcer disease has revolutionized the way we view and treat PUD. Most peptic ulcers are thought to be caused by either *H. pylori* or NSAIDs. Although infection with *H. pylori* appears to be common, most individuals with *H. pylori* do not develop ulcers. For this reason, empiric treatment of individuals with *H. pylori* is not recommended in the absence of a documented ulcer.[16] Treatment is also not recommended for individuals with NUD. Peptic ulcers may involve any portion of the UGI tract, but ulcers are most often found in the stomach and duodenum. Duodenal ulcers are approximately three times as common as gastric ulcers; perhaps 10% of the population suffers from duodenal ulcers at some time in their lives.[17] In the past PUD was considered a chronic disease, marked by periods of healing and recurrence. Successful treatment of ulcers associated with *H. pylori* infection greatly diminishes recurrences.

Presentation

Epigastric pain is the most common presenting problem of both duodenal and gastric ulcer disease. The pain may be described as gnawing, burning, boring, aching, or severe hunger pains. Patients with duodenal ulcers typically experience pain within a few hours after meals and complete or partial relief of pain with ingestion of food or antacids. Pain in gastric ulcer patients is more variable; pain may worsen with eating. Both duodenal and gastric ulcers may occur and recur in the absence of pain. Pain is variable among patients with both kinds of ulceration and correlates poorly with ulcer healing. Physical examination usually reveals epigastric tenderness midway between the xiphoid and umbilicus, but maximal tenderness is sometimes to the right of midline. Other findings may include a succussion splash due to a mixture of air and fluid in the stomach when gastric outlet obstruction results from an ulcer in the duodenum or pyloric channel or abdominal rigidity is apparent in the presence of perforation.

Diagnosis

The first priority is to document the ulcer, as only individuals with *H. pylori*-associated ulcers are to be treated with antibiotic therapy. Although duodenal and gastric ulcers can be diagnosed by UGI contrast studies, especially when double contrast studies are used, when available upper endoscopy is the investigation of first choice. In addition to the indicators listed earlier in the chapter, endoscopy should be considered in patients with negative radiographic studies, those with a history of deformed duodenal bulbs (thus making radiographic examination difficult), and in patients with GI bleeding.[17] As documented by contrast studies, gastric ulcers more than 3 cm in diameter or without radiating mucosal folds are more likely to be malignant.

Once an ulcer is documented, some form of testing for *H. pylori* is performed. If an ulcer is diagnosed endoscopically, a rapid *Campylobacter*-like organism urease test (CLO) is a quick, relatively inexpensive, sensitive test for determining the presence of *H. pylori*. False positives are uncommon, and false negatives occur in approximately 10% of cases. The use of proton pump inhibitors, bismuth preparations, and antibiotics can suppress *H. pylori* and lead to false-negative results. The presence of *H. pylori* can also be determined histologically and by culture. Culture with drug sensitivities is important when drug resistance is suspected. If an ulcer is diagnosed radiographically, testing for *H. pylori* can be problematic. Both qualitative and quantitative (enzyme-linked immunosorbent assay, or ELISA) serology tests are available, but a positive result does not necessarily mean active infection. A carbon isotope (^{13}C or ^{14}C) urea breath test can be used to determine the presence of *H. pylori*. Unfortunately, the test is still not widely available. To test for cure, a urea breath test (4 weeks after therapy), a falling ELISA titer (1, 3, and 6 months after therapy), or CLO at repeat endoscopy can be used.

Treatment

If PUD is associated with the use of an NSAID, the NSAID should be discontinued and traditional antiulcer therapy begun with either an H_2RA or PPI. Antibiotic treatment is given only to patients positive for *H. pylori* and a documented ulcer. A number of drug regimens have been shown to effective (Table 14.2). The addition of an H_2RA or PPI hastens relief of pain. If a PPI is already part of the antibiotic regimen, a second antiulcer agent is not necessary. Patients with *H. pylori*-negative ulcers are treated with traditional antacid agents alone for 4 to 6 weeks. There is no evidence that the use of two or more antiacid agents (e.g., sucralfate and an H_2RA) offers any advantage over the use of a single antacid agent.[19]

TABLE 14.2. Treatment for eradication of *Helicobacter pylori*-associated peptic ulcer disease

Regimen	Duration of therapy (days)	Eradication rate (%)
MOC	7	87–91
AOC	7	86–91
MOA	7–14	77–83
BMT	7–14	86–90
BMTO	7	94–98
BMA	7–14	75–86
OA	7–14	56–70
OC	14	83

Source: Adapted from Soll.[18] With permission.
O = omeprazole 20 mg bid; B = bismuth subsalicylate 2 tablets qid; T = tetracycline hydrochloride 500 mg qid; M = metronidazole 250 mg qid; A = amoxicillin 1000 mg bid or 500 mg qid; C = clarithromycin 500 mg bid–tid.

There are a number of problems with the current antibiotic regimens. First, compliance may be a problem because of cost, duration of therapy, and side effects. GI side effects can occur with metronidazole, amoxicillin, and clarithromycin. There is a trade-off between better compliance with the shorter duration of therapy and better eradication rate with longer duration of therapy. A second problem is the emergence of antibiotic resistance against both metronidazole and clarithromycin, which favors the use of triple drug regimens.

Antacids are used infrequently because patient compliance is poor with this regimen owing to the number of doses required. Side effects include constipation (common when aluminum hydroxide alone is used), diarrhea (common when magnesium hydroxide alone is used), phosphate depletion in malnourished patients, and hypermagnesemia in patients with chronic renal failure.

All H_2RAs effectively heal ulcers in equipotent doses (Table 14.1).[20] About 75% to 90% of ulcers are healed after 4 to 6 weeks of therapy. Cimetidine is the most inexpensive but appears to have the highest incidence of side effects and drug interactions.

The PPIs heal ulcers more quickly than H_2RAs, but healing rates at 6 weeks are not significantly improved over those with H_2RAs.[19] Omeprazole should be considered only for patients with severe symptoms, a potential for complications, or with refractory disease. Healing rates with sulcralfate are comparable to those with H_2RAs. There are no significant side effects, but the size of the tablet and frequency of administration (twice daily to four times daily) are possible drawbacks.

Prostaglandins protect the gastric mucosa, possibly by enhancing mucosal blood flow. Misoprostol, a prostaglandin E_1 analog, has been used to prevent ulcers due to NSAIDs. Misoprostol also heals ulcers at approximately the same rate as H_2RAs, but severe diarrhea may limit patient compliance. Stimulation of uterine contractions and induction of abortions are the most serious side effects of misoprostol.

Dietary therapy is now limited to the elimination of foods that exacerbate symptoms and the avoidance of alcohol and coffee (with or without caffeine) because alcohol and coffee increase gastric acid secretion. Cessation of cigarette smoking is also recommended to speed healing and prevent recurrence. NSAIDs should be withheld as well.

Refractory Ulcers and Maintenance Therapy

Most duodenal ulcers heal within 4 to 8 weeks of the start of therapy. After 12 weeks of therapy, 90% to 95% of ulcers are healed. Higher doses of H_2RAs (e.g., ranitidine 600–1200 mg/day) or omeprazole may be used to heal refractory ulcers. Gastric ulcers heal more slowly than duodenal ulcers, but 90% are healed after 12 weeks of therapy.[19]

Individuals with persistent or recurrent symptoms after therapy are reevaluated. Compliance with previous recommendations and a search for NSAID use are reviewed. Endoscopy should be performed to document healing. Drug resistance may be a factor in persistence of ulcers secondary to *H. pylori*. Gastric cancer should be excluded by biopsy if a gastric ulcer remains unhealed (see Gastric cancer, below). Zollinger-Ellison syndrome is also considered in the case of refractory ulcers.

The place of maintenance therapy is still unclear. Previous recommendations were made during the pre-*H. pylori* era. In patients successfully treated for *H. pylori* or who have discontinued the use of NSAIDs, maintenance treatment should not be needed. Patients with complications of PUD (e.g., bleeding or perforation), a history of refractory ulceration, age greater than 60 years, or a deformed duodenum are candidates for at least 1 year of maintenance therapy with H_2RAs or PPIs.

Gastritis

Gastritis, or inflammation of the gastric mucosa, is a collection of disorders most commonly grouped into acute and chronic forms.[17] Acute erosive gastritis is common with severe illness, such as sepsis, trauma or after surgery, or as a consequence of the administration of certain drugs (NSAIDs, aspirin, alcohol). Symptoms range from hematemesis and melena to anorexia, nausea, and vomiting. Pain is much less common than with peptic ulcer disease. Most patients are asymptomatic unless blood loss is appreciable. Patients may present with signs of massive blood loss (e.g., orthostatic hypotension, tachycardia, and pallor) or evidence of chronic blood loss (e.g., iron deficiency anemia).

Treatment consists of managing the underlying disease and removing possible gastric irritants. For management and treatment of bleeding due to gastritis, see Upper Gastrointestinal Bleeding, below. Administration of antacids or H_2RAs in sufficient quantities to keep the gastric pH above 4 are effective in reducing the incidence of stress gastritis, but whether these therapies help to stop bleeding is not clear. Surgery is a last resort but may be required if medical therapies fail.

Chronic gastritis has been classified into types A and B. Type A, commonly called atrophic gastritis, involves the body and fundus of the stomach, and may lead to pernicious anemia. Antibodies to parietal cells and to intrinsic factor are common.

Type B gastritis is much more common than type A. Stomach involvement ranges from only the antrum to the entire stomach. *H. pylori* is frequently found in patients with type B gastritis, and antibiotic treatment is suggested.

Upper Gastrointestinal Bleed

Upper gastrointestinal bleed is defined as GI blood loss above the ligament of Treitz. It may present in one of three ways. First, it may present as hematemesis, which may be bright red or coffee-ground-appearing material. Usually hematemesis means active bleeding. Second, UGI bleed may present as melena. Black, tarry stools signify that the blood has transited through the GI tract, causing digestion of blood. Melena may also be caused by lower GI bleeding. Third, UGI bleed may present as hematochezia if bleeding is brisk. Blood can have a cathartic effect on the bowel.

Causes

The four most common causes of UGI bleeding are peptic ulceration, gastritis, esophageal varices, and esophagogastric mucosal tear (Mallory-Weiss syndrome). Because bleeding due to peptic ulceration may present without pain, peptic ulceration should always be considered. The causes of gastritis are described above. Bleeding due to varices is usually abrupt and massive, and chronic blood loss is unusual. Varices may be due to alcohol cirrhosis or any other cause of portal hypertension such as portal vein thrombosis. Mallory-Weiss syndrome classically presents with retching followed by hematemesis. Other causes of UGI bleeding include gastric carcinoma, lymphoma, polyps, and diverticula.

Diagnosis and Management

The diagnosis and management of the patient with UGI bleeding depends on the site and extent of bleeding. Vomitus and stool should be tested to confirm the presence of blood. Initial management for all patients includes assessment of vital signs including orthostatic changes. Patients thought to have significant blood loss should also be typed and matched for blood replacement and a large-bore intravenous line placed for fluid and blood replacement.

A nasogastric tube should be placed to help determine the site and extent of the bleeding. The nasogastric aspirate is then tested for blood. If the aspirate consists of red blood or coffee-ground materials, the stomach is lavaged with saline. Blood products and intravenous fluids may be required. Iced saline has been used to halt bleeding, but the efficacy of this treatment has never been demonstrated. Once the patient is hemodynamically stable and the bleeding has stopped, upper endoscopy can be performed. Upper endoscopy can be both diagnostic and therapeutic. Sclerotherapy or ligation of esophageal varices can be performed through the endoscope. Active bleeding from a peptic ulcer can also be treated endoscopically.

If the patient has persistent bleeding, many physicians recommend endoscopy to locate the source of bleeding and possible therapy. Massive hemorrhage from varices can make endoscopy useless.

There are two additional therapies for bleeding varices. Peripherally administered vasopressin is as effective as intraarterially administered vasopressin. Balloon tamponade with a Sengstaken-Blakemore tube is another alternative for bleeding varices.

As always, prevention of GI bleeding is more effective than treatment. Maintenance therapy for PUD may decrease subsequent bleeding episodes. β-Adrenergic antagonists (propranolol, usual dose 20 mg tid) or isosorbide (20 mg tid) can prevent and reduce the mortality rate associated with GI bleeding in patients with cirrhosis, regardless of severity.[21,22]

Gastric Cancer

The incidence of gastric cancer has declined significantly since the 1930s,[23] but it still causes thousands of deaths each year. Ninety percent of the lesions are adenocarcinomas; non-Hodgkin's lymphomas and leiomyosarcomas constitute the remainder. Possible etiologic factors are ingestion of high nitrate foods, atrophic gastritis, and decreased gastric acidity.

Early gastric cancers are usually asymptomatic. As the cancer grows, patients may complain of anorexia or early satiety, vague discomfort, or steady pain. Weight loss, nausea and vomiting, and dysphagia may also be present. The physical examination is usually normal in patients with early disease, but a palpable abdominal mass, enlarged liver, ascites, or enlarged supraclavicular nodes may be present with metastatic disease.

Double-contrast radiographic studies can usually detect gastric cancer. However, if a benign-appearing ulcer is found, further workup may be necessary. Endoscopy with biopsy and brushings is advised by many, but others follow the healing of the ulcer by radiography. Benign ulcers are assumed if some degree of healing has been demonstrated by 6 weeks. Complete healing should have occurred within 12 weeks. Another study is done several months later to confirm that no new lesions have appeared. If healing has not occurred by 6 weeks, gastric cancer is suspected and biopsies and brushings should be obtained. Endoscopy should be repeated at 12 weeks to ensure that the ulcer has healed completely. An alternative approach is to recommend endoscopy with biopsy for all patients with gastric ulcers over the age of 50, as the incidence of gastric cancer peaks during the sixth decade.

Surgical treatment is the only definite chance for a cure. Unfortunately, only one-third of patients present early enough to achieve a cure through surgery. Five-year survival rates are about 25% for those with distal tumors and 10% for those with tumors of the proximal stomach. Surgery with or without radiation therapy may be given for palliation.

Chemotherapy has been successful in reducing tumor size, but responses are transient and the role of chemotherapy is still evolving. Adjuvant chemotherapy for patients undergoing complete resection is still investigational.

References

1. Lydeard S, Jones R. Factors affecting the decision to consult with dyspepsia: comparison of consulters and non-consulters. J R Coll Gen Pract 1989;39: 495–8.
2. Johnsen R, Bernersen B, Straume B, et al. Prevalences of endoscopic and histological findings in subjects with and without dyspepsia. BMJ 1991; 302: 749–52.
3. Health and Public Policy Committee, American College of Physicians. Endoscopy in the evaluation of dyspepsia. Ann Intern Med 1985;102:266–9.
4. Ebell MH, Warbasse L, Brenner C. Evaluation of the dyspeptic patient: A cost-utility study. J Fam Pract 1997;44:545–55.
5. Ofman JJ, Etchason J, Fullerton S, et al. Management strategies for *Helicobacter pylori*-seropositive patients with dyspepsia: Clinical and economic consequences. Ann Intern Med 1997;126:280–91.
6. Bytzer P, Hansen JO, deMuckadell OB. Empirical H_2-blocker therapy or prompt endoscopy in management of dyspepsia. Lancet 1994;343:811–16.
7. Fraser AG, Ali MR, McCullough S. Diagnostic tests for *Helicobacter pylori:* can they help select patients for endoscopy? NZ Med J 1996;109:95–8.
8. Mendall MA, Jazrawi RP, Marrero JM, et al. Serology for *Helicobacter pylori* compared with symptom questionnaires in screening before direct access endoscopy. Gut 1995;36:330–3.
9. Altorki NK, Skinner DB. Pathophysiology of gastroesophageal reflux. Am J Med 1989;86:685–9.
10. Klinkenber-Knol EC, Festen HP, Meuwissen SG. Pharmacological management of gastro-oesophageal reflux disease. Drugs 1995;49:695–710.
11. Cisapride for nocturnal heartburn. Med Lett 1994;36:11–13.
12. Robinson M. Prokinetic therapy for gastroesophageal reflux disease. Am Fam Physician 1995;52:957–66.
13. Roberts PJ, Cuschieri A. Laparoscopic and thorascopic antireflux surgery. Ann Chir Gynaecol 1995;84:130–7.
14. Richter JE. Surgery for reflux disease: reflections of a gastroenterologist. N Engl J Med 1992;326:825–6.
15. Spechler SJ, Department of Veterans Affairs Gastroesophageal Reflux Disease Study Group. Comparison of medical and surgical therapy for complicated gastroesophageal reflux disease in veterans. N Engl J Med 1992;326:786–92.
16. NIH Consensus Conference. *Helicobacter pylori* in peptic ulcer disease. NIH consensus development panel on *Helicobacter pylori* in peptic ulcer disease. JAMA 1994;272: 65–9.

17. McGuigan JE. Peptic ulcer and gastritis. In: Isselbacher KJ, Braunwald E, Wilson JDet al., editors. Harrison's principles of internal medicine. 13th ed. New York: McGraw-Hill, 1994:1363–82.
18. Soll AH, for the Practice Parameters Committee of the American College of Gastroenterology. Medical treatment of peptic ulcer disease: practice guidelines. JAMA 1996;275:622–9.
19. Hixson LJ, Kelley CL, Jones WN, Tuohy CD. Current trends in the pharmacotherapy for peptic ulcer disease. Arch Intern Med 1992;152:726–32.
20. Feldman M, Burton ME. Histamine$_2$-receptor antagonists: standard therapy for acid-peptic diseases. N Engl J Med 1990;323:1672–80.
21. Poynard T, Cales P, Pasta L, et al. Beta-adrenergic-antagonist drugs in the prevention of gastrointestinal bleeding in patients with cirrhosis and esophageal varices: an analysis of data and prognostic factors in 589 patients from four randomized clinical trials. N Engl J Med 1991;324:1532–8.
22. Angelico M, Carli C, Piat C, et al. Isosorbide-5-mononitrate versus propranolol in the prevention of first bleeding in cirrhosis. Gastroenterology 1993;104:1460–5.
23. Mayer RJ. Neoplasms of the esophagus and stomach. In: Isselbacher KJ, Braunwald E, Wilson JD, et al., editors. Harrison's principles of internal medicine. 13th ed. New York: McGraw-Hill, 1994:1382–6.

Case Presentation

Subjective

Patient Profile

Ralph Martino is a 45-year-old divorced white male attorney.

Presenting Problem

"Heartburn."

Present Illness

For the past 6 weeks, Mr. Martino has had a recurrent burning sensation in the upper abdomen, worse after meals, especially if the food is spicy or "acid." Antacids and milk afford some relief. There has been no nausea, vomiting, constipation, or diarrhea. He notes occasional upper abdominal pain that seems different from the "heartburn." Similar heartburn has occurred several times in the past, especially at the time of his divorce 10 years ago.

Past Medical History

The patient had hepatitis and a fractured femur as a teenager.

Social History

He is divorced and lives alone with two dogs. He is a partner in a law firm and specializes in labor relations.

Habits

He smokes one pack of cigarettes daily and takes one to two drinks of vodka each evening. He uses six to eight cups of coffee daily but takes no recreational drugs.

Family History

His father died at age 66 of colon cancer. His mother, aged 78, has had gallbladder surgery. One sister, aged 47, has Crohn's disease.

REVIEW OF SYSTEMS

He has a long history of recurrent headache and low back pain.

- What additional information regarding the medical history would you like to know? Why?
- What might the patient be trying to tell you?
- What questions might you ask to learn more about current stressors in his life?
- What is likely to be the patient's adaptation to his illness? Why might this be pertinent?

Objective

VITAL SIGNS

Height, 5 ft 11 in; weight 186 lb; blood pressure, 138/90; pulse, 70; respirations, 18.

EXAMINATION

The patient appears tense and "worried." The chest is clear to percussion and auscultation. The heart has a regular sinus rhythm, and no murmurs are heard. The abdomen is scaphoid, and active bowel sounds are present. There is mild epigastric tenderness, but no mass is found. On rectal examination, the prostate is normal and no rectal mass is palpable. There is a positive test for occult blood in the feces.

- What more data—if any—might be derived from the physical examination? Explain.
- Are there specific diagnostic maneuvers that might be helpful today?
- What—if any—laboratory studies might be useful in making the diagnosis?
- What—if any—diagnostic imaging or endoscopy would you recommend today? Why?

Assessment

- What is your diagnostic assessment at this time? How would you explain this to Mr. Martino?

- What is likely to be the meaning of this illness to Mr. Martino? Explain.
- What is the significance of the positive test for occult blood in feces?
- What are the possible contributions of alcohol and tobacco use to his current illness?

Plan

- Pending the results of further tests, what therapeutic recommendations would you make to Mr. Martino regarding diet, life style, and medication?
- Is consultation likely to be necessary? Under what circumstances? Explain.
- If the patient calls tonight describing the passage of large quantities of dark red blood from the rectum, what would be your concern? What would you do?
- What follow-up would you recommend for this patient?

15

Urinary Tract Infections

Boyd L. Bailey, Jr.

Urinary tract infection (UTI) is a cause of significant discomfort, acute and long-term morbidity, and loss of productivity, resulting in 7 million to 8 million office visits with an estimated 100,000 episodes annually of pyelonephritis requiring hospitalization.[1] Among children, 1 in 20 females and 1 in 50 males have a UTI each year.[2]

Four major risk groups[3] for community-acquired UTIs have been identified: school-age girls, young women in their sexually active years (including pregnancy), males with prostate obstruction, and the elderly. This chapter deals with important clinical issues in the following categories: UTI in children, UTI in pregnancy, acute uncomplicated lower UTI in young women, recurrent infection in women, acute uncomplicated pyelonephritis in young women, complicated UTIs, UTIs in young men, catheter-associated UTIs, asymptomatic bacteriuria without a catheter, chronic UTI in the elderly, and UTIs with spinal cord injuries. The primary aim of UTI diagnosis and management is the prevention of long-term complications or progressive events that affect later life morbidity or mortality.

UTIs in Children

For males and females the incidence of symptomatic infection during the first 6 months of life is similar, but after 6 months to a year it falls off rapidly for males. Among females, the first-year incidence is more evenly distributed through the year. During the first 3 months boys are infected more often.[2] In neonates the prevalence is threefold higher among premature infants.[4] For girls the incidence steadily rises with a small transient increase at preschool time and then remains level until sexual activity becomes a factor. Asymptomatic bacteriuria is absent in males until later in adult life when obstructive problems occur. In females asymptomatic bacteriuria is present early in infancy and remains fairly constant until the late teens.[1]

The primary host-related factors that lead to the development of UTI include infancy, female sex, abnormal defense mechanisms, the presence of urinary tract abnormalities, sexual activity, and instrumentation.[4] In children without urinary tract abnormalities, periurethral bacterial colonization, for unclear reasons, is a risk factor for UTI.[5]

Escherichia coli accounts for as much as 80% of cases of UTI.[2,4] In neonates and complicated cases, *Proteus mirabilis* (mainly in boys), *Klebsiella pneumoniae, Pseudomonas aeruginosa, Enterobacter* species, *Staphylococcus aureus* (mainly in older children), *Streptococcus viridans,* enterococci, and *Candida albicans* are to be considered.[4]

Diagnosis

URINALYSIS AND CULTURE

In any febrile infant or child the differential diagnosis should include UTI. Screening by urinalysis for pyuria and bacteriuria is not adequately sensitive to allow UTI to be ruled out without a culture.[4] In a properly collected specimen (urethral catheterization or suprapubic aspiration in infants), a presumptive diagnosis can be made with the presence of any bacteria and 5 leukocytes per high-power field (hpf).[6]

IMAGING EVALUATION

Imaging tests should be conducted after the first episode of UTI in girls younger than 5 years, boys of any age, older sexually inactive girls with recurrent UTI, and any child with pyelonephritis.[6] Debate continues about the best radiologic approach for evaluating UTI.[7] The issue centers around the role of radionuclide cystography (RNC) and renal cortical scintigraphy (RCS), and how these methods may replace or be used in conjunction with traditional ultrasonography (US), voiding cystourethrography (VCUG), and intravenous pyelography (IVP).

Radionuclide cystography, a method using scintigraphic imaging, gives accurate information similar to that of contrast-based VCUG, with the possible advantage of significantly less radiation exposure.[8] RCS, a scintigraphic study using technetium 99m dimercaptosuccinic acid (DMSA), provides an image and an estimate of the proportion contributed by each kidney to total renal function.[9] The renal image also reflects scarring to some degree. US has the obvious advantage of being a noninvasive test that is strong at ruling out obstruction. IVP gives comprehensive structural information, but transient swelling during infection weakens the predictive capability of the test. VCUG gives comprehensive lower tract information and allows grading the severity of reflux.[9]

The preferred workup for children has evolved so the process can be expressed in a series of four questions[10]: (1) Is there a structural abnormality of the urinary tract causing urinary stasis that predisposes to infection? US remains the test of choice for ruling out ureteral dilatation. If positive, then more specific testing is usually needed. (2) Does the patient have vesicoureteral reflux (VUR)? At this point, the choice is cystography by the traditional VCUG or RNC. RNC may be suitable for all cases, but the debate centers primarily on its utility in girls with signs of bladder dysfunction and boys with presumed abnormalities of the lower urinary tract. At this point, clinician and institutional preferences prevail. (3) Is there acute pyelonephritis? US and IVP are not sufficiently sensitive to rule out pyelonephritis. RCS is held to be more sensitive and specific, and it may give additional information regarding parenchymal involvement that could affect management. (4) Is there renal scarring? Small scars that elude both US and IVP can more likely be identified by RCS. It may be important to perform RCS at 4 months after infection to establish a small scar that later is shown to grow. RCS, in this instance, could prompt a cystogram that would uncover otherwise hidden VUR. RCS may play an important role in establishing the degree of previous injury where the history is unclear.[10]

MANAGEMENT

Early diagnosis and prompt treatment of UTI in infants and young children are crucial. With vesicoureteral reflux, or other urinary tract abnormalities, immediate treatment reduces the risk of renal scarring.

Symptomatic neonates should be treated for 7 to 10 days with a parenteral combination of ampicillin and gentamicin. Young infants with UTI, children with clinical evidence of acute pyelonephritis, and children with upper tract infection associated with urologic abnormalities or surgical procedures can be treated with a combination of an aminoglycoside and ampicillin, or an aminoglycoside and a cephalosporin.[4]

For uncomplicated UTI, oral agents may include amoxicillin, ampicillin, sulfisoxazole acetyl, trimethoprim-sulfamethoxazole, nitrofurantoin, or cephalosporins. Antibiotic treatment of asymptomatic bacteriuria in children is controversial based on certain issues: There is limited evidence that renal damage is prevented or function is reduced; replacement of a low-virulence organism with a more virulent one may occur; and the child may experience unknown long-term side effects of antibiotics.[4] A reasonable approach with asymptomatic bacteriuria is to treat children less than 5 years of age or ones who have urinary tract structural abnormalities.

UTI During Pregnancy

Pregnant women with UTIs are at greater risk of delivering infants with low birth weight, premature infants, preterm infants with low birth weight, and infants small for gestational age. In addition, the likelihood is greater for premature labor, hypertension/preeclampsia, anemia, and amnionitis. There is strong evidence that UTI causes low birth weight through premature delivery rather than growth retardation.[11]

The risk of pyelonephritis from antepartum bacteriuria may be as high as 30%. Identification and eradication reduces this risk to less than 5%. Antepartum bacteriuria has an estimated prevalence of 2% to 12%, with an increasing relation to age, parity, and lower socioeconomic status.[12]

An optimal time for screening all pregnancies has been suggested to be around 16 weeks (see Chapter 3). Although often the first prenatal visit is before 16 weeks, a practical approach to screening is to obtain a culture at the first visit. If negative, no further cultures are necessary unless there is a history of prior UTI, or the patient becomes symptomatic. If the screening culture result is 10^5 colony-forming units (CFU)/ml or higher, the test should be repeated to improve on the specificity of a single culture. If the repeat culture is positive, treatment for asymptomatic bacteriuria follows.[12]

As in nonpregnant females, *E. coli* is the most common cause of UTI during pregnancy, accounting for more than 80% of isolates. Other organisms include *Enterobacter* species, *Klebsiella* species, *Proteus* species, enterococci, and *Staphylococcus saprophyticus.*

The first concern regarding treatment during pregnancy is the safety of antibiotics. Considered reasonably safe are penicillins, cephalosporins, and methenamine. Cautious use can be considered with sulfonamides [allergic reaction, kernicterus, glucose-6-phosphate dehydrogenase (G6PD) deficiency], aminoglycosides (eighth nerve and renal toxicity), nitrofurantoin (neuropathy, G6PD deficiency), clindamycin (allergic reaction, pseudomembranous colitis), and erythromycin estolate (cholestatic hepatitis).[12,13]

For asymptomatic bacteriuria, a regimen of 3 to 7 days is used with antibiotics chosen with safety in mind. There is little support for single-dose therapy, although for a pregnant female with a history of recurrent UTIs, or who develops a UTI early in pregnancy, a single postcoital prophylactic dose may be considered. Appropriate postcoital single oral doses are either cephalexin 250 mg or nitrofurantoin 50 mg.[14] Pyelonephritis is managed the same as with nonpregnant females.[12]

Acute Uncomplicated Lower UTI in Young Women

The risk for UTI is increased by sexual intercourse, delayed postcoital voiding, diaphragm and spermicidal gel, and a history of recurrent UTIs.[15] One of three types of infection can account for these infections: acute cystitis; acute urethritis; or vaginitis.[16]

Cystitis pathogens include *E. coli, Staphylococcus saprophyticus, Proteus* species, or *Klebsiella* species. Symptoms are abrupt in onset, severe, and usually multiple: they include dysuria, increased frequency, and urgency. Suprapubic pain and tenderness and sometimes low back pain also occur. Pyuria is usually present and occasionally hematuria.

Urethritis pathogens include *Chlamydia trachomatis, N. gonorrhoeae,* and herpes simplex virus. Symptoms are more likely to be gradual in onset, mild (including dysuria and possibly vaginal discharge and bleeding from a concomitant cervicitis), and lower abdominal pain. Suspicion is raised if there is history of a new sexual partner or evidence of cervicitis on examination. Pyuria is usually present.

Vaginitis pathogens include *Candida* species and *Trichomonas vaginalis.* Symptoms include vaginal discharge or odor, pruritus, dyspareunia, and external dysuria without increased frequency or urgency. Pyuria and hematuria are rarely present (see Chapter 16).

With no complicating clinical factors, reasonable empiric treatment for presumed cystitis, prior to organism identification, is a 3-day regimen of any of the following: oral trimethoprim-sulfamethoxazole (TMP-SMX), trimethoprim, norfloxacin, ciprofloxacin, ofloxacin, lomefloxacin, or enoxacin (Table 15.1). With the complicating factors of diabetes, symptoms for more than 7 days, recent UTI, use of a diaphragm, or age over 65 years, a 7-day regimen can be considered using these same antibiotics.[16]

For cystitis during pregnancy, consider a 7-day regimen that includes oral amoxicillin, macrocrystalline nitrofurantoin, cefpodoxime proxetil, or TMP-SMX. Avoid using fluoroquinolones in pregnant women, and use gentamicin cautiously because of fetal eighth nerve threat. TMP-SMX has not been approved for use during pregnancy but is widely used. Once the causative organism(s) has been identified, the antibiotics can be modified.[16]

Recurrent Infections (Cystitis) in Women

Recurrent cystitis can be termed relapse or reinfection. *Relapse* is defined as a recurrence within 2 weeks of completing therapy for the same pathogen. *Reinfection* is defined as a recurrence after 2 weeks after completing therapy for a different species or strain. For relapse, efforts should be put to ruling out a urologic abnormality and treating for an extended time, such as 2 to 6 weeks. For reinfection, the following strategy is useful. If a spermicide and diaphragm are being used, changing the contraceptive method is recommended. For two or fewer incidents of UTI per year, physician- or patient-initiated therapy can be started based on symptoms, using either single-dose or 3-day therapy. For

TABLE 15.1. Antibiotic regimens for adult cystitis, pyelonephritis, and prophylaxis

Antibiotic	Oral (cystitis)	Oral (pyelonephritis and complicated UTIs)	Parenteral	Daily prophylaxis	Single dose postcoital
Amoxicillin	250 mg q8h	500 mg q8h			
Ampicillin			1 g q6h		
Trimethoprim	100 mg q12h			100 mg q24h	
Trimethoprim-sulfamethoxazole	160 plus 800 mg q12h	160 plus 800 mg q12h	160 plus 800 mg q12h	40 plus 200 mg q24h	
Norfloxacin	400 mg q12h	400 mg q12h		200 mg q24h	
Ciprofloxacin	250 mg q12h	500 mg q12h	200 to 400 mg q12h		
Ofloxacin	200 mg q12h	200 mg followed by 300 mg q12h			
Lomefloxacin	400 mg qd	400 mg qd			
Enoxacin	400 mg q12h	400 mg q12h			
Macrocrystalline nitrofurantoin	100 mg four times a day			100 mg q24h	50 mg
Cephalexin				250 mg q24h	250 mg
Cefpodoxime proxetil	100 mg q12h	200 mg q12h			
Cefixime	400 m qd	400 mg qd			
Ceftriaxone			1–2 qd		
Gentamicin			1mg/kg body weight q8h, or 3–5 mg/kg q24h		
Imipenem-cilastatin			250–500 mg q6–8h		
Ampicillin-sulbactam			1.5 g q6h		
Ticarcillin-clavulanate			3.2 g q6–8h		
Piperacillin-tazobactam			3.375 g q6–8h		
Aztreonam			1 g q8–12h		

Source: Adapted from Pfau and Sacks,[14] Stamm and Hooton,[16] and Johnson.[17]

three or more UTIs per year, the relation to coitus must be considered. If the UTI is not related to coitus, a low-dose antibiotic, daily or three times weekly, is recommended. This regimen is commonly continued for 6 months to 1 year. If the recurrent UTIs are related to coitus, a single low-dose postcoital treatment may be preferable (Table 15.1).

Usually not attributable to predisposing anatomic defects, recurrent UTIs in women most likely are related to an underlying biologic predisposition or to behavior-promoting urinary tract infection.[17] Although perineal cleansing methods are partially protective, oral antimicrobial therapy is probably most effective. It can be accomplished as chronic prophylaxis, postcoital prophylaxis, or intermittent self-administered therapy.

Acute Uncomplicated Pyelonephritis in Young Women

Uncomplicated pyelonephritis exhibits findings suggestive of upper tract tissue penetration and inflammation, such as fever and flank pain. Underlying factors that impede the response to natural host responses are minimized. The infecting organism should be highly susceptible to most antibiotics.

Characteristic pathogens in acute uncomplicated pyelonephritis in young women include *E. coli, Proteus mirabilis, Klebsiella pneumoniae,* and *Staphylococcus saprophyticus.* Outpatient management is reasonable for mild to moderate illness without nausea and vomiting. A 10- to 14-day regimen of the following is appropriate: oral TMP-SMX, norfloxacin, ciprofloxacin, ofloxacin, lomefloxacin, or enoxacin (Table 15.1). For severe illness or possible urosepsis requiring hospitalization, the following regimen can be followed: parenteral TMP-SMX, ceftriaxone, ciprofloxacin, gentamicin (with or without ampicillin), or ampicillin-sulbactam until afebrile; then oral TMP-SMX, norfloxacin, ciprofloxacin, ofloxacin, lomefloxacin, or enoxacin (Table 15.1) to complete a 14-day course of therapy.[16]

During pregnancy hospitalization is the optimal course, with the following suggested regimen: parenteral ceftriaxone, gentamicin (with or without ampicillin), aztreonam, ampicillin-sulbactam, or TMP-SMX until afebrile, then oral amoxicillin, amoxicillin-clavulanate, a cephalosporin, or TMP-SMX to complete a 14-day course of therapy.[16]

Complicated UTIs

Clinically, a complicated UTI may present the same as an uncomplicated one. A complicated infection occurs in urinary tracts that have a functional, metabolic, or anatomic derangement predisposing to a more difficult infectious process including more resistant organisms.

Characteristic organisms present in complicated urinary tract infections include *E. coli, Proteus* species, *Klebsiella* species, *Pseudomonas* species, *Serratia* species, enterococci, and staphylococci. Outpatient management is reasonable for mild to moderate illness without nausea or vomiting. The best oral antibiotic course, administered for 10 to 14 days, is norfloxacin, ciprofloxacin, ofloxacin, lomefloxacin, or enoxacin. TMP-SMX, amoxicillin, or cefpodoxime proxetil could also be used. For severe illness or possible urosepsis, hospitalization is necessary with treatment by parenteral ampicillin and gentamicin, ciprofloxacin, ofloxacin, ceftriaxone, aztreonam, ticarcillin-clavulanate, piperacillin-tazobactam, or imipenem-cilastatin until afebrile, then oral TMP-SMX, norfloxacin, ciprofloxacin, ofloxacin, lomefloxacin, or enoxacin for a total of 14 to 21 days.[16]

UTIs in Young Men

Without underlying structural urologic abnormalities, risk factors for UTIs in young men include homosexuality, lack of circumcision,[18] and a sex partner colonized with uropathogens.[16] Management of symptomatic cystitis without obvious complicating factors requires a urine culture to establish the pathogen. This step establishes sensitivity and helps define relapse or reinfection in the event of recurrence. Once the culture is obtained, a 7-day course of TMP-SMX, trimethoprim, or a fluoroquinolone is initiated.[16]

The traditional approach of undertaking a thorough post-UTI evaluation to rule out a urologic abnormality has been disputed.[19,20] If pursued in young men who have responded to treatment, the chance of finding a urinary tract defect is low.[17]

Catheter-Associated UTIs

Mortality from UTIs is increased threefold in hospitalized patients with an indwelling catheter. With short-term catheterization, *E. coli* is the most common organism, followed by *Pseudomonas aeruginosa, Klebsiella pneumoniae, Proteus mirabilis, Staphylococcus epidermidis,* and enterococci.[21] With long-term catheterization, significant infection may be due to the ordinarily nonuropathogenic *Providencia stuartii* or *Morganella morganii.* Yeast may become an isolated pathogen when antibiotics are in use.[21]

Treatment revolves around three modes of action: prevention, antimicrobials for acquired asymptomatic bacteriuria and symptomatic lower UTI, and antimicrobials for a symptomatic (complicated) upper UTI. Prevention focuses on avoiding catheterization if possible. If catheterization is a mandatory, minimize the duration and use a closed drainage system. For short-term catheterization of 3 to 14 days, daily prophylactic norfloxacin, ciprofloxacin, or amoxicillin has shown benefit.[17] For acquired asymptomatic bacteriuria and symptomatic lower UTI after short-term catheter use, a single-dose of TMP-SMX (320–1600 mg) has been shown to be as effective as a 10-day course.[22]

Asymptomatic Bacteriuria in Patients Without a Catheter

With the exception of pregnancy and prior to urologic surgery, screening for asymptomatic bacteriuria has no apparent value. Even among the elderly where there appears to be an association between asymptomatic bacteriuria and mortality, a causal link has not been demonstrated.[16]

Chronic UTI in the Elderly

Among males the incidence of bacteriuria essentially disappears after infancy and reappears during later adulthood as obstructive elements come into play. With aging, both symptomatic infection and asymptomatic bacteriuria occur. The incidence of UTI in both sexes steadily rises with age during the elderly years.[1] The place of residence helps predict incidence. For those over age 65, estimates of incidence have been (1) at home: women 20%, men 10%; (2) in nursing homes: women 25% and men 20%. In hospitals the incidence is high for both sexes.[23] The elderly behave in a dynamic fashion, with high turnover of those with bacteriuria and those with a UTI.[23]

Many factors come into play for elderly men and women that balance the incidence of UTI: lack of estrogen in women, prostatic secretion in men,[24] and bacterial adhesion factors in both sexes.[23]

Whereas *E. coli* and *Staphylococcus saprophyticus* are the most common cause of UTI in young adults, some significant shifts in causative organism occur with the elderly. Principally, *S. saprophyticus* does not occur. *E. coli* drops in frequency for females, and gram-positive organisms can dominate among men.[25] This shift to non-*E. coli* organisms can easily be attributed to an increased rate of hospitalization of the elderly.[23]

A debatable issue that has become somewhat clearer is that asymptomatic bacteriuria does not seem to influence mortality in elderly women.[26] Previous studies have pointed in both directions,[27] with some clearly showing increased functional disability even if an effect on mortality is not clear.[28]

Basically, a lower UTI presents with dysuria, urgency, and frequency. An upper UTI may present with clear signs of fever, chills, and flank pain with tenderness. In a fair percentage of cases, possibly 20%, these signs and symptoms can be absent or obscured by a presentation that might include altered mental status with variable gastrointestinal symptoms and signs (nausea and vomiting, abdominal tenderness), and even respiratory symptoms.[23] Alternatively, not all nonspecific "mental status" changes can be attributed to a UTI, and focusing on antibiotic therapy alone is inappropriate.[24] A difficult question is whether bacteriuria is really asymptomatic in the elderly. Laboratory screening is a little more direct in men than women but does not, unfortunately, substitute for a culture in the elderly, as it can in younger people.

The management of UTIs in the elderly is addressed in specific areas of this chapter: recurrent infection in females, complicated UTIs, and catheter-associated UTIs. Antibiotic choices are as shown in Table 15.1. Regular use of cranberry juice (300 ml/day) appears to reduce both bacteriuria and pyuria and leads to fewer symptomatic infections and less antibiotic use.[29]

UTIs and Spinal Cord Injuries

Special considerations for increased risk of UTI with spinal cord injuries include bladder overdistension, vesicoureteral reflux, high-pressure voiding, large postvoid residuals, stones in the urinary tract, and outlet obstruction.[30] Management of infection risks focuses primarily on proper drainage of the bladder. A turning point that occurred during the 1960s was the understanding of the value of intermittent catheterization in reducing the risk of significant bacteriuria.[31] Development of bacteriuria is certain with an indwelling catheter and suprapubic catheter. Although the reason is not fully understood, bacteriuria and the incidence of symptomatic UTIs are reduced by intermittent catheterization. In addition, intermittent catheterization performed by the affected person is preferable to having it done by a caretaker.[30] There are many variations in the technique of intermittent catheterization. The critical predictor for improved outcome is intermittent catheterization rather than having an indwelling catheter.

Diagnostic signs and symptoms are poorly sensitive and specific.[30] Estimation of pyuria is generally considered the best indication of UTI.

Laboratory Guides and Interpretation

The organisms that cause UTIs are few in number, but there are growing pressures for more efficient and timely screening measures to determine the likelihood of a UTI. Ideal screening for a UTI would involve a highly sensitive test that confidently excludes the disease, thereby eliminating the need to proceed to more costly follow-up tests of culturing and antibiotic sensitivity. The ideal screening test would be highly specific for detecting or identifying the disease for which empiric treatment has been initiated while uropathogen identity and antimicrobial sensitivity are pending. Unfortunately, the ideal screening test does not exist.

Pyuria

From a practical standpoint, pyuria represents readily measurable evidence of host injury. The most accurate method, or gold standard, of defining significant pyuria is the leukocyte excretion rate. There is evidence that the significant rate is 400,000 white blood cells (WBC)/hr.[32] Obviously, this measurement is cumbersome—hence the popularity of quicker, simpler, but less accurate screening tests. They include microscopic examination of unspun urine in a counting chamber (WBC/mm^3), spun urine under a coverslip (WBC/hpf), and leukocyte esterase.[33] In general, the WBC/hpf is approximately 11% of the WBC/mm^3.[34] Diagnostic information related to these tests is displayed in Table 15.2.[33–41]

TABLE 15.2. Diagnostic information on common urine screening tests, individually and in various combinations[a]

Screening test	Sensitivity	Specificity	Positive likelihood ratio	Negative likelihood ratio
Nitrite (present or absent)	0.5	0.95	10.00	0.53
Bacteria				
Unstained, spun (2+ on scale of 4+)	0.75	0.8	3.75	0.31
Gram stain, unspun (1/hpf)	0.8	0.85	5.33	0.24
Microscopic pyuria				
Spun (5 WBC/hpf)	0.6	0.85	4.00	0.47
Unspun (50 WBC/mm^3)	0.65	0.9	6.50	0.39
WBCs + bacteria				
Standard spun[b]	0.66	0.99	66.00	0.34
Enhanced unspun[c]	0.85	0.98	42.50	0.15
Leukocyte esterase (present or absent)	0.2	0.95	4.00	0.84
Leukocyte esterase + nitrite	0.5	0.98	25.00	0.51
Methylene blue (pyrine)	0.6	0.98	30.00	0.41
Uriscreen	0.9	0.9	9.00	0.11
Bac-T-Screen	0.9	0.7	3.00	0.14
Chemstrip LN	0.9	0.7	3.00	0.14

[a]Values have been taken from several sources,[34–41] were rounded by the authors, and represent reasonable numbers to use in clinical practice.
[b]5 WBC/hpf + any bacteria in spun urinalysis.
[c]10 WBC/mm^3 + any bacteria by Gram stain.

Bacteriuria

A UTI can be defined as the presence of significant numbers of pathogenic bacteria in appropriately collected urine.[33] Urine culture is considered the gold standard for defining significant bacteriuria. All other tests are simply screening devices chosen to balance immediate, simple results with accuracy. The most common tests are direct microscopy and the nitrite test. Many methods have been used with variable accuracy.[40] Commonly used screening tests with approximated diagnostic information are shown in Table 15.2.

Urine Culture

It is important to realize that even though the culture is universally used as a gold standard for significant bacteriuria in UTIs against which other tests are measured, it is not the perfect test and falls short of being 100% sensitive and specific. Bacterial culture methods include, in order of decreasing predictive accuracy, the quantitative culture (pour plate method), semiquantitative culture (surface streak procedure), and miniaturized culture (filter paper, roll tube, and dipslide methods). The colony count that

TABLE 15.3. Suggested culture colony count thresholds for significant bacteriuria

Clinical setting	Significant bacteriuria (CFU/ml)
Infants and children	
Voided	$\geq 10^3$
Catheter	$\geq 10^3$
Suprapubic aspirate (SPA)	$\geq 10^3$
External collection devices	$\geq 10^4$
Adults	
Midstream clean-catch	
Female	
Asymptomatic	$\geq 10^5$
Symptomatic	$\geq 10^2$
Male	$\geq 10^3$
In-and-out (straight) catheterization	$\geq 10^2$
Chronic indwelling catheter	$\geq 10^2$
Indwelling catheter or SPA in spinal injuries	Any detectable colony count
External collection devices	$\geq 10^5$
Condom collection device in spinal injuries	$\geq 10^4$

Source: Data are from Cardenas and Hooton[30] and Eisenstadt and Washington.[41]

represents significant bacteriuria varies with factors that include age, sex, anatomic location of the infection, and symptoms. Although the urine culture is considered the gold standard for defining significant bacteriuria, the level of significance is not uniform across the clinical spectrum of disease. Colony counts of what can currently be considered as significant bacteriuria for infection is shown in Table 15.3.[30,41]

References

1. Warren JW. Clinical presentations and epidemiology of urinary tract infections. In: Mobley LT, Warren JW, editors. Urinary tract infections: molecular pathogenesis and clinical management. Washington, DC: ASM Press, 1996:3–28.
2. Stull TL, LiPuma JJ. Epidemiology and natural history of urinary infections in children. Med Clin North Am 1991;75: 287–98.
3. Stamm WE, Hooton TM, Johnson JR, et al. Urinary tract infections: from pathogenesis to treatment. J Infect Dis 1989; 159:400–6.
4. Zelikovic I, Adelman RD, Nancarrow PA. Urinary tract infections in children: an update. West J Med 1992;157:554–61.
5. Shortliffe LM. The management of urinary tract infections in children without urinary tract abnormalities. Urol Clin North Am 1995;22:67–73.
6. Carmack MA, Arvin AM. Urinary tract infections—navigating complex currents [editorial]. West J Med 1992;157:587–8.
7. Hellerstein S. Evolving concepts in the evaluation of the child with a urinary tract infection [editorial comment]. J Pediatr 1994;124:589–92.
8. Conway JJ, Cohn RA. Evolving role of nuclear medicine for the diagnosis and management of urinary tract infection [editorial comment]. J Pediatr 1994;124:87–90.
9. Smellie JM, Rigden SP. Pitfalls in the investigation of children with urinary tract infection. Arch Dis Child 1995; 72:251–6.
10. Leonidas JC. The preferred workup of children or infants with urinary tract infection seems to change every year. AJR 1995;165:481.
11. Schieve LA, Handler A, Hershow R, et al. Urinary tract infection during pregnancy: its association with maternal morbidity and perinatal outcome. Am J Public Health 1994; 84:405–10.
12. Zinner SH. Management of urinary tract infections in pregnancy: a review with comments on single dose therapy. Infection 1992;20 Suppl 4:S280.
13. Chow AW, Jewesson PJ. Use and safety of antimicrobial agents during pregnancy. West J Med 1987;146:761–4.
14. Pfau A, Sacks TG. Effective prophylaxis for recurrent urinary tract infections during pregnancy. Clin Infect Dis 1992; 14:810.
15. Hooton TM, Hillier S, Johnson C, et al. *Escherichia coli* bacteriuria and contraceptive method. JAMA 1991;265:64–9.
16. Stamm WE, Hooton TM. Management of urinary tract infections in adults. N Engl J Med 1993;329:1328.
17. Johnson JR. Treatment and prevention of urinary tract infections. In: Mobley LT, Warren JW, editors. Urinary tract infections: molecular

pathogenesis and clinical management. Washington, DC: ASM Press, 1996: 95–118.

18. Spach DH, Stapleton AE, Stamm WE. Lack of circumcision increases the risk of urinary tract infection in young men. JAMA 1992;267:679.
19. Krieger JN, Ross SO, Simonsen JM. Urinary tract infections in healthy university men. J Urol 1993;149:1046–8.
20. Pfau A. Re: urinary tract infections in healthy university men [letter]. J Urol 1994;151:705–6.
21. Warren JW. The catheter and urinary tract infection. Med Clin North Am 1991;75:481–95.
22. Harding GKM, Nicolle LE, Ronald AR, et al. How long should catheter-acquired urinary infection in women be treated? A randomized controlled study. Ann Intern Med 1991;114:713.
23. Baldassarre JS, Kaye D. Special problems in urinary tract infection in the elderly. Med Clin North Am 1991;75:375–90.
24. Nicolle LE. Urinary tract infections in long-term care facilities. Infect Control Hosp Epidemiol 1993;14:220–5.
25. Lipsky BA, Ireton RC, Gihn SD, et al. Diagnosis of bacteriuria in men: specimen collection and culture interpretation. J Infect Dis 1987;155: 847–54.
26. Abrutyn E, Mossey J, Berlin JA, et al. Does asymptomatic bacteriuria predict mortality and does antimicrobial treatment reduce mortality in elderly ambulatory women? Ann Intern Med 1994;120:827–33.
27. Nordenstam GR, Brandberg CA, Oden AS, et al. Bacteriuria and mortality in an elderly population. N Engl J Med 1986; 314:1152–6.
28. Nicolle LE, Henderson E, Bjornson J, et al. The association of bacteriuria with resident characteristics and survival in elderly institutionalized men. Ann Intern Med 1987;106:682–6.
29. Avorn J, Monane M, Gurwitz JH, et al. Reduction of bacteriuria and pyuria after ingestion of cranberry juice. JAMA 1994;271:751–4.
30. Cardenas DD, Hooton TM. Urinary tract infection in persons with spinal cord injury. Arch Phys Med Rehabil 1995; 76:272–80.
31. Ronald AR, Pattullo ALS. The natural history of urinary tract infection in adults. Med Clin North Am 1991;75:299–312.
32. Stamm WE. Measurement of pyuria and its relation to bacteriuria. Am J Med 1983;75:53–8.
33. Pappas PG. Laboratory in the diagnosis and management of urinary tract infections. Med Clin North Am 1991;75:313–26.
34. Alwall N. Pyuria: deposit in high-power microscopic field—WBC/hpf—versus WBC/mm^3 in counting chamber. Acta Med Scand 1973;194:537–40.
35. Bailey BL. Urinalysis predictive of urine culture results. J Fam Pract 1995;40:45–50.
36. Hoberman A, Wald ER, Penchansky L, et al. Enhanced urinalysis as a screening test for urinary tract infection. Pediatrics 1993;91: 1196–9.
37. Bachman JW, Heise RH, Naessens JM, Timmerman MG. A study of various tests to detect asymptomatic urinary tract infections in an obstetric population. JAMA 1993;270: 1971–4.

38. Lockhart GR, Lewander WJ, Cimini DM, et al. Use of urinary gram stain for detection of urinary tract infection in infants. Ann Emerg Med 1995;25:31–5.
39. Carroll KC, Hale DC, Von Boerum DH, et al. Laboratory evaluation of urinary tract infections in an ambulatory clinic. Am J Clin Pathol 1994;101:100–3.
40. Jenkins RD, Fenn JP, Matsen JM. Review of urine microscopy for bacteriuria. JAMA 1986;255:3397–403.
41. Eisenstadt J, Washington JA. Diagnostic microbiology for bacteria and yeasts causing urinary tract infections. In: Mobley LT, Warren JW, editors. Urinary tract infections: molecular pathogenesis and clinical management. Washington, DC: ASM Press, 1996:29–68.

CASE PRESENTATION

Subjective

PATIENT PROFILE

Nancy Nelson is a 40-year-old married white female accountant.

PRESENTING PROBLEM

"It hurts when I pass urine."

PRESENT ILLNESS

For 2 days, Mrs. Nelson has had urinary burning, frequency, urgency, and nocturia. She reports some mild left flank pain. She has felt warm but has not taken her temperature.

PAST MEDICAL HISTORY

She has had two urinary tract infections over the past 18 months, and both responded promptly to medication.

SOCIAL HISTORY

She works 3 days a week as a bookkeeper in a large firm. Her husband, Ken, is a home builder, and they have two teenage children.

HABITS

She uses no tobacco and takes alcohol occasionally. She drinks six cups of coffee daily.

FAMILY HISTORY

Her father, aged 71, is living and well. Her mother died at age 68 of breast cancer. She has no siblings.

REVIEW OF SYSTEMS

She has occasional pain in the joints of her hands and low back pain after lifting and carrying.

- What additional medical history would be helpful? Why?
- What symptoms or past history—if present—would you consider especially worrisome? Explain.
- Might a vulvovaginitis be part of her problem? How would you inquire about this possibility?
- What are Mrs. Nelson's possible concerns about her symptoms? How would you address this issue?

Objective

VITAL SIGNS

Blood pressure, 112/64; pulse, 68; respirations, 18; temperature, 37.4°C.

EXAMINATION

The patient is ambulatory and does not appear acutely ill. There is no mass or organ enlargement in the abdomen. There is moderate suprapubic tenderness without bladder distension. There is equivocal left costovertebral angle tenderness. The examination of the vagina, cervix, fundus, and adnexa are normal except for a thin watery vaginal discharge.

LABORATORY

There is a positive nitrite reaction on urinary dipstick. Red blood cells, bacteria, and many white blood cells are present on microscopic examination of a spun urine specimen.

- What additional data—if any—from the physical examination might be useful, and why?
- What—if any—laboratory tests would you obtain today? Why?
- What—if any—diagnostic imaging would you obtain today?
- If the patient had a thick purulent vaginal discharge, what might you do differently? Explain.

Assessment

- What is the probable diagnosis? What is the likely etiologic cause?
- How would you explain your assessment to the patient and her husband?
- What is the possible significance of the prior urinary tract infections?
- What is the possible meaning of this illness to the patient? To her husband?

Plan

- Describe your therapeutic recommendations for the patient. How would you explain this plan to the patient?
- What is your advice regarding work, household duties, and sexual relations?
- Might this patient benefit from consultation with a urologist? Explain.
- What follow-up would you advise?

16

Vulvovaginitis and Cervicitis

MARY WILLARD

Although modern medical practice has often relegated vaginal symptoms to the realm of the specialist gynecologist, the range of symptoms and diagnoses covered under this category with the concomitant preventive health and risk management issues is ideally suited to the expertise of the family physician. Excellence in the diagnosis and management of these diseases is the standard of care and can be achieved with a minimal investment of equipment, time (a 1-minute slide examination), and cost to the patient. Patients with vaginal complaints account for an estimated 10% of office visits each year[1] and many more may be inaccurately diagnosed by phone. This chapter reviews the systematic approach to the evaluation and treatment of vaginal diseases as well as issues of particular interest to family physicians.

Diagnostic Assessment

It is critical for the family physician to remember that few complaints are more annoying to the female patient than vaginal itching and discharge. Tolerance of low-grade symptomatology is the norm for some patients until a flare turns the problem into a midnight emergency. Although the history and physical examination are helpful, the diagnosis can be made only by appropriate testing.

Laboratory Equipment and Technique

The equipment needed for accurate diagnosis of vaginal complaints is simple: saline in small containers, nonsterile cotton Q-tips, slides, coverslips, a good microscope with 10× and 40× capacity (i.e., low and high dry power), 10% potassium hydroxide solution (KOH preparation), diagnostic tests for *Chlamydia* and gonococci, and a small magnifying lens. Vaginal fluid should be examined as soon as possible after the fluid is obtained, as *Trichomonas vaginalis* is fragile and may die quickly.

The technique of examining vaginal fluid is straightforward. After inserting the vaginal speculum, a plain cotton-tipped applicator is swept into the vaginal fluid, withdrawn (preferably with a "clump" of discharge), and placed immediately into a small container with only 1 ml of saline. Small pediatric red-topped tubes containing saline can be kept in all rooms where pelvic examinations may be performed so they are immediately available. For maximal results, the smallest amount of saline and the largest sample of vaginal fluid should be used. Once the sample of vaginal fluid is obtained, cervical cultures can be prepared if necessary, the pelvic examination completed, and the saline examined.

The vaginal fluid in saline is examined microscopically using gloves as per universal precautions. Take the cotton applicator from the tube and place a drop of fluid on two slides, one for the saline examination and one for a KOH preparation. If a diagnosis of yeast is being entertained, it is critical to try to get a "clump" of the discharge onto the designated KOH slide. A drop of a 10% KOH solution (made by mixing 90 ml distilled water with 10 g KOH) is dropped on it and immediately smelled for a fishy odor, which may be an indicator of bacterial vaginosis. If further evaluation for hyphae is to be done, place a coverslip and allow the slide to sit until the saline slide is examined. The KOH destroys some of the vaginal epithelial and white blood cells (WBCs), leaving only hyphae for inspection.

Next examine the saline slide with coverslip under low power. Search for motion of cells, sheets of epithelial cells compatible with denuding of mucosa, or "clue cells" (Fig. 16.1). The latter are vaginal epithelial cells "studded" with bacteria that adhere for unknown reasons. These epithelial cells look dense and tend to "glitter" when the focus is varied. Although clue cells are present normally in up to 10% of the field, a preponderance of them, especially when combined with a fishy odor on the KOH preparation, supports the diagnosis of bacterial vaginosis.[2]

Once the examination under low power is completed, it is appropriate to scan the field under high dry power to check for *T.*

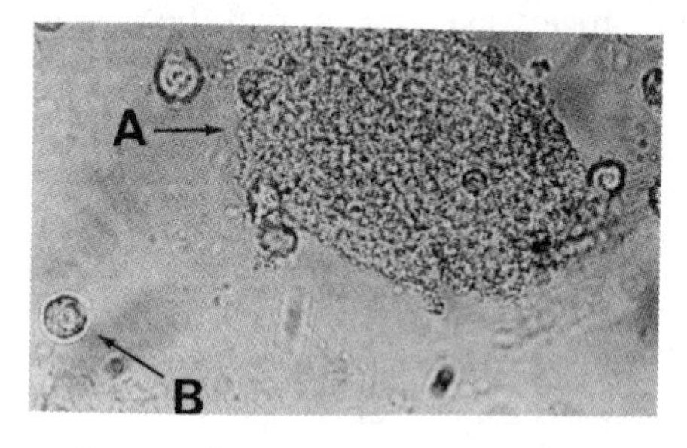

FIGURE 16.1. A = Clue cell. B = White blood cell in a vaginal wet preparation. Viewed under high dry objective. (From Fischer P. *The Office Laboratory.* Norwalk, CT: Appleton & Lange, 1983. With permission.)

vaginalis and to better examine the epithelial cells. Trichomonads appear as motile triangular cells, somewhat larger than WBCs, with long moving tails. Because many bacteria are part of the normal vaginal ecosystem and are nonpathogenic[3] Gram stains and routine cultures are not first-line tests for diagnosing vaginal diseases. If the high power field has more than 10 WBCs, consider the possibility of an upper genital tract infection.

If an examination for yeast is necessary, place the KOH preparation under the microscope. Hyphae and spores are best seen on this specimen by focusing under low power to find a "clumped" area and then going immediately to high dry power and focusing on the edges of the clump. The clumped material usually represents epithelial cells and hyphae tissue not desiccated by the KOH preparation; the edge of the clump is the best place to identify the hyphae. Certainly if the history so warrants and the cervical os reveals discharge from above, appropriate tests for *Chlamydia,* gonococci, or both are performed.

For analysis of vaginal complaints, few tests other than those noted above are needed except in specific circumstances or in refractory cases (which are discussed in relevant sections). One area of controversy is the role of vaginal pH tests. Because the premenopausal vaginal ecosystem keeps the pH under 4.5, assessment of change might be of some value. Although sensitive, this test is not specific and can be influenced greatly by fluids from the cervix, semen, or douching. It has therefore limited application in the office. There is also investigation into the use of monoclonal antibodies and DNA analysis. Unfortunately, none of these tests is of sufficient reliability to replace the simple slide evaluations.

History

As with any clinical problem, the history is a critical clue to diagnosis and must be obtained methodically from each patient. The ambiguous nature of the problem, however, means that the diagnosis cannot be made solely on historical clues, such as a "cheesy" discharge.

Most women can, with minimal clarification by the physician, reveal a clear history of their complaint. Because there is individual variation in the amount and character of the vaginal discharge that is "normal," the family physician role is to help patients distinguish a change from that pattern. Ask about skin lesions, internal or external itching, odor, dyspareunia, and the use (and frequency) of douching, new soaps, or deodorant sprays. Always inquire about previous similar episodes, but ask how these diagnoses were made, especially in the patient treated over the phone. Many patients who state that they "always get yeast infections" have never had an accurate diagnosis made and any vaginal cream has the potential of calming an inflamed mucosa (thereby diminishing the symptoms until the next flare).

One of the most commonly missed presentations of vaginitis is the complaint of dysuria (see Chapter 15). Treating all patients with dysuria as cystitis results in the inevitable phone call 48 to 72 hours later from a patient who is no better. Because women with vulvitis complain of pain externally with urination, clarification of the type of dysuria at the initial encounter assists in determining which patients require additional evaluation for vaginitis.

It is essential that the family physician obtain a complete sexual history from these patients and assess them for risk of sexually transmitted diseases. If the patient is sexually active, the physician should inquire about any new spermicidal agents or condoms, symptom complaints from a partner(s), a new sexual partner, and sexual practices. Moreover, the patient should be educated about sexual practices that minimize risk of disease.

Physical Examination

Although the pelvic examination can be tailored by the history, patients with vaginal complaints must be evaluated systematically. The external genitalia are thoroughly assessed for clues using a hand-held magnifying lens if necessary. The urethra, labia, and vulva are completely checked for ulcerations, warts, tears, cysts, abscesses, erythema, and edema. In addition, the vaginal mucosa itself must be inspected for color, lesions, and edema. Normal vaginal mucosa is pink with moist folds. A fiery red or weepy mucosa is a sign of inflammation. Any plaque-type lesions are scraped for adherence to vaginal mucosa, a sign of possible candidiasis.

As part of the complete evaluation, observe the cervical os for pus as a cause of discharge. Using a large cotton swab (e.g., one used for proctoscopic examinations), clean the cervix of all discharge, and observe the os for a short time, usually 10 seconds. If purulent fluid appears at the os opening from above, it is an indicator of upper pelvic infection for which *Chlamydia* and gonococci must be tested. At this point, a bimanual examination should also be performed to assess adnexal tenderness or masses.

Clinical Presentation

It is impossible, given the constraints of space, to discuss all possible forms of vaginitis or other vaginal diseases. Instead, the focus here is on the more common etiologies and important vaginal skin diseases that may masquerade as "itch." This approach assists in clarifying most vaginal complaints.

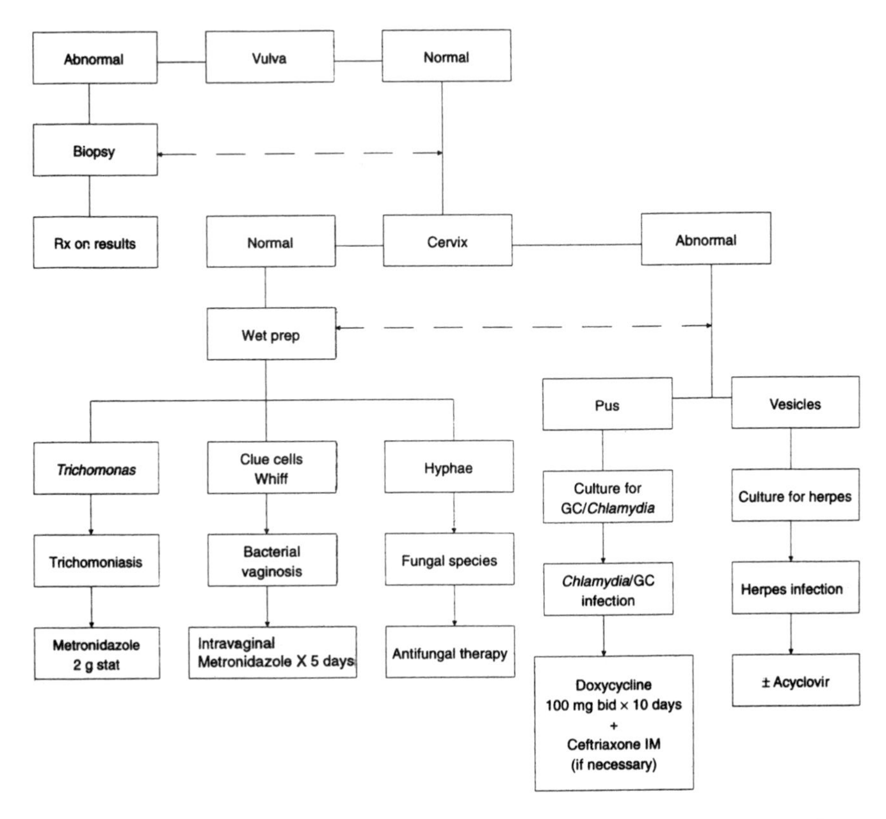

FIGURE 16.2. Diagnostic algorithm for vaginal symptoms. GC = gonococcus; Rx = treatment.

Traditional medical training clearly defined the "classic" presentations for vaginitis. Unfortunately, this "eyeball" method correctly diagnoses only one-third of the cases,[4] making thorough clinical evaluation necessary (Fig. 16.2). Nevertheless, an appreciation of the textbook presentations is necessary when teasing apart the significant historical details given by the patient. It is equally important to realize the change in epidemiology of vaginitis since the 1970s. The most common cause of vaginitis is now bacterial vaginosis, followed by mycotic diseases (e.g., *Candida* sp.), with trichomoniasis on the decline.[5] Whatever the reason for this shift, a knowledge of the probabilities is useful.

Contact and Chemical Dermatitides

Contact and chemical dermatitides are much overlooked diagnoses for the patient with vulvitis. Any topical agent used in the genital area (including nonoxynol-9 and rubber in condoms) can be an allergen.

Symptoms are characterized by a reddened, swollen vulva or a vaginal mucosa exuding a clear exudate. Equally important is the patient who has been douching repeatedly and with increasing frequency. This practice sets up a denuding phenomenon that inflames and strips the mucosa. The appropriate treatment for this category of inflammation is to discontinue the product and consider using a short-term course of topical external steroids for symptomatic relief.[6]

Mycotic Diseases

Although the incidence is rising,[5] contrary to popular belief among patients and physicians, true fungal infections probably account for approximately one-third of all vaginal infections. The textbook presentation is a patient complaining of a vaginal itch and cheesy exudate, with white plaques adherent to the vaginal wall and a KOH preparation showing multiple hyphae. The diagnosis should not be made unless hyphae are seen on the slide. Because as many as 20% of asymptomatic women have positive cultures,[7] it is obvious that culture methods are too sensitive and should be reserved for refractory cases,[8] frequent relapses, or when yeast is suspected clinically but the KOH preparation is negative. In this case, suspect *Candida glabrata,* which may present with vaginal burning and, as a spore former, can be diagnosed only on Gram stain. This infection is often refractory to the standard duration of treatment and may require protracted therapy.[6]

Yeast infections typified by *Candida albicans* have been erroneously ascribed to many causes. For example, yeast infections probably do not occur any more frequently in diabetic women but may be more difficult to eradicate.[6] Therefore consider diabetes in the patient with "chronic" infections, not frequent ones. There is also little proved association between yeast infection and use of birth control pills.[9] For frequent relapses, consider treating the sexual partner(s) to achieve full eradication and changing the patient's diet, as high calories and crude fiber have been associated with susceptibility to infection.[10] Remember, too, that women with human immunodeficiency virus (HIV) disease may manifest persistent or diffuse candidiasis as a presenting symptom (see Chapter 21).

Treatment is straightforward and consists of topical application of one of several groups of medication.[11] To date, no data prove oral routes to be superior and they are associated with side effects such as headache, drug reactions, and gastrointestinal (GI) toxicity.[12] In addition, there is no proved superiority of one drug over another or of creams over tablets, although general data show the azoles to be slightly more efficacious than nystatin.[12] Use of a cream allows external and internal application and may be more soothing acutely. Several forms of these medications are now available over the counter and are generally less expensive than most

TABLE 16.1. Examples of drugs to treat vaginal candidiasis

Generic drug and examples	Formulation	Dose	Cost to patient
Terconazole			
Terazol 7	Cream 4%	5 g hs × 7 days	$33.49
Terazol 3	Vaginal suppository 80 mg	1 hs × 3 days	11.59
Terazol 3	Cream 3%	5 g hs × 3 days	4.99
Nystatin	Vaginal tablet 100,000 U	1 hs × 14 days	8.99
Tioconazole (Vagistat)	Ointment 6.5%	4.5 g hs × 1	36.49
Fluconazole (Diflucan)	Oral tablet 150 mg	One tablet once	19.99
Clotrimazole			
Gyne-Lotrimin[a]	Vaginal tablet 100 mg	1 hs × 7 days	10.99[b]
	Cream 1%	5 g hs × 7–14 days	9.99
Mycelex[a]	Vaginal tablet 100 mg	1 hs × 7 days	8.99
	Cream 1%	5 g hs × 7 days	8.89
Miconazole			
Monistat 7[a]	Cream 2%	5 g hs × 7 days	13.99[b]
	Vaginal suppository 100 mg	1 hs × 7 days	12.99[b]
Monistat 3	Vaginal suppository 200 mg	1 hs × 3 days	28.69

[a]Available over the counter 1996.
[b]Example of over-the-counter cost at various chain pharmacies (not including generic discount drugs) in 1996.

prescription medications (Table 16.1). Physician and patient preferences dictate the specific drug and route, and there is no risk associated with treatment during pregnancy. Truly refractory cases may require longer treatment courses, and the patient with frequent relapses may benefit from oral ketoconazole (Nizoral) 100 mg/day or oral fluconazole 150 mg every week or month except during pregnancy.[12,13]

Trichomoniasis

The syndrome caused by *Trichomonas vaginalis* may cause severe itching or pain often accompanied by frequency of urination because of concomitant cystitis from the organism. On examination the vulva and the vaginal mucosa are fiery red with cervical petechiae ("strawberry cervix"). The typical discharge is yellow-green and bubbly in nature, but any range of color and texture may be seen, making slide examination critical. As noted above, the diagnosis is made by finding motile trichomonads on the saline smear. Because of the low positive predictive value of *Trichomonas* reported on Papanicolaou smears,[7] all of these results should be confirmed by a wet preparation before therapy is initiated. Although the culture methodology for *T. vaginalis* may have better sensitivity and specificity in theory, there is still debate over the ideal medium and methods, so the technique is not useful.[14]

The drug of choice in therapy is metronidazole (Flagyl, Prostat) with the best response noted after a 2 g immediate dose.[15] An alternative regimen of 250 mg tid for 7 days is best used for refractory cases only, as it produces no higher an initial cure than the one-time dose. Metronidazole has a significant Antabuse-type reaction, so patients must be cautioned to use no alcohol, including cough medicine, during the treatment. As a sexually transmitted disease, it is critically important for the patient's sexual partner(s) to be treated concurrently to prevent reinfection; and although there are some resistant cases, resistance is not an all-or-none phenomenon. Rather, resistance may range from mild (where treatment is effective) to severe, necessitating a treatment dose of 2.5 g/day in divided doses for 7 to 10 days.[16] At this time, no other medication available in the United States provides better therapeutic results.

Trichomoniasis during pregnancy is difficult to treat. Although the literature is scant, oral metronidazole may be teratogenic during the first trimester and is therefore contraindicated until the second trimester and reserved for severe infections only. Both intravaginal clotrimazole and clindamycin may be effective in controlling the symptoms during the first trimester, although may not produce eradication.[6,15]

Bacterial Vaginosis

Formerly known as *Gardnerella* or nonspecific vaginitis, bacterial vaginosis has been credited with as many as 50% of all diagnoses of vaginitis.[17] It represents an overgrowth in the vagina of anaerobic organisms classically known as *Gardnerella vaginalis* and now noted to be multiple organisms. It produces no vulvar symptoms, no change in vaginal mucosa, little itching, and no pain, unless the discharge is so profuse the vulvae are simply macerated. Because its course is usually indolent, it does not cause an acute change in symptoms. The patient may note only a slight change in normal discharge and an odor that may be more pronounced after intercourse. Patients are frequently inured to the symptoms until treatment is finished and the discharge gone. There may not be an odor immediately on examination, but KOH releases the amines in the epithelial cells and produces the classic fishy odor that is diagnostic when clue cells are present. Because *Gardnerella* bacteria may be normal inhabitants of the vagina, culture of the organisms for a diagnosis has poor specificity and so has not been recommended.[7]

Treatment for this syndrome is intravaginal metronidazole or clindamycin for 5 or 7 days, respectively (Fig. 16.2).[15,18] For refractory cases or as an alternate, oral metronidazole 500 mg bid for 7 days or clindamycin 300 mg bid for 7 days may be used.[15] Unfortunately, the one-time dose used to treat trichomoniasis is insufficient for vaginosis.

Because some association has been noted between bacterial vaginosis and premature rupture of membranes or postpartum endometriosis, therapy should be considered during pregnancy.[19] The recommended drug during pregnancy is a 2% clindamycin vaginal cream at night for 7 days or oral clindamycin 300 mg bid for 7 days.[15,19] There is a preliminary indication that screening and treatment for bacterial vaginosis early in pregnancy is efficacious.[20]

At this time, the role of sexual transmission of this disorder is unclear. Studies can be found to support either opinion, and partner therapy has not produced an improved cure rate, at least at conventional dosage.[18] Equally unclear is the role of treatment in the asymptomatic patient, but it may be considered in someone undergoing vaginal surgery because of a potential role in pelvic inflammation.[18]

Atrophic Vaginitis

A common cause of vaginal symptoms in the postmenopausal woman, atrophic vaginitis should be considered concomitantly with the evaluation for other etiologies. Lack of estrogen produces thin vaginal epithelium and cells deficient in the acids that provide the premenopausal woman with a balanced vaginal ecosystem. Therefore the mucosa easily denudes and becomes traumatized. Thus presenting symptoms may include lack of vaginal lubrication with coitus, pruritus, and dyspareunia, with or without discharge.

On examination the vaginal folds are flattened, and the mucosa is pale pink and shows lack of lubrication. The cervix is usually atrophic and frequently friable; and the wet preparation is negative. Hormone replacement therapy is the treatment of choice, but vaginal estrogen creams used nightly can provide short-term relief.[21] The patient must be reminded that a vaginal "discharge" may recur as the cells mature back to a premenopausal pattern.

Sexually Transmitted Diseases

The following are several sexually transmitted diseases (STDs) that present with predominantly vaginal symptoms.

CHLAMYDIA INFECTION

Even though *Chlamydia* does not produce vaginitis (except in adolescents), it does cause mucopurulent cervicitis. On examination, the cervix may be eroded and present a mucopurulent discharge that when wiped quickly re-forms at the os. When this condition is seen, the alert clinician performs appropriate tests, examining wet preparations for concomitant vaginal infections, as patients with one STD are at high risk of having more.

Once a diagnosis of *Chlamydia* is suspected, empiric treatment is warranted, especially in a high-risk patient (defined as sexually active, nonmonogamous, young). The standard treatment is doxycycline (Vibramycin) 100 mg PO bid for 7 to 10 days.[15] If the patient is allergic to tetracycline (rare) or pregnancy is suspected, an appropriate alternative is erythromycin 500 mg PO qid for 7 days. Partners should be treated aggressively, but a test of patient cure is considered unnecessary.

HERPESVIRUS INFECTION

Especially in the case of recurrences, patients with herpesvirus infection may present only with symptoms of external burning and minimal liquid discharge. Without ulcerations externally or on the cervix, this diagnosis should not be entertained unless there is a known history of a positive culture.

HUMAN PAPILLOMAVIRUS INFECTION

Current trends indicate that most human papillomavirus (HPV) disease presents as warts[22] either externally or internally. Therefore HPV is unlikely to be a cause of any symptoms unless the growth is large enough to cause an exudative process. Because HPV is associated with cervical dysplasia, a Papanicolaou smear must be examined regularly. No form of treatment has proved to be superior or to eradicate the virus. Topical podophyllin externally and cryotherapy internally remain widely used. Podofilox (0.5% solution) is available by prescription for patient home use.

Leukorrhea Secondary to Birth Control Pills

On some occasions, the only cause of leukorrhea is an eroded cervix secondary to the use of birth control pills. The hormones in birth control pills cause more endocervix to be exposed to the environment of the vagina, producing irritation and weeping of the mucosa. It is usually asymptomatic. If a patient is having symptoms, this diagnosis is excluded.

Vulvar Diseases

It is critical to remember that many skin diseases manifest with vaginal symptoms. Most, such as seborrheic dermatitis, psoriasis, tinea, and pediculosis, have unique characteristics that are obvious. Without these unique characteristics, the physician must perform a biopsy with a simple punch instrument for diagnosis and appropriate therapy. All patients must be educated that the treatment effect may take months to realize. In addition, any pigmented lesion should be biopsied and the patient referred if indicated by biopsy results.

Vestibulitis

With vestibulitis there is variable redness and edema of the vestibular glands, frequently with a lesion. The number of glands involved can range from 1 to 100, and the symptoms are vulvar pain with dyspareunia. The etiology is still hotly debated but probably HPV is involved. Treatment results are best with vestibular resection or intralesional interferon, but no therapy is 100% effective.[23]

Lichen Sclerosis

Lichen sclerosis is a hyperplastic condition with a white lesion seen predominantly in women over age 50. There is a typical "keyhole" pattern on both sides of the vulva. The lesion may eventually cover the entire vulva with adhesion and eventual obliteration of the labia minora to the majora. Treatment is a topical testosterone ointment (30 ml of testosterone in oil with 120 gm petrolatum) twice a day for 4 to 6 months and then 1 or 2 times a week for life.[21] If the patient cannot tolerate the side effects, alternative therapy of progesterone cream can be used. There is a high recurrence rate, even with surgery or laser, so dramatic treatment is best avoided.

Lichen Simplex Chronicus

Caused by chronic itching or irritation, lichen simplex chronicus is a thick, scaly condition with localized vulvar lesions without adhesions. Treatment is symptomatic with topical steroids for 1 to 2 months. Because the only recurrences are seen in patients treated by surgery, this intervention is no longer acceptable.[24]

Lichen Planus

Lichen planus may involve mucous membranes in other organ systems (see Chapter 19). There is vulvar burning, leukorrhea, and redness of the inner labia. Patients may have violaceous papules externally and small, lacy, gray, reticular patterns on the inner labia. Without these identifying marks, this lesion may appear similar to that of atrophic vaginitis; it should be entertained as a diagnosis whenever therapy for atrophic vaginitis fails. Treatment is topical with either a potent fluorinated steroid or a medium-potency steroid under occlusion.[24] The patient must be reminded that this condition flares and remits over long periods.

When the Tests Are Negative

A dilemma ensues when, despite the best efforts of the clinician, the examination and tests reveal no reason for the patient's symptoms. In such cases, mentally review the history, the adequacy of specimen collection, the performance of the laboratory test, and the possibility of *Chlamydia*. Obtain any history previously overlooked and consider the diagnosis of an acid-base change in the vaginal environment known as *cytolytic vaginosis*. Although not easily diagnosed, this entity is caused by an overgrowth of acidophilic Döderlein's lactobacilli, producing an increase in enzymes that degrade intracellular glycogen to lactic acid and causing massive desquamation and cytolysis and a watery discharge. Because the luteal phase epithelial cells are richer in lactic acid, this syndrome may be cyclic in nature. The hallmark for diagnosis is epithelial cells that have a motheaten appearance, often called pseudo-clue cells, and a few WBCs on the wet preparation. In addition, because this process is driven by an acidic environment, the symptoms worsen with douching using conventional acidic agents. Instead, these patients can be treated with a douching mixture of sodium bicarbonate and water (1–2 tablespoons in 500 ml water) used three times a week while symptomatic.[4]

If the workup was adequate, resist the urge to perform "shotgun" or even empiric treatment, as such treatment perpetuates old myths. Be supportive and understanding of the symptoms and encourage the patient to be checked with subsequent recurrences.

Special Considerations for the Family Physician

Much of the success of therapy depends on the unique relationship between the family physician and the patient.

Compliance

The trusting relationship between the patient and the family physician enhances compliance with often distasteful regimens. The patient is encouraged to finish the full course of therapy despite symptom resolution; and when the therapy demands partner compliance, the patient must be instructed to abstain from intercourse until therapy is completed. Role-playing this partner discussion with the patient may help allay anxiety. Choose the shortest regimen possible and make sure the patient understands side effects (including local irritation), route of usage, and use of medication during menses. Negotiate with the patient the best time to begin treatment and inform her of the possibility of recurrence or treatment failure. In addition, it is critical to assess the patients' attribution of disease in this condition. Clarity about sexual transmission is important; if possible, use printed information for the patient to read and give to her partner(s).

Issues of self-support and control of symptoms can be critical to compliance as well. These points can be reinforced through good patient education. Sources of self-help for the patient can be found in women's health literature such as *Our Bodies, Our Selves.*[25] These references may provide the patient with more detailed information on hygiene, as well as alternative remedies. The physician, however, should first read the relevant sections to be sure that the information is consonant with good care and to explain areas of disagreement. (For example, there is scant scientific evidence for the use of intravaginal yogurt.) Some patients work best with a combination of conventional medical therapy and time-honored suggestions.

Recurrent or Persistent Vaginitis

Nothing is more frustrating to the patient or physician than recurrence (defined as symptoms recurring after a 1-month disease-free interval) or persistence of symptoms. In this situation the physician should start over with the history, emphasizing compliance with previous therapy and focusing attention on details of diet, clothing, and irritants. Question the patient about high dairy intake, increased simple sugars, use of new deodorant tampons, pads, or other topical agents such as perfumes or home remedies. Explore the relation to tight clothing, exercise gear, the use of dildos or vibrators, and the use of hot tubs or pools.

The examination and basic tests should be repeated, but if the history reveals no further clues, culture the cervix for *Chlamydia* and the vaginal vault for bacteria and *Candida* and perform any necessary vulvar biopsies. In the diabetic patient the blood glucose must be controlled concomitantly with reinstituting therapy.

Results of the tests dictate therapy. Persistent *Candida* or *Trichomonas* may need prolonged (*Candida*) or increased (*Trichomonas*) therapy. Consider treating according to the results of the bacterial culture using an antibiotic[6] targeted to the dominant organism.

If tests are negative, emphasize your support and sympathy, educate the patient about good hygiene and sexual behaviors that minimize risk, and proscribe anything that might exacerbate symptoms. Encourage the patient to return to be examined when symptoms recur.

Management of the HIV-Positive Patient

Other than the fact that patients who are HIV-seropositive may have problems with HPV, treatment of vaginal disorders follows the same recommendations as for nonpositive patients. Although refractory candidiasis may be a clue for the physician to check a patient for HIV status, a normal vaginal infection should not be of concern. Flares of venereal warts can be treated conventionally, although at least one author suggested that flares may be a sign to check the patient's CD4 count.[26]

Role of Colposcopy

The role of colposcopy is not well defined regarding vaginal symptoms. It may be a useful tool in the future, but its current usage is in the evaluation of an abnormal Papanicolaou smear or cervix. Therefore use it in a patient with persistent cervicitis only to screen for abnormal areas to biopsy. In addition, conventional wisdom dictates that patients with HPV undergo colposcopy to detect a precancerous state of the cervix.

Prevention of Vaginitis

When an STD has caused the vaginitis, the family physician must educate the patient about the difference between a disease that can arise de novo and then be propagated between partners and one acquired *from* someone else. Patients are understandably concerned about *where* they got the disease, but you can help focus the patient on treatment, give basic relevant information, and plan a subsequent visit to continue pursuing their concerns. Clarity about sexual transmission is important, as the patient may also need to be concerned about hepatitis and HIV risk. Acquisition of an STD is certainly threatening to partners who thought of themselves as mutually monogamous, and relationship issues are frequently topics for subsequent visits.

In addition to concerns about sexual transmission, the physician should educate the patient about the causative or associative factors found to be significant in the history. Use of local irritants, clothing, and other offending behaviors must be prevented. Above all, encouraging the patient to come in for evaluation of subsequent infections is critical, as the etiology may differ from the current one.

References

1. Paavonen J, Stamm WE. Lower genital tract infections in women. Infect Dis Clin North Am 1987:1179–98.
2. Bump RC, Zuspan FP, Buesching WJ, et al. The prevalence, six-month persistence and predictive values of laboratory indicators of bacterial vaginosis (nonspecific vaginitis). Am J Obstet Gynecol 1984; 150:917–23.
3. Faro S. Bacterial vaginitis. Obstet Gynecol 1991;34:582–6.
4. Cibley LJ, Cibley LJ. Cytolytic vaginosis. Am J Obstet Gynecol 1991; 165:1245–8.
5. Kent HL. Epidemiology of vaginitis. Am J Obstet Gynecol 1991;165:1168–76.
6. Horowitz BJ, Mardh PA, editors. Vaginitis and vaginosis. New York: Wiley Liss, 1991.
7. Eschenbach DA, Hiller SL. Advances in diagnostic testing for vaginitis and cervicitis. J Reprod Med 1989;34 Suppl 18:555–64.
8. Horowitz BJ. Mycotic vulvovaginitis: a broad overview. Am J Obstet Gynecol 1991;165:1188–92.
9. Roy S. Vulvovaginitis: causes and therapies: nonbarrier contraceptives and vaginitis and vaginosis. Am J Obstet Gynecol 1991;165:1240–4.
10. Reed B, Slatery M, French T. Diet and vaginitis. J Fam Pract 1989;29:509–15.
11. Topical treatment for bacterial vaginosis. Med Lett Drugs Ther 1992; 34:109.
12. Reef SE, Levine WC, McNeil MM, et al. Treatment option for vulvovaginal candidiasis 1993. Clin Infect Dis 1995;20 Suppl 1:580–90.
13. Soble JD. Recurrent vulvovaginal candidiasis: a prospective study of the efficacy of maintenance ketoconazole therapy. N Engl J Med 1986;315: 1455–8.
14. Lossick JG. The diagnosis of trichomoniasis [editorial]. JAMA 1988;259:1230.
15. MMWR 1998 guidelines for treatment of sexually transmitted diseases. MMWR Weekly Report vol 47, Jan 23, 1998.
16. Lossick JG, Kent HL. Trichomoniasis: trends in diagnosis and management. Am J Obstet Gynecol 1991;165:1217–22.
17. Eschenbach DA, Hiller S, Critchlow C, et al. Diagnosis and clinical manifestations of bacterial vaginosis. Am J Obstet Gynecol 1988;158: 819–23.
18. Joesoef MR, Schmid GP. Bacterial vaginosis: review of treatment options and potential clinical indications for therapy. CID 1995;20 Suppl 1:572–9.
19. McCoy MC, Katz VL, Kuller JA, et al. Bacterial vaginosis in pregnancy: an approach for the 1990's. Obstet Gynecol Surg 1995;50:482–8.
20. McGregor JA, French L, Parker R, et al. Prevention of premature birth by screening and treatment for common genital tract infections: results of a prospective controlled evaluation. Am J Obstet Gynecol 1995;173:157–67.
21. Byyny RL, Speroff L. A clinical guide for the care of older women. Baltimore: Williams & Wilkins, 1990.

22. Reid R, Greenberg MD. Human papillomavirus-related diseases of the vulva. Clin Obstet Gynecol 1991;3:630–50.
23. McKay M, Frankman O, Horovitz BJ, et al. Vulvar vestibulitis and vestibular papillomatoses: report of the ISSVD committee on vulvodynia. J Reprod Med 1991;36:413–5.
24. McKay M. Vulvar dermatoses. Clin Obstet Gynecol 1991;34: 614–29.
25. Boston Women's Health Book Collective. The New Our Bodies, Our Selves. New York: Simon & Schuster, 1992.
26. Hammill HA, Murtagh CP. Gynecologic care of the human immunodeficiency virus-positive woman. Clin Obstet Gynecol 1991;34:599–604.

CASE PRESENTATION

Subjective

PATIENT PROFILE

Ellen McCarthy Harris is a 26-year-old married white female secretary.

PRESENTING PROBLEM

Vaginal discharge.

PRESENT ILLNESS

There is a 10-day history of vaginal discharge with intense itching that began after her last menstrual period. The symptoms have not responded to an over-the-counter vaginal cream.

PAST MEDICAL HISTORY

No serious illnesses or hospitalizations.

SOCIAL HISTORY

She has worked at her secretarial job for 4 years. She and her husband, Andrew, have two children.

HABITS

She does not use tobacco, coffee, or recreational drugs.

FAMILY HISTORY

Her father has diabetes mellitus and coronary artery disease. Her mother is living and well. Her brother, aged 28, is HIV-positive.

REVIEW OF SYSTEMS

No symptoms in other areas.

- What additional information regarding the history of present illness might be important? Explain.
- Why might the over-the-counter medication not have worked?
- Over the past 10 days, what might the patient be doing differently because of her illness? Why might this be pertinent?
- What might the patient be trying to tell you today?

Objective

VITAL SIGNS

Blood pressure, 112/64; pulse, 68; temperature, 37.0°C.

EXAMINATION

The abdomen is scaphoid with no mass, tenderness, or organ enlargement. The vaginal introitus is moderately inflamed. There is a frothy vaginal discharge. The cervix is mildly injected, and there are a few punctate hyperemic areas. The fundus and adnexa are normal. The rectal examination is normal, and the test for occult blood in the feces is negative.

- What other data—if any—regarding the physical examination might be important?
- What office diagnostic test(s) might you perform, and what are you likely to find?
- What specimens—if any—might you send to the laboratory?
- If the vaginal discharge were thick and purulent, what might you do differently? Explain.

Assessment

- What is the probable etiologic diagnosis? How will you explain this to the patient?
- What—if any—is the likely relationship to her menses?
- What are some concerns that the patient might like to address? How would you give "permission" to address these issues?
- What are the possible family issues in this case? How might you address these?

Plan

- What are your specific therapeutic recommendations? How will you explain these to Mrs. Harris?
- What is your advice regarding her activities, including sexual intercourse?
- Mrs. Harris asks what she can do to prevent recurrence. How would you reply?
- What follow-up would you advise?

17

Disorders of the Back and Neck

WALTER L. CALMBACH

Disorders of the Back

Low back pain occurs in 60% to 80% of adults at some point in their lives and is second only to upper respiratory infections as a cause for absence from work.[1] Each year 2% of all American workers have a compensable back injury, and 14% lose at least one work day due to low back pain.[2] Among chronic conditions, back problems are the most frequent cause for limitation of activity (work, housekeeping, school) among patients under 45 years of age.[3] Nonsurgical low back pain is the fourth most common admission diagnosis for patients over 65.[4] Although low back pain is usually a self-limited problem, it still costs approximately $24 billion per year in direct medical expenses and another $27 billion per year in lost productivity and compensation.[5] In most cases, low back pain is treated successfully with a conservative regimen, supplemented by selective use of neuroradiologic imaging and appropriate surgical intervention for a few patients.[6]

Epidemiology

Estimates of the lifetime prevalence of low back pain range from 60% to 80%, and the annual incidence is estimated at 5% per year.[5,7] At any moment, 15% to 20% of the population report symptoms of back pain.[5] Risk factors for low back pain include age, occupation, and psychosocial issues such as job satisfaction.[4] In cases of more severe back pain, occupational exposures are much more significant, including repetitive heavy lifting, pulling, or pushing, and exposures to industrial and vehicular vibrations. If even temporary work loss occurs, additional important risk factors include job dissatisfaction, supervisor ratings, and job environment (i.e., boring, repetitive tasks).[5] Factors associated with recurrence of low back pain include traumatic origin of first attack, sciatic pain, radiographic changes, alcohol abuse, specific job situations, and psychosocial stigmata.

Of patients with acute low back pain, only 1.5% develop sciatica (i.e., painful paresthesias or motor weakness in the distribution of a nerve root). The lifetime prevalence of sciatica is 40%, and sciatica afflicts 11% of patients with low back pain that lasts more than 2 weeks.[8,9] Sciatica is associated with long-distance driving, truck driving, cigarette smoking, and repeated lifting in a twisted posture. It is most common during the fourth and fifth decades of life, peaking during the fourth decade. Most patients with sciatica, even those with significant neurologic abnormalities, recover without surgery.[10,11] Only 5% to 10% of patients with persistent sciatica require surgery.[4,5]

Despite the incidence and prevalence of low back pain and sciatica, the major factor responsible for its societal impact is disability.[5] The National Center for Health Statistics estimates that 5.2 million Americans are disabled with low back pain, and of these 2.6 million are permanently disabled.[12] Between 70% and 90% of the total costs due to low back pain are incurred by the 4% to 5% of patients with temporary or permanent disability.[5] Risk factors for disability due to low back pain include poor health habits, job dissatisfaction, unappealing work environments, poor ratings by supervisors, psychological disturbances, compensable injuries, and a history of prior disability.[5] These same factors are associated with high failure rates for treatments of all types.

Natural History

Low back pain is usually a benign, self-limited condition.[13] For most patients with acute low back pain a definitive diagnosis is not possible.[14] Approximately 90% of cases of acute low back pain are due to musculoskeletal sprains and strains.[4,9] Acute disc herniation has changed little from its description in the classic article of Mixter and Barr: the annulus fibrosus begins to deteriorate by age 30, which leads to partial or complete herniation of the nucleus pulposus, causing irritation and compression of adjacent nerve roots.[4,14,15] Usually this herniation is in the posterolateral position, producing unilateral symptoms. Occasionally, the disc herniates in the midline, and a large herniation in this location can cause bilateral symptoms. More than 95% of lumbar disc herniations occur at the L4–5 or L5–S1 levels. Involvement of the L5 nerve root results in weakness of the great toe extensors and dorsiflexors of the foot, and sensory loss at the dorsum of the foot and in the first web space. Involvement of the S1 nerve root results in a diminished ankle reflex, weakness of the plantar flexors, and sensory loss at the posterior calf and lateral foot.

Although 60% to 80% of the population experiences low back pain during any one year, most people do not present for medical treatment. Of those who do, 90% recover within 6 weeks with or without therapy.[1,16] Even in industrial settings, 75% of patients with symptoms of acute low back pain return to work within 1 month.[1] Only 2% to 3% of patients continue to have symptoms at 6 months and only 1% at 1 year. However, symptoms of low back pain recur in approximately 60% of cases over the next 2 years. Demographic characteristics such as age, gender, race, or ethnicity do not appear to influence the natural history of low back pain. Obesity, smoking, and occupation, however, are important influences.[13] Adults in the upper fifth quintile of height and weight are more likely to report low back pain lasting for 2 weeks or more.[8,13] Cigarette smoking delays recovery from acute low back pain, either through a direct effect of smoking on the nutrition of the lumbar intervertebral disc or through an indirect mechanical effect on coughing; alternatively, smoking may simply be a marker for differences in the health behavior and physical fitness of smokers.[13,17] Occupational factors that prolong or delay recovery from acute low back pain include heavier job requirements, job dissatisfaction, repetitious or boring jobs, poor employer evaluations, and noisy or unpleasant working conditions.[15] Psychosocial factors play an important role in the natural history of low back pain, modulating response to pain and promoting illness behavior. The generally favorable natural history of acute low back pain is significantly influenced by a variety of medical and psychosocial factors with which the practicing physician must be familiar in order to counsel patients regarding prognosis and treatment.

Clinical Presentation

HISTORY

Low back pain is a symptom that has many causes. The onset of symptoms may be sudden or insidious. For example, 70% of patients with noncompensation injuries are unable to identify the specific injury that initiated their back pain.[18] Useful items on the history include age, fever, weight loss, adenopathy, steroid use, and previous tuberculosis or cancer. Factors that aggravate or alleviate low back pain should be elicited. Nonmechanical back pain is usually continuous, whereas mechanical back pain is aggravated by motion and relieved by rest. Low back pain that worsens with cough has traditionally been associated with disc herniation, although data now indicate that mechanical low back pain also worsens with cough.[18] The presence of leg weakness or leg paresthesias in a nerve root distribution is consistent with disc herniation. Bowel or bladder incontinence with or without saddle paresthesias suggests the cauda equina syndrome, which is a surgical emergency and requires immediate referral to a surgeon. Hip pain can mimic low back pain and is often referred to the groin, anterior thigh, or knee and is worsened with ambulation. Patients with osteoarthritis or degenerative joint disease report morning stiffness that improves as the day progresses. Patients with spinal stenosis report symptoms suggestive of spinal claudication, that is, neurologic symptoms in the legs that worsen with ambulation. Spinal claudication is differentiated from vascular claudication in that the symptoms of spinal claudication have a slower onset and slower resolution. A history of pain at rest, pain in the recumbent position, or pain at night suggests infection or tumor as a cause for low back pain. Osteoporosis is a consideration among postmenopausal women or women who have undergone oophorectomy. These patients report severe, localized, unrelenting pain after even "minor" trauma. Patients who present writhing in pain suggest the presence of an intraabdominal process or vascular cause for the pain, such as abdominal aortic aneurysm.

PHYSICAL EXAMINATION

The initial examination is fairly detailed. With the patient standing and appropriately gowned, the examining physician notes the stance and gait, as well as the presence or absence of the normal curvature of the spine (e.g., thoracic kyphosis, lumbar lordosis, splinting to one side, scoliosis). The range of motion of the back is documented, including flexion, lateral bending, and rotation. Intact dorsiflexion and plantar flexion of the foot is determined by observing heel-walk and toe-walk. Intact knee extension is determined by observing the patient squat and rise while keeping the back straight.

With the patient seated, a distracted straight-leg raising test is applied. With the hip flexed at 90 degrees, the flexed knee is brought to full extension. A positive straight-leg raising test reproduces the patient's paresthesias in the distribution of a nerve root at less than 60 degrees of knee extension. Sensation to light touch and pinprick are examined, and the motor strength of the hip and knee flexors is tested. The deep tendon reflexes are tested [knee jerk (L4), ankle jerk (S1)], and long tract signs are elicited by applying Babinski's maneuver (Table 17.1).

With the patient in the supine position, the straight-leg raising test is repeated. With the hip and knee extended, the leg is raised (i.e., the hip is flexed). A positive test reproduces the patient's paresthesias in the distribution of a nerve root. Isolated low back pain does not indicate a positive straight-leg raising test. The crossed straight-leg raising test (i.e., reproduction of the patient's symptoms by straight-leg raising of the contralateral leg) is specific for acute disc herniation and suggests a large central disc herniation. Hip range of motion is then tested, and pain radiation to the groin, anteromedial thigh, or knee is documented.

A more detailed examination may be necessary in selected patients. If significant pathology is suspected in a male patient, the cremasteric reflex is tested (i.e., application of a sharp stimulus at the proximal medial thigh

TABLE 17.1. Motor, sensory, and deep tendon reflex patterns associated with commonly affected nerve roots

Nerve root	Motor reflexes	Sensory reflexes	Deep tendon reflexes
C5	Deltoid	Lateral arm	Biceps jerk (C5, C6)
C6	Biceps, brachioradialis, wrist extensors	Lateral forearm	Brachioradialis
C7	Triceps, wrist flexors, MCP extensors	Middle of hand, middle finger	Triceps jerk
C8	MCP flexors	Medial forearm	—
T1	Abductors and adductors of fingers	Medial arm	—
L4	Quadriceps	Anterior thigh	Knee jerk
L5	Dorsiflex foot and great toe	Dorsum of foot	Hamstring reflex (L5, S1)
S1	Plantarflex foot	Lateral foot, posterior calf	Ankle jerk

MCP = metacarpophalangeal.

normally causes retraction of the ipsilateral scrotum). With the patient in the prone position, the femoral stretch test is applied. While the hip and knee are in extension the knee is flexed, placing increased stretch on the femoral nerve, which includes elements from the L2, L3, and L4 nerve roots.[12] The hamstring reflex is tested by striking the semitendinosus and semimembranosus tendons at the medial aspect of the popliteal fossa. The hamstring reflex involves both the L5 and S1 nerve roots. Thus an absent or decreased hamstring reflex in the presence of a normal ankle jerk response (S1) implies involvement of the L5 nerve root (Table 17.1). Sensation in the area between the upper buttocks is tested, as is the anal reflex and anal sphincter tone (S2, S3, S4).

The clinical diagnosis of acute disc herniation requires repeated physical examination demonstrating pain or parasthesias localized to a specific nerve root, with reproduction of pain on straight-leg raising tests, and muscle weakness in the nerve appropriate root distribution.

Diagnosis

RADIOLOGY

Plain Radiographs. Plain radiographs are usually not useful for diagnosing acute low back pain because they cannot demonstrate soft tissue sprains and strains or an acute herniated disc. However, plain radiographs are useful for ruling out conditions such as vertebral fracture, spondylolisthesis, spondylolysis, infection, tumor, or inflammatory spondyloarthropathy[4,19] (Fig. 17.1). In the absence of neurologic deficits, plain radiographs in the evaluation of low back pain should be reserved for patients over 50 years of age, temperature over 38°C, anemia, a history of

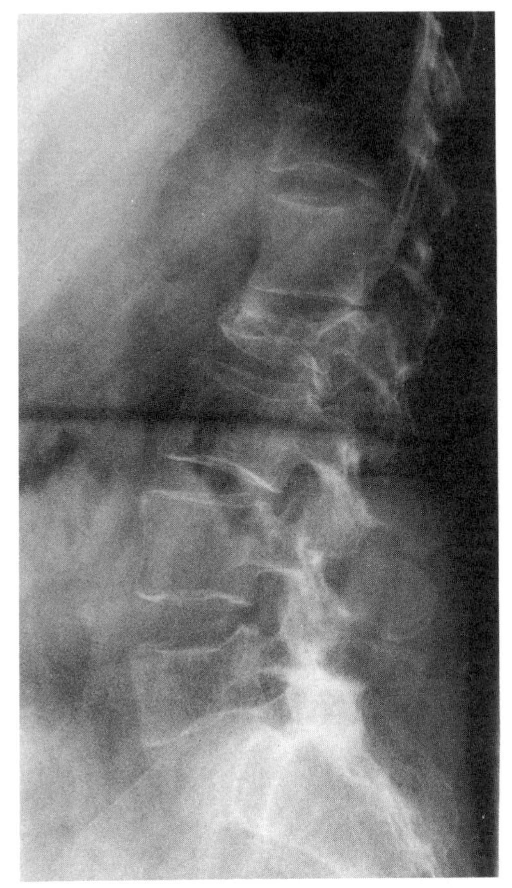

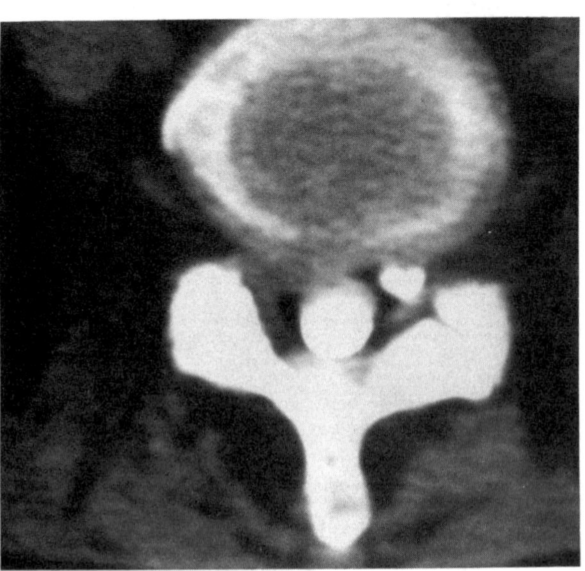

FIGURE 17.1. Radiologic studies of the lumbar spine. (A) Plain radiograph demonstrating a compression fracture of the L2 vertebral body due to multiple myeloma. (B) CT scan demonstrating nucleus pulposus herniating posteriorly into the spinal canal.

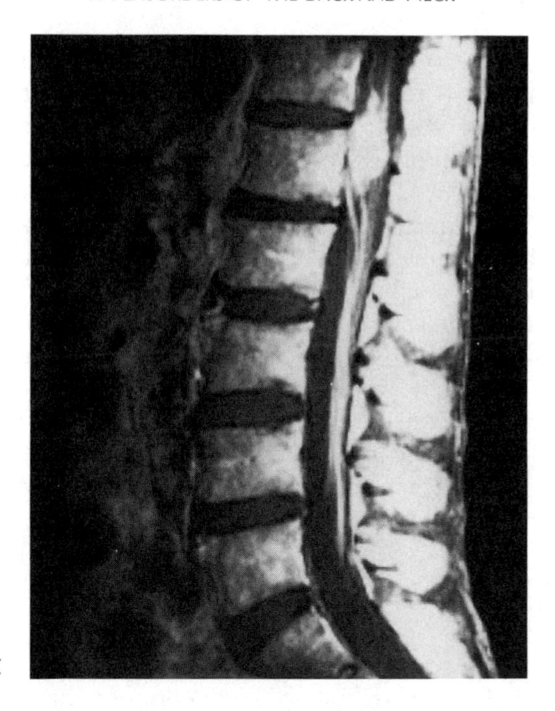

FIGURE 17.1. (continued) (C) MRI demonstrating an enhancing intramedullary metastatic lesion in the cauda equina at the L-1 level.

trauma, previous cancer, pain at rest, or unexplained weight loss, drug or alcohol abuse, steroid use, diabetes mellitus, or any other reason for immunosuppression.[20] For selected patients, initial plain radiographs of the spine during the early evaluation of acute low back pain should include anteroposterior and lateral views of the lumbar spine.[14] Oblique views are used to rule out spondylolysis, particularly when evaluating acute low back pain in young athletic patients active in sports such as football, wrestling, gymnastics, diving, or ballet.[21] Radiographic abnormalities are nonspecific and are observed equally in patients with and without symptoms of low back pain.[22] Clinical correlation is essential before symptoms of low back pain can be attributed to radiographic abnormalities.

Computed Tomography, Magnetic Resonance Imaging, Myelography. Computed tomography (CT), myelography, and magnetic resonance imaging (MRI) each has a specific role in evaluating a select subset of patients with low back pain. Physicians must be aware that many asymptomatic patients demonstrate disc bulging, protrusion, and even extrusion.[4,23] For example, 30% to 40% of CT scans and 64% of MRIs demonstrate abnormalities of the intervertebral disc in asymptomatic patients.[6,23] CT or

MRI should be reserved for patients with neurologic findings who show no response after a 4- to 6-week course of conservative therapy.[4] Earlier imaging should be considered if the patient demonstrates the cauda equina syndrome, a progressive neurologic deficit, or if tumor or infection are suspected.[4,6,14] The CT scan is best used for evaluating bony abnormalities (e.g., fracture or spinal stenosis) or the intervertebral disc (Fig. 17.1). Myelography is useful for differentiating significant disc herniation from incidental disc bulging not responsible for the patient's signs or symptoms but it has largely been replaced by noninvasive techniques such as MRI or CT.[14] MRI is particularly useful for examining the soft tissues of the central nervous system, assessing the postoperative spine, delineating postoperative scarring, recurrent disc disease, and fusion stability (Fig. 17.1). Some investigators believe that MRI is the procedure of choice for lumbar spine imaging, but others recommend judicious use of CT and myelography as well.[19,24]

Differential Diagnosis

OSTEOARTHRITIS

Osteoarthritis of the vertebral spine is common in later life and is especially prevalent in the cervical and lumbar spine. Typically, the pain of osteoarthritis of the spine is worse in the morning, increases with motion, and is relieved by rest. It is associated with morning stiffness and decreased range of motion of the spine in the absence of systemic symptoms. The severity of symptoms does not correlate well with radiographic findings, and patients with severe degenerative changes on plain radiographs may be asymptomatic, whereas patients with symptoms suggestive of osteoarthritis of the spine may have minimal radiologic findings. In some patients extensive osteophytic changes may lead to compression of lumbar nerve roots or may even cause cauda equina syndrome.

SPINAL STENOSIS

Spinal stenosis is most common in older adults and can occur at a single or multiple levels. The pain of spinal stenosis is aggravated by standing, increases during the day, and is relieved by rest. Symptoms usually begin during the sixth decade, and over time the patient's posture becomes progressively flexed forward. The mean age of patients at the time of surgery for spinal stenosis is 55 years, with an average symptom duration of 4 years.[9] Plain radiographs often show osteophytes at several levels, but as mentioned earlier, caution must be used when ascribing back pain to these degenerative changes. The neurogenic claudication of spinal stenosis is described as pain or even neurologic deficits in the legs that occur after walking.[9] Spinal claudication is differentiated from vascular claudication in that spinal claudication has a slower onset and a slower resolution of symptoms.[6]

OSTEOPOROSIS

Osteoporosis is a common problem among seniors, affecting up to 25% of women over age 65. Decreased bone mineral density in the vertebral body is associated with an increased risk for spinal compression fractures. In primary care settings, 4% of patients who present with acute low back pain have compression fractures as the cause.[12] Pain symptoms are worse with prolonged sitting or standing and usually resolve over 3 to 4 months as compression fractures heal.[6] African American and Mexican American women have only one-fourth as many compression fractures as European American women.[4] Patients with compression fractures due to osteoporosis usually have no neurologic complaints and do not suffer from neural compression. Plain radiographs document a loss of vertebral body height due to compression fractures. Laboratory tests are normal in patients with primary osteoporosis; any abnormalities should prompt a search for secondary causes of osteoporosis. The diagnosis of primary osteoporosis is made on clinical grounds (i.e., diffuse osteopenia, compression fractures, and normal laboratory findings.[25,26]

NEOPLASIA

Multiple myeloma is the most common primary malignancy of the vertebral spine. Metastatic lesions are the most common cause of cancers of the spine, arising from breast, lung, prostate, thyroid, renal, or gastrointestinal tract primary tumors. Hodgkin's and non-Hodgkin's lymphomas frequently involve the vertebral spine. Because the primary site of the tumor is often overlooked, back pain is the presenting complaint for many cancers. In primary care settings, 0.7% of patients who present with low back pain have cancer as the cause.[9,27] Findings significantly associated with cancer as the cause of low back pain include age 50 years or older, history of cancer, pain lasting more than 1 month, failure to improve with conservative therapy, elevated erythrocyte sedimentation rate (ESR), and anemia.[27] Patients report a dull, constant pain that is worse at night and not relieved by rest or the recumbent position. Typical radiographic changes may be absent early in the course of vertebral body tumors. A technetium bone scan is usually positive owing to increased blood flow and reactive bone formation, although with multiple myeloma and metastatic thyroid cancer, the bone scan may be negative.[28] Symptomatic cancer of the lumbar spine is an ominous sign with a potential for devastating morbidity due to spinal cord injury.[29] Early recognition and treatment are essential if irreversible cord damage is to be avoided.

POSTERIOR FACET SYNDROME

The posterior facet syndrome is caused by degenerative changes in the posterior facets, which are true diarthrodial joints that sometimes develop degenerative joint changes visible on plain radiographs. Degenerative changes in the posterior facet joints cause a dull, achy pain that radiates to the groin, hip, or thigh and is worsened with twisting or hyperextension of the spine.[30] Steroid injection into the posterior facet joints to relieve presumed posterior facet joint pain is a popular procedure, but the placebo effect of injection in this area is significant and controlled studies have failed to demonstrate benefit from steroid injections.[31,32] The presence of degenerative changes in the facet joints on plain radiographs does not imply that the posterior facets are the cause of the patient's pain. Caution must be used when ascribing the patient's symptoms to these degenerative changes. Historically, the posterior facet syndrome was diagnosed by demonstrating pain relief after injecting local anesthetic into the posterior facet joints, but more recent studies cast doubt on the validity of this procedure.[6,30]

ANKYLOSING SPONDYLITIS

Ankylosing spondylitis is a spondyloarthropathy most commonly affecting young men. Patients present with mild to moderate low back pain centered in the back and radiating to the posterior thighs. At its initial presentation the symptoms are vague, and the diagnosis is often overlooked. Pain symptoms are intermittent, but decreased range of motion in the spine remains constant. Early signs of ankylosing spondylitis include limitation of chest expansion, tenderness of the sternum, and decreased range of motion and flexion contractures at the hip. The radiologic hallmarks of ankylosing spondylitis include periarticular destructive changes, obliteration of the sacroiliac joints, development of syndesmophytes on the margins of the vertebral bodies, and bridging of these osteophytes by bone between vertebral bodies, the so-called bamboo spine. Laboratory analysis is negative for rheumatoid factor, but the ESR is elevated early in the course of the disease. Tests for HLA-B27 antigen are not recommended because as many as 6% of an unselected population test positive for this antigen.[14]

VISCERAL DISEASES

Several visceral diseases may present with back pain as a chief symptom,[4] including nephrolithiasis, endometriosis, and abdominal aortic aneurysm. Abdominal aortic aneurysm causes low back pain by compression of surrounding tissues or by extension or rupture of the aneurysm. Patients report dull, steady back pain unrelated to activity that radiates to the hips or thighs. Patients with an acute rupture or extension of the aneurysm report severe tearing pain, diaphoresis, or syncope; and they demonstrate signs of circulatory shock.[25]

PSYCHOSOCIAL FACTORS

Psychological factors are frequently associated with complaints of low back pain, influencing both patient pain symptoms and therapeutic outcome.[33] Features that suggest psychological causes of low back pain include nonorganic signs and symptoms, dissociation between verbal and nonverbal pain behaviors, compensable cause of injury, joblessness, disability-seeking, depression, anxiety, requests for narcotics or other psychoactive drugs, or repeated failure of multiple treatments.[34]

Management

Most patients with low back pain should initially be treated conservatively.[3,4] A 4- to 6-week trial of conservative therapy is appropriate in the absence of cauda equina syndrome or a rapidly progressive neurologic deficit (Table 17.2).

BED REST

One of the mainstays of treatment for acute low back pain is a brief course of bed rest. Two days of bed rest are as effective and may be superior to 7 days of bed rest.[35] Prolonged immobilization leads to muscle weakness, cardiovascular deconditioning, and bone mineral loss. For initial management, physicians should recommend a 2- to 3-day course of bed rest on a firm mattress or padded floor.[34] Sitting in bed should be avoided because the sitting position increases intradiscal pressures.[4] Patients with neuromotor deficits may require longer and stricter periods of bed rest.

MEDICATIONS

Nonsteroidal anti-inflammatory drugs (NSAIDs) are effective in the treatment of low back pain. Therapy is titrated to provide pain relief at a minimal dose and is continued for 4 to 6 weeks. NSAIDs should not be continued indefinitely but, rather, prescribed for a specific period.[3]

Narcotics. Mild narcotic analgesics are useful, especially for acute disc herniations with sciatica. They should be used for brief periods and prescribed in a strictly time-limited fashion (i.e., narcotics should not be prescribed on the basis of persistent symptoms), usually for less than 2 weeks.

Muscle Relaxants. Although evidence for the effectiveness of muscle relaxants is scant, the main value of muscle relaxants is less for muscle

TABLE 17.2. Nonoperative treatment considerations for low back pain and sciatica

Treatment	Acute low back pain	Acute sciatica	Subacute low back pain and leg pain	Chronic low back pain and leg pain
Bed rest	2–7 days	2–7 days	Avoid	Avoid, short-term for flare-ups only
NSAIDs	Minimum 5–10 days; optimal 2–6 weeks	Minimum 5–10 days; optimal 2–6 weeks	Selected cases if effective	Avoid long-term
Muscle relaxants	Optimal 1 week; maximum 2–4 weeks	Optimal 1 week; maximum 2–4 weeks	Selected cases if effective	Avoid long-term
Opioids	Optimal 1–3 days; maximum 2–3 weeks	Optimal 1–3 days; maximum 2–3 weeks	Selected presurgical cases; avoid	Avoid
Antidepressants	No	No	Selected cases	Yes
Local injections	Short-term benefit if effective	No	Selected cases as an adjunct	Flare-ups
Facet injections	Avoid	No	Selected cases but no long-term benefit alone	Avoid; no long-term effect alone
Epidural corticosteroids	No	Yes	Flare-ups, if effective	Flare-ups only; avoid
Orthoses	Adjunctive	No	Adjunctive	Adjunctive
Cryotherapy (ice)	Adjunctive	Adjunctive	Flare-ups	Flare-ups; self-applied
Thermotherapy	Adjunctive	Adjunctive	Adjunctive	Flare-ups; self-applied
Traction	Yes, if effective	Yes, if effective	Self-applied; if effective	Self-applied; if effective
Joint manipulation	Yes, if effective	Not with neural signs	If effective; maximum 2–4 months	Flare-ups; time-contingent if effective
Joint mobilization	Yes, if effective	Yes, if effective	If effective; maximum 2–4 months	Flare-ups; time-contingent if effective
Soft tissue techniques (massage, myofascial release, mobilization)	Yes, if effective	Yes, if effective	If effective; maximum 2–4 months	Flare-ups; time-contingent if effective
McKenzie exercises	Yes, if effective	Yes, if effective	Flare-ups, if effective	Flare-ups, if effective
Dynamic lumbar stabilization	Yes	Yes	Yes	Yes
Back school	Yes	Yes	Yes	Yes
Functional restoration	No	No	Yes	Optimal 3–4 months; maximum 4–6 months
Pain clinic	No	No	No	Yes

Source: Adapted from Wheeler.[34,70] With permission.

relaxation than for their sedative effect. Diazepam (Valium), cyclobenzaprine (Flexeril), and methocarbamol (Robaxin) are commonly used as muscle relaxants; and carisoprodol (Soma) has documented effectiveness.[3] Muscle relaxants are prescribed in a time-limited fashion, usually for less than 2 weeks. Muscle relaxants and narcotics are not recommended for patients who present with complaints of chronic low back pain (i.e., low back pain of more than 3 months' duration).[4]

UNPROVED TREATMENTS

The use of traction, corsets, or braces is not recommended for treatment of acute low back pain.[4] No scientific evidence supports the efficacy of these treatments. Transcutaneous electrical nerve stimulation (TENS) has been shown to be ineffective for treating low back pain.[36]

EXERCISE

Exercise is commonly used to treat acute low back pain. Even in the setting of acute herniation, patients should avoid prolonged inactivity and the debilitation that results from prolonged bed rest.[4] After a short 2- to 3-day course of bed rest, patients should begin standing and walking by the third day of treatment. Within the first week of therapy, patients should walk 20 minutes for every 3 hours in the supine position. A moderate exercise program increases activity levels and decreases both pain scores and pain frequency.[37]

Flexion Exercises. Flexion exercises strengthen the abdominal muscles that protect the lumbar disc from excessive loads and are useful in the subacute setting once acute symptoms have resolved. These exercises must be performed in the proper position to avoid further injury to the lumbar spine. The patient, supine on a firm surface with knees flexed, begins with knee-to-chest exercises to stretch the hamstrings, followed by head and shoulder raises (not "sit-ups") to strengthen the abdominis rectus, elbow-to-opposite-knee rotational raises to strengthen the abdominis oblique, and pelvic tilt or thrust to strengthen the lower abdominal musculature. Flexion exercises are contraindicated in the setting of acute disc herniation, immediately after a prolonged period of rest (the disc is hyperhydrated and prone to injury), in cases of postural low back pain (where flexion should be relieved), and in cases of a lateral trunk shift or lift.[3,37,38]

Extension Exercises. Back extension exercises are useful and often reduce the pain and paresthesias due to acute disc herniation. McKenzie described a set of hyperextension exercises for the spine as a means of treating chronic back pain,[39] and another study documented the safety and efficacy of these maneuvers.[40] Extension-to-neutral exercises, with the patient in the prone position, strengthen the paravertebral muscles that support the spine and promote endurance and full function.[41] Proper extension exercises are best performed under the supervision of a qualified physical therapist.

Aerobic Fitness. Aerobic fitness training is an effective means of preventing low back injury and rehabilitating patients in whom low back pain has developed.[42] For example, in patients with acute low back pain, bed rest for 2 to 3 days can be prescribed. After a pain-free interval of 2 weeks, the patient begins aerobic training, gradually increasing the duration, frequency, and intensity. A typical prescription includes 30 to 40 minutes of aerobic exercise three to five times a week, including warm-up and cool-down. Exercises should be aerobic in nature, involving large muscle groups. Adequate footgear and exercise on a level surface are necessary to avoid further injury to the lumbar spine. Typical exercises include walking, jogging, or aerobics; swimming is a useful alternative when weight-bearing exercise is painful.[34] Cycling is not recommended because the sitting position increases the biomechanical workload on the lumbar spine. Jumping rope should be avoided because it places a high compression load on the spine and requires a high level of intensity before aerobic benefit is achieved.[41]

BACK SCHOOL

Patients should be taught about common causes of low back pain and have a basic understanding of proper sitting, standing, and lifting techniques. Patients receiving such education return to work earlier than controls and have fewer low back injuries in the workplace.[43,44] Some investigators have found that "back school" is less effective than McKenzie extension exercises and fails to improve outcome at 1 year.[45,46] However, even in cases of low back pain that has persisted for 6 months or more, enrollment in a "back school" leads to improved function and fewer pain symptoms.[47] A structured educational program promoting effective "back hygiene" is probably of benefit to most patients with low back pain.[8]

SURGERY

The rate of lumbar surgery in the United States is 40% higher than in most developed nations and five times higher than in England and Scotland.[48] The lifetime prevalence of lumbar spine surgery ranges between 1% and 3%, and 2% to 3% of patients with low back pain may be surgical candidates on the basis of sciatica alone.[5] Surgery rates vary widely by geographic region in the United States and have risen dramatically since the mid-1980s.[49] Psychological factors influence postsurgical outcomes more strongly than initial physical examination or surgical findings. Prior to surgery, patients should be evaluated with standard pain indices, activities of daily living scales, and psychometric testing. Surgical results for treating symptomatic lumbar disc herniation unresponsive to conservative therapy are excellent in well-selected patients.[50]

Indications. The major benefit and primary indication for surgery is relief of sciatica. In well-selected patients, 75% have complete relief of sciatic symptoms after surgery, and an additional 15% have partial relief. Patients with clear symptoms of radicular pain have the best surgical outcome, whereas those with the least evidence of radiculopathy have the poorest surgical outcome.[51] Relief of back pain itself is less consistent. Surgery is indicated in cases of cauda equina syndrome, progressive neurologic deficit, or disc herniation documented by neuroradiologic imaging, with symptoms of pain and weakness in a nerve root distribution, unresponsive to a 4- to 6-week trial of conservative therapy. Surgical treatment is a consideration in cases of spinal stenosis, degenerative changes, or spinal instability. Appropriate patient selection is key to successful surgical outcome.

Options. *Standard discectomy* is the most common procedure used to relieve symptomatic disc herniation. A posterior longitudinal incision is made over the involved disc space, a variable amount of bone is removed, the ligmentatum flavum is incised, and herniated disc material is excised. This procedure allows adequate visualization and yields satisfactory results among 65% to 85% of patients.[11,52,53] Standard discectomy provides improved pain relief and functional ability at 1-year follow-up, but these advantages over conservative therapy are reduced at 4 years and absent at the 10-year follow-up.

Microdiscectomy allows smaller incisions, little or no bony excision, and removal of disc material under magnification. This procedure has fewer complications, fewer unsuccessful outcomes, and permits faster recovery. However, rates of reoperation are significantly higher in patients initially treated with microdiscectomy, presumably due to missed disc fragments or operating at the wrong spinal level.[53]

Percutaneous discectomy is an outpatient procedure performed under local anesthesia in which the surgeon uses an automated percutaneous cutting and suction probe to aspirate herniated disc material. The procedure results in lower rates of nerve injury, postoperative instability, infection, fibrosis, and chronic pain syndromes. However, patients undergoing percutaneous discectomy sustain unacceptably high rates of recurrent disc herniation. This procedure is not recommended for patients with previous back surgery, sequestered disc fragments, bony entrapment, or multiple herniated discs.[53,54]

Chemonucleolysis is a procedure in which a proteolytic enzyme (chymopapain) is injected into the disc space to dissolve herniated disc material. In a randomized trial comparing chemonucleolysis with chymopapain to standard discectomy, 63% of chymopapain-treated subjects had satisfactory outcomes. However, the rate of reoperation was significantly higher for the chymopapain-treated group (25% versus 3%). Although chemonucleolysis produces initial results comparable to those with standard discectomy, requires shorter hospital stays, and incurs lower costs, it has fallen into disfavor owing to anaphylactic reactions and neurologic complications.[6,55]

Complications. Complications of surgery on the lumbar spine are largely related to patient age, gender, diagnosis, and type of procedure.[56] Mortality rates increase substantially with age, but are less than 1% even among patients over 75 years of age. Mortality rates are higher for men, but morbidity rates and the likelihood of discharge to a nursing home are significantly higher for women, particularly those over 75. With regard to underlying diagnosis, complications and duration of hospitalization are highest after surgery to correct spinal stenosis, degenerative changes, or instability and are lowest for procedures to correct a herniated disc. With regard to type of procedure, complications and duration of hospitalization are highest for procedures involving arthrodesis with or without laminectomy, followed by laminectomy alone or with discectomy; they are lowest for discectomy alone. Other surgical complications include thromboembolism (1.7%) and infection (2.9%).[4]

SUMMARY

The physician's goal of treating patients with low back pain is to promote activity and an early return to work. Although it is important to rule out significant pathology as the cause of low back pain, most patients can be reassured that symptoms are due to simple muscular strain. Patients should be counseled that they will improve with time, usually quickly. Patients may require a brief period of bed rest during the acute phase, usually no more than 2 to 3 days, as well as adequate pain relief. Physicians should encourage early mobilization, usually within a few days and certainly within 2 weeks. Patients are encouraged to return to work, usually within 1 to 2 weeks and almost always by 6 weeks.[14] Work activities may be modified at first, but avoiding iatrogenic disability is key to successful management of acute low back pain.[4,34]

Chronic Low Back Pain

Chronic low back pain (i.e., pain persisting for more than 3 months) is a special problem that deserves careful consideration. Patients presenting with a history of chronic low back pain require an extensive diagnostic workup on at least one occasion, including an in-depth history, physical examination, and the appropriate imaging techniques (plain radiographs, CT scan, myelogram, or MRI). Therapy is directed at strengthening the musculature supporting the spine, including aerobic fitness and flexion and extension exercises, as well as an educational program on proper sitting, standing, and working techniques[6] (Table 17.2). Functional restoration programs combine intense physical therapy with cognitive-behavioral interventions and increasing levels of task-oriented rehabilitation and work simulation.[34,57] Antidepressants have been used to treat chronic low back pain, but a literature review has cast doubt on the effectiveness of this therapy.[58] Decompressive laminectomy is reserved for patients with persistent spinal claudication, significant nerve root or spinal cord compression, or progressive loss of bowel or bladder control.

Prevention

Prevention of low back injury and consequent disability is an important challenge in primary care. Preemployment physical examination screening is not effective in reducing the occurrence of job-related low back pain. Worker strength assessment and job or workplace modification are effective ways to decrease the occurrence of job-related low back pain.[6,17,42] Active, aerobically fit individuals have fewer back injuries, miss fewer workdays, and report fewer back pain symptoms.[59] Worksite exercise interventions produce significant decreases in reported low back pain. Similarly, education about basic lumbar biomechanics, back care, and proper standing, sitting, and lifting techniques result in fewer workdays missed and fewer episodes of lower back pain. Evidence to support smoking cessation and weight loss as means of reducing the occurrence of low back pain is sparse but these behavior modifications should be recommended for other health reasons.[59]

Disorders of the Neck

Cervical Radiculopathy

Cervical radiculopathy is a common cause of neck pain and can be caused by a herniated cervical disc, osteophytic changes, compressive pathology, or hypermobility of the cervical spine. The lifetime prevalence of neck and arm pain among adults may be as high as 51%. Risk factors associated with neck pain include heavy lifting, smoking, diving, working with vibrating heavy equipment, and possibly riding in cars.[60]

Cervical nerve roots exit the spine above the corresponding vertebral body (e.g., the C5 nerve root exits above C5). Therefore, disc herniation at the C4–5 interspace causes symptoms in the distribution of C5.[61] Radicular symptoms may be caused by a "soft disc" (i.e., disc herniation) or a "hard disc" (i.e., osteophyte formation and foraminal encroachment).[61] The most commonly involved interspaces are C5–6, C6–7, C4–5, C3–4, and C7–T1.[60]

The symptoms of cervical radiculopathy may be single or multiple, unilateral or bilateral, symmetric or asymmetric.[62] Acute cervical radiculopathy is commonly due to a tear of the annulus fibrosus with prolapse of the nucleus pulposus, and it is usually the result of mild to moderate trauma. Subacute symptoms are usually due to long-standing spondylosis accompanied by mild trauma or overuse. Most patients with subacute cervical radiculopathy experience resolution of their symptoms within 6 weeks with rest and analgesics. Chronic radiculopathy is more common in middle age or old age, and patients present with complaints of neck or arm pain due to heavy labor or unaccustomed activity.[62–64]

Cervical radiculopathy rarely progresses to myelopathy, but as many as two-thirds of patients treated conservatively report persistent symptoms. In severe cases of cervical radiculopathy in which motor function has been compromised, 98% of patients recover full motor function after decompressive laminectomy.[65]

CLINICAL PRESENTATION

Among patients with cervical radiculopathy, sensory symptoms are much more prominent than motor changes. Typically, patients report proximal pain and distal paresthesias.[61] The fifth, sixth, and seventh nerve roots are most commonly affected. Referred pain caused by cervical disc herniation is usually vague, diffuse, and lacking in the sharp quality of radicular pain. Pain referred from a herniated cervical disc may present as pain in the neck, at the top of the shoulder, or around the scapula.[62]

On physical examination, radicular pain increases with certain maneuvers such as neck range of motion, Valsalva maneuver, cough, or sneeze. Active and passive neck range of motion is tested, examining flexion, rotation, and lateral bending. Spurling's maneuver is useful for assessing neck pain: The examining physician flexes the patient's neck, then rolls the neck into lateral bending, and finally extends the neck. This maneuver narrows the cervical foramina posterolaterally and may reproduce the patient's radicular symptoms.

DIAGNOSIS

The differential diagnosis of cervical nerve root pain includes cervical disc herniation, spinal canal tumor, trauma, degenerative changes, inflammatory disorders, congenital abnormalities, toxic and allergic conditions, hemorrhage, and musculoskeletal syndromes (e.g., thoracic outlet syndrome, shoulder pain).[61,65] In cases of cervical radiculopathy unresponsive to conservative therapy or in the presence of progressive motor deficit, investigation for other pathologic processes is indicated. Plain radiographs are usually not helpful because abnormal radiographic findings are equally common among symptomatic and asymptomatic patients. CT scans, myelography, and MRI each has a role to play in the diagnosis of cervical radiculopathy.[63,64]

MANAGEMENT

Immobilization. The purpose of neck immobilization is to reduce any intervertebral motion that may cause compression, mechanical irritation, or stretching of the cervical nerve roots.[66] The soft cervical collar or the more rigid Philadelphia collar both hold the neck in slight flexion. The collar is useful in the acute setting, but prolonged use leads to deconditioning of the paracervical musculature. Therefore the collar is prescribed in a time-limited manner, and patients are instructed to begin isometric neck exercises early in the course of therapy.

Bed Rest. Bed rest is another form of immobilization that modifies the patient's activities and eliminates the axial compression forces of gravity.[66] Holding the neck in slight flexion is accomplished by arranging two standard pillows in a V, with the apex pointed cranially, and then placing a third pillow across the apex. This arrangement provides mild cervical flexion and internally rotates the shoulder girdle, thereby relieving traction on the cervical nerve roots.

Medications. NSAIDs are particularly beneficial in relieving acute neck pain. However, side effects are common, and usually two or three medications must be tried before a beneficial result without unacceptable side effects is achieved. Muscle relaxants help relieve muscle spasm in some patients; alternatives include carisoprodol, methocarbamol, and diazepam (Valium). Narcotics may be useful in the acute setting but should be prescribed in a strictly time-limited manner.[66] The physician should be alert to the possibility of addiction or abuse.

Physical Therapy. Moist heat (20 minutes three times daily), ice packs (15 minutes four times daily or even hourly), ultrasound therapy, and other modalities also help relieve the symptoms of cervical radiculopathy.[66]

Surgery. Surgical intervention is reserved for patients with cervical disc herniation confirmed by neuroradiologic imaging and radicular signs and symptoms that persist despite 4 to 6 weeks of conservative therapy.[61]

Cervical Myelopathy

The cause of pain in cervical myelopathy is not clearly understood but is presumed to be multifactorial, including vascular changes, cord hypoxia, changes in spinal canal diameter, and hypertrophic facets. Therefore patients with cervical myelopathy present with a variable clinical picture. The usual course is one of increasing disability over several months, usually beginning with dysesthesias in the hands, followed by weakness or clumsiness in the hands, and eventually progressing to weakness in the lower extremities.[62]

CLINICAL PRESENTATION

In cases of cervical myelopathy secondary to cervical spondylosis, symptoms are usually insidious in onset, often with short periods of worsening followed by long periods of relative stability. Acute onset of symptoms or rapid deterioration suggests a vascular etiology.[61] Unlike cervical radiculopathy, cervical myelopathy rarely presents with neck pain; instead, patients report an occipital headache that radiates anteriorly to the frontal area, is worse on waking, but improves through the day.[62] Patients also report deep, aching pain and burning sensations in the hands, loss of hand dexterity, and vertebrobasilar insufficiency, presumably due to osteophytic changes in the cervical spine.[61,62]

On physical examination, patients demonstrate motor weakness and muscle wasting, particularly of the interosseous muscles of the hand. Lhermitte's sign is present in approximately 25% of patients (i.e., rapid flexion or extension of the neck causes a shock-like sensation in the trunk or limbs). Deep tendon reflexes are variable. Involvement of the anterior horn cell causes hyporeflexia, whereas involvement of the corticospinal tracts causes hyperreflexia. The triceps jerk is the reflex most commonly lost owing to frequent involvement of the sixth nerve root (i.e., the C5–6 interspace). Almost all patients with cervical myelopathy show signs of muscular spasticity.[64]

DIAGNOSIS

Intrathecal contrast-enhanced CT scan is a highly specific test that allows evaluation of the intradural contents and the disc margins; it also helps differentiate an extradural defect due to disc herniation from that due to osteophytic changes.[63] MRI allows visualization of the cervical spine in both the sagittal and axial planes. Resolution with MRI is sharp enough to identify lesions of the spinal cord and differentiate disc herniation from spinal stenosis.[63] CT scanning is preferred for evaluating osteophytes, foraminal encroachment, and other bony changes. CT and MRI complement one another, and their use is individualized for each patient.[64] Clinical correlation of abnormal neuroradiologic findings is essential because degenerative changes of the cervical spine and cervical disc are common even among asymptomatic patients.[63,64]

MANAGEMENT

Conservative Therapy. Most patients with cervical myelopathy present with minor symptoms and demonstrate long periods of nonprogressive disability. Therefore these patients are initially treated conservatively: rest with a soft cervical collar, physical therapy to promote range of motion, and judicious use of NSAIDs.[67] Only 30% to 50% of patients improve with conservative management.

Surgery. Early surgical decompression is appropriate for patients with cervical myelopathy who present with moderate or severe disability, or in the presence of rapid neurologic deterioration.[67] Anterior decompression with fusion, posterior decompression, laminectomy, or laminoplasty are each appropriate to particular clinical situations.[68] The best surgical prognosis is achieved by careful patient selection. Obviously, accurate diagnosis is essential, and patients with symptoms of relatively short duration have the best prognosis.[61] If surgery is considered, it should be performed early in the course of the disease, before cord damage becomes irreversible.

Cervical Whiplash

Cervical whiplash is a valid clinical syndrome with symptoms consistent with the anatomic site(s) of injury and a potential for significant impairment.[69] Symptoms of cervical whiplash injuries are due to soft tissue trauma, particularly musculoligamentous sprains and strains to the cervical spine. After a rear-end impact in a motor vehicle accident, the patient is accelerated forward and the neck is thrown into hyperextension, which centers on the C5–6 interspace, followed by flexion of the neck, which is limited by the chin striking the chest. Hyperextension commonly causes an injury to the anterior longitudinal ligament of the cervical spine and other soft tissue injuries of the anterior neck, including muscle tears, muscle hemorrhage, esophageal hemorrhage, or disc disruption. Muscles most commonly injured include the sternocleidomastoid, scalenus, and longus colli muscles. Patients may also develop visual disturbances, possibly due to vertebral, basilar, or other vascular injury or injury to the cervical sympathetic chain.

CLINICAL PRESENTATION

Patients describe a typical rear-end impact motor vehicle accident with hyperextension of the neck followed by hyperflexion. Pain in the neck may be immediate or may be delayed hours or even days after the accident. Pain is usually felt at the base of the neck and increases over time. Patients report pain and decreased range of motion in the neck that is worsened by motion or activity, as well as paresthesias or weakness in the upper extremities, dysphagia, or hoarseness.

Physical examination may be negative if the patient is seen within hours of the accident. Over time, however, patients develop tenderness in the cervical spine area, decreased range of motion, and muscle spasm. Neurologic examination of the upper extremity should include assessment of motor function and grip strength, sensation, deep tendon reflexes, and range of motion (especially of the neck and shoulder).

DIAGNOSIS

Findings on plain radiographs are usually minimal. Five views of the cervical spine are obtained: anteroposterior, lateral, right and left obliques, and odontoid. Straightening of the cervical spine or loss of the normal cervical lordosis may be due to positioning in radiology, muscle spasm, or derangement of the skeletal alignment of the cervical spine. Films are also examined for soft tissue swelling anterior to the C3 vertebral body, osteophytic changes, disc space narrowing, or narrowing of the cervical foramens. Electromyography and nerve conduction velocity tests are considered if paresthesia or radicular pain is present. MRI is indicated in patients unresponsive to conservative therapy or in the presence of a progressive neurologic deficit. Technetium bone scan is sensitive for detecting occult injuries. However, whiplash injuries usually cause soft tissue injuries that are not demonstrable with most of these studies.

MANAGEMENT

Rest. Initially, patients are treated with rest and protection of the cervical spine, usually with a soft cervical collar. The collar holds the neck in slight flexion, so the widest part of the cervical collar is worn posteriorly. The cervical collar is especially useful for alleviating pain if worn at night or when driving. If used during the day, it is worn 1 to 2 hours and then removed for a similar period in order to preserve paracervical muscle conditioning. The cervical collar is prescribed for a specific duration, usually a few weeks, and then discontinued.

Medications. NSAIDs are effective treatment for the pain and muscle spasm caused by whiplash injuries. Muscle relaxants are a useful adjunct, especially when used nightly, and are prescribed in a time-limited manner. Narcotics are usually not indicated for treatment of whiplash injuries.

Physical Therapy. Physical modalities alleviate symptoms of pain and muscle spasm. Early in the course of whiplash injuries, heat modalities for 20 to 25 minutes every 3 to 4 hours are useful, although excessive use of heat can delay recovery. Later in the course of whiplash injury, usually 2 to 3 days after injury, cold therapy is indicated to decrease muscle spasm and pain. Range of motion exercises followed by isometric strengthening exercises are initiated early in the therapy of whiplash injuries, even immediately after injury. Patients are given specific instructions regarding neck exercises and daily activities. Patient education programs regarding exercises, daily activities, body mechanics, and the use of heat and cold modalities are also helpful.

Prognosis. Most patients with whiplash injuries have negative diagnostic studies but improve, although slowly and irregularly. Patients benefit from a program of rest, immobilization, neck exercises, and return to function. A few patients do more poorly, and many factors contribute to a poor prognosis, including chronic symptoms for 12 months or more, loss of employment, persistent neurologic symptoms (e.g., pain radiation, paresthesias, altered reflexes, and muscle weakness or atrophy), osteophytic changes on plain radiographs, and neuroradiologic findings on CT or MRI.

References

1. Spitzer WO, LeBlanc FE, Dupuis M, et al. Scientific approach to the assessment and management of activity related spinal disorders: a monograph for clinicians: report of the Quebec Task Force on Spinal Disorders. Spine 1987;12 Suppl 1:S1–59.
2. Loeser JD, Volinn E. Epidemiology of low back pain. Neurosurg Clin North Am 1991;2:713.
3. Deyo RA. Conservative therapy for low back pain. JAMA 1983;250:1057–62.
4. Deyo RA, Loeser JD, Bigos SJ. Herniated lumbar inter-vertebral disc. Ann Intern Med 1990;112:598–603.
5. Frymoyer JW, Cats-Baril WL. An overview of the incidences and costs of low back pain. Orthop Clin North Am 1991; 22:263–71.
6. Frymoyer JW. Back pain and sciatica. N Engl J Med 1988; 318:291–300.
7. Frymoyer JW, Pope MH, Clements JH, et al. Risk factors in low back pain: an epidemiological survey. J Bone Joint Surg Am 1983;65:213–18.
8. Deyo RA, Tsui-Wu YJ. Descriptive epidemiology of low back pain and its related medical care in the United States. Spine 1987;12:264–8.
9. Deyo RA, Rainville J, Kent DL. What can the history and physical examination tell us about low back pain? JAMA 1992;268:760–5.
10. Hazard RG, Fenwick JW, et al. Functional restoration with behavioral support: a one-year prospective study of patients with chronic low back pain. Spine 1989;14:157–69.

11. Weber H. Lumbar disc herniation: a controlled prospective study with ten years of observation. Spine 1983;8:131–40.
12. National Center for Health Statistics. Prevalence of selected impairments. U.S., 1977. Series 10, No. 132. Hyattsville, MD: DHHS, 1981. Publ. (PHS) 81-1562.
13. Frymoyer JW, Nachemson A. Natural history of low back disorders. In: Frymoyer JW, editor. The adult spine: principles and practice. New York: Raven, 1991:1537–50.
14. Wipf JE, Deyo RA. Low back pain. Med Clin North Am 1995;79:231–46.
15. Mixter WJ, Barr JS. Rupture of inter-vertebral disc with involvement of the spinal canal. N Engl J Med 1934;211:210–15.
16. Nachemson A. Newest knowledge of low back pain: a critical look. Clin Orthop 1992;279:8–20.
17. Deyo RA, Bass JE. Lifestyle and low back pain: the influence of smoking and obesity. Spine 1989;14:501–6.
18. Fairbank JCT, Hall H. History taking and physical examination: identification of syndromes of back pain. In: Weinstein JN, Wiesel SW, editors. The lumbar spine. Philadelphia: Saunders, 1990:88–106.
19. Modic MT, Ross JS. Magnetic resonance imaging in the evaluation of low back pain. Orthop Clin North Am 1991;22: 283–301.
20. Deyo RA, Diehl AK. Lumbar spine films in primary care: current use and effects of selective ordering criteria. J Gen Intern Med 1986;1:20–5.
21. Hensinger RN. Spondylolysis and spondylolisthesis in children and adolescents. J Bone Joint Surg Am 1989;71:1098–1107.
22. Frymoyer JW, Newberg A, Pope MH, et al. Spine radiographs in patients with low back pain: an epidemiological study in men. J Bone Joint Surg Am 1984;66:1048–55.
23. Jensen MC, Brant-Zawadzki MN, Obuchowski N, et al. Magnetic resonance imaging in people without back pain. N Engl J Med 1994; 331:69–73.
24. Modic MT, Masaryk T, Boumphrey F, et al. Lumbar herniated disc disease and canal stenosis: prospective evaluation by surface coil MR, CT, and myelography. AJR 1986;147:757–65.
25. McCowin PR, Borenstein D, Wiesel SW. The current approach to the medical diagnosis of low back pain. Orthop Clin North Am 1991;22:315–25.
26. Barth RW, Lane JM. Osteoporosis. Orthop Clin North Am 1988;19:845–58.
27. Deyo RA, Diehl AK. Cancer as a cause of back pain: frequency, clinical presentation, and diagnostic strategies. J Gen Intern Med 1988;3:230–8.
28. Bates DW, Reuler JB. Back pain and epidural spinal cord compression. J Gen Intern Med 1988;3:191–7.
29. Perrin RG. Symptomatic spinal metastases. Am Fam Physician 1989;39: 165–72.
30. Jackson RP. The facet syndrome: myth or reality? Spine 1992; 279:110–21.
31. Carette S, Marcoux S, Truchon R, et al. A controlled trial of corticosteroid injections into facet joints for chronic low back pain. N Engl J Med 1991;325:1002–7.
32. Lilius G, Laasonen EM, Myllynen P, et al. Lumbar facet joint syndrome: a randomized clinical trial. J Bone Joint Surg Br 1989;71:681–4.

33. Frymoyer JW, Rosen JC, Clements J, Pope MH. Psychologic factors in low back pain disability. Clin Orthop 1985;195: 178–84.
34. Wheeler AH. Diagnosis and management of low back pain and sciatica. Am Fam Physician 1995;52:1333–41.
35. Deyo RA, Diehl AK, Rosenthal M. How many days of bedrest for acute low back pain? A randomized clinical trial. N Engl J Med 1986;315:1064–70.
36. Deyo RA, Walsh NE, Martin DC, Schoenfeld LS, et al. A controlled trial of transcutaneous electrical nerve stimulation (TENS) and exercise for chronic low back pain. N Engl J Med 1990;322:1627–34.
37. Kendall PH, Jenkins JM. Exercises for backache: a double blind controlled trial. Physiotherapy 1968;54:154–9.
38. Williams PC. Lesions of lumbo-sacral spine. Part 2. J Bone Joint Surg 1937;19:690–703.
39. McKenzie RA. Prophylaxis in recurrent low back pain. N Z Med J 1979;89:22–3.
40. Elnaggar IM, Nordin M, Sheikhzadeh A, et al. Effects of spinal flexion and extension exercises on low back pain and spinal mobility in chronic mechanical low-back pain patients. Spine 1991;16: 967–72.
41. Jackson CP, Brown MD. Analysis of current approaches a practical guide to prescription of exercise. Clin Orthop 1983; 179:46–54.
42. Cady LD, Bischoff DP. Strength and fitness and subsequent back injuries in firefighters. J Occup Med 1979;21:269–73.
43. Berquist-Ullman M, Larsson U. Acute low back pain in industry: a controlled prospective study with special reference to therapy and confounding factors. Acta Orthop Scand Suppl 1977;170:1–117.
44. Hall H, Iceton JA. Back school: an overview with specific reference to the Canadian back education units. Clin Orthop 1983;179:10–17.
45. Stankovic R, Johnell O. Conservative treatment of acute low back pain. Spine 1990;15:120–3.
46. Cohen JE, Goel V, Frank JW, et al. Group education interventions for people with low back pain. Spine 1994;19: 1214–22.
47. Klaber-Moffett JA, Chase SM, Portek I, Ennis JR. A controlled prospective study to evaluate the effectiveness of a back school in the relief of chronic low back pain. Spine 1986;11:120–2.
48. Cherkin DC, Deyo RA, Loeser JD, et al. An international comparison of back surgery rates. Spine 1994; 19:1201–6.
49. Taylor VM, Deyo RA, Cherkin DC, Kreuter W. Low back pain hospitalization: recent U.S. trends and regional variations. Spine 1994;19:1207–13.
50. Hurme M, Alaranta H. Factors predicting the results of surgery for lumbar inter-vertebral disc herniation. Spine 1987; 12:933–8.
51. Abramovitz JN, Neff SR. Lumbar disc surgery: results of the prospective lumbar discectomy study. Neurosurgery 1991;29: 301–8.
52. Van Alphen HAM, Braakman R, Bezemer PD, et al. Chemonucleolysis vs. discectomy: a randomized multicenter trial. J Neurosurg 1989;70: 869–75.
53. Hoffman RM, Wheeler KJ, Deyo RA. Surgery for herniated lumbar discs: a literature synthesis. J Gen Intern Med 1993; 8:487–96.

54. Revel M, Payan C, Vallee C, et al. Automated percutaneous lumbar discectomy vs. chemonucleolysis in the treatment of sciatica. Spine 1993;18:1–7.
55. Nordby EJ, Wright PH. Efficacy of chymopapain in chemonucleolysis: a review. Spine 1994;19:2578–83.
56. Deyo RA, Cherkin DC, Loeser JD, et al. Morbidity and mortality in association with operations on the lumbar spine: the influence of age, diagnosis, and procedure. J Bone Joint Surg Am 1992;74:536–43.
57. Mayer TG, Gatchel RJ, Mayer H, et al. A prospective 2-year study on functional restoration in industrial low back injury: an objective assessment procedure. JAMA 1987;258:1763–7.
58. Turner JA, Denny MC. Do antidepressant medications relieve chronic low back pain? J Fam Pract 1993;37:545–53.
59. Lahad A, Malter AD, Berg AO, Deyo RA. The effectiveness of four interventions for the prevention of low back pain. JAMA 1994;272:1286–91.
60. Kelsey JL, Githens PB, Walter SD, et al. An epidemiological study of acute prolapsed cervical intervertebral disc. J Bone Joint Surg Am 1984;66:907–14.
61. Clark CR. Degenerative conditions of the spine. In: Frymoyer JW, editor. The adult spine: principles and practice. New York: Raven, 1991:1145–64.
62. Lestini WF, Wiesel SW. The pathogenesis of cervical spondylosis. Clin Orthop 1989;239:69–93.
63. Jahnke RW, Hart BL. Cervical stenosis, spondylosis, and herniated disc disease. Radiol Clin North Am 1991;29:777–91.
64. Russell EJ. Cervical disk disease. Radiology 1990;177:313–25.
65. Dillin W, Booth R, Cuckler J, et al. Cervical radiculopathy: a review. Spine 1986;11:988–91.
66. Murphy MJ, Lieponis JV. Non-operative treatment of cervical spine pain. In: Sherk HH, editor. The cervical spine. Philadelphia: Lippincott, 1989: 670–7.
67. La Rocca H. Cervical spondylotic myelopathy: natural history. Spine 1988; 13:854–5.
68. White AA III, Panjabi MM. Biomechanical considerations in the surgical management of cervical spondylotic myelopathy. Spine 1988;13:856–69.
69. Hirsch SA, Hirsch PJ, Hiramoto H, Weiss A. Whiplash syndrome: fact or fiction? Orthop Clin North Am 1988;19:791–5.
70. North American Spine Society's Ad Hoc Committee on Diagnostic and Therapeutic Procedures. Common diagnostic and therapeutic procedures of the lumbosacral spine. Spine 1991;16:1161–7.

Case Presentation

Subjective

Patient Profile

Andrew Harris is a 27-year-old white male married truck driver.

Presenting Problem

"Back strain."

Present Illness

Mr. Harris describes a 4-day history of low back pain that began when he lifted a heavy box while unloading his truck. The pain occasionally radiates to the right leg and foot. He has difficulty walking and is unable to work despite 3 days of rest.

Past Medical History

He has had several episodes of back strain over the past 5 years, but none as severe as the current illness.

Social History

Mr. Harris has been employed by a national freight line for 8 years. He lives with his wife and their two young children.

Habits

He uses no alcohol, tobacco, or recreational drugs. He drinks four cups of coffee daily.

Family History

His father had surgery for prostate enlargement 2 years ago and is now living and well at age 61. His mother died at age 60 of a stroke. There is one 32-year-old brother who has had lumbar disc surgery.

REVIEW OF SYSTEMS

Mr. Harris has an occasional tension headache and some pain in his shoulders and knees during cold damp weather.

- Discuss the possible reasons for Mr. Harris' visit today.
- What additional historical information might be useful? Why?
- What more would you like to know about the previous instances of back strain?
- What further information about the patient's job might be useful? Explain.

Objective

VITAL SIGNS

Height, 5 ft 10 in; weight, 232 lb; blood pressure, 140/84; pulse, 74.

EXAMINATION

The patient is ambulatory but moves carefully owing to low back pain. He has difficulty climbing onto the examination table. There is mild tenderness of the lumbosacral spine with adjacent right paraspinal muscle tenderness. Straight leg raising is positive on the right but not on the left. Deep tendon reflexes are +2 and symmetrical. There is decreased perception of pinprick on the lateral right lower leg and foot.

- What further information obtained from the physical examination might be helpful? Why?
- What is the relationship of the patient's weight to his ideal weight and height?
- What—if any—diagnostic maneuvers might help clarify the problem?
- What—if any—diagnostic imaging would you obtain today?

Assessment

- Describe your diagnosis. What is the likely anatomical cause?
- How will you explain your assessment to Mr. Harris?
- What might be the meaning of this illness to the patient? How would you ask about this concern?

- What is the potential economic impact of this illness on the family? How would you address this issue?

Plan

- What would be your therapeutic recommendation? How would you explain this to the patient?
- What would you advise regarding Mr. Harris's weight? How might you persuade him to lose weight?
- Is a subspecialist consultation appropriate at this time? If so, how would you explain this to the patient?
- What follow-up would you plan for Mr. Harris?

18

Osteoarthritis

Alicia D. Monroe and John B. Murphy

Osteoarthritis (OA) is the most common rheumatic disease affecting humans and the third most common principal diagnosis recorded by family practitioners for office visits made by older patients.[1,2] Population-based studies of OA demonstrate that the prevalence of radiographic OA is much higher than is symptomatic OA, and that there is a progressive increase in the prevalence of OA with advancing age.[2,3] The prevalence of OA and pattern of joint involvement varies with gender and ethnic and racial background. Knee OA is twice as prevalent in women (18.0%) as men (8.3%) ages 65 through 74.[4] Europeans have a higher prevalence of hip OA than do the Chinese and most black populations; U.S. Native Americans have higher rates of OA than U.S. Caucasians; African American women have higher rates of knee OA than Caucasians; and Caucasians have a higher prevalence of polyarticular OA of the hands compared to black Africans and Malaysians.[4,5]

Pathophysiology

Although OA is much more common with advancing age, the changes seen in osteoarthritic cartilage are clearly distinct from those seen with normal aging.[6] The pathologic and biochemical changes found in osteoarthritic cartilage appear to be mediated by complex remodeling interactions, the precise mechanism of which is not fully understood, but the net result includes increasing water content and disorganization of the cartilage matrix. As the disease advances, disorganization gives way to erosion and ulceration, and eventually cartilage is irreversibly destroyed. As the cartilage degenerates, joint stresses are increasingly transmitted to the underlying bone, initiating the bony remodeling process, which results in marginal osteophytes, subchondral sclerosis, and cysts.

Clinical Presentation and Diagnosis

Symptoms and Signs

Osteoarthritis, classified as primary (idiopathic) or secondary, represents a "final common pathway" for a number of conditions of diverse etiologies.[1,4] Primary OA is further classified as (1) localized (e.g., hands, feet, knees, or other single sites) or (2) generalized including three or more local areas. Secondary OA is classified as (1) posttraumatic; (2) congenital or developmental; (3) metabolic (e.g., hemochromatosis, crystal deposition diseases); (4) endocrine (e.g., hyperparathyroidism, acromegaly); (5) other bone and joint diseases (infection, avascular necrosis); (6) neuropathic (e.g., tabes dorsalis, syringomyelia); (7) miscellaneous (e.g., frostbite). Commonly affected joints include the interphalangeal, knee, hip, acromioclavicular, subtalar, first metatarsophalangeal, sacroiliac, temporomandibular, and carpometacarpal joint of the thumb. Joints usually spared include the metacarpophalangeal, wrist, elbow, and shoulder.

Early during the symptomatic phase of OA, pain is often described as a deep, aching discomfort. It occurs with motion, particularly with weight-bearing, and is relieved by rest. As the disease progresses, pain can occur with minimal motion and at rest. OA pain is typically localized to the joint, although pain associated with OA of the hip is often localized to the anterior inguinal region and the medial or lateral thigh regions, but it may also radiate to the buttock, anterior thigh, or knee. OA pain of the spine may be associated with radicular symptoms including pain, paresthesias, and muscle weakness. Although joint stiffness can occur, it is usually of short duration (< 30 minutes).

Physical examination of an affected joint may show decreased range of motion, joint deformity, bony hypertrophy, and occasionally an intraarticular effusion. Crepitance and pain on passive and active movement and mild tenderness may be found. Inflammatory changes including warmth and redness are usually absent. During late stages there may be demonstrable joint instability. Physical findings associated with hand OA include Heberden's nodes of the distal interphalangeal joints, representing cartilaginous and bony enlargement of the dorsolateral and dorsomedial aspects. Bouchard's nodes are similar findings at the proximal interphalangeal joints.

Quadriceps muscle atrophy, marginal bony overgrowth, joint crepitance, effusion, and mediolateral joint instability are possible physical findings with OA of the knee. Limitation of joint motion, initially with extension, and varus angulation can also develop as a result of degenerative cartilage in the medial compartment of the knee. The patient with OA of the hip often holds the hip adducted, flexed, and internally rotated, which may result in functional shortening of the leg and the characteristic limp (antalgic gait).

Radiographic Features and Laboratory Findings

During early stages of OA radiographs may be normal. Joint space narrowing becomes evident as articular cartilage is lost. Subchondral bony sclerosis (eburnation) appears radiographically as increased bone density. Subchondral bone cysts develop and vary in size from several millimeters to several centimeters. These appear as translucent areas in periarticular bone. Bony deformity, joint subluxation, and loose bodies may be seen in advanced cases. Marginal osteophyte formation is seen as a result of bone proliferation. The newer imaging modalities—computed tomography, magnetic resonance imaging, ultrasonography—provide potentially powerful tools for the assessment of OA, although the diagnosis of OA rarely requires such expensive modalities.

There are no specific laboratory tests for OA. Unlike with the inflammatory arthritides (e.g., rheumatoid arthritis) the erythrocyte sedimentation rate (ESR) and hemogram are normal and autoantibodies are not present. If there is joint effusion, the synovial fluid is noninflammatory, with fewer than 2000 white blood cells (WBCs), a predominance of mononuclear WBCs, and a good mucin clot. The diagnosis of OA is usually based on clinical and radiologic features with the laboratory assessment being useful for excluding other arthritic conditions or secondary causes of OA.

Management

The management of OA focuses on pain relief, the prevention of progressive joint damage, and maximization of functional ability. Maximizing nonpharmacologic measures and employing adjunctive drug therapy and surgical interventions are important for the comprehensive management of patients with OA.

Nonpharmacologic management strategies for OA include periods of rest (1–2 hours) when symptoms are at their worst, avoidance of repetitive movements or static body positions that aggravate symptoms, heat (or cold) for the control of pain, weight loss if the patient is obese, adaptive mobility aids to diminish the mechanical load on joints, adaptive equipment to assist in activities of daily living (ADL) skills, range of motion exercises, strengthening exercises, and endurance exercises.[7,8] Immobilization should be avoided because of the deleterious effects on muscle strength, exercise capacity, and joint range of motion with the associated risk of contracture development. The use of adaptive mobility aids (e.g., canes, walkers) is an important strategy, but care must be taken to ensure that the mobility aid is the correct device, properly used, appropriately sized, and in good repair. Medial knee taping to realign the patella in patients with patellofemoral OA and the use of 5- to 10-degree wedged insoles for patients with medial compartment OA may help reduce joint symptoms.[9]

Pharmacologic approaches to the treatment of OA include acetaminophen, salicylates, nonsteroidal antiinflammatory drugs (NSAIDs), and intraarticular steroids (Table 18.1). Acetaminophen is advocated for use as a first line therapy by some authors based on clinical experience, short-term intervention studies, and the gastric toxicity associated with NSAIDs including gastric and duodenal ulceration and perforation.[10,11] Salicylates and NSAIDs are, however, still the most commonly used first line medications for the relief of pain related to OA. Compliance with salicylates can be a major problem given their short duration of action and the need for frequent dosing; thus NSAIDs are commonly used preferentially over salicylates. There is no justification for choosing one NSAID over another based on efficacy, but it is clear that a patient who does not respond to an NSAID from one class may well respond to an NSAID from another. Intraarticular steroids are generally reserved for the occasional instance when there is a single painful joint or a large effusion in a single joint, and the pain is unresponsive to

TABLE 18.1. Pharmacologic Treatment of Osteoarthritis

Drug	Dosage range/frequency	Relative cost for 30 days[a]
Acetaminophen	650–1000 mg qid	$
Aspirin, enteric coated	1000 mg qid	$
Extended release aspirin	1600 mg bid	$
Magnesium salicylate (Magan)	1090 mg tid to qid	$$$$
Choline salicylated (Arthropan)	4.8–7.2 g/day	$$$
Salicylsalicylic acid (Salsalate)	3–4 g/day in 2 or 3 doses	$$
Diclofenac (Voltaren)	150–200 mg/day in 2 or 3 doses	$$$$
Diflunisal (Dolobid)	500–1000 mg/day in 2 doses	$$
Fenoprofen (Nalfon)	300–600 mg tid–qid	$$
Flurbiprofen (Ansaid)	200–300 mg/day in 2, 3, or 4 doses	$$
Ibuprofen	1200–3200 mg/day in 3 or 4 doses	$
Indomethacin	25–50 mg tid–qid	$
Ketoprofen (Orudis)	50–75 mg tid–qid	$$$$
Meclofenamate sodium	50–100 mg qid	$$$ to $$$$
Nabumetone (Relafen)	1000 mg once/day to 2000 mg/day	$$$$
Naproxen (Naprosyn)	250–500 mg bid–tid	$$$
Naproxen sodium (Anaprox)	275–550 mg bid	$$$
Oxaprozin (Daypro)	1200 mg once/day to 1800 mg/day	$$$$
Piroxicam (Feldene)	20 mg once/day	$$$$
Sulindac (Clinoril)	150–200 mg bid	$$$
Tolmetin (Tolectin)	600–800 mg/day in 3 or 4 doses	$$$

[a]$ = < $10 to < $20; $$ = $20 to $35; $$$ = $36 to $60; $$$$ = range of > $60.[12]

other modalities. Systemic steroids and narcotics are avoided if possible. Topical capsaicin may improve knee OA symptoms when added to the usual treatment; however, its use may be limited by cost and the delayed onset of effect requiring sustained use for up to 4 weeks of multiple applications daily.[12]

Total joint replacement is the primary surgical approach for OA of the knee and the hip. Candidates for arthroplasty are individuals with severe pain, impaired joint function, or who have experienced declines in functional status that do not improve with nonpharmacologic and pharmacologic measures.

Prevention and Family Issues

Osteoarthritis affects the entire family. The costs of OA can be substantial.[12] The direct costs for drug therapy (which can easily exceed $60 per month) are added to lost income related to time spent on physician and physical therapy visits, disability-related work absences, and absences related to surgery. OA can preclude an individual from performing his or her previous occupation, and so vocational rehabilitation is considered an important component of OA management. The pain and functional disability associated with OA can contribute to social isolation and depression. Sexual intercourse can become difficult and painful, thereby adding to family stress. Emphasis should be placed on educating the patient and family (see Chapter 5).

Potentially modifiable risk factors include obesity, mechanical stress/repetitive joint usage, and joint trauma.[10] Weight reduction, avoidance of traumatic injury, prompt treatment of injury, and work site programs designed to minimize work-related mechanical joint stress may be effective interventions for preventing OA. Early treatment of congenital and developmental disorders known to be associated with the development of secondary OA have the potential for preventing OA.

References

1. Facts about family practice. Kansas City, MO: AAFP, 1987:30–7.
2. Lawrence RC, Hochberg MC, Kelsey JL, et al. Estimates of the prevalence of selected arthritic and musculoskeletal diseases in the US. J Rheumatol 1989;16:427–41.
3. Croft P. Review of UK data on the rheumatic diseases: osteoarthritis. Br J Rheumatol 1990;29:391–5.
4. Sack KE. Osteoarthritis a continuing challenge. West J Med 1995;163:579–86.
5. Jones A, Doherty M. Osteoarthritis. BMJ 1995;310:457–60.
6. Hamerman D. The biology of osteoarthritis. N Engl J Med 1989;320:1322–30.

7. Dunning RD, Materson RS. A rational program of exercise for patients with osteoarthritis. Semin Arthritis Rheum 1991; 21 Suppl 2:33–43.
8. Kovar PA, Allegrante JP, MacKenzie CR, et al. Supervised fitness walking in patients with osteoarthritis of the knee: a randomized controlled trial. Ann Intern Med 1992;116:529–34.
9. Brandt KD. Nonsurgical management of osteoarthritis, with an emphasis on nonpharmacologic measures. Arch Fam Med 1995;4:1057–64.
10. Bradley J, Brandt K, Katz B, et al. Comparison of an inflammatory dose of ibuprofen, an analgesic dose of ibuprofen and acetominophen in the treatment of patients with osteoarthritis. N Engl J Med 1991;325:87–91.
11. Griffin MR, Brandt KD, Liang MH, et al. Practical management of osteoarthritis: integration of pharmacologic and nonpharmacolic measures. Arch Fam Med 1995;4: 1049–55.
12. Med Lett 1994;36:101–6.

CASE PRESENTATION

Subjective

PATIENT PROFILE

Harold Nelson is a 76-year-old married white male retired welder.

PRESENTING PROBLEM

"My knees and hands hurt."

PRESENT ILLNESS

Mr. Nelson has a 20-year history of "arthritis" involving multiple joints, especially the hands and knees. The symptoms seem worse for the past 6 to 8 weeks, especially since the weather turned cold and snowy. He currently takes six to eight aspirin a day but is afraid to use other medication because of his diabetes, especially since he had an episode of incontinence after taking an over-the-counter cold remedy in the past.

PAST MEDICAL HISTORY, SOCIAL HISTORY, HABITS, AND FAMILY HISTORY

These are all unchanged since his previous visit 7 months ago (see Chapter 5).

REVIEW OF SYSTEMS

Mild constipation present for the past 4 to 6 weeks.

- What additional historical data might be useful? Why?
- What might be causing the increasing joint pain, and how would you inquire about these possibilities?
- What more would you like to know about his constipation? Why might this be significant?
- What might Mr. Nelson be doing differently because of his joint pain? How would you address this issue?

Objective

VITAL SIGNS

Height 5 ft 7 in; weight, 166 lb (This is a 10-lb weight gain in the past 7 months); blood pressure, 152/82; pulse, 72; temperature, 37.2°C.

EXAMINATION

There are Heberden's nodes of the distal joints of the fingers. There is a knobby deformity of multiple joints of the hands, wrists, and knees. The involved joints are not hot, but grip strength is decreased and the knees lack about 10 degrees of flexion and extension. The low back is not tender, and no muscle spasm is present. He lacks about 20 degrees of flexion at the waist.

LABORATORY

A blood glucose test performed in the office reveals a level of 110 mg/dl.

- What—if any—additional information might be derived from the physical examination? Why?
- What other areas of the body should be examined? Why?
- What—if any—laboratory determinations should be ordered today?
- What—if any—diagnostic imaging should be obtained?

Assessment

- What is your diagnostic assessment? How would you describe this to the patient?
- What might be the significance of the weight gain over the past 7 months?
- What might be the meaning of the joint pain to the patient? How would you ask about this?
- What would be your thoughts if the patient developed warm swollen tender joints? What would you do differently?

Plan

- What would be your therapeutic recommendation today? How would you explain this to Mr. Nelson?
- How would you approach the patient's concern about medication use?
- What life-style and activity recommendations would you make today?
- What continuing care would you advise?

19

Common Dermatoses

DANIEL J. VAN DURME

Acne Vulgaris

Acne is the most common dermatologic condition presenting to the family physician's office. It is usually found in patients between the ages of 12 and 25, with about 80% of teenagers affected.[1] It can present with a wide range of severity and may be the source of significant emotional and psychological, as well as physical, scarring. As adolescents pass through puberty and develop their self-image, the physical appearance of the skin can be critically important. Despite many effective treatments for this disorder, patients (and their parents) often view acne as a normal part of development and do not seek treatment. The importance of early treatment to prevent the physical and emotional scars cannot be overemphasized.

The pathogenesis of acne is important to understand, as most treatments are not curative but, rather, are directed at disrupting selected aspects of development. Acne begins with abnormalities in the pilosebaceous unit. There are four key elements involved in acne development: (1) keratinization abnormalities; (2) increased sebum production; (3) bacterial proliferation; and (4) inflammation. Each may play a greater or lesser role and manifests as a different type or presentation of acne. Initially, there is an abnormality of keratinization. Cohesive hyperkeratosis in the pilosebaceous unit causes blocking of the follicular canal by "sticky" epithelial cells and the development of a microcomedo. This blocked canal leads to a buildup of sebum behind the plug. Sebum production can be increased by androgens and other factors. This plugged pilosebaceous unit is seen as a closed comedone ("whitehead"), or as an open comedone ("blackhead") when the pore dilates and the fatty acids in the sebaceous plug become oxidized. The normal bacterial flora of the skin, especially *Proprionybacterium acnes,* proliferates in this plug and releases chemotactic factors drawing in leukocytes. The plug may also cause rupture of the unit under the skin, which in turn causes an influx of leukocytes. The resulting inflammation leads to the development of papular or pustular acne. This process can be marked and accompanied by hypertrophy of the entire pilosebaceous unit, leading to the formation of nodules and cysts. Many factors can aggravate or trigger acne, from the increase in androgens of puberty to cosmetics, mechanical trauma, medications, and others.[2]

Diagnosis

Diagnosis is straightforward and is based on the finding of comedones, papules, pustules, nodules, or cysts primarily on the face, back, shoulders, or chest, particularly in an adolescent patient. The presence of comedones is considered a necessity for the proper diagnosis of acne vulgaris. Without comedones, one must consider rosacea, steroid acne, or other acneiform dermatoses. It is important for choice of therapy and for long-term follow-up to describe and classify the patient's acne appropriately. Both the quantity *and* the type of lesions are noted. The number of lesions indicates whether the acne is mild, moderate, severe, or very severe (sometimes referred to as grades I–IV). The predominant type of lesion should also be noted (i.e., comedonal, papular, pustular, nodular, or cystic).[3] Thus a patient with hundreds of comedones on the face may have "very severe comedonal acne," whereas another patient may have only a few nodules and cysts and have "mild nodulocystic acne."

Management

Prior to pharmacologic management it is important to review and dispel some of the misperceptions that many patients (and parents) have about acne. This condition is not due to poor hygiene. Aggressive and frequent scrubbing of the skin may actually aggravate the condition. Mild soaps should be used regularly, and the face should be washed gently and dried well prior to the application of topical medication. Several studies have failed to implicate diet as a significant contributor to acne,[4,5] and fatty foods and chocolates have not been found to be significant causative agents. Nevertheless, if patients are aware of something in their diet that triggers a flare-up, they should obviously avoid it.

All patients should be taught that acne can be suppressed or controlled when medicines are used regularly, but that the initial therapy usually takes several weeks to show significant benefit. As the current lesions heal, the medications work to prevent the eruption of additional lesions. Typically, a noticeable response to medication is seen in about 6 weeks, and patients must be informed of this time lapse so they do not "give up" too soon. Some patients may have some initial worsening in the appearance of the skin when they first start treatment as well.

The treatment options for acne are based on the individual patient and the classification of his or her acne. Benzoyl peroxide serves as the foundation of most acne therapy. This antibacterial agent is available as cleansing liquids and bars and as gels or creams, with strengths ranging from 2.5% to 10%. The increase in strength increases the drying (and often the irritation) of the skin. It does not provide additional antibacterial activity. This agent should be used once or twice daily as basic therapy in most patients.

Because all acne starts with some degree of keratinization abnormality and microcomedone formation, it is prudent to start with a comedolytic agent. Currently, the most effective agent is tretinoin (Retin-A, Avita, and others), which is started at the lowest dose possible (0.025% cream) and applied nightly. Mild erythema and irritation are common at first, and if it is severe the frequency can be decreased to three times per week or less, then slowly increased to every night. The strength of the preparation can also be gradually increased as needed and as tolerated over several months. It is available as a cream, a liquid, and a gel. The liquid and gel have more alcohol, which can dry the skin (thus making them preferable for the patient with oily skin) and make the preparation somewhat stronger. Patients should be warned about some degree of photosensitivity with tretinoin and should use sun blocks as needed. If benzoyl peroxide is also used, it is crucial to separate the application of these compounds by several hours. When applied close together, these preparations cause more irritation to the skin while inactivating each other, rendering treatment ineffective.

Antibiotics are recommended for papular or pustular (papulopustular) acne. They act by decreasing the proliferation of *P. acnes* and by inactivating the neutrophil chemotactic factors released during the inflammatory process. Topical agents include erythromycin (A/T/S 2%, Erycette solution, T-Stat 2%), clindamycin (Cleocin T), tetracycline (Topicycline), and sodium sulfacetamide with sulfur (Novacet, Sulfacet-R). These agents are available in a variety of delivery vehicles and are applied once (sometimes twice) a day in conjunction with benzoyl peroxide. With both topical and oral antibiotics, some degree of trial and error is necessary. Some patients respond well to clindamycin, whereas another patient may respond only to erythromycin.

Oral antibiotics are indicated for patients with severe or widespread papulopustular acne or patients with difficulty reaching the affected areas on their body (i.e., on the back). The most commonly used oral antibiotics are tetracycline and erythromycin, which are started at 1 g/day in divided doses. Tetracycline patients are warned of the photosensitivity side effect and advised to take the medicine on an empty stomach, without dairy products. Erythromycin patients are warned of potential gastrointestinal (GI) upset. Other options for oral medications are doxycycline (50–100 mg twice a day), minocycline (50–100 mg twice a day), and occasionally trimethoprim-sulfamethoxazole (Bactrim DS or Septra DS 1 tablet once daily) for the refractory cases. As the acne improves, the dose of the oral medications can often be gradually decreased to about one-half the original dose for long-term maintenance therapy.

Nodulocystic acne requires initial therapy with benzoyl peroxide, tretinoin, and antibiotics. If these agents fail to control the acne adequately, oral isotretinoin (Accutane) may be used. This agent has been extremely effective in decreasing the production of sebum and shrinking the hypertrophied sebaceous glands of nodulocystic acne. In most patients it induces a remission for many months or cures the condition. If lesions remain, they are usually more susceptible to conventional therapy as described above. Treatment consists of a 16- to 20-week course at 0.5 to 2.0 mg/kg/day. Although this medicine can be profoundly effective, it has "black box" warnings about its teratogenicity and its association with pseudotumor cerebri. There are also numerous less severe side effects, including xerosis, cheilitis, epistaxis, myalgias, arthralgias, elevated liver enzymes, and others. Liver function tests, triglyceride levels, and complete blood counts should be frequently monitored. The high teratogenic potential must be made clear to all female patients, and this medicine must be used with extreme caution in all women with childbearing potential. Patient selection guidelines for women have been proposed, including (negative) serum pregnancy tests before starting, maintenance of highly effective methods of contraception throughout therapy and for 1 to 2 months after therapy, and finally signed forms for informed consent by the patient.[6]

Atopic Dermatitis

Atopic dermatitis (AD) is a common, chronic, relapsing skin condition with an estimated incidence of 10% in the United States. It usually arises during childhood, with about 85% of patients developing it during the first 5 years of life.[7] The disease presents with severe pruritus, followed by various morphologic features. It has been described as "the itch that rashes." Although AD can be found as an isolated illness in some individuals, it is often a manifestation of the multisystemic process of atopy, which includes asthma, allergic rhinitis, and atopic dermatitis. A family or personal history of atopy can be a key element in making the diagnosis.

There is some controversy over the role of the immune system and allergies in AD. There is some type of abnormality in the cell-mediated immune system (a T cell defect) in these patients, as they have an increased susceptibility to cutaneous viral (and fungal) infections, especially herpes simplex, molluscum contagiosum, and papillomavirus.[8,9] However, even though about 80% of patients with AD have an elevated immunoglobulin E

(IgE) level, there is not enough evidence to conclude that allergies play the key role in the development of this disease.[10] Thus even though many people are under the misperception that their skin is allergic to just about everything, they should be taught that the process is not a true allergy but, rather, a reaction of genetically abnormal skin to environmental stressors.

The eruption is eczematous and usually symmetric. It is erythematous, may have papules and plaques, and often has secondary changes of excoriations and lichenification. The persistent excoriations can lead to secondary bacterial infection, which may be noted by more exudative and crusting lesions. In infants and children, AD is commonly seen on the face and the extensor areas, whereas in older children and adults it is more commonly seen in flexural areas of the popliteal and antecubital fossae and the neck and wrists (Fig. 19.1). Patients with AD may also have numerous other features including generalized xerosis, cheilitis, hand dermatitis, palmar hyperlinearity, and sensitivity to wool and lipid solvents (e.g., lanolin).[8]

Treatment of atopic dermatitis begins with attempts at moisturizing the skin. Bathing is done only when necessary and then with cool or tepid water and a mild soap (e.g., Dove or Purpose) or a soap substitute (e.g., Cetaphil). Immediately after bathing and gently patting the skin dry, an emollient is applied to the skin to help seal in the moisture. This emollient should have no fragrances, no alcohol, and no lanolin (e.g., Aquaphor, Keri lotion, Lubriderm) and should be used daily to maintain well-lubricated skin. If the affected areas are particularly severe in an acute outbreak, wet dressings with aluminum acetate solution (Burow's

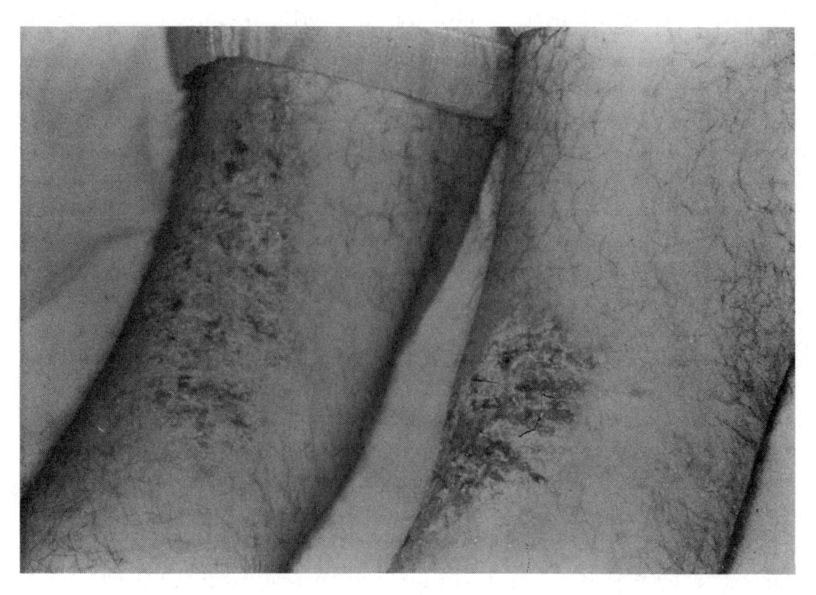

FIGURE 19.1. Atopic dermatitis in the popliteal fossae.

solution) can be applied two or three times daily.[8] If the affected area has dry, noninflamed skin, a moisturizer with lactic acid (e.g., Lac-hydrin) can be of such help that steroids can be avoided.

Controlling the intense pruritus is important. Keeping the nails trimmed short and the use of mittens at night can decrease the excoriations in children. Topical steroids can control the inflammatory process. Generally the lowest possible potency should be used, but often high-potency creams may be needed on lichenified areas. In infants and children, one can often maintain good control with 0.25% to 2.5% hydrocortisone cream or ointment, applied two or three times a day. For more severe cases and in adults, 0.1% triamcinolone cream or ointment (or an equivalent-strength steroid) may be needed. Only rarely should fluorinated steroid preparations be used. The intense pruritus can be controlled with the use of antihistamines such as diphenhydramine (Benadryl) or hydroxyzine (Atarax, Vistaril) titrated to balance the antipruritic effect with the sedating effect. Doxepin hydrochloride 5% cream (Zonalon) has potent H_1- and H_2-blocking effects and can control pruritus without the problems of long-term topical steroid use; however, absorption of this agent leads to drowsiness in some patients, particularly if a large amount of the skin is treated.[11] The nonsedating antihistamines are helpful if drowsiness becomes a problem. Such agents include astemizole (Hismanal), loratidine (Claritin), fexofenadine (Allegra), and the newer agent cetirizine (Zyrtec). If the AD suddenly becomes much worse, development of a secondary infection or a possible contact dermatitis must be considered.[12] If there is secondary infection, antibiotics directed at *Staphylococcus aureus* are used. Dicloxacillin, erythromycin, cephalexin, and topical mupirocin (Bactroban) are good choices. If these measures fail to provide adequate control, it may be reasonable to pursue possible specific provocative factors such as foods, contact allergens or irritants, dust mites, molds, or possible psychological stressors.[13]

This condition can produce a great deal of anxiety and frustration in both patients and parents, and the stress can further aggravate the condition. Although psychological factors aggravate the condition, it is important to emphasize that the condition is not "caused by nerves." It is an inherited condition that can be aggravated by emotional stress. This supportive counseling for the patient and the family can be crucial. Furthermore, although affected children may appear "fragile," they are not; and they may desperately need some affectionate handling to help ease their own anxieties about their condition.[14]

Miliaria

Miliaria (heat rash) is a common condition resulting from the blockage of eccrine sweat glands. There is an inflammatory response to the sweat that leaks through the ruptured duct, and papular or vesicular lesions result. It usually occurs after repeated exposure to a hot and humid environment. Miliaria can occur at any age but is especially common in infants and children.[15]

One of the most common forms of miliaria is miliaria crystallina, in which the blockage occurs near the skin surface and the sweat collects below the stratum corneum. A thin-walled vesicle then develops, but there is little to no erythema. This situation is often seen in infants or bedridden patients and can be treated with cool compresses and good ventilation to control perspiration.

Miliaria rubra (prickly heat or "heat rash") is more commonly seen in susceptible patients of any age group when exposed to sufficient heat. In this case the occlusion is at the intraepidermal section of the sweat duct. As a result there is more erythema, sometimes a red halo, or just diffuse erythema with papules and vesicles. Occasionally, the eruptions become pustular, resulting in miliaria pustulosa. There is usually more of a mild stinging or "prickly" sensation than real pruritus. The condition is self-limited but can be alleviated by cool wet to dry soaks. A low-strength steroid lotion (e.g., 0.025% or 0.1% triamcinolone lotion) is often helpful for alleviating the symptoms in these patients.[8]

Pityriasis Rosea

Pityriasis rosea (PR) is a benign, self-limited condition primarily found between the ages of 10 and 35; it is more common in women (1.5:1.0). The cause is unknown, but a viral etiology is suspected as some patients have a prodrome of a viral-like illness with malaise, low grade fever, cough, and arthralgias; there is an increased incidence in the fall, winter, and spring.[16]

This disorder often starts with a single, 2- to 10-cm, oval, papulosquamous, salmon-pink patch (or plaque) on the trunk or proximal upper extremity. This "herald patch" is followed by a generalized eruption of discrete, small, oval plaques on the trunk and proximal extremities, sparing the palms and soles and oral cavity. These plaques align their long axis with the skin lines, thus giving the rash a characteristic "Christmas tree" appearance. (Fig. 19.2) The plaques often have a fine, tissue-like "collarette" scale at the edges.

The differential diagnosis includes tinea corporis, as the initial herald patch can be confused with "ringworm." The diffuse eruption of PR may resemble secondary syphilis but can often be distinguished by the sparing of the palms and soles in PR. It may also give the appearance of psoriasis (especially guttate psoriasis) but has much finer plaques that are not clustered on the extensor areas. Finally, the eruption may be confused with tinea versicolor. Skin scrapings for a KOH preparation should be

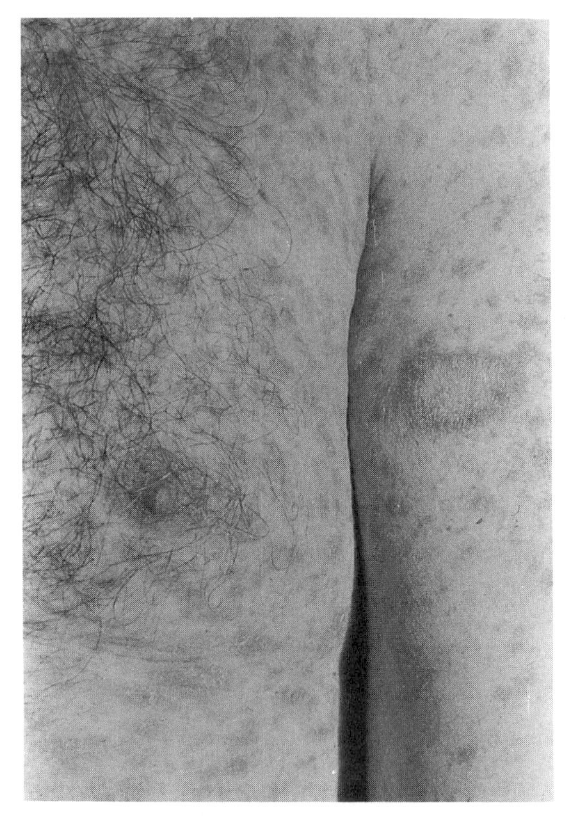

FIGURE 19.2. Pityriasis rosea. (Note herald patch on arm.)

strongly considered in any patient with apparent PR, as well as serologic testing for syphilis in any sexually active patient.

The management of PR is fairly easy. Pruritus is generally mild and can be controlled with oral antihistamines or topical low-potency steroid preparations. The patient can be reassured that the lesions will fade within about 6 weeks. They should be warned, however, that postinflammatory hypo- or hyperpigmentation (especially in blacks) is possible.[17]

Psoriasis

Psoriasis is a chronic, recurrent disorder characterized by an inflammatory, scaling, hyperproliferative papulosquamous eruption. Lesions are well-defined plaques with a thick, adherent, silvery white scale. If the scale is removed, pinpoint bleeding can be seen (Auspitz's sign). Psoriasis occurs in about 1% to 3% of the population worldwide.[18] The etiology is unknown, although some genetic link is suspected, as one-third of patients have a positive family history for the disease. It may start at any age, with the mean age of onset during the late twenties.[19]

Lesions most commonly occur on the extensor surfaces of the knees and elbows but are also typically seen on the scalp and the sacrum and can affect the palms and soles as well. The nails may show pitting, onycholysis, or brownish macules ("oil spots") under the nail plate. Finally, about 7% of these patients develop psoriatic arthritis, which can be severe, even crippling.[19,20]

Although psoriasis is usually not physically disabling and longevity is not affected, the patient's physical appearance can be profoundly affected and may cause significant psychological stress as the patient withdraws from social activities. Attention to the psychosocial implications of this chronic disease is crucial for every family physician.

The classic presentation with its erythematous plaques and thick, silvery scales on elbows or knees (Fig. 19.3) is usually easy to diagnose, but there are numerous morphologic variants. Discoid, guttate, erythrodermic, pustular, flexural (intertriginous), light-induced, and palmar-plantar psoriasis are among the many clinical presentations of this condition. The plaques may be confused with seborrheic or atopic dermatitis, and the guttate variant may resemble pityriasis rosea or secondary syphilis. If the diagnosis is unclear, referral to a dermatologist or a biopsy (read by a dermatopathologist, if possible) is in order.

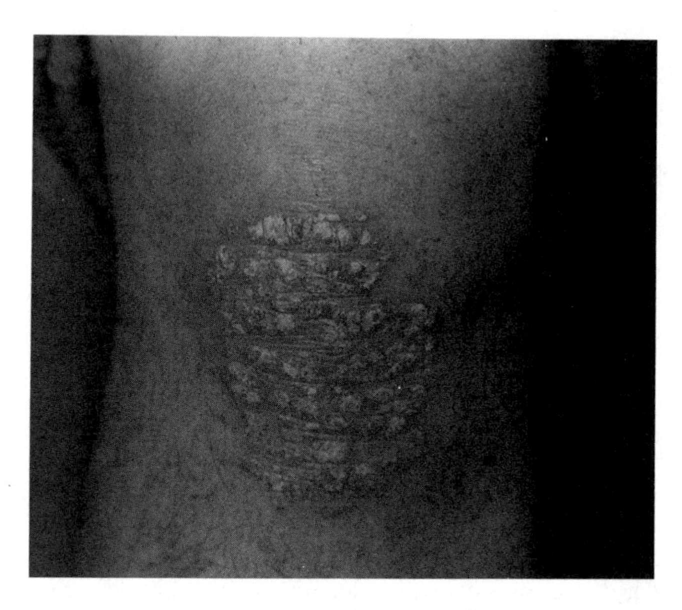

FIGURE 19.3. Typical psoriatic plaque.

The lesions often appear on areas subjected to trauma (Koebner phenomenon.) Other precipitating factors include infections, particularly upper respiratory infections, and stress. Several drugs, particularly lithium, β-blockers, angiotensin-converting enzyme (ACE) inhibitors, and antimalarial agents are well known to exacerbate psoriasis in some patients.[18] The NSAIDs used for psoriatic arthritis may worsen the skin manifestations. Systemic corticosteroids can initially clear the psoriasis, but a "rebound phenomenon," or worsening of the lesions, even after slowly tapering the dose is common.

Management

Patients must understand that there is no cure for psoriasis. All treatments are suppressive (i.e., designed to control the manifestations, improve the cosmetic appearance for the patient, and hopefully induce a remission). Therapy can start with liberal use of emollients (to keep the skin as moist as possible) and mild soaps. Moderate exposure to sunlight, while avoiding sunburn, can also improve the condition. After this start, treatment modalities are divided into topical agents and systemic therapies. The decision to use systemic agents is usually based on the percent of body surface area involved, with 20% often being used as the cutoff for changing to systemic treatment. In practice, however, the decision to use systemic therapy is based on the severity of the disease, the resistance to topical treatments, the availability of other agents, and a complex of social and psychological factors.[18,21] This decision is usually best made by an experienced dermatologist in consultation with the patient and the family physician.

Keratolytic preparations such as those with salicylic acid (e.g., Keralyt gel) can soften plaques and increase the efficacy of other topical agents. Topical steroid preparations can provide prompt relief, but it is often temporary. Tolerance to these agents is common (tachyphylaxis), and one must remain vigilant for the long-term side effects of thinning of the skin, hypopigmentation, striae, and telangiectasia. The lowest effective strength is used, always using caution with higher strengths on the face, groin, and intertriginous areas. Increased efficacy is seen when ointments are used under occlusion, but this practice can also lead to enough systemic absorption to suppress the pituitary-adrenal system.[18]

The topical agent calcipotriene 0.005% (Dovonex) has shown good results with mild to moderate plaque psoriasis. It is a derivative of vitamin D and works by inhibiting keratinocyte and fibroblast proliferation. It is is applied as a thin layer twice a day with most improvement noted within 1 month. Side effects include itching or burning in 10% to 20% of patients and rare cases of hypercalcemia (< 1%), particularly when large amounts are used (> 100 g/week).[22,23]

Chronic plaques are often best managed by using the antimitotic agents anthralin or coal tar. Anthralin preparations (e.g., Anthra-Derm, Drithocreme, Dritho-scalp) can be applied to thick plaques in the lowest dose possible for about 15 minutes a day and then showered off. Care must be taken to avoid the face, genitalia, and flexural areas. The duration and strength of the preparation is gradually increased as tolerated until irritation occurs. This preparation is messy and can stain normal skin, clothing, and bathroom fixtures. Coal tar preparations can be used alone or, more successfully, in combination with ultraviolet B (UVB) light therapy (Goeckerman regimen).[19] Coal tar may be found in both crude and refined preparations, such as bath preparations, gels, ointments, lotions, creams, solutions, soaps, and shampoos. In general, the treatment is similar to that with anthralin; high concentrations are used until irritation or improvement results. The preparations are left on overnight, and staining can be a problem.

When systemic therapy is needed, treatment with UV light can be extremely effective. There are two basic regimens: One uses UVB (alone or with coal tar or anthralins) and the other uses ultraviolet A light therapy with oral psoralens (PUVA) therapy). The psoralen acts as a photosensitizer, and the UVA is administered in carefully measured amounts via a specially designed unit. Phototherapy or photochemotherapy can be expensive and carcinogenic. Thus they are administered only by an experienced dermatologist. Other systemic agents include methotrexate, etretinate (Tegison), and cyclosporine.[18]

The lesions of psoriasis may disappear with treatment, but residual erythema, hypopigmentation, or hyperpigmentation is not uncommon. Patients must be instructed to continue treatment until there is near or complete resolution of the induration and not to always expect complete disappearance of the lesions.

Family and Community Issues

Proper patient and family education is crucial for managing the physical and psychosocial manifestations of this disease. The patient should be allowed to participate in the decision of which treatment modalities will be used and must be carefully instructed on the proper use of the one(s) chosen. The ongoing emotional support the family physician provides can help prevent the emotional scars that psoriasis may leave behind. The National Psoriasis Foundation is a nonprofit organization dedicated to supporting research and education in this field. They provide newsletters and other educational material for patients and their families. A written prescription with their address (National Psoriasis Foundation, 6600 SW 92nd, Suite 300, Portland, OR 97223; phone 503-244-7404) can be one of the most effective long-term "treatments" for these patients.

Poison Ivy, Poison Oak, and Sumac (Rhus Allergy)

Plant-related contact dermatitis can be triggered by numerous plant compounds, but the most common allergen is the urushiol resin found in the genus *Toxicodendron* (formerly *Rhus*) containing the plants poison ivy, poison oak, and poison sumac. These three plants cause more allergic contact dermatitis than that from all other contact materials combined.[8] The oleoresin urushiol, which serves as the allergen (and rarely as a primary irritant), is located within all parts of the plant.[24]

The clinical presentation varies with the amount of the allergen and the patient's own degree of sensitivity. About 70% to 80% of Americans are mildly to moderately sensitive to the allergen, with about 10% to 15% at each end of the spectrum: either very sensitive or completely tolerant.[25] The eruption is erythematous with papules, wheals, and often vesicles. In severe cases large bullae or diffuse urticarial hives are seen. The distribution is often linear or streak-like on exposed skin from either direct contact with the plant or by inadvertent spreading of the resin by the patient.

A history of exposure to the plant or to any significant activities outdoors helps in the diagnosis. It must be remembered, however, that the resin adheres to animal hair, clothing, and other objects and can then cling to the patient's skin after this indirect contact. Thus the patient may not be aware of any direct exposure. The thick, calloused skin on the hands often prevents eruption on the palms while the resin is transferred to another part of the body, where an eruption does occur. Outbreaks may occur within 8 hours of the exposure. Alternatively, the initial exposure may sensitize the patient so the rash occurs a couple of weeks after exposure in response to the resin remaining on or in the skin.[24] The ability of the resin to remain on the skin (even after washing) and cause a later eruption has led to the mistaken belief that the fluid of the vesicles can cause spreading of the lesions.

Treatment begins with removal of any remaining allergen by thorough skin cleansing with soap and water as soon after exposure as possible. Rubbing (isopropyl) alcohol can be even more effective in dispersing the oily resin. Any clothing that may have come in contact with the plant should also be washed. If the affected area is small, and there is no significant vesicular formation, topical steroids (medium to high potency, such as triamcinolone 0.1–0.5%) are sufficient. The blisters can be relieved by frequent use of cool compresses with water or with Burow's solution (one packet or tablet of Domeboro in 1 pint of water). Oral antihistamines (e.g., diphenhydramine 25–50 mg or hydroxyzine 10–25 mg, four times a day) can help relieve the pruritus. If the outbreak is severe or widespread, or it involves the face and eyes, oral steroids may be needed. A tapering dose of prednisone (starting at 0.5–1.0 mg/kg/day) can be used over 5 to 7 days if the outbreak started a week or more after exposure. A longer, tapering course should be used (10–14 days) if treating an outbreak that started within 1 to 2 days of exposure. This regimen treats the lesions that are present and should suppress further development of lesions as the skin is sensitized.[26]

Prevention is best done by avoidance, but the U.S. Food and Drug Administration (FDA) has approved the first medication proved to prevent outbreak, bentoquatum (IvyBlock). This nonprescription lotion is applied before potential exposure and dries on the skin to form a white protective barrier. Desensitization attempts have not been successful and are not recommended.

Seborrheic Dermatitis

Seborrheic dermatitis, a recurrent scaling eruption, is common (incidence 3–5%) and typically occurs on the face and scalp. It is usually seen in two age groups: infants during the first few months of life (may present as "cradle cap") and adults ages 30 to 60 ("dandruff"). It causes mild pruritus, is generally gradual in onset, and is fairly mild in its presentation. An increased incidence (up to 80%) has been described in patients with acquired immunodeficiency syndrome (AIDS), and these patients often present with a severe, persistent eruption[27] (see Chapter 21). The etiology is unknown, but there is some link to the proliferation of the fungus *Pityrosporum ovale.*

The lesions are scaling macules, papules, and plaques. They may be yellowish, thick and greasy, or sometimes white, dry, and flaky. Thick, more chronic lesions occasionally crust and then fissure and weep. Secondary bacterial infection leading to impetigo is not uncommon. The differential diagnosis includes atopic dermatitis, candidiasis, or a dermatophytosis. When the scalp is involved, the plaques are often confused with psoriasis, and the two conditions may overlap, referred to as *seboriasis* or *sebopsoriasis.* When the trunk is involved, the lesions may appear similar to those of pityriasis rosea.

Treatment of hair-bearing areas consists of periodic use of shampoos containing selenium sulfide (Selsun, Selsun Blue), pyrithione zinc (Sebulon, Head and Shoulders), salicyclic acid and sulfur combinations (Sebulex), or coal tar (Denorex, Neutrogena T-Gel). The antifungal agent ketoconazole (Nizoral) is also available as a shampoo and can be highly effective (which supports the *Pityrosporum ovale* theory). These shampoos are used two or three times a week and must be left on the skin (scalp) for about 5 minutes prior to rinsing. They are used alternating with regular shampoos as needed. This regimen may prevent the tachyphylaxis that can occur with daily use. After about 1 month the frequency of use can be decreased as tolerated to maintain control. Low-potency topical steroid creams or lotions (e.g., 2.5% hydrocortisone or 0.01% fluocinolone) can be used once or twice a day in the scalp or in other areas such as the face, groin, and chest. Topical ketoconazole cream (Nizoral) twice daily can also be helpful. Thick scales, such as may be found on the scalps of infants, can be gently scrubbed off with a soft toothbrush after soaking the area for 5 minutes with warm mineral oil or a salicyclic acid shampoo.

Rosacea (Acne Rosacea)

A chronic facial dermatosis, acne rosacea typically appears in patients between the ages of 30 and 60. It is characterized by acneiform lesions such as papules, pustules, and occasionally nodules (Fig. 19.4). Patients

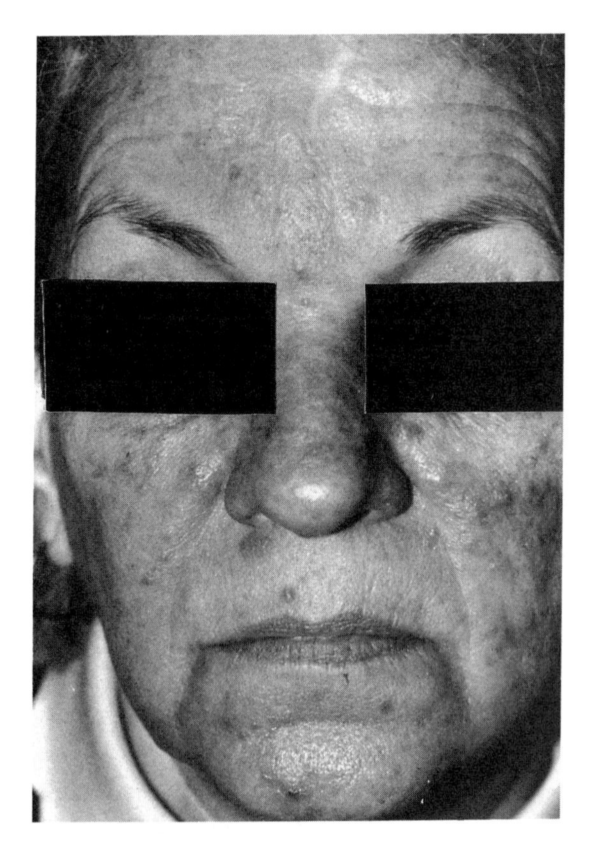

FIGURE 19.4. Acne rosacea.

also have facial flushing, generalized erythema, and telangiectasias; and they may have moderate to severe sebaceous gland hyperplasia. Ocular manifestations such as conjunctivitis, blepharitis, and episcleritis can be found in about half of the patients. Severe involvement of the nose can lead to soft-tissue hypertrophy and rhinophyma. Otherwise, most lesions are on the forehead, cheeks, and nose. The pathogenesis is unknown, but increasing evidence suggests that it is primarily a cutaneous vascular disorder that leads to lymphatic damage followed by edema, erythema, and finally papules and pustules.[28] Despite popular conception, alcohol is not known to play a causative role, but the vasodilatory effects of alcohol may make the condition appear worse. There is also some vasomotor instability in response to hot liquids and spicy foods, and these entities should be avoided.[8]

Treatment with oral erythromycin or tetracycline 1 g/day in divided doses or with minocycline or doxycycline at 50 to 100 mg twice a day can help alleviate both the facial and ocular manifestations of the disease. Response is variable, with some patients showing a prompt response followed by weeks or months of remission and others requiring long-term suppression with antibiotics. If long-term treatment is needed, the dose is titrated down to the minimal effective amount. Topical agents include clindamycin and erythromycin, but some of the better responses are seen with metronidazole gel or cream in mild to moderate cases.[29] Topical sodium sulfacetamide and sulfur lotion is available in a unique preparation (Sulfacet-R) that includes a color blender for the patient to add tint to the lotion to match their own skin coloration. This agent is popular with women in particular who may wish to "hide" the erythema and lesions. Oral metronidazole (Flagyl) may be used with caution in resistant cases. Topical tretinoin (Retin-A) and oral isotretinoin (Accutane) have shown promising results in patients with severe, refractory rosacea.[30]

Pomphylox (Dyshidrotic Eczema)

Pomphylox, a recurrent eczematous dermatosis of the fingers, palms, and soles, is more common in the young population (under age 40) and presents with pruritic, often tiny, deep-seated vesicles. The etiology is unknown, but despite the name and the fact that many patients may have associated hyperhidrosis, it is not a disorder of sweat retention. Many of these patients have a history of atopic dermatitis, and it is considered a type of hand/foot eczema. Emotional stress plays a role in some cases, as does ingestion of certain allergens (e.g., nickel and chromate).[8]

The onset is typically abrupt and lasts a few weeks, but the disorder can become chronic and lead to fissuring and lichenification. Secondary bacterial infection can also occur. The vesicles are usually small but can be bullous and may give the appearance of tapioca. The most common site is the sides of the fingers in a cluster distribution (Fig. 19.5). The nails can also show involvement with dystrophic changes such as ridging, pitting, or thickening.

Controlling this disorder can be difficult and frustrating for the physician and patient alike. Attempts should be made to remove the inciting stressor whenever possible. Further treatment is similar to that for atopic dermatitis: Cool compresses may provide relief, and topical steroids can alleviate the inflammation and pruritus. It is one of the dermatoses in which high-potency fluorinated or halogenated steroids (in the gel or ointment formulation) are often needed to penetrate the thick stratum corneum of the hands. If secondary infection is present, erythromycin or cephalexin can be helpful. Rarely, oral steroids may be needed, but these drugs are reserved for the more severe, recalcitrant cases.

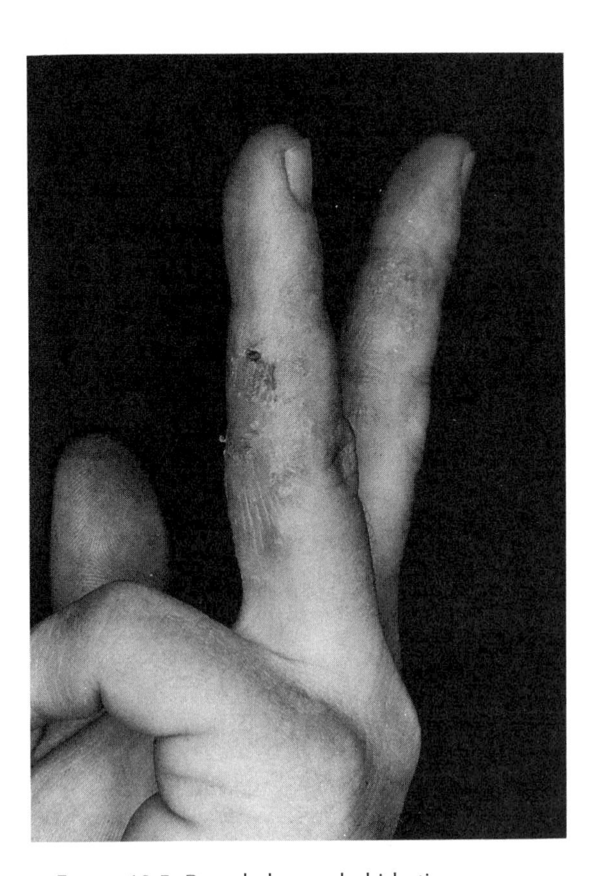

FIGURE 19.5. Pomphylox or dyshidrotic eczema.

Drug Eruptions

Rashes of various types are common reactions to medications. The dermatologic manifestations can be highly variable: maculopapular (or morbilliform) eruptions; urticaria; fixed, hyperpigmented lesions; photosensitivity reactions; vesicles and bullae; acneiform lesions; and generalized pruritus, among others. Serious and even life-threatening dermatologic reactions can occur as well, such as Stevens-Johnson syndrome, toxic epidermal necrolysis, hypersensitivity syndrome, and serum sickness.[31,32]

Definitively assigning a diagnosis of a particular eruption to a single agent can be difficult, as patients may take multiple medications, they may have coexistent illnesses, and the drug eruption may not manifest until the patient has been taking it for several days (sometimes weeks). Only when the eruption follows the administration a particular agent, resolves with removal of the agent, recurs with readministration, and other causes have been excluded can one say that the eruption is definitely due to a specific drug. Obviously, caution must be used prior to any rechallenge with an agent, and so readministration is often not recommended. Subsequently, many patients mistakenly believe they have dermatologic reactions or allergies to certain medications when their rash may have had nothing to do with their medication.

Table 19.1 is a listing of several of the typical drug reactions to some of the more common drugs in clinical practice.[8,14,26,33] Treatment consists of stopping the offending (or suspected) medication. Topical low-potency to mid-potency steroids and oral antihistamines can relieve the pruritus that accompanies many eruptions.

Contact Dermatitis

Contact dermatitis is the clinical response of the skin to an external stimulant. It is an extremely common condition. Chemically caused dermatitis is responsible for an estimated 30% of all occupational illness.[34] The condition is such a problem with a wide variety of mechanisms of pathogenesis and potential products involved that an international journal, *Contact Dermatitis,* is devoted specifically to this topic. By suspecting virtually everything and anything and taking a thorough history, the family physician nevertheless should be able to diagnose and manage most of these patients.

There are a few subtypes of contact dermatitis, the most common type being irritant contact dermatitis, which accounts for 70% to 80% of cases of contact dermatitis.[35] It is the result of a break in the skin's integrity and subsequent local absorption of an irritant. There is no true demonstrable

TABLE 19.1. Common reactions to common drugs

Anaphylaxis
- Aspirin
- Sulfonamides
- NSAIDs
- Serum (animal derived)
- Penicillins

Fixed drug eruptions
- Aspirin
- Phenolphthalein
- Barbiturates
- Sulfonamides
- NSAIDs
- Tetracyclines

Lupus-like eruptions
- Hydralazine
- Methyldopa
- Hydrochlorothiazide
- Procainamide
- Isoniazid
- Quinidine

Maculopapular (morbilliform)
- Barbiturates
- Isoniazid
- Phenothiazines
- Sulfonamides
- Diflunisal (Dolobid)
- Meclofenamate (Meclomen)
- Phenytoin
- Thiazides
- Gentamicin
- Penicillin compounds
- Quinidine

Photosensitivity
- Carbamazepine
- Methotrexate
- Piroxicam
- Sulfonylureas
- Furosemide
- Naproxen
- Quinidine
- Tetracyclines
- Griseofulvin
- Phenothiazines
- Sulfonamides
- Thiazides

Serum sickness
- Aspirin
- Penicillin
- Sulfonamide

Urticaria
- Antibiotics
- Opiates
- Blood products
- Radiocontrast agents
- NSAIDs

Vesicular eruption
- Barbiturates
- Clonidine
- Naproxen
- Sulfonamides
- Captopril
- Furosemide
- Penicillin
- Cephalosporins
- Nalidixic acid
- Piroxicam

allergen present. A single exposure can induce an inflammatory response if the agent is caustic enough or if the there is a marked degree of exposure. Often the response is the result of prolonged exposure with repeated minor damage to the skin, such as in those who must wash their hands frequently. Common offending agents include soaps, industrial solvents, and topical medications (e.g., benzoyl peroxide, tretinoin, lindane, benzyl benzoate, anthralin).[34–36]

The second most common type is allergic contact dermatitis. It is a delayed hypersensitivity reaction that occurs after the body is sensitized to the offending agent. The reaction is thus often delayed somewhat from the time of exposure. The response varies depending on the individual's sensitivity, the amount and concentration of the allergen, and the degree of penetration. Poison ivy dermatitis is perhaps the most common form of allergic contact dermatitis (discussed earlier in the chapter). Other common offenders are nickel, fragrances, rubber chemicals, neomycin, parabens (found in sunscreens and lotions), and benzocaine (topical anesthetic).[36,37] Even topical steroid preparations have been reported to cause allergic contact dermatitis in some patients.[36]

Physical findings vary somewhat with different forms of contact dermatitis. The irritant type causes an erythematous scaling eruption with a typically indistinct margin (Fig. 19.6). The allergic type usually causes more erythema, edema, vesicular formation, and weeping. These erup-

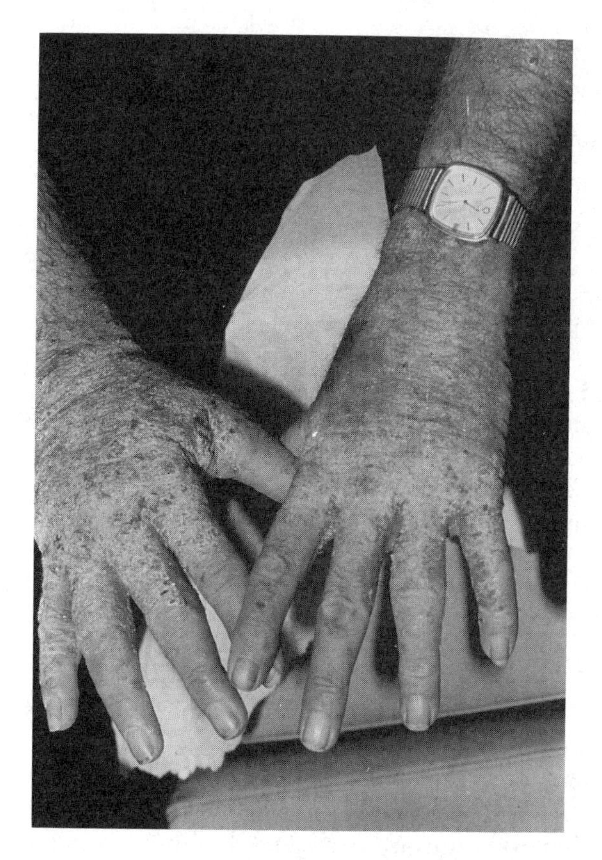

FIGURE 19.6. Contact dermatitis, irritant type.

tions are typically better defined and may correspond to the shape of the offending agent (e.g., a watchband or the elastic band of some article of clothing).

Treatment is symptomatic after removal of the irritant or allergen. Cool compresses can provide relief from the pruritus, particularly if there is any weeping. Oral antihistamines may be needed along with topical steroids. Ointment compounds are recommended, as they are less irritating and sensitizing than most creams or lotions. The patient should avoid any topical preparations with benzocaine or other "-caines," as they may aggravate the condition. In severe cases a tapering course of oral steroids over 1 to 2 weeks is necessary. Subacute and chronic cases may also be colonized with *Staphylococcus aureus,* and an oral antibiotic (e.g., dicloxacillin, erythromycin, or cephalexin) may speed resolution.[37]

Avoidance of the irritant or allergen is sometimes difficult for patients. Their job may require some exposure, or it may be difficult to verify the specific agent. Patch testing may be reasonable to determine the likely candidate(s) and thus assist in a long-term plan of avoidance.

Urticaria

Urticaria, a common skin condition affecting about 20% of the population, is characterized by transient wheals or hives.[38] It is typically a type I immunologic reaction (mediated by IgE) but may be from physical or environmental exposure (pressure- or cold-induced). Urticaria can be acute (lasting less than 6 weeks) or chronic. Perhaps the most frustrating issue for the patient and physician faced with urticaria is that the underlying cause is often difficult to ascertain. In only about 20% of cases of chronic urticaria can the specific etiology be determined.[38,39]

A generalized eruption of pruritic wheals with erythema and localized edema and lesions lasting less than 24 hours establishes the diagnosis. Angioedema is a closely related process in which deeper tissues may be involved, particularly mucus membranes. Severe generalized urticaria can be a systemic illness leading to cardiac problems and even death.

One should search carefully to find the underlying etiology by doing a thorough comprehensive history and physical examination. Common causes include medications (antibiotics, NSAIDs, narcotics, radiocontrast dyes), illnesses (viral hepatitis, streptococcal, parasitic), connective tissue disorders (lupus, juvenile rheumatoid arthritis), endocrine disorders (hyper- or hypothyroidism), neoplastic disorders (lymphoma, leukemia, carcinoma), physical agents (pressure, cold, heat, exercise, menstruation), skin contacts (chemicals, fragrances, dyes, soaps, lotions, feathers, animal dander), insect bites and bee stings, foods (chocolate, shellfish, strawberries, nuts), and psychological stress.[8,14,39,40] The amount of laboratory work and other testing recommended can be highly variable and depends in part on the clinical utility of finding the underlying trigger(s). In general, an extensive workup is not advised during the early weeks and is begun only when the urticaria becomes chronic (> 6 weeks), when the patient seems otherwise ill or is pressing hard for an etiology, or other signs and symptoms point to another cause.[40]

Treatment consists of avoidance of any known or suspected precipitant and the use of medications as needed for comfort. The H_1-blockers such as astemizole (Hismanal), cetirizine (Zyrtec), loratadine (Claritin), diphenhydramine, or hydroxyzine can be used alone or in combination with an H_2-blocker such as cimetidine (Tagamet). Doxepin, a tricyclic antidepressant, can also be helpful at 25 mg once or twice a day. For severe, acute urticaria, a tapering dose of prednisone over 2 weeks can be helpful. Chronic urticaria may require a great deal of maintenance emotional support, as the condition can make normal activities difficult. Patients must be reassured, and medications may be needed on a long-term daily basis.

References

1. Leydon JJ. Therapy for acute acne vulgaris. N. Engl J Med 1997;336: 1156–63.
2. Nguyen QH, Kim YA, Schwartz RA. Management of acne vulgaris. Am Fam Physician 1994;50:89–96.
3. Pochi PE, Shalita AR, Strauss JS, et al. Report on the Consensus Conference on Acne Classification. Washington, D.C., March 24 and 25, 1990. J Am Acad Dermatol 1991;24:495–500.
4. Rosenberg EW. Acne diet reconsidered. Arch Dermatol 1981; 117:193–5.
5. Rasmussen JE. Diet and acne. Int J Dermatol 1977;16:488–92.
6. Anonymous. American Academy of Dermatology. Guidelines of care for acne vulgaris. J Am Acad Dermatol 1990; 22:676–80.
7. Hanifin JM. Atopic dermatitis in infants and children. Pediatr Clin North Am 1991;38:763–89.
8. Habif TP. Clinical dermatology: a color guide to diagnosis and therapy. 3rd ed. St. Louis: Mosby-Year Book, 1996.
9. Kolmer HL, Platts-Mills TAE. Atopic dermatitis: new knowledge and new approaches. Hosp Pract 1995;10:63–72.
10. Halbert AR, Weston WL, Morelli JG. Atopic dermatitis: is it an allergic disease? J Am Acad Dermatol 1995;33:1008–18.
11. Doxepin cream for pruritus. Med Lett 1994;36:99–100.
12. McHenry PM, Williams HC, Bingham EA. Management of atopic eczema. BMJ 1995;310:843–7.
13. Przybilla B, Eberlein-Konig B, Rueff F. Practical management of atopic eczema. Lancet 1994;343:1342–6.
14. Goldstein BG, Goldstein AO. Practical dermatology. St. Louis: Mosby-Year Book, 1992.
15. Feng E, Janniger CK. Miliaria. Cutis 1995;55:213–6.
16. Allen RA, Janniger CK, Schwartz, RA. Pityriasis rosea. Cutis 1995;56:198–202.
17. Bjornberg A. Pityriasis rosea. In: Fitzpatrick TB, Eisen AZ, Wolff K, et al, editors. Dermatology in general medicine. 4th ed. New York: McGraw-Hill, 1993:1117–23.
18. Greaves MW, Weinstein GD. Treatment of psoriasis. N Engl J Med 1995; 332:581–8.
19. Gibson LE, Peary HD. Papulosquamous eruptions and exfoliative dermatitis. In: Moschella SL, Hurley HJ, editors. Dermatology. 3rd ed. Philadelphia. Saunders, 1992:607–51.
20. Christophers E, Sterry W. Psoriasis. In: Fitzpatrick TB, Eisen AZ, Wolff K, et al, editors. Dermatology in general medicine. 4th ed. New York: McGraw-Hill, 1993:489–514.
21. Anonymous. Guidelines for the management of patients with psoriasis: workshop of the research unit of the Royal College of Physicians of

London: Department of Dermatology, University of Glasgow: British Association of Dermatologists. BMJ 1991;303:829–35.
22. Kirsner RS, Federman D. Treatment of psoriasis: role of calcipotriene. Am Fam Physician 1995;52:237–43.
23. Calcipotriene for psoriasis. Med Lett 1994;36:70–1.
24. Baer RL. Poison ivy dermatitis. Cutis 1990;40:34–6.
25. Epstein WL. Occupational poison ivy and oak dermatitis. Dermatol Clin 1994;12:511–5.
26. Pariser RJ. Allergic and reactive dermatoses. Postgrad Med 1991;89:75–85.
27. Janniger CK, Schwartz RA. Seborrheic dermatitis. Am Fam Physician 1995;52:149–59.
28. Wilkin JK. Rosacea: pathophysiology and treatment. Arch Dermatol 1994; 130:359–62.
29. Thiboutot DM. Acne rosacea. Am Fam Physician 1994;50: 1691–1702.
30. Ertl GA, Levine N, Kligman AM. A comparison of the efficacy of topical tretinoin and low dose oral isotretinoin in rosacea. Arch Dermatol 1994; 130:319–24.
31. Roujeau JC, Stern RS. Severe adverse cutaneous reactions to drugs. N Engl J Med 1994;33:1272–85.
32. Manders SM. Serious and life-threatening drug eruptions. Am Fam Physician 1995;51:1865–72.
33. Kalish RS. Drug eruptions: a review of clinical and immunologic features. Adv Dermatol 1991;6:221–37.
34. Anonymous. Contact dermatitis and urticaria from environmental exposures: Agency for Toxic Substances and Disease Registry. Am Fam Physician 1993;48:773–80.
35. Oxholm A, Maibach MI. Causes, diagnosis, and management of contact dermatitis. Compr Ther 1990;16:18–24.
36. Adams RM. Recent advances in contact dermatitis. Ann Allergy 1991; 67:552–66.
37. Whittington C. Clinical aspects of contact dermatitis. Prim Care 1989;16: 729–38.
38. Huston DP, Bressler RB. Urticaria and angioedema. Med Clin North Am 1992;76:805–40.
39. Mahmood T. Urticaria. Am Fam Physician 1995;51:811–6.
40. Greaves MW. Chronic urticaria. N Engl J Med 1995;332: 1767–72.

CASE PRESENTATION

Subjective

PATIENT PROFILE

Ruth Nelson McCarthy is a 51-year-old married white female restaurant operator.

PRESENTING PROBLEM

"Rash on hands."

PRESENT ILLNESS

For 8 to 10 months, the patient has noticed a rash on her hands. It occurs especially between the fingers and, when present, is red, irritated, and scaling. The itching of the rash prompts scratching, especially during her sleep at night.

PAST MEDICAL HISTORY

She has been taking estrogen replacement therapy since her previous visit 8 months ago (see Chapter 2).

FAMILY HISTORY, SOCIAL HISTORY, AND HABITS

All are unchanged since her previous visit.

- What additional information would you like regarding the history of present illness? Explain.
- What more would you like to know about her work?
- What might the patient be doing to treat her rash? Why might this be important?
- What are possible reasons for the patient's visit today? How would you address this issue?

Objective

VITAL SIGNS

Blood pressure, 136/88; pulse, 72; respirations, 18; temperature, 37°C.

EXAMINATION

There is dermatitis of both hands, worse on the right. The rash especially involves the fingers and the interdigital folds. The skin is cracked and bleeding in places, and there is evidence of excoriation.

- What additional data about the examination of the hands might be useful?
- Are there additional areas of the body that you might examine? Why?
- What—if any—laboratory tests might be useful? Why?
- What physical findings might suggest that the problem is other than a localized dermatitis? Explain.

Assessment

- What is the probable diagnosis and its cause? How will you explain this to the patient?
- How might this relate to activities in her life?
- What are some implications of the diagnosis for Mrs. McCarthy and her family?
- If a similar rash were also present on other areas of the body, what diagnostic possibilities would you consider?

Plan

- What specific therapy would you recommend? How would you explain this to Mrs. McCarthy?
- How might this problem be prevented in the future? What changes in her work would you advise?
- If the rash became infected, with purulent drainage and crusting, what might you do differently?
- What continuing care would you recommend?

20
Diabetes Mellitus

CHARLES KENT SMITH, JOHN P. SHEEHAN, AND MARGARET M. ULCHAKER

Diabetes mellitus (DM) affects 12 million to 15 million individuals in the United States, incurring an immense cost in terms of morbidity and premature death. The most common form is type II, or adult-onset, DM, which has racial preponderances, female predilection, and strong associations with obesity. There was a revolution in DM management during the 1980s with the advent of home blood glucose monitoring devices, human insulin, and reliable laboratory markers of long-term glycemic control. In addition, published national and international standards of care have been disseminated directly to patients and physicians, heightening the importance of adequate care and glycemic control to minimize devastating long-term complications.[1,2] Table 20.1 describes diagnostic criteria for diabetes mellitus, impaired glucose tolerance, and gestational diabetes.

Heightened clinical awareness of the genetics and predisposing factors should foster early diagnosis and adequate metabolic control of the type II patient. In contrast, the type I DM patient generally presents with a more precipitous clinical picture of ketoacidosis. Declining islet cell secretory function is more gradual, however, and can evolve over a 10-year period. Understanding the autoimmune nature of islet destruction has led to experimental protocols attempting to interrupt this process. Occasionally there is diagnostic confusion owing to a lack of a family history, the absence of significant ketosis, and the absence of significant obesity and other diagnostic hallmarks. The measurement of C-peptide levels and islet cell antibodies provides useful diagnostic clarification.[3] Careful clinical follow-up can clarify evolving absolute insulin deficiency even in the absence of these laboratory markers.

Pathophysiology

Previously, type I DM was considered to be an acute event. Viral associations were invoked with regard to the seasonal trends in its

TABLE 20.1. Diagnostic criteria for diabetes mellitus, impaired glucose tolerance, and gestational diabetes

Nonpregnant adults

Criteria for diabetes mellitus: Diagnosis of diabetes mellitus in nonpregnant adults should be restricted to those who have *one* of the following:

Fasting plasma glucose ≥ 126 mg/dl. Fasting is defined as no caloric intake for at least 8 hours.

Symptoms of diabetes mellitus (such as polyuria, polydipsia, unexplained weight loss coupled with a casual plasma glucose level ≥200 mg/dl. Casual is defined as any time of day, without regard to time interval since the last meal.

2-hour postprandial plasma glucose ≥ 200 mg/dl during an oral glucose tolerance test. The test should be performed by World Health Organization criteria using a glucose load containing the equivalent of 75 g anhydrous glucose dissolved in water.

Note: In the absence of unequivocal hyperglycemia with acute metabolic decompensation, these criteria should be confirmed by repeat testing on a second occasion. The oral glucose tolerance test is not recommended for routine clinical use.

Criterion for impaired glucose tolerance: 2-hour postprandial plasma glucose greater than or equal to 140 mg/dl and less than or equal to 200 mg/dl during an oral glucose tolerance test. The test should be performed by World Health Organization criteria using a glucose load containing the equivalent of 75 g anhydrous glucose dissolved in water.

Pregnant Women

Criteria for gestational diabetes: After an oral glucose load of 100 g, gestational diabetes is diagnosed if two plasma glucose values equal or exceed:

Fasting:	105 mg/dl
1 Hour:	190 mg/dl
2 Hour:	165 mg/dl
3 Hour:	145 mg/dl

Source: Report of the Expert Committee on the Diagnosis and Classification of Diabetes Mellitus. *Diabetes Care* 1997 July. 20(7):1183–1197.

incidence. However, patients can have markers of islet destruction in the form of islet cell antibodies for up to 10 years prior to the development of overt DM. Islet and insulin autoantibodies along with the loss of first-phase insulin secretion in response to an intravenous glucose tolerance test are highly predictive of evolving type I DM.[4] Attempts to interrupt this autoimmune process with immunosuppressive agents have been tried with some encouraging results, but toxicity remains a concern. Clinical trials are ongoing in this area, as are trials with early insulin replacement therapy. Insulin has been given to experimental animals that have autoimmune islet destruction without overt DM in an attempt to suppress the autoimmune process. A pilot study of 12 patients holds exciting promise for clinical applicability of this approach in humans.[5] From the clinical perspective, only patients who have newly diagnosed DM can be offered early aggressive insulin replacement treatment unless they are willing to participate in research protocols at specialized centers.

Type II DM is associated with genetic predispositions, advancing age, obesity, and lack of physical exercise. The importance of caloric intake and energy expenditure has been clearly established.[6] Although type II

DM is a syndrome of insulin resistance and islet secretory defects, in any given individual it is not possible to define the degree of insulin resistance versus secretory defects with any precision. The earliest metabolic defect found in first-degree relatives of individuals with type II DM is defective skeletal muscle glucose uptake with later increased insulin resistance at the level of the liver and resultant uncontrolled hepatic glucose output. The ensuing hyperglycemia can have a toxic effect called glucotoxicity on the islets, resulting in secondary secretory defects with declining insulin secretion and self-perpetuating hyperglycemia. Hyperglycemia may also down-regulate glucose transporters. It is unclear whether secretory defects or insulin resistance is the primary defect even for type II DM; they appear to coexist in patients with established disease. Patients may exhibit many abnormalities, including loss of first-phase insulin secretion and loss of the pulsatility of insulin secretion.[7–10] In addition, both men and women tend to have abdominal obesity, which is associated with hyperinsulinemia and insulin resistance.[11] Type II DM is a syndrome not only of disordered glucose metabolism but also of lipid metabolism; many patients have a concurrent dyslipidemia manifesting elevations in serum triglycerides, depressions in high-density lipoprotein (HDL)-cholesterol, and marginal increases in total cholesterol. This dyslipidemia results from uncontrolled hepatic very-low-density lipoprotein (VLDL) secretion and defective clearance of lipoprotein molecules. The associations of hyperinsulinemia and insulin resistance with essential hypertension have been documented[12] along with the marked tendency for patients with essential hypertension to develop DM and the converse: patients with type II DM developing essential hypertension. A central unifying hypothesis focuses on hyperinsulinemia and insulin resistance being primary metabolic aberrations that result not only in hyperglycemia but also hypertension and dyslipidemia. Thus our current understanding of type II DM and syndrome X[13] (hyperinsulinemia, dyslipidemia, hypertension, and hyperglycemia) highlight the important issue not only of primary prevention of type II DM but also secondary prevention.

Importance of Glycemic Control

The relation between microvascular complications of DM and glycemic control has been debated for decades. Many studies suggest an association between poor long-term glycemic control and retinopathy, neuropathy, and nephropathy. Unfortunately, many of these studies were not randomized, and the role of genetic factors was unclear. However, positive trends with glycemic control have been described. Small human studies and several animal studies link sustained metabolic control to the prevention of complications. One study showed, however, that early poor control despite later good control results in diabetic complications.[14] The Diabetes Control and Complications Trial (DCCT) proved the profound impact of intensive therapy on reducing the risk of microvascular complications.[15] Decades of questions about the glucose hypothesis are therefore finally answered, with the obvious recommendation that most individuals with type I diabetes mellitus be treated with intensive therapy. The major negative aspect of attempts to achieve optimum glycemic control by intensive insulin therapy is the potential for severe hypoglycemia. Careful screening of individuals with a history of severe unconscious reactions is necessary to redefine realistic treatment goals. Many individuals, though, can safely achieve excellent metabolic control as defined by normal glycohemoglobin levels without significant hypoglycemia.

Defining Control

The definition of DM control has varied. During the era of urine testing, predominantly negative urine tests were indicative of good glycemic control. However, because blood glucose can be twice normal in the absence of glycosuria, urine glucose monitoring is now outmoded. Home blood glucose monitoring (HBGM) provides positive feedback of daily glycemic control to patients and physicians. Patients engaged in intensive insulin therapy can monitor themselves four to seven times per day and make adjustments in their regimen to optimize blood glucose control. The precision and accuracy of the home units has improved considerably, as has the simplicity and duration of the test (Table 20.2). Each system has its inherent weaknesses and limitations in such areas as blood volume, timing, hematocrit, temperature, and humidity. It is important that patients adhere strictly to the manufacturers' guidelines because attention to proper calibrations, strip handling, and ongoing maintenance are critical. Noninvasive HBGM with infrared technology may be the wave of the future. Markers of long-term control such as the glycohemoglobin assays are also available. These tests measure the degree of glycosylation of hemoglobin either as total glycosylated hemoglobin (TGH) or glycosylation of subfractions such as the A_1 or A_{1c}. Hemoglobinopathies can affect all of these tests except the TGH. Glycohemoglobins reflect the average blood glucose over the previous 60 to 90 days. They are useful not only for confirming the degree of glycemic control but also for identifying possible falsification or errors in HBGM results. Glycohemoglobins are useful motivating tools for the patient; it often becomes a perceived challenge to reduce the result within the constraints of hypoglycemia. It is recommended that this test be done at least two to four times per year in all patients. Given that the

TABLE 20.2. Home blood glucose monitoring units

Meter	Manufacturer	Test time (seconds)	Blot/wipe required	Telephone no.
Companion 2 Pen 2	MediSense	20	No	800-537-3575
Exactech Companion/Pen	MediSense	30	No	800-537-3575
Accu-chek III	Boehringer-Mannheim	120	Yes	800-858-8072
Tracer II	Boehringer-Mannheim	120	Yes	800-858-8072
Accu-chek Easy	Boehringer-Mannheim	[a]	No	800-858-8072
Glucometer III	Ames	60	Yes	800-348-8100
One Touch II	Lifescan	45	No	800-227-8862
Answer	Wampole	90	No	800-525-6718
Precision qid	MediSense	20	No	800-537-3575
Accu-chek Advantage	Boehringer-Mannheim	< 40	No	800-858-8072
Accu-chek Instant	Boehringer-Mannheim	12	No	800-858-8072
One Touch Profile	Lifescan	45	No	800-227-8862

[a]Test time is dependent on blood glucose level.

DCCT demonstrated a linear relationship between the glycohemoglobin (all the way into the normal, nondiabetic range) and microvascular complication risk, the ideal is therefore normalization of the TGH within the constraints of hypoglycemia. In addition to markers of glycemic control, it is critical to monitor other clinical parameters. Annual lipid profiles are an integral part of overall DM care in view of the high prevalence of dyslipidemia especially in the patient with type II DM. In type I DM patients, lipid disturbances are uncommon unless patients are in poor glycemic control, have a familial dyslipidemia, or have renal insufficiency. Markers of nephropathy are also important to measure. The earliest marker, microalbuminuria, is not only a forerunner of overt clinical nephropathy but also a marker for greatly increased cardiovascular risk in both type I and type II patients.[16,17] Microalbuminuria can be conveniently measured in spot urine specimens or by overnight albumin excretion rates.[18]

Patient Education

Patient attention to management principles decidedly affects short-term metabolic control and ultimately has an impact on long-term complications. The interactions of nurse educators and dietitians are important. The presence of family members and significant others during the educational sessions is vital to a successful outcome. Education must encompass a comprehensive understanding of the pathophysiology of DM and its complications and the importance of attaining and sustaining metabolic control. Accurate HBGM is critical; after initial instruction, periodic reassessment of performance technique helps to ensure continued accuracy.

Education should also focus on dietary principles. For individuals with diabetes, the current dietary recommendations are a diet containing at least 50% carbohydrate, less than 30% fat, and 20% or less protein. Caloric requirements are based on ideal body weight (IBW)—not actual body weight. We calculate IBW by the Hamwi formula.[19]

Women

100 pounds for 5 feet
5 pounds for every additional inch
Example: Woman 5′3" = 115 pounds IBW

Men

106 pounds for 5 feet
6 pounds for every additional inch
Example: Man 5′8" = 154 pounds IBW

Based on anthropometric measures, 10% may be subtracted or added based on small body frame or large body frame, respectively.

Basal caloric requirements then are as follows.

Woman 5′3": IBW = 115 pounds
115 × 10 kcal = 1150 kcal/day

Add 300 to 400 kcal/day for moderate to strenuous activity. Subtract 500 kcal/day for 1 pound per week weight loss.

Because individuals with DM type II are generally hyperinsulinemic, diet prescriptions for weight loss and maintenance require a lower caloric level than previously mentioned. The activity factor in kilocalories (300–400 kcal/ day) can be modified in these individuals. For the type II DM patient, caloric restriction is of major importance. In contrast, diet for the type I DM patient should involve careful consistency of carbohydrate intake. Achieving this degree of dietary education generally requires several sessions with a nutrition specialist. Dietary principles are an ongoing exercise, and eradication of myths and misconceptions is a major task. Unfortunately, many patients still perceive that "sugar-free" implies carbohydrate-free and that "sugar-free" foods cannot affect blood glucose control. This belief, of course, fails to recognize the monomer/ polymer concept and the fact that most carbohydrates are ultimately digested into glucose. In addition to maintaining carbohydrate consistency, patients must learn carbohydrate augmentation for physical activity in the absence of insulin reduction. Patients also need instruction on carbohydrate strategies for dealing with intercurrent illness during which the usual complex carbohydrate may be substituted with simple carbohydrate. Although it has long been said that diet is the cornerstone of DM management,[20] effective DM dietary education is still problematic owing to time constraints and reimbursement problems.

Insulin-requiring patients must be aware of the many facets of insulin therapy. Accurate drawing-up and mixing of insulin is an assumption that is often not founded in reality. Site selection, consistency, and rotation are crucial. Insulin absorption is most rapid from the abdomen; the arms, legs, and buttocks, respectively, are next. We find that administering the premeal insulin in the abdomen optimizes postmeal control (assuming the use of Regular insulin). In contrast, the buttocks, as the slowest absorption site, is not a good choice for premeal injections. However, the lower buttocks is an ideal site for bedtime injections to minimize nocturnal hypoglycemia. Haphazard site selection and rotation can lead to erratic glycemic control. Because of the variability in absorption among sites, we suggest site consistency, that is, using the same site at the same time of day (all breakfast injections in the abdomen, all dinner injections in the arms, all bedtime injections in the lower buttocks). Broad rotation within the sites is important to eliminate local lipohypertrophy.[21] Careful premeal timing of insulin injections (generally 30 minutes) is also required for optimal postprandial glycemic control. Patients need a comprehensive perspective on insulin adjustments[22] for hyperglycemia, altered physical activity, illness management, travel, and alcohol consumption.

Patients need education on the pathophysiology, prevention, and treatment of microvascular complications. Education on macrovascular risk factors and their modification for prevention of cardiovascular, cerebrovascular, and peripheral vascular disease is also critical. Patients can have a considerable impact on decreasing foot problems and amputations with simple attention to hygiene (avoidance of foot soaks), daily foot inspection, and the use of appropriate footwear. These measures can greatly reduce the incidence of trauma, sepsis, and ultimately amputations.[23]

Diabetic Complications

Complications of DM include those that are specific to DM and those that are nonspecific but are accelerated by the presence of DM. The specific complications of DM are microvascular, the triad of retinopathy, neuropathy, and nephropathy. Atherosclerosis, a common complication in patients with DM, is not specific to DM but is greatly accelerated by its presence. A major misconception among patients and even physicians is that the complications of DM tend to be less severe in patients with type II DM. In terms of macrovascular disease, patients with type II DM or impaired glucose tolerance have greatly accelerated macrovascular disease; patients with type II also suffer significant morbidity from microvascular complications.

Retinopathy

Retinopathy, the commonest cause of new-onset blindness during middle life, is classified as background, preproliferative, and proliferative. The need for early diagnosis and treatment with laser cannot be overemphasized for the preservation of vision. Several studies clearly document the importance of annual examinations by an ophthalmologist for all patients.[24] Good visual acuity does not exclude significant retinal pathology; unfortunately, many patients believe good visual acuity implies an absence of significant retinal disease.

Neuropathy

The clinical spectrum of diabetic neuropathy is outlined in Table 20.3.

Nephropathy/Hypertension

Diabetic nephropathy may first manifest as microalbuminuria, detected on a spot urine determination or by the timed overnight albumin excretion rate. The presence of microalbuminuria should alert the patient and

TABLE 20.3. Classification of diabetic neuropathy

Type	Signs and symptoms
Sensory peripheral polyneuropathy	Pain and dysesthesia Glove and stocking sensory loss Loss of reflexes Muscle weakness/wasting
Autonomic	Orthostatic hypotension Gastroparesis, diarrhea, atonic bladder, impotence, anhidrosis, gustatory sweating, cardiac denervation on ECG
Mononeuropathy	Cranial nerve palsy Carpal tunnel syndrome Ulnar nerve palsy
Amyotrophy	Acute anterior thigh pain Weakness of hip flexion Muscle wasting
Radiculopathy	Pain and sensory loss in a dermatomal distribution

physician to the need for stringent glycemic control; such control has been shown to decrease the progression from microalbuminuria to clinical proteinuria and attendant evolution of hypertension. Hypertension increases the rate of deterioration of renal function in patients with DM, and aggressive treatment is mandatory. The Captopril Diabetic Nephropathy Study demonstrated that treatment with the angiotensin-converting enzyme (ACE) inhibitor captopril was associated with a 50% reduction in the risk of the combined endpoints of death, dialysis, and transplantation in macroproteinuric (> 500 mg/24 hr) type I diabetic patients. Overall, the risk of doubling the serum creatinine was reduced by 48% in captopril-treated patients. The beneficial effects were seen in both normotensive and hypertensive patients such that captopril at a dose of 25 mg PO tid is approved for use in normotensive proteinuric (> 500 mg/24 hr) type I diabetic patients.[25] We also favor the use of ACE inhibitors and calcium channel blockers in light of data that show decreasing proteinuria with many of these agents over and above that achievable with conventional antihypertensive therapy. In addition, α-blockers have a favorable metabolic and side effect profile. Avoidance of excessive dietary protein intake is also important, as excessive dietary protein may be involved in renal hypertrophy and glomerular hyperfiltration. Strict glycemic control even over a 3-week period can decrease renal size (as seen on ultrasonography) and decrease the hyperfiltration associated with amino acid infusions to levels comparable to those of normal, non-DM individuals.[26] Nationwide clinical trials with pimagedine (an inhibitor of protein glycosylation and cross-linking) are ongoing for both type I and type II diabetes and hopefully will demonstrate slowing of progression of not only nephropathy but also other diabetic complications.

Patients with DM in general are salt-sensitive, having diminished ability to excrete a sodium load with an attendant rise in blood pressure; therefore avoidance of excessive dietary sodium intake is important. Hyperinsulinemia and insulin resistance are also important in the genesis of hypertension, with insulin-resistant patients having higher circulating insulin levels to maintain normal glucose levels. Associated with this insulin resistance and hyperinsulinemia is the occurrence of elevated blood pressures even in nondiabetic individuals. Insulin is antinatriuretic and stimulates the sympathetic nervous system; both mechanisms may be important in the genesis of hypertension. Hypertension exacerbates retinopathy, nephropathy, and macrovascular disease and must be diagnosed and managed aggressively. When life style modifications fail to control blood pressure, the pharmacologic agent chosen should be not only efficacious but kind to the metabolic milieu. β-Blockers and diuretics should be avoided whenever possible, as they worsen insulin resistance. ACE inhibitors are a good choice in the proteinuric patient; calcium channel blockers are a good choice for the angina patient; and α-blockers are a good choice in the patient with benign prostatic hyperplasia. Monotherapy is frequently unsuccessful, especially in the setting of nephropathy, such that combination therapy is frequently needed with special attention to underlying concomitant medical problems.

Macrovascular Disease

Macrovascular disease is the major cause of premature death and considerable morbidity in individuals with DM, especially those with type II DM. Conventional risk factors for macrovascular disease deserve special attention in DM; they include smoking, lack of physical activity, dietary fat intake, obesity, hypertension, and hyperlipidemia. Correction and control of hyperlipidemia through improved metabolic control and the use of diet or pharmacotherapy is mandatory for the DM patient. The National Cholesterol Education Program guidelines[27] are of special importance to the diabetic, as are the American Diabetes Association guidelines[28] for the treatment of hypertriglyceridemia, with pharmacotherapy now being indicated for patients with persistent elevation in triglycerides above 250 mg/dl. LDL-cholesterol lowering has been demonstrated to confer greater coronary event risk reduction and mortality reduction in diabetic patients than in nondiabetic patients. DM is one of the few diseases in which women have greater morbidity and mortality than men, especially in terms of macrovascular disease, with the black woman bearing the greatest load.

Foot Problems

Foot problems in the diabetic are a major cause of hospitalization and amputations. They generally constitute a combination of sepsis, ischemia, and neuropathy. The presence of significant neuropathy facilitates repetitive trauma without appropriate pain and ultimately nonhealing. In addition, neuropathy may mask manifestations of peripheral vascular disease (PVD) (e.g., claudication and rest pain) such that patients may have critical ischemia with minimal symptoms. Therefore PVD may be difficult to diagnose on usual clinical grounds alone. Not only may neuropathy mask clinical symptoms, the clinical signs may be somewhat confusing. Patients with less severe neuropathy may exhibit cold feet related to arteriovenous shunting, and patients with more severe neuropathy may exhibit cutaneous hyperemia related to autosympathectomy. Noninvasive vascular testing along with clinical evaluation is helpful for the diagnosis and management of PVD. Calcific medial arterial disease is common and can cause erroneously high blood pressure recordings in the extremities, confusing the assessment of the severity of

PVD. Severe ischemia with symptoms and nonhealing wounds generally require surgical intervention. Milder symptoms and disease may respond favorably to enhanced physical activity and the use of the hemorrheologic agent pentoxifylline. Appropriate podiatric footwear and management are important to both ulcer healing and prevention of repetitive trauma.[23–29] A reduced ankle-brachial index at the posterior tibial artery in isolation has been demonstrated to be an important marker, conferring a 3.8-fold increased risk of cardiovascular death.

Achieving Glycemic Control

Type I DM

Optimal management of type I DM requires an educated, motivated patient and a physiologic insulin regimen. The major challenge is physiologic insulin replacement matched to dietary carbohydrate with appropriate compensation for variables such as exercise. Physiologic insulin replacement involves intensive insulin therapy with multiple injections (three or more per day) or the use of continuous subcutaneous insulin infusion (CSII) pumps. Several regimens have been utilized to achieve glycemic control (Table 20.4). The conventional split-mix regimen combining regular and an intermediate-acting insulin in the morning before breakfast and in the evening before supper has the major limitation of nocturnal hypoglycemia from the presupper intermediate-acting insulin when stringent control of the fasting blood glucose is sought. Dividing the evening insulin dose—delivering Regular insulin before supper and the intermediate-acting insulin at bedtime—can afford a significant reduction in the risk of nighttime hypoglycemia.[30] Most patients require 0.5 to 0.8 U/kg body weight to achieve acceptable glycemic control. It is generally distributed as two-thirds in the morning and one-third in the evening, with (1) one-third of the morning dose being Regular and two-thirds being intermediate-acting insulin; (2) 50% of the evening insulin as Regular insulin before supper; and (3) the remaining 50% as intermediate-acting insulin at bedtime (10 p.m. to

TABLE 20.4. Multiple injection regimens

Breakfast	Lunch	Dinner	Bed (10 p.m.–1 a.m.)
R + N or L	0	R	N or L
R + U	R	R + U	0
R	R	R	N or L

R = regular; N = NPH; L = lente; U = ultralente.

1 a.m.). These doses are modified according to individual dietary preferences and carbohydrate distribution.

In addition, patients need algorithms to adjust their insulin for hyperglycemia, varying physical activity, and intercurrent illnesses. Many episodes of severe hypoglycemia occur in the context of unplanned physical activity and dietary errors; likewise, many episodes of ketoacidosis occur during episodes of intercurrent illness. For physical activity, a reduction in insulin dosage of 1 to 2 units per 20 to 30 minutes of activity generally suffices depending on the intensity of the activity. The other option is to augment carbohydrate intake (i.e., 15 g carbohydrate prior to every 20–30 minutes of activity). During illness it is important that patients appreciate the fact that illness is a situation of insulin resistance and that all of the routine insulin should be administered. Carbohydrate from meals and snacks may be substituted for by simple carbohydrate in the form of liquids such as juices and regular ginger ale. It is important that all treatment regimens be individualized and therapeutic options for insulin administration be discussed. In this way, patients' life styles can be accommodated and appropriate insulin regimens tailored.[22] For example, using a basal-bolus regimen with Ultralente, it is possible to delay the lunchtime injection depending on the patient's time constraints; furthermore, the insulin dose can be adjusted depending on carbohydrate intake and physical activity. In some individuals, a noontime injection is not feasible. A schoolchild or a person engaged in construction work might find it difficult to accommodate a prelunch insulin injection and might be better off with a morning intermediate-acting insulin to cover the lunchtime carbohydrate intake, with regular insulin being taken to cover the breakfast carbohydrate intake as a combined prebreakfast dose.

Severe hypoglycemia in the well-educated, adherent, motivated patient on a physiologic insulin regimen is uncommon. Most severe hypoglycemic episodes are explained on the basis of diet or exercise and insulin-adjustment errors.[31] The individual who is attempting to achieve true euglycemia, however, is at risk for periodic easily self-treated hypoglycemia. See Table 20.5 for management strategies. For the individual with type I DM who has been educated thoroughly, is on a physiologic insulin regimen with an agreed diet plan, and has algorithms for illness and physical activity, failure to attain the desired degree of glycemic control is largely related to psychosocial variables. Lispro (Humalog) is a new fast-acting insulin analog created by a two-amino-acid substitution in the insulin molecule. Lispro, like Regular insulin, forms stable hexamers in the insulin vial. However, after injection Lispro dissociates much faster to the rapidly absorbed monomeric form. This rapid onset of action allows patients to inject Lispro at the beginning of the meal rather that the traditional 30 minute premeal injection of Regular insulin. In addition, the peak action of Lispro closely matches the postprandial blood

TABLE 20.5. Hypoglycemia management strategies

Causes	Signs and symptoms	Treatment
Insulin/OHA overdose	Sympathomimetic	Conscious—15-g
Carbohydrate omission	Coldness	Simple carbohydrate
Missed/late meal	Clamminess	Juice 4 oz
Missed/late snack	Shaking	Regular soda 6 oz
	Diaphoresis	3 B-D glucose tablets
	Headaches	7 Lifesavers
Uncompensated activity/exercise	Neuroglycopenic	Unconscious
	Confusion	Glucagon S.C.[a]
	Disorientation	D_{50} 50 cc
	Loss of consciousness	

OHA = oral hypoglycemic agent.
[a]We do not recommend the use of gel products (e.g., Monojel) for treatment of unconscious hypoglycemia, as aspiration is a potential hazard.

glucose peak, which in theory potentially reduces the risk of hypoglycemia and eliminates the need for a carbohydrate snack 3 hours after injection of Regular insulin. On the negative side, patients who hitherto used a regimen of pre-meal Regular insulin coupled with a bedtime (11 p.m.) injection of intermediate-acting insulin may experience insulin run-out before meals (lunch, dinner, bedtime) owing to the shorter duration of action of the Lispro. This problem may be circumvented by adding a small dose of intermediate-acting (NPH/Lente) insulin or long-acting (Ultralente) insulin in the morning.

Type II DM

In most instances, type II DM is a syndrome of insulin resistance coupled with variable secretory defects, both of which can be compounded by glucotoxicity. As insulin resistance is related to genetic factors, obesity, and sedentary life style, the mainstay of treatment for the type II diabetic patient is correction of insulin resistance through diet and exercise and reversal of glucotoxicity acutely through reestablishment of euglycemia. Many patients still perceive themselves to be more absolutely insulin-deficient than insulin-resistant and are willing to accept insulin therapy as a compromise in the context of failed weight loss efforts. In addition, many patients perceive pharmacotherapy to be equivalent to a diet and exercise regimen alone, assuming the desired degree of glycemic control is achieved. Chronic nonadherence to a diet regimen with resultant failure of weight loss or progressive obesity frequently leads to mislabeling the patient as a "brittle diabetic." It is important to avoid premature and unnecessary insulin therapy in these individuals and to stress to them the importance of diet and exercise as the most physiologic approach to controlling their metabolic disorder.

Pharmacotherapy for type II DM (Table 20.6) can be directed at (1) decreasing insulin resistance and increasing insulin sensitization (metformin hydrochloride troglitazone), (2) augmentation of insulin secretion and action (sulfonylureas), and (3) interference with the digestion and absorption of dietary carbohydrate (α-glucosidase inhibitors). Metformin hydrochloride (Glucophage) is a true insulin sensitizer, enhancing peripheral glucose utilization and decreasing hepatic glucose production. As it has no effect on insulin secretion, when used as monotherapy it cannot induce hypoglycemia. Ideal candidates for treatment are overweight or obese type II diabetic patients. The potentially fatal side effect of lactic acidosis generally occurs only when metformin is used in contraindicated patients: those with renal insufficiency, liver disease, alcohol excess, or underlying hypoxic states.

Sulfonylureas enhance insulin secretion and action. The second and third generation agents are preferred owing to their increased potency, shorter duration of action, and better side effects profile. Concern about possible cardiotoxicity of sulfonylureas related to the University Group Diabetes Program (UGDP) study has largely disappeared, given the emergence of data to support the safety of these agents from the cardiovascular perspective.

α-Glucosidase inhibition by acarbose primarily decreases postprandial blood glucoses by direct interference on digestion and absorption of dietary carbohydrate. This agent is most commonly used as an adjunct to metformin hydrochloride or sulfonylurea therapy. Monotherapy with acarbose is indicated in the newly diagnosed, mildly hyperglycemic patient. Increased intestinal gas formation is the most common adverse effect and does improve with time. Gradual dose titration to 100 mg tid minimizes this problem.

Insulin therapy in type II diabetic patients is indicated in situations where patients are acutely decompensated and are more insulin-resistant due to intercurrent illnesses. Clearly, short-term insulin therapy can reestablish glycemic control acutely in many individuals. However, reevaluation of endogenous insulin production with C-peptide determinations is important. Most obese patients with type II DM have considerable elevation in their C-peptide levels, assuming they are not glucotoxic from antecedent chronic hyperglycemia. The initiation of insulin therapy in a type II patient remains controversial in terms of indications and optimum insulin regimen. The dilemma revolves around the obese C-peptide–positive patient who was achieving good glycemic control in the short term with insulin. This individual often suffers progressive obesity and worsening glycemic control owing to worsening insulin resistance, thereby increasing requirements for exogenous insulin. Thus frequently insulin therapy in an obese C-peptide–positive patient fails to achieve its primary goal of sustained improved glycemic

TABLE 20.6. Oral agent summary

Parameter	Metformin/ troglitazone	Sulfonylureas	Acarbose	Repaglinide
Mode of action	↓ Hepatic glucose ↑ Glucose utilization	↑ Insulin secretion ↓ Hepatic glucose production	α-Glucosidase inhibition → ↓ CHO absorption from GI tract	↑ Insulin secretion
Glucose effects	Fasting and postprandial	Fasting and postprandial	Postprandial	Fasting and postprandial
Hypoglycemia when used as monotherapy	No	Yes	No	Yes; lower risk than that with sulfonylureas
Weight gain	No/possible	Yes	No	Yes; less than that seen with sulfonylureas
Insulin levels	↓	↑	↔	↑
Side effects	GI (self-limiting sx of nausea, anorexia, diarrhea)/none comparable to placebo ↑ LFTs/serious liver injury (troglitazone)	Potential allergic reaction if sulfa allergy, SIADH, drug interactions with first generation agents	GI (flatulence, diarrhea, abdominal distension)	Similar to placebo
Lipid effects	↓	↓ or ↔	↓	↓ or ↔
Starting dose for a 70-kg man	500 mg bid with meals/ 200 mg/d	Varies with each agent Glyburide 2.5 mg qd Glucotrol XL 5 mg qd Glynase 3 mg qd Amaryl 2 mg qd	25 mg tid with first bite of meal	0.5 mg immediately prior to each meal and snack
Maximum dose	850 mg tid/ 600 mg/d	Varies with each agent Glyburide 10 mg bid Glucotrol XL 20 mg qd Glynase 6 mg bid Amaryl 8 mg qd	100 mg tid with first bite of meal	4 mg with each of three meals and one snack; 16 mg/day maximum
Contraindications	Renal dysfunction/ Hepatic dysfunction History of EtOH abuse Chronic conditions associated with hypoxia (CHF, AMI, COPD, asthma) Acute conditions associated with potential for hypoxia (CHF, AMI, surgery) Conditions associated with renal dysfunction (IV contrast)/hepatic dysfunction	Hepatic dysfunction Significant renal dysfunction	Type I DM Cirrhosis Inflammatory bowel disease Bowel obstruction Chronic conditions with maldigestion or malabsorption	Type I DM Careful dose titration in renal and/or hepatic dysfunction

control. In addition, perpetuation of the obese state, or indeed worsening thereof, in conjunction with progressive hyperinsulinemia raises concerns about the impact of this worsened metabolic milieu on hypertension, dyslipidemia, and the atherosclerotic process. Initiation of insulin therapy should therefore be undertaken cautiously in most patients and their progress carefully monitored in terms not only of glycemic control but also of hypertension, dyslipidemia, and obesity.

Many insulin regimens have been used to treat type II DM, many being similar to those used in the type I setting. Trends have focused on the use of bedtime insulin therapy in these individuals on the grounds that it can maximally affect the dawn hepatic glucose output/disposal and peak insulin resistance, thereby achieving the best possible fasting blood glucose and minimizing glucotoxicity. Minimizing glucotoxicity facilitates daytime islet secretory function and minimizes the need for daytime insulin therapy.[32] Combination therapy with insulin and oral hypoglycemic agents (OHAs) seems theoretically sound, with OHAs presumably enhancing insulin sensitivity and reducing the need for exogenous insulin. The data, however, support only modest improvements in glycemic control and modest reduction in insulin requirements at best. One such regimen has been the use of an intermediate-acting insulin at bedtime at a dose of 0.2 U/kg coupled with a daytime second-generation OHA. Unlike the situation in the type I diabetic patient, hypoglycemia tends to be uncommon in type II patients owing to their fundamental insulin resistance. Hypoglycemia can occur in the type II patient on either insulin or OHAs. OHAs should be used with caution in patients with hepatic or renal impairment and the elderly.

Troglitazone, a thiazolidinedione, is a unique antihyperglycemic agent that binds to the PPAR nuclear receptor, amplifies the insulin signal, and reduces insulin requirements in insulin type II patients. In addition to glucose-lowering properties, this insulin sensitizing agent has beneficial effects on the other components of Syndrome X.[33] Serious liver injury has been reported with troglitazone, including one death and one patient requiring liver transplantation. Liver enzymes should be monitored within 1–2 months of initiating therapy and every 3 months thereafter. Uniquely, troglitazone can be safely used in patients with renal insufficiency without the need for dosage adjustment. Bioavailability is significantly enhanced by ingestion with food, however the onset of glucose lowering is very gradual such that individualized downward dose titration of insulin therapy may not be needed for at least 2 weeks. The initial recommended starting dose is 200 mg qd, the maximum 600 mg qd, with the mean dose in clinical trials being 400 mg qd. Currently troglitazone is approved for a broad range of type 2 diabetes mellitus patients, either as monotherapy or combined with sulfonylureas or with insulin.

Repaglinide (Prandin) is a benzoic acid derivative unrelated to sulfonylureas. Repaglinide causes rapid insulin release from pancreatic islets in response to hyperglycemia. Repaglinide is rapidly absorbed from the gastrointestinal tract. It acts via closure of ATP-dependent potassium channels in the islet cells with resultant insulin release. Peak plasma drug levels occur in approximately 1 hour; the drug is rapidly cleared with a $t_{1/2}$ of 1 hour. The lack of sustained elevation in insulin levels that is seen with sulfonylurea use results in improved postprandial glucose control, less hypoglycemia, less weight gain, and possibly better long-term preservation of islet function. Repaglinide is approved for use as monotherapy or in combination with Metformin.

Gestational Diabetes Mellitus

Gestational DM (GDM) is an important entity in terms of maternal morbidity, fetal macrosomia, associated obstetric complications, and neonatal hypoglycemia. GDM should be sought in all patients using current screening and diagnostic guidelines (Table 20.1). Early, aggressive management can significantly improve outcome. The initial strategy for the patient with GDM is dietary control; when the goals of pregnancy are not being achieved (i.e., premeal and bedtime glucose < 90 mg/dl and 1 hour postprandial glucose < 120 mg/dl), insulin therapy is initiated. Given the data linking postprandial blood glucose levels to macrosomia, it is important that postprandial glucose levels are controlled adequately and that target glucose levels are achieved.[34,35] In our center this goal is most readily and predictably reached with premeal regular insulin and overnight intermediate-acting insulin. Most women with GDM have reestablishment of euglycemia immediately postpartum. These individuals, however, should be counseled on the long-term risks of prior GDM for developing overt type II DM, which may occur in as many as 70% of these individuals.[36] In addition, the hazards of uncorrected obesity, associated insulin resistance, dyslipidemia, hypertension, and potential for premature cardiovascular death must be addressed.[37]

Individuals with type I DM who are contemplating pregnancy should be in optimal glycemic control prior to conception to decrease the risk of congenital malformations and the incidence of maternal-fetal complications. The achievement of two consecutive glycosylated hemoglobin levels in the nondiabetic range is recommended before conception. A regimen of premeal Regular insulin and overnight intermediate-acting insulin (alternatively, CSII) may readily achieve these goals. Careful follow-up by a skilled management team is essential to an optimum outcome.[35]

Contraception and DM

The use of oral contraceptives (OCs) in women with type I or type II DM has been an area of controversy,[35] with many believing that significant elevations occur in blood glucose along with an increased risk of vascular complications. In our experience the incidence of such problems is minimal given a woman who is normotensive and has an absence of vascular disease; therefore we believe OCs can be safely used. Even for a woman in poor glycemic control, OCs are still the most effective form of contraception.

Diabetic Ketoacidosis

Diabetic ketoacidosis (DKA) is the ultimate expression of absolute insulin deficiency resulting in uncontrolled lipolysis, free fatty acid delivery to the liver, and ultimately accelerated ketone body production. Insulin deficiency at the level of the liver results in uncontrolled hepatic glucose output via gluconeogenesis and glycogenolysis; and with insulin-mediated skeletal muscle glucose uptake being inhibited, hyperglycemia rapidly ensues. The attendant osmotic diuresis due to hyperglycemia results in progressive dehydration and a decreasing glomerular filtration rate. Dehydration may be compounded by gastrointestinal fluid losses (e.g., emesis from ketones or a primary gastrointestinal illness with concurrent diarrhea). Insensible fluid losses from febrile illness may further compound the dehydration.

Diagnosis of DKA is fairly characteristic in the newly presenting or established type I diabetic patient. The history of polydipsia, polyuria, weight loss, and Kussmaul's respirations are virtually pathognomonic. Physical examination is directed at assessing the level of hydration (e.g., orthostasis) and possibly the underlying and precipitating illness. Measurement of urine ketone, urine glucose, and blood glucose levels can rapidly confirm the clinical suspicion, with arterial pH, serum bicarbonate, and ketones validating the diagnosis. A thorough search for an underlying precipitating illness remains axiomatic (e.g., urosepsis, respiratory tract infection, or silent myocardial infarction). Treatment is directed at correcting: (1) dehydration/hypotension; (2) ketonemia/acidosis; (3) uncontrolled hepatic glucose output/hyperglycemia; and (4) insulin resistance of the DKA/underlying illness. Of course specific treatment is directed to any defined underlying illnesses.

Dehydration and hypotension require urgent treatment with a 5- to 6-liter deficit to be anticipated in most individuals. Initial treatment is 0.9% NaCl, with 1 to 2 L/hr being given for the first 2 hours and flow rates thereafter being titrated to the individual's clinical status. Use of a

Swan-Ganz catheter is prudent in the individual with cardiac compromise. Potassium replacement at a concentration of 10 to 40 mEq/L is critical to replace the usual deficits of more than 5 mEq/kg once the patient's initial serum potassium level is known and urine output is documented. Giving 50% of the potassium as KCl and 50% as KPO_4 appears theoretically sound, but phosphate replacement has not been shown to alter the clinical outcome. Bicarbonate therapy is generally reserved for patients with a pH of less than 7.0, plasma bicarbonate less than 5.0 mEq/L, severe hyperkalemia, or a deep coma. Bicarbonate is administered by slow infusion 50 to 100 mEq over 1 to 2 hours with the therapeutic endpoint being a pH higher than 7.1 rather than normalization of the pH. Overzealous use of bicarbonate can result in severe hypokalemia with attendant cardiac arrhythmogenicity, paradoxic central nervous system acidosis, and possible lactic acidosis due to tissue hypoxia. Intravenous insulin therapy is initiated at a dose of 0.1 U/kg/hr with rapid titration every 1 to 2 hours should a 75 to 100 mg/dl/hr decrease in glucose not be achieved. Insulin therapy at this relatively high dose is needed to combat the insulin resistance of the hormonal milieu of DKA (i.e., high levels of glucagon, cortisol, growth hormone, and catecholamines). Given that hepatic glucose output is more rapidly controlled than ketogenesis, the insulin infusion rate can be maintained by switching the intravenous infusion to dextrose 5% to 10% when blood glucose is less than 250 mg/dl. The insulin infusion is continued until the patient is ketone-free, clinically well, and able to resume oral feeding. It is of paramount importance that subcutaneous insulin be instituted promptly at the time of refeeding.

Flow sheets should be generated documenting the following:

1. Patient admission weight relative to previous weights with serial weights every 6 to 12 hours, urine ketones, and fluid balance
2. Vital signs and mental status every 1 to 2 hours
3. Bedside glucose monitoring every 1 to 2 hours
4. Urine ketones every 1 to 2 hours
5. Fluid balance
6. Blood gases and arterial pH on admission, repeating until pH is over 7.1
7. Serum potassium on admission and then every 2 to 4 hours
8. Serum ketones on admission and then every 2 to 4 hours
9. Complete blood count, serum chemistries, chest roentgenogram, electrocardiogram, and appropriate cultures on admission
10. Abnormal chemistries other than potassium repeated every 4 hours until normal[38,39]

References

1. Clinical practice recommendations: 1990–1991. Diabetes Care 1991.14 Suppl 2:1–81.

2. The European patient's charter. Diabet Med 1991;8:782–3.
3. Landin-Olsson M, Nilsson KO, Lernmark A, Sunkvist G. Islet cell antibodies and fasting C-peptide predict insulin requirement at diagnosis of diabetes mellitus. Diabetologia 1990;33:561–8.
4. Zeigler AG, Herskowitz RD, Jackson RA, et al. Predicting type I diabetes. Diabetes Care 1990;13: 762–75.
5. Keller RJ, Eisenbarth GS, Jackson RA. Insulin prophylaxis in individuals at high risk of type I diabetes. N Engl J Med 1993;341:927–8.
6. Helmrich SP, Ragland DR, Leung RW, Paffenbarger RS. Physical activity and reduced occurrence of non-insulin-dependent diabetes mellitus. N Engl J Med 1991;325:147–52.
7. DeFronzo RA. The triumvirate: B-cell, muscle. and liver: a collusion responsible for NIDDM. Diabetes 1988;37:667–87.
8. Erikkson J, Franssila-Kallunki A, Ekstrand A. Early metabolic defects in persons at increased risk for non-insulin-dependent diabetes mellitus. N Engl J Med 1989;321:337–43.
9. DeFronzo RA, Bonadonna RC, Ferrannini E. Pathogenesis of NIDDM. Diabetes Care 1992;15:318–68.
10. Clark PM, Hales CN. Measurement of insulin secretion in type 2 diabetes: problems and pitfalls. Diabet Med 1992; 9:503–12.
11. Bjornstorp P. Metabolic implications of body fat distribution. Diabetes Care 1991;14:1132–43.
12. Ferrannini E, Buzzigoli G, Bonadonna B, et al. Insulin resistance in essential hypertension. N Engl J Med 1987;317:350–7.
13. Zavaroni I, Bonora E, Pagliara M, et al. Risk factors for coronary artery disease in healthy persons with hyperinsulinemia and normal glucose tolerance. N Engl J Med 1989;320:703–6.
14. Kern TS, Engerman RL. Arrest of glomerulonephropathy in diabetic dogs by improved glycemic control. Diabetologia 1990;33:522–5.
15. Diabetes Control and Complications Trial Research Group. The effect of intensive treatment of diabetes on the development and progression of long-term complications in insulin-dependent diabetes mellitus. N Engl J Med 1993;329:977–86.
16. Viberti GC. Etiology and prognostic significance of albuminuria in diabetes. Diabetes Care 1988;11:840–8.
17. Deckert T, Feldt-Rasmussen B, Borch-Johnson K, et al. Albuminuria reflects widespread vascular damage: the Steno hypothesis. Diabetologia 1989;32: 219–26.
18. Marshall SM. Screening for microalbuminuria: which measurement? Diabet Med 1991;8:706–11.
19. Hamwi GL. Changing dietary concepts in therapy. In: Danowski TS, editor. Diabetes mellitus: diagnosis and treatment. New York: American Diabetes Association, 1964:73–8.
20. Wood FC, Bierman EL. Is diet the cornerstone in management of diabetes? N Engl J Med 1986;1244–7.
21. Zehrer C, Hansen R, Bantl J. Reducing blood glucose variability by use of abdominal injection sites. Diabetes Educator 1990;16:474–7.

22. Skyler JS, Skyler DL, Seigler DE, O'Sullivan M. Algorithms for adjustment of insulin dosage by patients who monitor blood glucose. Diabetes Care 1981;4:311–8.
23. Frykberg RG. Management of diabetic foot problems (Joslin Clinic). Philadelphia: Saunders, 1984.
24. Singerman LJ. Early-treatment diabetic retinopathy study: good news for diabetic patients and health care professionals [editorial]. Diabetes Care 1986;9:426–9.
25. Lewis EJ, Hunsicker LG, Bain RE, Rohde RD. The effect of angiotenisin-converting enzyme inhibition on diabetic nephropathy. N Engl J Med 1993;329:1456–62.
26. Tuttle KR, Bruton JL, Perusek MC, et al. Effect of strict glycemic control on renal enlargement in insulin-dependent diabetes mellitus. N Engl J Med 1991;324:1626–32.
27. Report of the National Cholesterol Education Program expert panel on detection, evaluation, and treatment of high blood cholesterol in adults. Arch Intern Med 1988;148:36–69.
28. Role of cardiovascular risk factors in prevention and treatment of macrovascular disease in diabetes. Diabetes Care 1992;15:68–74.
29. Flynn MD, Tooke JE. Aetiology of diabetic foot ulceration: a role for the microcirculation? Diabet Med 1992;9:320–9.
30. Skyler JS. Insulin treatment: therapy for diabetes mellitus and related disorders. Alexandria, VA: American Diabetes Association, 1991:127–37.
31. Bhatia V, Wolfsdorf JI. Severe hypoglycemia in youth with insulin-dependent diabetes mellitus: frequency and causative factors. Pediatrics 1991;88: 1187–93.
32. Groop LC, Widèn E, Ekstrand A, et al. Morning or bedtime NPH insulin combined with sulfonylureas in treatment of NIDDM. Diabetes Care 1992;15:831–4.
33. Saltiel AR, Olefsky JM. Thiazolidinediones in the treatment of insulin resistance and type 2 diabetes. Diabetes 1966; 45:1661–9.
34. Proceedings of the Third International Workshop-Conference on Gestational Diabetes Mellitus. Diabetes 1991;40 Suppl 2:1–201.
35. Jovanovic-Peterson L, Peterson CM. Pregnancy in the diabetic woman: guidelines for a successful outcome. Endocrinol Metab Clin North Am 1992;33:433–56.
36. Kaufmann RC, Amankwah KS, Woodrum J. Development of diabetes in previous gestational diabetic [abstract]. Diabetes 1991;40:137A.
37. Kaufmann RC, Amankwah KS, Woodrum J. Serum lipids in former gestational diabetics. [abstract]. Diabetes 1991;40:192A.
38. Kozak GP, Rolla AR. Diabetic comas. In: Kozak GP, editor. Clinical diabetes mellitus. Philadelphia: Saunders, 1982:109–45.
39. Siperstein MD. Diabetic ketoacidosis and hyperosmolar coma. Endocrinol Metab Clin North Am 1992;33:415–32.

CASE PRESENTATION

Subjective

PATIENT PROFILE

Harold Nelson is a 76-year-old married white man.

PRESENTING PROBLEM

"Blood sugar going up and down."

PRESENT ILLNESS

Mr. Nelson has been diabetic for 24 years. He was initially diet-controlled but has taken glyburide, 5 mg daily, in the morning for the past 3 years. For about 2 months, he has noted wide swings in his blood sugar levels from 60 to more than 300 mg/dl on home blood glucose monitoring. He has had no shakiness or sweating at times of low blood sugar, although sometimes he feels inappropriately weak and sleeps more than usual. His appetite is fair, and he has lost some weight in the past few weeks.

PAST MEDICAL HISTORY, SOCIAL HISTORY, AND FAMILY HISTORY

All are unchanged since his previous visits 2 and 9 months ago (see Chapters 5 and 18).

HABITS

Unchanged except that he reports drinking alcoholic beverages "a little more than usual."

REVIEW OF SYSTEMS

Occasional constipation. Sometimes he has lower leg pain after walking.

- What additional medical history might be important? Why?
- What might you ask to clarify his alcohol use?
- What might you ask to further evaluate the leg pain?

- Have you listened carefully to what Mr. Nelson is trying to tell you?

Objective

VITAL SIGNS

Height, 5 ft 7 in; weight, 160 lb (a decrease of 6 lb in 2 months); blood pressure, 162/84; pulse, 74; respirations, 20; temperature, 37.0°C.

EXAMINATION

The patient is ambulatory and alert. The eyes, ears, nose, and throat—including a funduscopic examination—are normal. The chest is clear to percussion and auscultation. The heart has a regular sinus rhythm, and no murmurs are present. On the abdominal examination, there is no mass or tenderness, and the liver is palpable about 1 cm below the right costal margin. There are Heberden's nodes of both hands and osteoarthritic swelling of other joints, especially the knees. The deep tendon reflexes are normal, and there is no decreased perception of pinprick in the lower extremities.

LABORATORY

An office determination reveals a blood sugar of 270 mg/dl approximately 2 hours after breakfast.

- What more data could you obtain from the physical examination, and why?
- What might you do to help clarify the patient's lower leg pain?
- What—if any—laboratory tests would you order today? Explain.
- What—if any—diagnostic imaging would you order today? Why?

Assessment

- What are possible causes of Mr. Nelson's problems with blood sugar control? How would you explain this to the patient?
- Could the presenting complaint be related to problems in the family? How might you assess this possibility?
- What are possible causes of the weight loss? Of the leg pain?

- What might be the meaning of these problems to the patient? How might you address this issue?

Plan

- Describe your therapeutic recommendations for the patient. How would you explain this to Mr. Nelson?
- Describe your advice regarding diet, alcohol use, and exercise.
- How might you involve other family members in dealing with the problem?
- What continuing care would you advise?

21

Human Immunodeficiency Virus Infection and Acquired Immunodeficiency Syndrome

RONALD H. GOLDSCHMIDT AND JILL J. LEGG

Care for patients with human immunodeficiency virus (HIV) infection requires excellence in all aspects of family practice. The family physician's roles include providing patient education to prevent uninfected persons from becoming infected, identifying and counseling infected persons, delivering comprehensive medical care (including antiretroviral treatment), prophylaxis against opportunistic infections, management of the acquired immunodeficiency syndrome (AIDS), and providing support and care for the family. New manifestations of HIV disease, diagnostic protocols, and drug recommendations for HIV disease[1] change on a regular basis. Epidemiologic, social, and community trends also have important effects on clinical care.

The striking benefits of combination antiretroviral therapy, especially with protease inhibitor drugs, have changed the implications of HIV dramatically. Although long-term outcomes remain unknown, the demonstrated effectiveness of combination therapies has made the hope of prolonged suppression of HIV disease a real possibility. In addition, the ability of antiretroviral therapy to decrease transmission from mother to infant and among health care workers sustaining occupational exposures further establish the efficacy of drug intervention against HIV.

Acute HIV infection usually produces a flu-like syndrome about 2 weeks after transmission. This acute illness is followed by an asymptomatic phase, usually lasting more than 5 years. Immunodeficiency, characterized by progressive destruction of $CD4^+$ (T-helper) lymphocytes, results in susceptibility to opportunistic infections and malignancies. Early symptomatic disease (oral candidiasis, oral hairy leukoplakia, and lymphadenopathy) is followed by the opportunistic infections and malignancies that characterize AIDS[2] (Table 21.1). The average time from infection to AIDS-defining illnesses appears to be about 8 to 11 years.

TABLE 21.1. Identifier diseases for AIDS surveillance case definition

Candidiasis of bronchi, trachea, or lungs
Candidiasis, esophageal
Cervical cancer, invasive
Coccidioidomycosis, disseminated or extrapulmonary
Cryptococcosis, extrapulmonary
Cryptosporidiosis, chronic intestinal (> 1 month duration)
Cytomegalovirus disease (other than liver, spleen, or nodes)
Cytomegalovirus retinitis
HIV encephalopathy
Herpes simplex: chronic ulcer (> 1 month duration); or bronchitis, pneumonitis, or esophagitis
Histoplasmosis, disseminated or extrapulmonary
Isosporiasis, chronic intestinal (> 1 month duration)
Kaposi's sarcoma
Lymphoma, Burkitt's
Lymphoma, immunoblastic
Lymphoma, primary in brain
Mycobacterium-avium intracellularae complex or *M. kansasii* infection, disseminated or extrapulmonary
Mycobacterium tuberculosis infection, any site (pulmonary or extrapulmonary)
Mycobacterial disease, other species or unidentified species, disseminated or extrapulmonary
Pneumocystis carinii pneumonia
Pneumonia, recurrent
Progressive multifocal leukoencephalopathy
Salmonella septicemia, recurrent
Toxoplasmosis of brain
Wasting syndrome due to HIV

Source: Adapted from Centers for Disease Control.[2] With permission.

Risk Factors, Risk Reduction, and Patient Education

The HIV is usually transmitted from person to person by the passage of blood or body fluids such as semen and vaginal secretions. Urine, sweat, and saliva are not considered to be infectious. Persons engaging in unsafe sexual activity and intravenous drug use with needle-sharing account for most cases of HIV infection. Transfusion-related infection now occurs in only about 1 of every 500,000 units of donated blood. Vertical transmission occurs in 25% of children of infected mothers; zidovudine therapy can decrease this transmission by two-thirds. Casual transmission (in the absence of sexual contact or passage of blood) from person to person does not seem to occur. Transmission from infected patients to health care workers occurs at a rate of 0.3% (one sero-conversion for every 333 needlesticks or similar injury) and constitutes an uncommon but important transmission category. Antiretroviral therapy can decrease needlestick transmission.[3,4] The use of universal blood and body fluid precautions are essential for minimizing health care worker risk.

Physicians should assess their patients' risk for HIV infection by obtaining a sexual and drug history. Education about the use of condoms is essential for all persons who do not remain celibate or in a mutually monogamous relationship. Intravenous drug users can be encouraged to enter a drug treatment program. Those who do not abstain from intravenous drug use must be educated about safe needle use through a needle exchange program or by cleaning their injection equipment with bleach. Physicians' offices should have health education materials about HIV and sexually transmitted diseases openly available for patients and families to read and take with them.

Counseling and Testing

Counseling about HIV is the beginning of a critical medical intervention.[5,6] During the pretest counseling sessions(s), the physician and patient need to discuss the patient's risk of being infected, ongoing activities that put the patient or others at risk, and methods of future risk reduction. Before offering testing, the physician should assess whether the patient appears psychologically and socially prepared for results and if support from friends and family is available. A discussion of the risks of testing (including false-positive results, false-negative results, the possible loss of confidentiality, and family and social disruption) precedes obtaining informed consent for testing.

The difference between confidential and anonymous testing needs to be discussed. Although confidential testing can be done in the physician's office, it results in charted documentation that can reveal HIV status to health care workers and others who process medical records. To avoid possible breaches of confidentiality and to ensure anonymity, the patient can be referred to an anonymous test site or obtain home testing. Testing to establish the diagnosis of HIV infection usually requires an enzyme-linked immunosorbent assay (ELISA) screening test followed by either a Western blot (WB) or immunofluorescent antibody (IFA) confirmatory test.

A "window period" of 6 weeks to 3 months exists between the time of infection and seroconversion. During this time patients can be infected but do not have a sufficient antibody response to result in positive serologic testing. For seronegative patients with recent at-risk activities, retesting at 3 to 6 months is advised. In a few patients, serologic evidence of HIV infection may not occur for 6 months to 1 year or longer and, rarely, not at all.

Posttest counseling is likely a turning point in the HIV-positive patient's life. The patient should be told clearly that the test is positive, and that he or she is infected with the HIV virus. It is important to reassure the patient that HIV positivity does not mean he or she has AIDS. Because there is a long asymptomatic phase of HIV infection and because advances in treatment of HIV infection and opportunistic infections continue, there may be many years before problems arise. Upon hearing an HIV-positive result, however, most patients are in some degree of psychological shock and might not be able to assimilate much information. A commitment to ongoing care should be the focus of the first posttest counseling session. Perhaps the most important intervention the family physician can make is to provide reassurance that he or she will remain the patient's personal physician while assembling a multidisciplinary team to meet problems should they arise. Offering to meet with the family and members of the patient's social network can be helpful.

Health Care Maintenance

The seropositive patient requires routine health care maintenance and special attention to specific signs, symptoms, and laboratory markers for HIV disease progression. Routine health care maintenance includes a comprehensive history and physical examination with special attention to a history of sexually transmitted diseases and physical findings of skin and oral conditions. Laboratory evaluation includes a routine complete blood count including platelet count, chemistry panel, and syphilis serology. A chest roentgenogram is required for persons with a history of cardiopulmonary problems but is not required for all HIV-infected persons. Influenza, pneumococcal, and hepatitis B vaccination is recommended. Polio vaccination for HIV-infected persons and their family members should be with the inactivated (intramuscular) preparation.

Tuberculin skin testing should be performed with the recognition that in HIV-infected persons a 5 mm (rather than the usual 10 mm) reaction to an intermediate-strength purified protein derivative (PPD) is considered indicative of tuberculous infection.[7,8] For HIV-infected persons known to be at high risk for tuberculosis (injection drug users, homeless persons, and persons from countries with a high incidence of tuberculosis) even a negative tuberculin skin test cannot eliminate the possibility of coinfection with tuberculosis. Patients with positive tuberculin skin tests and those with a high risk of tuberculosis require a chest roentgenogram to exclude active tuberculosis.

Laboratory Markers of HIV Disease

The most widely employed surrogate marker for HIV disease progression is the $CD4^+$ lymphocyte count. The normal range for $CD4^+$ lymphocyte counts is broad and variable, so multiple measurements are required to detect trends. In general, $CD4^+$ lymphocyte counts decrease by about

85 cells/mm^3/year from an average baseline level of about 800–1000 cells/mm^3. CD4$^+$ cell counts should be determined every 6–12 months until the count is fewer than 500 cells/mm^3. Thereafter CD4$^+$ cell counts should be performed every 3 to 4 months to help guide decisions about antiretroviral therapy and prophylaxis against opportunistic infections.

The viral load should be quantified to assess prognosis and guide antiretroviral therapy. Both CD4$^+$ cell counts and viral load measurements correlate with disease progression. Low or undetectable viral loads are associated with a better prognosis. Viral loads should be measured along with CD4$^+$ cell counts and when changing drug regimens.

Antiretroviral Therapy

Guidelines for antiretroviral drug therapy[9,10] should be expected to change periodically with increasing experience with new drug combinations (Table 21.2). Combination drug therapy is more effective than monotherapy. No long-term clinical endpoint studies are available to establish the superiority of any specific regimen. The most widely recommended drug regimens include dual reverse transcriptase inhibitors (zidovudine plus lamivudine, didanosine, or zalcitabine ; lamivudine plus stavudine; didanosine plus stavudine; and possibly lamivudine plus didanosine or zalcitabine). When patients can adhere to and tolerate protease inhibitor drugs, they should be offered these very effective drugs. The protease inhibitors can be difficult to take, requiring strict adherence to medication regimens. Departures from the regimen for periods as short as one week can render patients resistant to this class of drugs permanently. The nonnucleoside reverse transcriptase inhibitors can be used in combination when patients cannot take other drug combinations; they should not be used as monotherapy, as resistance develops rapidly.

When to initiate therapy remains controversial. Advocates of early, aggressive therapy believe that treatment should be initiated at any CD4$^+$ level when viral loads are high, based on the hope that early treatment might decrease viral proliferation and produce better survival. Antiretroviral therapy is generally recommended for persons with fewer than 500 CD4$^+$ cells/mm^3 unless the virus is undetectable in the blood.

Changing regimens, other than for drug toxicity, is also an inexact science. If disease progression occurs, the CD4$^+$ count drops precipitously, or the viral load increases 0.5 log or more, the treatment regimen should be changed. The full effects of antiretroviral regimens, as measured by viral loads, can take 2–3 months to be demonstrated. Frequent regimen changes, and possibly drug resistance, can be avoided by waiting 2–3 months before evaluating efficacy. When changing

TABLE 21.2. Treatment regimens for HIV disease

Problem	Drug	Comments
Antiretroviral therapy		
Reverse transcriptase inhibitors	Zidovudine (AZT; Retrovir) 200 mg PO tid or 300 mg PO bid	Hematologic toxicity
	Didanosine (ddI; Videx) 200 mg PO bid: 125 mg PO bid for patients < 60 kg	Pancreatitis; painful peripheral neuropathy
	Zalcitabine (ddC; Hivid) 0.75 mg PO tid	Peripheral neuropathy
	Stavudine (d4T; Zerit) 20 mg PO bid	Peripheral neuropathy
	Lamivudine (3TC; Epivir) 150 mg PO bid	Approved for use with zidovudine
Protease inhibitors	Saquinavir (Fortovase) 1200 mg PO tid	Better oral absorption than the Invirase formulation of saquinavir
	Indinavir (Crixivan) 800 mg PO q8h on empty stomach	Hyperbilirubinemia, nephrolithiasis
	Ritonavir (Norvir) 600 mg PO bid with meals	Nausea, vomiting, diarrhea
	Nelfinavir (Viracept) 750 mg PO tid with meals	Diarrhea
	Combination saquinavir 400–600 mg PO bid plus ritonavir 400–600 mg PO bid	
Non-nucleoside reverse transcriptase inhibitors	Nevirapine (Viramune) 200 mg PO qd for 2 weeks; if no rash, increase to 200 mg PO bid	Use with reverse transcriptase inhibitor. Rash
	Delavirdine (Rescriptor) 400 mg PO tid	Use with reverse transcriptase inhibitor. Rash
Opportunistic infections		
Mycobacterium avium complex (MAC)	Ethambutol 15 mg/kg PO qd Clarithromycin (Claricid) 500 mg PO bid Azithromycin (Zinthromax) 500 mg PO qd Rifabutin (Mycobutin) 300 mg PO qd Ciprofloxacin (Cipro) 500–750 mg PO qd-bid	Use two or three drugs in combination—for lifetime if tolerated. Use ethambutol and clarithromycin or azithromycin whenever possible. Treatment indicated for patients with signs, symptoms, and laboratory abnormalities consistent with MAC disease who can tolerate multidrug regimen
Prophylaxis against MAC disease	Azithromycin 500 mg PO qd or 1200 mg PO once weekly *or* Clarithromycin 500 mg PO bid	

	or	
	Rifabutin 300 mg PO qd	Multiple drug interactions
Cytomegalovirus (CMV) retinitis	Ganciclovir (Cytovene) *Induction:* 5 mg/kg IV q12h for 2 weeks *Maintenance:* 5 mg/kg IV as 1-hour infusion daily for lifetime	Neutropenia, dosage modification in renal failure. Oral ganciclovir might be adequate
	or	
	Foscarnet (Foscavir) *Induction:* 90 mg/kg/dose IV q12h for 2 weeks as 2–hour infusion *Maintenance:* 90 mg/kg IV qd as 2–hour infusion daily for lifetime	Nephrotoxicity common
Mucocutaneous herpes simplex (localized)	Acyclovir (Zovirax) 200–400 mg PO 5 times/day until lesions healed	Chronic maintenance therapy (200–400 mg PO 2–3 times/day) may be necessary when repeated episodes occur
Disseminated, extensive, or persistent herpes simplex	Acyclovir 5 mg/kg/dose IV q8h until lesions healed	Chronic maintenance therapy (200–400 mg PO 3–5 times/day) may be necessary
Herpes zoster: shingles, disseminated, extensive, or persistent infection	Acyclovir 10 mg/kg/dose IV q8h until lesions healed; acyclovir 800 mg PO 5 times/day sometimes effective	Chronic maintenance therapy may be necessary
Acute *Pneumocystis carinii* pneumonia (PCP)	TMP-SMX (Septra, Bactrim) 15 mg TMP/kg daily given in 3–4 divided doses PO or IV	TMP-SMX first-line therapy; treatment is for 3 weeks. Add corticosteroid therapy for $PO_2 \leq 70$ mm Hg
	or	
	Pentamidine isethionate (Pentam) IV, dapsone plus trimethoprim PO, clindamycin plus primaquine IV and PO, or trimetrexate plus leucovorin IV and PO	Second-line therapies. Add corticosteroid therapy for $PO_2 \leq 70$ mm Hg

(*Table continues on next page*)

TABLE 21.2. (*continued*)

Problem	Drug	Comments
Prophylaxis or suppression of PCP for patients with $CD4^+ < 200$ cells/mm^3 or prior episode of PCP or other opportunistic infections	TMP-SMX 1 DS tablet PO qd or qod or 3 times weekly	TMP-SMX most effective for prophylaxis or suppression
	or	
	Inhaled pentamidine (Aeropent) 300 mg q4wk	Less effective than TMP-SMX
	or	
	Dapsone 100 mg PO daily with or without TMP or pyrimethamine 25–75 mg PO q1wk	Less effective than TMP-SMX
	or	
	Clindamycin 450–600 mg PO bid–tid plus primaquine 15 mg PO qd	Less effective than TMP-SMX
Toxoplasma gondii	Sulfadiazine 1 g PO q6h or clindamycin 600–900 mg PO or IV qid	Maintenance required for lifetime
	plus	
	Pyrimethamine 75–100 mg PO qod	
	plus	
	Leucovorin calcium (folinic acid) 10–25 mg PO qd	
Cryptococcus neoformans	Amphotericin B 0.7–1.0 mg/kg/day IV over 4–6 hours	Fluconazole maintenance required
	or	
	Fluconazole *Acute:* 400–800 mg PO qd *Maintenance:* 200–400 mg PO qd	Maintenance required for lifetime

Source: Adapted from Goldschmidt and Dong.[1] With permission.
TMP-SMX = trimethoprim-sulfamethoxazole.

antiretroviral regimens, at least two new drugs should be added, as adding one drug to a failing regimen is considered to be equivalent to changing to monotherapy.

Prophylaxis Against Opportunistic Infections

Preventing *Pneumocystis carinii* pneumonia (PCP) and other opportunistic infections[11] (Table 21.3) decreases morbidity and mortality. When $CD4^+$ lymphocyte counts fall to fewer than 200 cells/mm^3 or when patients develop symptoms of advanced HIV disease, prophylaxis against PCP should be initiated. Prophylaxis has been shown to delay or prevent the development of PCP and improve the survival and health of HIV-infected persons. Trimethoprim-sulfamethoxazole (TMP-SMX), one double-strength tablet daily, is the drug of choice. For patients unable to tolerate TMP-SMX, alternative regimens are available. Prophylaxis against *Toxoplasmosis gondii* disease for patients with fewer than 100 $CD4^+$ cells/mm^3 is generally recommended. Standard TMP-SMX regimens for PCP prophylaxis provide toxoplasmosis prophylaxis, as does dapsone plus pyrimethamine.

Prophylaxis against *Mycobacterium avium* complex (MAC) disease has been recommended for all patients with fewer than 50 $CD4^+$ lymphocytes/mm^3. Azithromycin or clarithromycin are the drugs of choice. Because MAC disease is a late-stage disease, some providers do not recommend prophylaxis when drug toxicity is of concern, preferring to treat patients who develop symptomatic MAC disease. Routine prophylaxis against systemic or serious fungal diseases, herpes simplex or zoster infections, and cytomegalovirus disease is not recommended routinely.

TABLE 21.3. Prophylaxis against opportunistic infections

Organism	USPHA/IDSA guidelines threshold
Pneumocystis carinii	< 200 $CD4^+$ or AIDS
Toxoplasma gondii	< 100 $CD4^+$
Mycobacterium tuberculosis	Any $CD4^+$
Mycobacterium avium complex (MAC)	< 50 to 75 $CD4^+$

Source: Adapted from Centers for Disease Control and Prevention.[11] With permission.
USPHS = U.S. Public Health Service; IDSA = Infectious Disease Society of America.

Clinical Presentations of HIV Disease

Virtually every organ system can be affected by opportunistic infections and malignancies. The Centers for Disease Control (CDC) 1993 surveillance case definition for AIDS includes the identifier diseases listed in Table 21.1. A $CD4^+$ lymphocyte count less than 200 cells/mm^3 also fulfills the case definition requirement for AIDS. Some guidelines for prophylaxis and treatment of the most common opportunistic infections are listed in Tables 21.2. and 21.3.

Nonspecific Symptoms and Signs

Nearly all patients with HIV disease develop weight loss,[12] weakness, malaise, and anorexia. Unexplained fevers are common with advanced HIV disease. Investigation for specific organ system disease and opportunistic infections and malignancies is the first step in evaluating these symptoms and signs. This investigation includes evaluations for pulmonary disease including PCP and disseminated MAC infection.[13] Treatable sepsis caused by bacteria and fungi (including cryptococcal sepsis) can also be identified. Fevers can be treated with nonsteroidal antiinflammatory drugs (NSAIDs), but these drugs appear to be especially nephrotoxic in AIDS patients and should be used only for persistent symptomatic fevers. Vigorous nutritional programs, including hyperalimentation, can increase the daily caloric intake; but they have not been shown to alter the course of advanced HIV disease.

Skin and Oral Cavity

Skin and oral cavity lesions are the most frequent first manifestations of HIV disease.[14,15] A form of seborrheic dermatitis is the most common skin condition found in HIV-infected persons. This condition is readily treated with a combination of low-strength hydrocortisone cream plus ketoconazole cream. Drug rashes can be bothersome and serious. Careful investigation to identify and discontinue the offending drug (including nonprescription drugs the patient may be taking without the physician's knowledge) is essential.

Kaposi's sarcoma (KS) is an AIDS-defining condition. The violaceous to brown lesions can occur anywhere on the body. A biopsy is required to establish the diagnosis of AIDS (when KS is the initial manifestation) and when bacillary angiomatosis (a bacterial condition that can produce lesions similar to those of KS) or other conditions are possible. KS does not require treatment unless the lesions are cosmetically bothersome, bulky, or painful or the patient wishes the lesions to be treated. Localized lesions can be treated successfully with cryotherapy, intralesional injections of chemotherapeutic agents or interferon, or radiation therapy. Extensive KS can be treated with systemic chemotherapeutic agents. Other skin conditions include bacterial folliculitis, fungal rashes, and molluscum contagiosum. Herpes zoster infections (shingles) can antedate the diagnosis of AIDS or can occur during the course of AIDS. Intravenous acyclovir (Zovirax) is usually required for disseminated disease.

Herpes simplex infections of the perioral and perirectal areas can be extensive and persistent. Treatment with oral acyclovir is usually effective, but extensive lesions require intravenous acyclovir. Disseminated herpes simplex and zoster infections usually require intravenous acyclovir treatment.

Oral candidiasis (thrush) is not an AIDS-defining condition. Thrush takes the form of white plaques that can be scraped from the tongue or other areas of the oral mucosa. Oral candidiasis can also present in an inflammatory form with erythema and atrophy but without white plaques. Treatment with topical or systemic antifungal agents is effective. Oral hairy leukoplakia is a viral lesion that appears on the lateral borders of the tongue. Because this condition is asymptomatic and recedes spontaneously, no treatment is required. Other oral conditions include KS, angular cheilitis secondary to candidal infection, and periodontal disease.

Eyes

Cytomegalovirus (CMV) retinitis[16] usually occurs late during the course of AIDS, when $CD4^+$ lymphocyte counts are lower than 50 cells/mm^3. Hemorrhages, perivascular exudates, and white, gray, or yellow discoloration of the peripheral retina are characteristic. When CMV retinitis is identified, treatment with gancyclovir (Cytovene) or foscarnet (Foscavir) should be instituted, as progression to blindness can occur rapidly and without warning. Cotton-wool spots are nonspecific signs of ischemia that are frequently noted on funduscopic examination of many AIDS patients. These small white lesions with indistinct margins can come and go and do not threaten vision.

Lymph Nodes and Hematopoietic System

Generalized lymphadenopathy caused by HIV-induced nodal hyperplasia is common and does not require biopsy or specific treatment. Treatable causes of lymphadenopathy, including lymphoma, tuberculosis, fungal infections, and KS, should be considered when suspicious clinical syndromes are present, lymphadenopathy is asymmetric, or prominent hard lymph nodes are present. Biopsy may be required in these instances.

All blood cell lines can be affected by HIV infection. Neutropenia is common, with reductions in the absolute neutrophil count to fewer than 300 to 500 neutrophils/mm3 frequently occurring in the patient with AIDS. Granulocyte/macrophage-stimulating factors can help raise the neutrophil count to noncritical levels in the presence of drug-induced granulocytopenia. Anemia caused by HIV disease can require transfusions or erythropoietin therapy. Macrocytosis is a normal hematologic response to zidovudine therapy and does not require or respond to treatment. Some patients receiving zidovudine develop a severe anemia with or without macrocytosis, requiring discontinuation of the drug or blood transfusion. Thrombocytopenia[17] can occur early in the course of HIV infection and does not appear to constitute a major prognostic risk factor, nor is it a condition that requires treatment. Thrombocytopenia late in the course of HIV disease does not require treatment unless bleeding is present.

Heart and Pericardium

Congestive cardiomyopathy has been described in patients with AIDS but is infrequent. More common is fluid overload and congestive heart failure caused by large-volume intravenous fluid administration required for the treatment of opportunistic infections and other AIDS-associated-problems. Fungal, bacterial, and tuberculous infections of the heart and pericardium can occur, requiring standard therapy.

Lungs

Pulmonary disease[18] is the most common cause of morbidity and mortality in HIV-infected persons. Pulmonary symptoms and signs can vary from only minimal shortness of breath or nonproductive cough to severe respiratory distress. The physical examination usually reveals tachypnea. Rales and cough with purulent sputum are not usually present unless bacterial pneumonia or pulmonary tuberculosis is present. Evaluation is based on the findings of the chest radiograph and arterial blood gas measurements. The chest film of PCP and many other pulmonary processes in AIDS typically shows diffuse interstitial infiltrates or alveolar infiltrates. Thoracic and mediastinal lymphadenopathy and pleural effusions, when present, may indicate fungal disease, *M. tuberculosis* infection, lymphoma, or pulmonary KS. Pleural effusions usually do not occur with PCP alone. The chest film is normal in 5% of patients with PCP. Arterial blood gas measurements usually show substantial hypoxemia with hypocarbia. Lactic dehydrogenase levels are frequently elevated in patients with AIDS pulmonary disease but do not provide sufficient information on which to base differential diagnostic decisions. Abnormalities of chest radiographs or arterial blood gases require further diagnostic investigation to establish the pathologic diagnosis.

The most common pulmonary disease in HIV-infected persons is PCP.[19] Examination of pulmonary specimens for *P. carinii* requires sputum induction or bronchoscopy; patients with PCP do not spontaneously expectorate sputum containing *P. carinii* organisms. *P. carinii* cysts can be detected for at least 3 weeks after initiation of therapy. Therefore patients seriously ill with presumptive PCP should be treated empirically, with diagnostic procedures performed later.

First-line treatment of PCP is with intravenous or oral TMP-SMX. The duration of PCP therapy is 3 weeks. TMP-SMX has the added advantage of treating possible concurrent bacterial pneumonia. Patients with PaO_2 less than 70 mm Hg should receive concurrent corticosteroids.[20] Patients with moderate to severe PCP are usually hospitalized to provide monitoring and ensure proper medication administration. Marked clinical worsening after 1 week or failure to respond after 2 weeks of therapy are reasonable indications for changing to an alternative agent. Patients with mild PCP who have adequate home support services can be treated as outpatients with oral medications. Oral treatment of PCP is with TMP-SMX or with dapsone plus trimethoprim. PCP recurrences can be treated with the same agent that was successful on previous episodes.

Other pulmonary pathogenic processes to be considered include pneumonia (most commonly caused by *Haemophilus influenzae, Streptococcus pneumoniae, Legionella pneumophila,* and *Mycoplasma pneumoniae*), tuberculosis,[21] MAC, and KS.

Gastrointestinal Tract

Esophagitis with dysphagia, odynophagia, and retrosternal pain can be caused by *Candida albicans,* CMV, or herpes simplex virus. Candidal esophagitis, which is an AIDS-defining disease, is most common. Systemic treatment with fluconazole or ketoconazole should be initiated as an empiric trial. If the patient does not respond, esophagoscopy with biopsies and cultures is advised to establish the diagnosis and direct therapy. Treatment of CMV esophagitis with gancyclovir or foscarnet and of herpes esophagitis with acyclovir is usually effective.

Diarrhea and weight loss are common. Bacterial cultures and parasite determination should be performed to identify treatable causes such as *Shigella, Salmonella,* and *Campylobacter* infections or cryptosporidial or other parasitic infestations. *Clostridium difficile* titers should be determined.

Perianal disease, most commonly caused by herpes simplex virus infections, requires prolonged therapy with oral acyclovir. Extensive perianal disease requires intravenous therapy.

Liver disease can be the result of drug toxicity, viral hepatitis, or other infections and malignancies. Patients with laboratory findings suggesting a predominantly obstructive pattern (elevated alkaline phosphatase) should undergo ultrasound examination to rule out hepatic masses or biliary tract obstruction. An AIDS-associated cholangiopathy with strictures and papillary stenosis can be identified by upper endoscopy with retrograde cholangiography. Sphincterotomy can effectively palliate symptoms of a biliary tract obstruction. When the ultrasound examination is negative, MAC disease, tuberculosis, fungal diseases, or other infiltrative hepatic processes should be considered.

Gynecologic Problems

Women with HIV infection[22] can have severe, persistent vaginal candidiasis (see Chapter 16). Prolonged or repeated antifungal treatment is often necessary. Cervical dysplasia and cancer are also reported to be more frequent and more aggressive than in women not infected with HIV. Papanicolaou smears should be examined every 6 months initially; and dysplasia should be evaluated by colposcopy.

Renal and Adrenal Disease

The most common renal problem is drug toxicity. Special attention is required when patients are taking TMP-SMX, NSAIDs, or other drugs known to cause nephrotoxicity. HIV-associated nephropathy with renal failure can occur, most commonly among patients who have been intravenous drug users, hypertensive patients, or those who have coexisting intrinsic renal disease. Adrenal insufficiency, characterized by hypotension and blunted stress response, can occur.

Musculoskeletal System

Polyarthralgias, Reiter syndrome, and other arthritis syndromes have been described in HIV-infected persons. A myopathy caused by zidovudine can be asymptomatic or can present with weakness and pain. The diagnosis is established by noting marked elevation of muscle enzymes in serum chemistry determinations. Discontinuation of zidovudine is required.

Neurologic Problems

Neurologic problems[23,24] include peripheral neuropathies, myelopathies, and central nervous system (CNS) disorders. Most common are the

CNS disorders, including dementia caused by HIV encephalopathy and other pathogenic processes.

The AIDS–dementia complex is usually a late manifestation of HIV disease. It can present with cognitive impairment, motor disturbances, or behavioral dysfunction. The most typical presentation is confusion, forgetfulness, and lethargy. Predominant features can also include ataxia and clumsiness. Behavioral changes are dominated by apathy, listlessness, and withdrawal. The major cause of the AIDS–dementia complex is HIV infection of the brain. The diagnosis is one of exclusion of other treatable causes of CNS disease. Treatment with high dosage (1200 mg/day PO) zidovudine has been reported to be successful in some cases.

The differential diagnosis of CNS disorders includes cryptococcal meningitis and toxoplasmic encephalitis. Cryptococcal meningitis can present with the AIDS–dementia complex, fever, photophobia, headache, or stiff neck. Serum and cerebrospinal fluid cryptococcal antigen tests are positive more than 95% of the time. Treatment with amphotericin B or fluconazole is usually effective.[25] Toxoplasmic encephalitis[26] can present as the AIDS–dementia complex but also can cause seizures and focal neurologic signs. Empiric treatment is usually given when suspicious lesions on computed tomography or magnetic resonance imaging scans are noted. Failure to respond clinically or radiologically within 2 weeks can be an indication for a brain biopsy to rule out lymphoma and other CNS problems.

Kaposi's Sarcoma and Lymphomas

Multisystem involvement by KS can present with mass lesions or disseminated disease. Most patients with systemic KS also have involvement of the skin or oral mucosa. Involvement of the lungs, pleura, and gastrointestinal tract can be associated with bleeding and other problems. Systemic chemotherapy has been used for widespread KS with variable results. Non-Hodgkin's lymphoma can occur in the brain, thoracic and abdominal lymph nodes, gastrointestinal tract, bone marrow, and elsewhere. Systemic disease can be treated with combination chemotherapy.

HIV Disease in Children

Infection with HIV can occur transplacentally, at the time of delivery, and at breast-feeding. Without peripartum antiretroviral treatment 25% of children born to mothers with HIV infection are infected.[27] When mothers are treated with zidovudine during pregnancy and during delivery, and the baby is treated for the first 6 weeks of life, transmission can be reduced to 8.3%.[27,28] Cesarean section is not recommended on a routine basis. Establishing the diagnosis of HIV infection in infants can be problematic, because testing for antibodies measures maternal antibodies until approximately 15 months of age. Special testing can identify infected infants as early as 1 month of age. The diagnosis in infants is confirmed by viral culture or clinical syndromes.

Children infected with HIV should receive routine diphtheria/pertussis/tetanus (DPT), *H. influenzae* (HiB), mumps/measles/rubella (MMR), and inactivated (intramuscular) poliovirus vaccine at standard intervals. Oral poliovirus vaccine should not be given to HIV-infected children or to household members living with immunocompromised persons. Influenza and one-time pneumococcal vaccines are recommended for children with symptomatic HIV infection.

In children, AIDS usually presents with constitutional symptoms (e.g., fever and failure to thrive), oral candidiasis, lymphadenopathy, hepatosplenomegaly, and persistent or recurrent bacterial infections. Viral infections can also be severe and persistent. Pulmonary manifestations include PCP and lymphocyte interstitial pneumonitis. Gastrointestinal complications include diarrheal syndromes and candidial esophagitis. Neurologic and developmental problems also occur and must be evaluated thoroughly. Antiretroviral treatment and prophylaxis against PCP with TMP-SMX have shown to improve outcomes, so these measures are recommended routinely.

References

1. Goldschmidt RH, Dong BJ. Treatment of AIDS and HIV-related conditions—1997. J Am Board Fam Pract 1997;10:144–67.
2. Centers for Disease Control. 1993 Revised classification system for HIV infection and expanded surveillance case definition for AIDS among adolescents and adults. MMWR 1992;41 RR-17:1–19.
3. Public Health Service statement on management of occupational exposure to human immunodeficiency virus, including considerations regarding zidovudine postexposure use. MMWR 1990;39 RR-1:1–14.
4. Centers for Disease Control and Prevention. Update: provisional Public Health Service recommendations for chemoprophylaxis after occupational exposure to HIV. MMWR 1996;45:468–72.
5. Centers for Disease Control. Public Health Service guidelines for counseling and antibody testing to prevent HIV infection and AIDS. MMWR 1987;36:509–15.
6. Goldschmidt RH, Legg JJ. Counseling patients about HIV test results. J Am Board Fam Pract 1991;4:361–3.
7. Centers for Disease Control. Tuberculosis and human immunodeficiency virus infection: recommendations of the Advisory Committee for the Elimination of Tuberculosis (ACET). MMWR 1989;38:236–8, 243–50.

8. Centers for Disease Control. Purified protein derivative (PPD)-tuberculin anergy and HIV infection: guidelines for anergy testing and management of anergic persons at risk of tuberculosis. MMWR 1991; 40 RR-5:27–33.
9. Carpenter CC, Fischl MA, Hammer SM, et al. Antiretroviral therapy for HIV infection in 1997: updated recommendations of the International AIDS Society—USA Panel. JAMA 1997;227:1962–9.
10. BHIVA Guidelines Co-ordinating Committee. British HIV Association guidelines for antiretroviral treatment of HIV seropositive individuals. Lancet 1997;349:1086–92.
11. Centers for Disease Control and Prevention. USPHS/IDSA guidelines for the prevention of opportunistic infections in persons infected with human immunodeficiency virus: a summary. MMWR 1995;44 RR-8:1–34.
12. Grunfeld C, Feingold KR. Metabolic disturbances and wasting in the acquired immunodeficiency syndrome. N Engl J Med 1992;327:329–37.
13. Horsburgh CR Jr. Mycobacterium avium complex infection in the acquired immunodeficiency syndrome. N Engl J Med 1991;324:1332–8.
14. Berger TG, Obuch ML, Goldschmidt RH. Dermatologic manifestations of HIV infection. Am Fam Physician 1990; 41:1729–42.
15. Cohen PR, Grossman ME. Recognizing skin lesions of systemic fungal infections in patients with AIDS. Am Fam Physician 1994;49:1627–34.
16. Holland GN, Tufail A. New therapies for cytomegalovirus retinitis. N Engl J Med 1995;333:658–9.
17. Glatt AE, Anand A. Thrombocytopenia in patients infected with human immunodeficiency virus: treatment update. Clin Infect Dis 1995;21:415–23.
18. Miller R. HIV-associated respiratory disease. Lancet 1996; 348:307–12.
19. Masur H. Prevention and treatment of *Pneumocystis* pneumonia. N Engl J Med 1992;327:1853–60.
20. Consensus statement on the use of corticosteroids as adjunctive therapy for *Pneumocystis carinii* pneumonia in the acquired immunodeficiency syndrome: the National Institutes of Health–University of California Expert Panel for Corticosteroids as Adjunctive Therapy for *Pneumocystis carinii* pneumonia. N Engl J Med 1990;323:1500–4.
21. Centers for Disease Control. Initial therapy for tuberculosis in the era of multidrug resistance: recommendations of the Advisory Council for the Elimination of Tuberculosis. MMWR 1993;42 RR-7:1–8.
22. Legg JJ. Women and HIV. J Am Board Fam Pract 1993;6:367–77.
23. Simpson DM, Tagliati M. Neurologic manifestations of HIV infection. Ann Intern Med 1994;121:769–85.
24. Newton HB. Common neurologic complications of HIV-1 infection and AIDS. Am Fam Physician 1995;51:387–98.
25. Saag MS, Powderly WG, Cloud GA, et al. Comparison of amphotericin B with fluconazole in the treatment of acute AIDS-associated cryptococcal meningitis. N Engl J Med 1992;326:83–9.
26. Luft BJ, Hafner R, Korzun AH, et al. Toxoplasmic encephalitis in patients with the acquired immunodeficiency syndrome. N Engl J Med 1993; 329:995–1000.

27. Connor EM, Sperling RS, Gelber R, et al. Reduction of maternal-infant transmission of human immunodeficiency virus type 1 with zidovudine treatment. N Engl J Med 1994; 331:1173–80.
28. Centers for Disease Control and Prevention. Recommendations of the US Public Health Service Task Force on the use of zidovudine to reduce perinatal transmission of human immunodeficiency virus. MMWR 1994;43 RR-11:1–20.

Case Presentation

Subjective

Patient Profile

Mark McCarthy is a 28-year-old single white male waiter.

Presenting Problem

"Cough and HIV-positive."

Present Illness

Mark has had a cough for 3 weeks with a recurrent low-grade fever. His cough has been productive of gray-yellow sputum with an occasional fleck of blood. He was found 10 months ago to be HIV-positive when he requested the test after several worrisome sexual contacts.

Past Medical History

Unremarkable since tonsillectomy, age 5.

Social History

The patient dropped out of college to organize a rock group that disbanded 2 years ago. He now works as a waiter in his parents' restaurant.

Habits

Smokes one and a half packs of cigarettes daily. He uses no alcohol. He drinks four cups of coffee a day and occasionally smokes marijuana.

Family History

His father, aged 54, is diabetic and has coronary artery disease. His mother, aged 51, and sister are living and in good health.

REVIEW OF SYSTEMS

Over the past month, he has had a poor appetite and believes that he has lost 3 to 5 pounds.

- What additional information about the history of present illness would be pertinent?
- What additional information about his HIV history might be pertinent? How would you elicit this information?
- What information about his current life style and work might be important? How would you frame this inquiry?
- What might be Mr. McCarthy's unstated reasons for the visit today? Why might this be important?

Objective

VITAL SIGNS

Height, 5 ft 9 in; weight, 145 lb; blood pressure, 110/72; pulse, 78; respirations, 24; temperature, 38.2°C.

EXAMINATION

The patient is a thin white man who does not appear acutely ill but coughs from time to time while speaking. The eyes, ears, nose, and throat are unremarkable except for mild pharyngeal injection. There are a few enlarged cervical nodes bilaterally. The chest has scattered rhonchi at both bases. The heart has a normal sinus rhythm with no murmurs. The skin has a few dark, slightly elevated areas of pigmentation on the dorsum of the hands.

- What other information obtained from the physical examination might be important? Why?
- Are there other areas of the body that you might examine? Why?
- What—if any—laboratory tests should be ordered today?
- What—if any—diagnostic imaging should be ordered today?

Assessment

- Pending the outcome of the tests you have ordered, what is your diagnostic assessment? How would you explain this to the patient?
- How would you assess Mr. McCarthy's knowledge of his health status and prognosis?

- What might be the meaning of the current illness to the patient? How would you address this issue?
- Describe the family implications of the illness.

Plan

- What are your specific recommendations for this patient? How would you explain this to the patient?
- What—if any—changes would you advise in his future work responsibilities?
- Mr. McCarthy's parents ask for an explanation of their son's illness. How would you respond?
- What are your recommendations for continuing care?

22

Anxiety Disorders

DAVID A. KATERNDAHL

This chapter deals with "high impact" anxiety disorders: (1) panic disorder with agoraphobia; (2) generalized anxiety disorder; (3) obsessive compulsive disorder; and (4) posttraumatic stress disorder. These four disorders are associated with considerable morbidity to the patient and family, and they frequently overlap.

Panic Disorder and Agoraphobia

Panic attacks are intense periods of fear that peak within 10 minutes of onset; they include at least four autonomic symptoms (e.g., palpitations, sweating, trembling, dyspnea, choking, chest pain, nausea, dizziness, depersonalization, paresthesias, hot and cold flashes, and fear of dying). The diagnosis of panic disorder (PD) requires recurrent panic attacks with 1 month of either secondary behavior change or persistent worry of additional attacks or their consequences (e.g., "going crazy"). PDs are not due to a general medical problem or the direct effect of a substance (e.g., amphetamines). Although patients frequently use multiple health care sites, 35% of panic attack patients seek care for their symptoms from their family physician, the most frequent site of presentation.[1] As many as 20% of family practice patients have a history of panic attacks. Because PD patients believe they have a physical disorder that is causing their symptoms, they prefer general health providers to mental health providers. Consequently, emergency room usage is frequent for PD patients.[1] Although anxiety is not a frequent presenting complaint in patients with PD, panic-related symptoms (Table 22.1) such as chest pain, dizziness, palpitations, and dyspnea often cause them to seek help.

Consequences and Complications

The longitudinal course of PD is one of persistent or recurring disability, with quality of life frequently being impaired. As many as 90% of PD patients have a history of major depression, and 20% of PD

TABLE 22.1. Criteria for panic attack

A discrete period of intense fear or discomfort, in which four (or more) of the following symptoms developed abruptly and reached a peak within 10 minutes.
Palpitations, pounding heart, or accelerated heart rate
Sweating
Trembling or shaking
Sensations of shortness of breath or smothering
Feeling of choking
Chest pain or discomfort
Nausea or abdominal distress
Feeling dizzy, unsteady, lightheaded, or faint
Derealization (feelings of unreality) or depersonalization (being detached from one's self)
Fear of losing control or going crazy
Fear of dying
Paresthesias (numbness or tingling sensations)
Chills or hot flushes

Source: American Psychiatric Association.[2] With permission.

patients report previous suicide attempts, irrespective of the presence of depression. Up to 20% of PD patients abuse alcohol. When patients associate their panic attacks with the situations in which they occurred, fear and avoidance of those situations may develop as the patient attempts to prevent another panic attack. When this phobic avoidance becomes severe enough to restrict the patient's life, agoraphobia has developed. Up to two-thirds of PD patients have some degree of phobic avoidance.

Diagnosis

Diagnosis of PD is based on the clinical history and the application of *Diagnostic and Statistical Manual of Mental Disorders, Fourth Edition* (DSM-IV) criteria (Table 22.2). Although screening systems exist [Symptom Driven Diagnostic System (SDDS-PC) and Primary Care Evaluation of Mental Disorders (Prime-MD)], their sensitivities for PD are inadequate.[2,3] Evaluation should consist of a thorough history and physical examination with assessment of possible complications. Because panic attacks are associated with a variety of organic pathology, patients must be evaluated for hyperthyroidism, cardiac arrhythmias, medication effects (stimulant use, sedative withdrawal), and partial complex epilepsy. However, without supporting evidence in the history and physical examination, routine laboratory screening is probably inappropriate.

Management

Management begins with patient education. The latter is especially important when dealing with patients with PD because they frequently

TABLE 22.2. Diagnostic criteria for 300.21 panic disorder with agoraphobia

A. Both (1) and (2).
  (1) Recurrent unexpected panic attacks
  (2) At least one of the attacks has been followed by 1 month (or more) of one (or more) of the following:
    (a) Persistent concern about having additional attacks
    (b) Worry about the implications of the attack or its consequences (e.g. losing control, having a heart attack, "going crazy")
    (c) Significant change in behavior related to the attacks

B. Presence of agoraphobia

C. Panic attacks are not due to the direct physiologic effects of a substance (e.g., drug abuse, medication) or a general medical condition (e.g., hyperthyroidism).

D. Panic attacks are not better accounted for by another mental disorder, such as Social Phobia (e.g., occurring on exposure to feared social situations), Specific Phobia (e.g., on exposure to a specific phobic situation), Obsessive-Compulsive Disorder (e.g., on exposure to dirt in someone with an obsession about contamination), Posttraumatic Stress Disorder (e.g., in response to stimuli associated with a severe stressor), or Separation Anxiety Disorder (e.g., in response to being away from home or close relatives).

Source: American Psychiatric Association.[2] With permission.

believe that a physical disorder is causing their symptoms. An explanation of the role of neurotransmitters in psychiatric disease and "labeling" their symptoms as "panic disorder" frequently reassures these patients. If an organic cause for the panic attacks is found, management begins with treatment directed at this condition. Dietary measures such as the avoidance of caffeine and other stimulants is important. Dietary inositol (found in poultry, fish, and dairy products), 12 g/day, decreases the frequency and severity of panic and phobias.[4] Also, patients should be encouraged to discontinue use of tobacco and marijuana. The goal of therapy is for the patient to be panic-free.

BEHAVIORAL THERAPY

Behavioral therapy can be successful. Individual psychotherapy and insight therapy are probably not helpful, but applied relaxation and cognitive therapy are appropriate in the PD patient. Also, patients with agoraphobia eventually need some form of behavioral therapy following resolution of their panic attacks. Systematic desensitization in which agoraphobic patients are progressively exposed to their situational fears is effective when coupled with physician and family support. Even if drug therapy is used, exposure to phobic situations should be encouraged in all patients with PD. Housebound agoraphobics can be treated with telephone-administered behavioral therapy.[5] Group therapy using cognitive-behavioral methods is also effective.[6]

DRUG THERAPY

A variety of medications successfully prevent recurrent panic attacks in susceptible individuals. No medication is effective in aborting a panic attack once it has begun. Tricyclic antidepressants are effective in up to 90% of PD patients. Although imipramine (Tofranil) is used in most studies, other tricylics such as desipramine (Norpramin) and clomipramine (Anafranil) are also effective. Because patients may respond to subantidepressant dosages and may be highly sensitive to imipramine, the initial starting dose should be low: 25 to 50 mg at bedtime. Patients should be warned that a sense of "jitteriness" may be seen early in the course of imipramine therapy. Maintenance of imipramine dosage usually results in resolution of this symptom. The dosage may be increased at regular intervals up to 300 mg per day. Optimal imipramine plasma levels for panic and phobias is 110 to 140 ng/ml.[7] Three weeks of treatment may be necessary before panic suppression is achieved.

The efficacy of selective serotonin reuptake inhibitors (SSRIs) is similar to that of tricyclic antidepressants. Paroxetine (Paxil) at 20 to 60 mg/day, fluoxetine (Prozac) at 20 to 40 mg/day, sertraline (Zoloft) at 50 to 100 mg/day, and fluvoxamine (Luvox) at 50 to 200 mg/day are effective but require 3 to 4 weeks for panic suppression. As with tricyclic antidepressants, hyperexcitation may be noted by patients early in therapy.[8]

Although neuroleptics are contraindicated for PD, certain benzodiazepines are highly effective. The high-potency benzodiazepines have efficacy similar to that of the tricyclics. The literature recommends high doses of these benzodiazepines [alprazolam (Xanax) 3–10 mg/day, clonazepam (Klonopin) 2 to 6 mg/day, and lorazepam (Ativan) 4 to 8 mg/day], but experience in primary care settings suggests that lower doses are effective in primary care patients. Based on plasma levels and balancing the side effects and remission rates, the optimal alprazolam dose may be 2 to 3 mg/day. Clonazepam may have less sedation and fewer withdrawal side effects. PD patients without a history of abuse rarely increase their alprazolam dose and do not abuse it.[9]

Monoamine oxidase inhibitors (MAOIs) such as phenelzine (Nardil) may be even more effective than the tricyclics. Beginning with a dose of 15 mg at bedtime, the dose can be increased to 60 mg/day. Due to the dietary restrictions, these drugs are not the first line of therapy. Other medications may also be effective for management of PD. There is evidence to support the antipanic efficacy of sodium valproate (Depakene), clonidine (Catapres), and verapamil (Calan). β-Blockers, bupropion (Wellbutrin), and buspirone (BuSpar) are not effective for management of PD.

Combination of behavioral therapy and drug therapy has been used. Although combining alprazolam with exposure therapy produces minimal enhancement over either alone,[10] combining exposure therapy with imipramine or fluvoxamine is effective in reducing phobias.[11,12] The value of combining medications (e.g., alprazolam, sertraline and imipramine) has not been shown. Although alprazolam, sertraline, and paroxetine are the only medications with U.S. Food and Drug Administration (FDA) approval for treatment of PD, drug selection depends on the patient's age, concurrent medications, and comorbid states. Elderly patients and those with a history of substance abuse should not be started on benzodiazepines. In the presence of major depression, an antidepressant would be appropriate. Treatment should be continued until patients are panic-free for at least 6 to 12 months. Medication should be tapered slowly to avoid withdrawal symptoms. Relapse is common especially when drug therapy is used.

Point of Referral

Because these patients are frequently seen by family physicians and treated with medications with which most family physicians are familiar, there is no immediate need for referral. Family physicians who make home visits can diagnose and manage agoraphobic patients more readily than other specialists. Referral is appropriate if the physician is uncomfortable with an indicated therapy (e.g., MAOIs). Referral is also considered in patients who are potentially suicidal or are actively abusing drugs or alcohol.

Family Issues

Studies have shown a strong familial pattern for both PD and agoraphobia. Children of PD patients frequently have behavioral problems associated with avoidance behavior in the parents.[13] PD has been linked to domestic violence; the prevalence of childhood sexual abuse is increased in those with PD, as is the frequency of current violence.[14]

Family members can be helpful in the management of agoraphobia, providing support at home while patients begin to confront their fears. PD and agoraphobia are stressful on the marital relationship, but the family frequently adapts to the agoraphobic's fears. Successful therapy implies changes in the family situation and dynamics. Hence successful treatment of agoraphobia generates stress on the family unit.

Generalized Anxiety Disorder

The hallmark of generalized anxiety disorder (GAD) is excessive or unrealistic worry, out of proportion to the problems that exist. More than 85% of patients state that they spend more than half of their time being anxious.

Generalized anxiety disorder is frequently associated with other anxiety disorders: social phobia, panic disorder, simple phobia, and obsessive compulsive disorder. More than 70% of patients claim to have had at least one panic attack previously.[15] The lifetime prevalence of major depressive episodes is 67%. This relation is particularly important because depression may represent a predisposing factor for GAD, and its presence frequently alters management.

Although patients rarely seek psychiatric help, they do frequently seek help from family physicians, cardiologists, and pulmonologists. They often present to their family physicians with multiple nonspecific complaints.

Differential Diagnosis

The diagnosis of GAD is based on DSM-IV criteria (Table 22.3). Not only must the patient have experienced excessive anxiety for at least a 6-month period, they must have at least three symptoms related to motor

TABLE 22.3. Diagnostic criteria for 300.02 generalized anxiety disorder

A. Excessive anxiety and worry (apprehensive expectation), occurring more days than not for at least 6 months, about a number of events or activities (such as work or school performance).

B. The person finds it difficult to control the worry.

C. The anxiety and worry are associated with three (or more) of the following six symptoms (with at least some symptoms present for more days than not for the past 6 months). Note: Only one item is required in children.
  (1) Restlessness or feeling keyed up or on edge
  (2) Being easily fatigued
  (3) Difficulty concentrating or mind going blank
  (4) Irritability
  (5) Muscle tension
  (6) Sleep disturbance (difficulty falling or staying asleep, or restless unsatisfying sleep)

D. The focus of the anxiety and worry is not confined to features of an axis I disorder, e.g., the anxiety or worry is not about having a panic attack (as in Panic Disorder), being embarrassed in public (as in Social Phobia), being contaminated (as in Obsessive-Compulsive Disorder), being away from home or close relatives (as in Separation Anxiety Disorder), gaining weight (as in Anorexia Nervosa), having multiple physical complaints (as in Somatization Disorder), or having a serious illness (as in Hypochondriasis); and the anxiety and worry do not occur exclusively during Posttraumatic Stress Disorder.

E. The anxiety, worry, or physical symptoms cause clinically significant distress or impairment in social, occupational, or other important areas of functioning.

F. The disturbance is not due to the direct physiologic effects of a substance (e.g., drug of abuse, medication) or a general medical condition (e.g., hyperthyroidism) and does not occur exclusively during a Mood Disorder, a Psychotic Disorder, or a Pervasive Developmental Disorder.

Source: American Psychiatric Association.[2] With permission.

tension, autonomic hyperactivity, and vigilance and scanning. Because of the association between GAD and other anxiety disorders, GAD can be diagnosed only when the anxiety is unrelated to the focus of the other anxiety disorder, such as panic attacks. If depression is present, the anxiety must be present when the depression is not. Organic factors known to be associated with anxiety must not be responsible for initiating *and* maintaining the anxiety. Hence hyperthyroidism, drugs such as cocaine and amphetamines, and general stimulants such as caffeine and tyramine must be excluded as the cause of the anxiety. Screening tests (SDDS-PC and Prime-MD) have been used. The SDDS-PC is more sensitive (85–90%) for detecting GAD than Prime-MD.[2,3] Because of the symptomatic similarity, adjustment disorder with anxious mood must be excluded. This disorder differs from GAD in that a psychosocial stressor is present, the duration of the disorder is less than 6 months, and the full symptomatic picture of GAD is usually not present.

Management

Elimination of dietary stimulants is recommended. Exercise reduces anxiety levels and should also be advocated.[16]

BEHAVIORAL THERAPY

A variety of modalities exist to help the GAD patient cope with stress and anxiety. Progressive relaxation, stress management, and assertiveness training with or without hypnosis are frequently used, as are family and group therapy and other forms of supportive psychotherapy. Studies with cognitive behavioral therapy, during which anxious thoughts are identified and then changed, suggest that such cognitive therapy may be superior to other forms of behavioral therapy.[17]

DRUG THERAPY

At least 70% of GAD patients respond to benzodiazepines (Table 22.4). Such response is more likely if a precipitating stress exists, significant depression is lacking, patients are aware of the psychological nature of their symptoms, there has been a prior response to benzodiazepines, and the patient expects recovery. Most patients who respond to benzodiazepines note improvement within the first week of therapy. Unfortunately, benzodiazepines frequently decrease alertness and performance. Although it is unusual for GAD patients without prior substance abuse to abuse benzodiazepines, physical dependence frequently develops. Tapering of the benzodiazepine dosage by reducing the dose by 10% per week can be tried after

TABLE 22.4. Commonly used benzodiazepines

Drug	Rate of onset	Usual daily dosage (mg)	Half-life (hours)
Alprazolam (Xanax)	Intermediate	0.5–4.0	12–15
Chlordiazepoxide (Librium)	Intermediate	15–100	5–30
Clonazepam (Klonopin)	Intermediate	1–10	30–60
Clorazepate (Tranxene)	Rapid	7.5–60.0	30–200
Diazepam (Valium)	Rapid	2–60	20–100
Lorazepam (Ativan)	Intermediate	2–6	10–20
Oxazepam (Serax)	Intermediate	30–120	5–15
Prazepam (Centrax)	Slow	20–60	30–200

2 months of therapy. Relapse is not uncommon and requires reinstituting the benzodiazepine or attempting intermittent therapy. Tricyclic antidepressants may reduce the chance of relapse.

Patients with respiratory disease, dementia, or prior substance abuse or who are on central nervous system (CNS) depressants may benefit from buspirone. Buspirone is helpful in patients in whom psychomotor impairment may be life-threatening. Owing to its delayed onset of anxiolytic activity, buspirone is useful only in patients with chronic anxiety. Adequate doses of buspirone may be required for 2 to 3 weeks before patients note a response. GAD patients on benzodiazepines can be switched to buspirone without rebound anxiety or withdrawal symptoms.[18] Because there is no potential for dependence, buspirone does not need to be tapered once therapy is completed.

There is no evidence that β-blockers are effective for management of GAD. Tricyclic antidepressants may be of some benefit in patients with GAD.[17] If present, depression must be treated aggressively. Hence the drug of choice for management of GAD with major depression is a tricyclic antidepressant. Buspirone is the next alternative. Because benzodiazepines may worsen depression, they should not be first-line agents in patients with GAD and depression.

Point of Referral

Referral is considered in the presence of comorbid anxiety or depressive disorders if the physician lacks comfort in management. Patients with current substance abuse or those requiring behavioral techniques unfamiliar to the physician may also be referred to appropriate mental health providers. Because some patients indeed require chronic benzodiazepine therapy, the recurrence of symptoms or difficulty of tapering benzodiazepines does not necessarily indicate the need for referral.

Family Issues

Although there is no reported familial pattern to GAD, family issues may be important. As mentioned before, many patient worries focus on family problems. Involvement of the family in therapy is helpful. Specifically, family and friends should be enlisted to encourage socialization and confrontation of fears. Although not frequently recognized, the presence of GAD within a family has serious implications. Not only can GAD produce functional impairment and affect quality of life, it represents a serious stress for the family. GAD in parents may be a risk factor for the development of autism in children.[19]

Obsessive-Compulsive Disorder

The hallmark of obsessive-compulsive disorder (OCD) is the presence of recurrent obsessions or compulsions (or both) that markedly distress or significantly interfere with the patient's life. *Obsessions*—intrusive ideas or thoughts—occur in more than half of OCD patients. Fears of contamination are common, as are thoughts of harming others, counting, praying, and blasphemous or sexual thoughts. *Compulsions*—repetitive intentional behaviors designed to neutralize discomfort—also occur in more than half of these patients. Rituals such as cleaning and hand washing, arranging items, and "checking" are common. Compulsions include acts to control the behavior of others, hoarding behaviors, and hair pulling. Fewer than 10% of patients have both obsessions and compulsions, but the presence of multiple obsessions or multiple compulsions is common. Delusions occur in as many as 12% of patients, but they are usually transient and their absurdity is realized by the patient. Although patients frequently consider themselves "crazy," they do not always believe that their obsessions are senseless, and their compulsions are not always resisted.

Obsessive-compulsive disorder is a continuous disorder in about 85% of patients; in only 5% is it episodic. Although 35% of OCD patients seek mental health care from general health physicians,[20] most of the cases are not recognized by the primary care physician. When such patients do present, they may expect extensive laboratory testing to assess what they consider serious physical problems.[21]

Comorbidity and Complications

Up to 80% of OCD patients have evidence of depression, anxiety, substance abuse, or work disability. Between 32% and 67% of patients have major depressive disorder, usually beginning after the onset of OCD.

Substance abuse is seen in 14% to 24% of patients, again usually beginning after the onset of OCD. Although panic disorder is seen in fewer than 15% of patients, almost 40% of patients do report panic attacks; 19% of these patients note panic attacks triggered only by OCD symptoms.[22] Usually beginning before the onset of OCD, phobias are present in almost half the patients. Although more than 50% of patients have at least one personality disorder, fewer than 15% of patients have an obsessive compulsive personality.[23]

With an obsession to body parts, it is not surprising that a high rate of eating disorders are seen in these patients. CNS disease is also common; abnormal scans are frequently seen, with more than 90% of patients having some abnormality on neurologic testing.[24] In addition to a high degree of psychosocial disability, OCD patients frequently have behavioral problems and find it difficult to maintain employment. Their social involvement is usually poor, and half of OCD patients have some marital distress.

Differential Diagnosis

Patients with OCD frequently use primary care physicians for their mental health care. The physician must therefore have a high index of suspicion because embarrassment usually prevents patients from spontaneously revealing their obsessions or compulsions. The diagnosis of OCD is based on *DSM-IV* criteria (Table 22.5). Although the SDDS-PC screens for OCD, it is not adequately sensitive.[2] Two screening questions can be useful for identifying possible OCD patients[21]: (1) Are you bothered by thoughts coming into your mind that make you anxious and that you are unable to get rid of? (2) Are there certain behaviors you do over and over that may seem silly to you or to others but that you feel you just have to do?

Physical examination can provide clues to the physician. Such clues are important because patients often do not voluntarily describe their obsessions or compulsions. Dermatologic changes may be due to compulsive hand-washing or self-mutilation. Similarly, hoarding behaviors may lead to collecting garbage, which can result in poor hygiene or infections. Hair-pulling behaviors (trichotillomania) may be evidenced by areas of alopecia. Similarly, a normal physical examination in the presence of repeated evaluations for somatic symptoms suggests OCD. Evidence of plastic surgery may reflect patients' obsessions with their bodies. Routine laboratory testing is not helpful for differentiating OCD from other disorders unless specifically indicated by the history or physical examination.

Several physical disorders simulate OCD. CNS infections such as encephalitis, head trauma, brain tumors involving the frontal or prefrontal cortex or residing near the basal ganglia, Huntington's chorea, and

TABLE 22.5. Diagnostic criteria for 300.3 obsessive-compulsive disorder

A. **Obsessions or compulsions**

Obsessions as defined by (1), (2), (3), and (4)

(1) Recurrent and persistent thoughts, impulses, or images that are experienced, at some time during the disturbance, as intrusive and inappropriate and that cause marked anxiety or distress.

(2) The thoughts, impulses, or images are not simply excessive worries about real-life problems.

(3) The person attempts to ignore or suppress such thoughts, impulses, or images or to neutralize them with some other thought or action.

(4) The person recognizes that the obsessional thoughts, impulses, or images are a product of his or her own mind (not imposed from without, as in thought insertion).

Compulsions as defined by (1) and (2):

(1) Repetitive behaviors (e.g., hand-washing, ordering, checking) or mental acts (e.g., praying, counting, repeating words silently) that the person feels driven to perform in response to an obsession, or according to rules that must be applied rigidly.

(2) The behaviors or mental acts are aimed at preventing or reducing distress or preventing some dreaded event or situation; however, these behaviors or mental acts either are not connected in a realistic way with what they are designed to neutralize or prevent or are clearly excessive.

B. At some point during the course of the disorder, the person has recognized that the obsessions or compulsions are excessive or unreasonable. *Note:* This does not apply to children.

C. The obsessions or compulsions cause marked distress, are time-consuming (take more than 1 hour a day), or significantly interfere with the person's normal routine, occupational (or academic) functioning, or usual social activities or relationships.

D. If another axis I disorder is present, the content of the obsessions or compulsions is not restricted to it (e.g., preoccupation with food in the presence of an eating disorder; hair pulling in the presence of trichotillomania; concern with appearance in the presence of body dysmorphic disorder; preoccupation with having a serious illness in the presence of hypochondriasis; preoccupation with sexual urges or fantasies in the presence of a paraphilia; or guilty ruminations in the presence of major depressive disorder).

E. The disturbance is not due to the direct physiologic effects of a substance (e.g., a drug of abuse, a medication) or a general medical condition.

Specify if:

With poor insight: If, for most of the time during the current episode, the person does not recognize that the obsessions and compulsions are excessive or unreasonable.

Source: American Psychiatric Association.[2] With permission.

diabetes insipidus should be considered in the differential diagnosis. A variety of psychiatric disorders may also be suggested. The content of the obsessions suggests the true diagnosis. For example, the realization by OCD patients that delusions are not real differentiate them from schizophrenics. Specific personality disorders such as obsessive compulsive and schizotypal personality should also be considered.

Management

BEHAVIORAL THERAPY

Whereas flooding therapy—sudden intense exposure to objects of fear until anxiety dissipates—may be helpful for OCD patients, insight therapy, dynamic psychotherapy, and systematic desensitization are not. Exposure therapy with response prevention is the behavioral technique of choice. Office-based, with homework assignments, exposure therapy involves exposure to stimuli associated with the patient's obsessions until the discomfort diminishes, within about 30 to 35 minutes. This therapy is coupled with response prevention in which patients are asked to refrain from rituals for progressively longer periods until their discomfort diminishes. If performed as directed, this therapy produces a 70% reduction in symptoms for at least 50% of patients. Unfortunately, 25% of patients either refuse or cannot comply. Patients who do comply report improvement in their work and social adjustment, and they experience diminished OCD symptoms and depression. Persistence of benefit is related to the duration of therapy and compliance with homework activities.

DRUG THERAPY

Drug therapy is helpful in patients who are purely obsessional, have a history of substance abuse, or cannot comply with behavioral therapy. Clomipramine in doses of up to 250 mg/day is more effective than other tricyclic antidepressants in OCD patients. Although there may be improvement in the ability to function, and alleviation of symptoms, clomipramine-treated patients are rarely symptom-free. OCD tends to relapse quickly after discontinuance of clomipramine. Although up to 10 weeks of therapy may be required before improvement is seen, once improvement occurs the clomipramine dose can frequently be reduced without exacerbation of the obsessive compulsive symptoms. Fluoxetine in doses up to 80 mg/day, sertraline (Zoloft) in doses of at least 50 mg/day, and fluvoxamine in doses up to 300 mg/day may also be effective in OCD patients.[25] Poor response to SSRIs is predicted by the presence of compulsions or schizotypal personality as well as a long duration of illness.[26] MOAIs and benzodiazepines are not helpful; in fact, benzodiazepines may interfere with behavioral therapy. Buspirone and lithium carbonate (Eskalith, Lithobid) may be useful for augmenting a response to clomipramine or fluoxetine.

The presence of co-morbid conditions affects the choice of therapeutic agents. In the presence of other anxiety disorders or major depressive disorder, the agent of choice is probably clomipramine. Depressed patients may also respond to fluoxetine or fluvoxamine to a lesser extent (see Chapter 23). Buspirone may also be appropriate in the depressed patient. When using drug therapy, patients should be treated for at least 1 year. Clomipramine and fluoxetine should be tapered every 2 months in decrements of 50 mg and 20 mg, respectively.

In general, patients with purely obsessional disorders should be treated with drug therapy first, followed by a variety of behavioral techniques—cognitive therapy, assertiveness training, flooding—if necessary. Drug therapy causes a reduction in symptoms in 30% to 42% of patients. Although behavioral therapy reduces symptoms in up to 50% of patients, OCD patients must have some ritual behavior for it to be effective. Although self-exposure techniques are the most potent, therapist-aided techniques are of marginal value but may be necessary. Behavioral therapy is less likely to succeed in patients who are depressed, delusional, or noncompliant because covert rituals may undermine therapy.[27] Although OCD is treatable, a poor response is more likely in patients who have personality disorders (especially schizotypal personality), patients who have overvalued ideas (a strong belief in the value of their rituals), and patients with a family history of psychiatric problems.[28]

Electroconvulsive therapy has not been shown to be helpful for OCD, but patients refractory to behavioral and drug therapy can be improved with surgery. Techniques that interrupt the connections between the frontal cortex and the limbic system result in marked improvement in 28% of patients, with an additional 37% becoming symptom-free. Only 12% of patients show no improvement.[27]

Point of Referral

There is no reason a family physician cannot use the medications or behavioral techniques mentioned. Therefore referral usually depends on physician comfort with the therapeutic program. Consider referral of patients who do not respond to adequate therapy or those with complicating medical or psychiatric problems.

Family Issues

The patient's family is important in OCD. Not only is the disorder a familial one, but OCD patients frequently have marital problems. Behavioral therapy can produce improvement in OCD patients despite these marital problems. Also, the spouse improves as the patient responds, regardless of whether the family has been involved in the treatment.[29] Unfortunately, because of the embarrassing nature of the disorder, evaluation is sometimes viewed as "taboo" by the family, thus presenting an obstacle to the help-seeking of the patient. Family members frequently accommodate the OCD patient in an attempt to reduce patient anxiety or anger directed at the family.[30] If the family is involved as cotherapist in family-based therapy, OCD patients have lower levels of anxiety, depression, and OCD symptoms; and they increase their social adjustment. If family members are to be involved in such therapy, they must have low levels of anxiety themselves and be able to tolerate the frustrating nature of this therapy.

Posttraumatic Stress Disorder

Posttraumatic stress disorder (PTSD) occurs in people experiencing a stressful event that is particularly distressing to that person. It is associated with persistent reexperiencing of the event, avoidance of stimuli associated with the event, and symptoms of increased arousal. Because of the dissociative nature of some of the symptoms, it has been suggested that PTSD should be classified as a dissociative disorder. Although the stressful event itself is the precipitant of the disorder, several factors have been identified as important in its development: factors present before the stressful event, characteristics of the stressor, and poststress factors. Patient factors that predispose to the development of PTSD include poor school performance, a rigid or immature personality, the lack of preparedness for the stressor, a disruptive environment before the stress, and preexisting psychiatric problems such as anxiety or depression.[31] The patient's family of origin may also be important. PTSD is more likely to develop in patients who come from families with low cohesion and expressiveness; early parental separation; familial history of depression, alcoholism, or anxiety; parental neglect; and intrafamilial conflict.[32]. Although the severity of the trauma itself does not predict development of PTSD, its duration and intensity does.[33] If the stress occurs during a vulnerable time in the patient's life or bears a similarity to an earlier traumatic event, PTSD is more likely. In rape victims PTSD is more likely to develop if the rape is done by a stranger, involves physical force or injury, includes the display of weapons, or is associated with a sense of helplessness by the victim.[34] After the stress has occurred, the subjective level of distress and weekly alcohol intake predict the development of PTSD.[35] Lack of support during recovery, financial and emotional, is also an important factor.

Symptoms and Course

Although symptoms usually begin immediately after the stressor, there may be a delayed onset. Once established, PTSD frequently persists for years. Left untreated, half of those with PTSD after a motor vehicle accident no longer meet criteria 6 months later.[36] Symptomatically, 90% of patients note sleep disturbance, loss of interest, emotional detachment, avoidance behavior of situations associated with the stressor, and reexperiencing the event.

Although patients with PTSD frequently develop depression, generalized anxiety disorder, and violent behavior, criminality without a prior predilection is uncommon.[31] In general, men are at greater risk for developing depression and drug abuse, whereas women are at greater risk of developing panic disorder and phobias. An increased risk of alcoholism and OCD appears similarly in both genders.

Diagnosis

Because patients frequently present with vague complaints, diagnosis of PTSD can be challenging. In addition to experiencing a traumatic stressor, *DSM-IV* criteria (Table 22.6) require evidence that the traumatic event is persistently reexperienced (e.g., flashbacks or nightmares). To be diagnosed with PTSD, a patient must also have persistent avoidance of stimuli associated with the stressor or a generalized numbing of emotions. Finally, patients must have persistent symptoms of increased arousal. Although the *DSM-IV* requires symptoms of at least 1 month duration, some authors recommend increasing this criterion to 3 months duration because of the observation that more than half of rape victims recover in less than 3 months.[37] When considering the differential diagnosis, adjustment disorder can usually be ruled out by the lack of severity of symptoms and the fact that the stressor is usually not extreme. In the presence of head trauma, postconcussive disorder and organic aggressive disorder must be considered. The presence of comorbid conditions such as depression and substance abuse frequently makes the diagnosis difficult. Depression and substance abuse themselves must be considered in the differential diagnosis. Finally, because of the publicity surrounding PTSD and its potential for financial compensation, malingering must be considered. Certain *DSM-IV* symptoms appear to be more specific for PTSD and may therefore have diagnostic implications. For example, the existence of many triggers for reexperiencing the event suggests the presence of PTSD, as does avoidance of stimuli through the loss of interest, estrangement, or a numbing effect. The presence of a startle response, sleep disturbance, memory disturbance, or disturbed concentration are specific for PTSD. Finally, if patients are either predominantly angry or avoid getting upset, PTSD should be considered.

Management

The disorder is not easily treated. Although two-thirds of patients completing a 4-week inpatient treatment program improved, 55% of them required hospitalization within 2 years.[38] Early treatment is important

TABLE 22.6. Diagnostic criteria for 309.81 posttraumatic stress disorder

A. The person has been exposed to a traumatic event in which both of the following were present:
  (1) The person experienced, witnessed, or was confronted with an event or events that involved actual or threatened death or serious injury, or a threat to the physical integrity of self or others.
  (2) The person's response involved intense fear, helplessness, or horror. *Note:* In children, this may be expressed instead by disorganized or agitated behavior.

B. The traumatic event is persistently reexperienced in one (or more) of the following ways:
  (1) Recurrent and intrusive distressing recollections of the event, including images, thoughts, or perceptions. *Note:* In young children repetitive play may occur in which themes or aspects of the trauma are expressed.
  (2) Recurrent distressing dreams of the event. *Note:* In children there may be frightening dreams without recognizable content.
  (3) Acting or feeling as if the traumatic event were recurring (includes a sense of reliving the experience, illusions, hallucinations, and dissociative flashback episodes, including those that occur on awakening or when intoxicated). *Note:* In young children trauma-specific reenactment may occur.
  (4) Intense psychological distress at exposure to internal or external cues that symbolize or resemble an aspect of the traumatic event.
  (5) Physiologic reactivity on exposure to internal or external cues that symbolize or resemble an aspect of the traumatic event.

C. Persistent avoidance of stimuli associated with the trauma and numbing of general responsiveness (not present before the trauma), as indicated by three (or more) of the following.
  (1) Efforts to avoid thoughts, feelings, or conversations associated with the trauma
  (2) Efforts to avoid activities, place, or people that arouse recollections of the trauma
  (3) Inability to recall an important aspect of the trauma
  (4) Markedly diminished interest or participation in insignificant activities
  (5) Feeling of detachment or estrangement from others
  (6) Restricted range of affect (e.g., unable to have loving feelings)
  (7) Sense of foreshortened future (e.g., does not expect to have a career, marriage, children, or a normal life-span)

D. Persistent symptoms of increased arousal (not present before the trauma), as indicated by two (or more) of the following.
  (1) Difficulty falling or staying asleep
  (2) Irritability or outbursts of anger
  (3) Difficulty concentrating
  (4) Hypervigilance
  (5) Exaggerated startle response

E. Duration of the disturbance (symptoms in criteria B, C, and D) is more than 1 month.

F. The disturbance causes clinically significant distress or impairment in social, occupational, or other important areas of functioning.

Specify if:
Acute: if duration of symptoms is less than 3 months
Chronic: if duration of symptoms is 3 months or more

Specify if:
With delayed onset: if onset of symptoms is at least 6 months after the stressor

Source: American Psychiatric Association.[2] With permission.

and depends heavily on the attitudes of the family and the physician. Also, the presence of predisposing factors, substance abuse, and subsequent stressors may impede recovery. Unfortunately, the presence of secondary gain, litigation, and encouragement from others to assume a sick role represent further obstacles to recovery.

BEHAVIORAL THERAPY

Negative symptoms such as avoidance behavior, loss of interest, and emotional numbing respond better to psychotherapy than to medication.[39] In general terms, the goals of psychotherapy are to encourage the patients to express their emotions and explore earlier events. Evaluation begins by exploring the stressor itself and the patient's status before the stressor. A detailed understanding of the problems experienced and the stressor are important. A variety of methods have been found to be successful in treating PTSD. Psychodynamic therapy, hypnotherapy, and desensitization to the stressor decrease symptoms. Although flooding therapy has been successful, it has also produced increased depression, panic attacks, and relapse of alcoholism. The use of PTSD groups may be helpful.

DRUG THERAPY

Although all PTSD patients require psychotherapy, medication frequently has a positive effect on the results of psychotherapy, particularly with hyperarousal and the reexperiencing of the event.[40] Although response to major tranquilizers is poor, both imipramine in doses sufficient to produce blood levels higher than 150 mg/ml and phenelzine in doses from 15 to 75 mg/day alleviate symptoms over an 8-week period. A variety of other medications may also augment the medication response.

Two approaches can be applied to selection of a drug regimen. Medication can be selected based on comorbid states. Hence in the presence of panic disorder or depression, the PTSD patient should be started on a tricyclic antidepressant. In the presence of generalized anxiety disorder, the patient should receive buspirone or a benzodiazepine. Finally, in the presence of outbursts, the patient should be prescribed propranolol (Inderal). The second approach to drug therapy is to begin the patient on a tricyclic antidepressant for a 6- to 8-week period. At the end of the 8 weeks the patient is reevaluated for response. In the presence of refractory depression or anger, the tricyclic antidepressant is changed to an MAOI, or lithium is added. Similarly, symptoms of autonomic arousal such as vigilance or a startle response can be treated with propranolol in doses of 60 to 640 mg/day or clonidine in doses of 0.2 to 0.6 mg/day. Persistent flashbacks respond to carbamazepine (Tegretol), and distress on reexposure to stimuli responds to propranolol. Finally, persistent aggression can be treated with propranolol, carbamazepine, or lithium.[39]

Point of Referral

Because family physicians are generally not trained in the psychodynamic techniques used for PTSD, most patients require referral for comanagement. Also, if an MAOI or lithium is indicated, some physicians are more comfortable referring those patients to a psychiatrist.

Family Issues

Family members often had PTSD-like symptoms during childhood, suggesting a familial predisposition.[41] The family is an important factor in the evaluation and treatment of the PTSD patient. The family should be included in the interview process because the patients are often incapable of revealing their own feelings or describing their behavior. Moreover, the family's attitude is important for treatment. It can help minimize secondary gain by the patient by discouraging the development of a sick role. Through patience and support the family can provide a positive setting for the patient's recovery.

References

1. Katerndahl DA, Realini JP. Where do panic attack sufferers seek care? J Fam Pract 1995;40:237–43.
2. American Psychiatric Association. Diagnostic manual of mental disorders. 4th ed. Washington, DC: APA, 1994.
2. Broadhead WE, Leon AC, Weissman MM, et al. Development and validation of the SDDS-PC screen for multiple mental disorders in primary care. Arch Fam Med 1995; 4:211–19.
3. Spitzer RL, Williams JBW, Kroenke K, et al. Utility of a new procedure for diagnosing mental disorders in primary care. JAMA 1994;272:1749–56.
4. Benjamin J, Levine J, Fux M, et al. Double-blind, placebo-controlled, crossover trial of inositol treatment for panic disorder. Am J Psychiatry 1995;152: 1084–6.
5. Swinson RP, Fergus KD, Cox BJ, Wickwire K. Efficacy of telephone-administered behavioral therapy for panic disorder with agoraphobia. Behav Res Ther 1995;33:465.
6. Bowen R, South M, Fischer D, Looman T. Depression, mastery, and number of group sessions attended predict outcome of patients with panic and agoraphobia in a behavioural/medication program. Can J Psychiatry 1994;39: 283–8.
7. Mavissakalian MR, Perel JM. Imipramine treatment of panic disorder with agoraphobia. J Psychiatry 1995;152:673–82.
8. Sheehan DV, Raj BA, Trehan RR, Knapp EL. Serotonin in panic disorder and social phobia. Int Clin Psychopharmacol 1993;8 Suppl 2:63.
9. Shelton RC, Harvey DS, Stewart PM, Loosen PT. Alprazolam in panic disorder. Prog Neuropsychopharmacol Biol Psychiatry 1993;17:423–34.

10. Marks IM, Swinson RP, Basoglu M, et al. Alprazolam and exposure alone and combined in panic disorder with agoraphobia. Br J Psychiatry 1993; 162:776–87.
11. Mavissakalian M. Combined behavioral therapy and pharmacotherapy of agoraphobia. J Psychiatr Res 1993;27 Suppl 1:179–91.
12. DeBuers E, van Balkonm AJLM, Large A, et al. Treatment of panic disorder with agoraphobia. Am J Psychiatry 1995;152:683–91.
13. Silverman WK, Cerny JA, Nelles WB, Burke AE. Behavior problems in children of parents with anxiety disorders. J Am Acad Child Adolesc Psychiatry 1988;27:779–84.
14. Pribor EF, Dinwiddie SH. Psychiatric correlates of incest in childhood. Am J Psychiatry 1992;149:52–6.
15. Sanderson WC, Barlow DH. Description of patients diagnosed with DSM-III-R GAD. J Nerv Ment Dis 1990;178:588–91.
16. Taylor CB, Sallis JF, Needle R. Relation of physical activity and exercise to mental health. Public Health Rep 1985;100: 195–202.
17. Butler G, Fennell M, Robson P, Gelder M. Comparison of behavior therapy and cognitive behavior therapy in the treatment of GAD. J Consult Clin Psychol 1991;59:167–75.
18. Chiaie RD, Pancheri P, Casacchia M, et al. Assessment of the efficacy of buspirone in patients affected by generalized anxiety disorder, shifting to buspirone from prior treatment with lorazepam. J Clin Psychopharmacol 1995;15:12–19.
19. Piven J, Chase GA, Landa R, et al. Psychiatric disorders in the parents of autistic individuals. J Am Acad Child Adolesc Psychiatry 1991;30:471–8.
20. Karno M, Golding JM, Sorenson SB, Burnam A. Epidemiology of OCD in five U.S. communities. Arch Gen Psychiatry 1988;45:1094–9.
21. Alarcon RD. How to recognize OCD. Postgrad Med 1991;90: 131–43.
22. Austin LS, Lydiard RB, Fossey MD, et al. Panic and phobic disorders in patients with OCD. J Clin Psychiatry 1990;51:456–8.
23. Riddle MA, Scahill L, King R, et al. OCD in children and adolescents. J Am Acad Child Adolesc Psychiatry 1990;29: 766–22.
24. Hollander E, Schiffman E, Cohen B, et al. Signs of central nervous system dysfunction in OCD. Arch Gen Psychiatry 1990;47:27–32.
25. Griest J, Chouinard G, DuBoff E, et al. Double-blind parallel comparison of three dosages of sertraline and placebo in outpatients with obsessive-compulsive disorder. Arch Gen Psychiatry 1995;52:289–95.
26. Ravizza L, Barzega G, Bellino S, et al. Predictors of drug treatment response in obsessive-compulsive disorder. J Clin Psychiatry 1995;56:368–73.
27. Greist JH. Treatment of OCD. J Clin Psychiatry 1990;51 Suppl 8:44–50.
28. Jenike MA. Approaches to the patient with treatment-refractory OCD. J Clin Psychiatry 1990;51 Suppl 2:15–21.
29. Emmelkamp PMG, de Haan E, Hoogduin CAL. Marital adjustment and OCD. Br J Psychiatry 1990;156:55–60.
30. Calvocoressi L, Lewis B, Harris M, et al. Family accommodation in obsessive-compulsive disorder. Am J Psychiatry 1995;152:441–3.
31. Pary R, Lippmann SB, Turns DM, Tobias CR. Post-traumatic stress disorder in Vietnam veterans. Am Fam Physician 1988; 37:145–50.

32. Silven SM, Iacono C. Symptom groups and family patterns of Vietnam veterans with PTSD. In: Figley CR, editor. Trauma and its wake. Vol II. New York: Brunner-Mazel, 1986.
33. Buydens-Branchey L, Noumair D, Branchey M. Duration and intensity of combat exposure and PTSD in Vietnam veterans. J Nerv Ment Dis 1990; 178:582–7.
34. Bownes IT, O'Gorman BC, Sayers A. Assault characteristics and PTSD in rape victims. Acta Psychiatr Scand 1991;83:27–30.
35. Feinstein A, Dolan R. Predictors of PTSD following physical trauma. Psychol Med 1991;21:85–91.
36. Blanchard EB, Hickling EJ, Vollmer AJ, et al. Short-term follow-up of post-traumatic stress symptoms in motor vehicle accident victims. Behav Res Ther 1995; 33:369–77.
37. Davidson JRT, Foa EB. Refining criteria for PTSD. Hosp Commun Psychiatry 1991;42:259–61.
38. Perconte ST, Griger ML, Belucci G. Relapse and rehospitalization of veterans two years after treatment for PTSD. Hosp Commun Psychiatry 1989;40:1072–3.
39. Silver JM, Sandberg DP, Hales RE. New approaches in the pharmacotherapy of PTSD. J Clin Psychiatry 1990;51 Suppl 10:33–8.
40. Friedman MJ. Toward rational pharmacotherapy for PTSD. Am J Psychiatry 1988;145:281–5.
41. Watson CG, Anderson PED, Gearhart LP. Posttraumatic stress disorder (PTSD) symptoms in PTSD patients' families of origin. J Nerv Ment Dis 1995; 183:633–8.

CASE PRESENTATION

Subjective

PATIENT PROFILE

Nancy Nelson is a 40-year-old white female accountant.

PRESENTING PROBLEM

"Feeling nervous."

PRESENT ILLNESS

Mrs. Nelson reports a long history of recurrent anxiety, becoming worse over the last 3 years. Her hands are often moist and tremulous, and she has trouble falling asleep at night. Her symptoms are worse with new people and when with clients at work. She is fearful of making mistakes on the job, especially on clients' tax returns. She has trouble relaxing even on weekends and vacations. She feels some relief when she takes a drink of alcohol.

PAST MEDICAL HISTORY

She has had three urinary tract infections over the past year; the last was treated 4 months ago.

SOCIAL HISTORY, HABITS, AND FAMILY HISTORY

Are unchanged since her last visit 4 months ago (see Chapter 15).

REVIEW OF SYSTEMS

She reports occasional urinary frequency and one- to two-time nocturia.

- What additional medical history would you like to know? Why?
- What is a likely reason for today's visit?
- What more would you like to know about her symptoms at work?
- What might Mrs. Nelson be trying to tell you today?

Objective

General

The patient appears tense and fidgets with her hair and fingers during the interview.

Vital Signs

Blood pressure, 118/60; pulse, 74 and regular; respirations, 18.

Examination

The eyes, ears, nose, and throat are normal; the neck and thyroid are unremarkable; the hands are cool with slightly moist palms. No tremor is present.

- What additional information—if any—might you include in the physical examination, and why?
- Are there other areas of the body that should be examined today? Why?
- What physical diseases might cause Mrs. Nelson's symptoms? How might you eliminate these as diagnostic possibilities?
- What laboratory tests or diagnostic imaging—if any—would you obtain today? Why?

Assessment

- What is your diagnostic assessment? How would you explain this to Mrs. Nelson?
- Might today's complaint be a "ticket of admission" to discuss other problems? Explain.
- Might her symptoms be related to life events that have not yet been discussed, and how would you elicit this information?
- What might be the impact of this illness on the family? On coworkers?

Plan

- Describe your therapeutic recommendation. How would you explain this to Mrs. Nelson?
- What—if any—life-style changes would you advise?
- Would you recommend consultation or referral? Explain.
- What continuing care would you recommend?

23 Depression

RUPERT R. GOETZ, SCOTT A. FIELDS, AND
WILLIAM L. TOFFLER

To effectively treat patients with depression, physicians need a clear understanding of the current systems of classification for depressive disorders. The *Diagnostic and Statistical Manual of Mental Disorders (DSM IV)* divides affective disorders into 10 categories: major depression; bipolar I, bipolar II, dysthymic, and cyclothymic disorders; mood disorders due to medical conditions and due to substance abuse; and depressive, bipolar, and mood disorders not otherwise specified.[1] We first explore diagnostic and therapeutic concepts, highlighting the structure behind the current understanding of these disorders. Then we discuss the application of these concepts to the process of evaluation and treatment of patients, including special populations.

Epidemiology

Almost half of all office visits resulting in a mental disorder diagnosis are to nonpsychiatrists, mostly physicians in primary care.[2] Patients seen in this setting may be in an earlier, less organized stage of illness.[3] Table 23.1 summarizes the prevalence of affective disorders. Generally, women are at higher risk than men, as are patients with other medical or psychiatric conditions.

Etiology

Mechanisms of depression in three main areas have been investigated: abnormalities in neurotransmission, neurophysiology, and neuroendocrine function. The ultimate causes of these disorders remain unclear. Clinically, etiologic differentiation and specific biologic tests remain limited in their usefulness. The biopsychosocial model described by Engel in 1980[4] underscores the interrelation of biologic, psychological,

Table 23.1. Epidemiology of affective disorders in the general population

Disorder	Current prevalence (%)	Lifetime prevalence (%)
Major depression	3–6	10–20
Dysthymia	1	2–3
Bipolar disorder	< 0.5	0.5–1.0

and social issues in illness and may be used to better understand the possible origins of depression. Genetic factors may play a role in increased susceptibility. First-degree relatives of a patient with affective disorder have about a 25% to 30% likelihood of major depression or bipolar disorder. Twin studies have shown concordance for major depression of 50% for monozygotic twins and 25% for dizygotic twins.[5] The variation in risk makes unlikely a single affective disorder gene with predictable penetrance for specific disorders.

Psychological factors have long been considered important in depression. Behavioral theorists[6] argue that impaired social skills lead to dysphoria and the addition of secondary gain leads to clinical depression. Cognitive-behavioral theory[7] holds that cognitive distortions, activated by a stressor, lead some individuals to unrealistically negative and demeaning views of themselves, the world, and the future. Some theories of depression place a high value on the patient's function within society. That is, patients cannot be understood outside their social context.

Diagnosis

Diagnostic Criteria

A *major depressive disorder* requires the patient to have a major depressive episode (Table 23.2), and there should never have been a manic, hypomanic, or mixed episode. Either depressed mood or loss of interest or pleasure is required. Once the diagnosis is made, the severity (mild, moderate, severe), result of treatment (partial or full remission), and presence or absence of psychotic features are noted. These features may be either mood congruent (depressive in character) or incongruent. Catatonic, melancholic, or atypical features, as well as postpartum onset or longitudinal course (seasonal, rapid cycling), can be described.

Dysthymia is used to describe a specific disorder rather than a "mild depression." It is diagnosed when two of six criteria (Table 23.3) are met over a period of 2 years, uninterrupted by more than a 2-month period and not initiated by a major depression.

TABLE 23.2. *DSM-IV* diagnostic criteria for a major depressive episode

A. Five of the following nine symptoms are present for at least 2 weeks
   1. Depressed mood
   2. Diminished interest or pleasure
   3. Significant appetite or weight change
   4. Sleep disturbance (insomnia or hypersomnia)
   5. Psychomotor agitation or retardation
   6. Fatigue or loss of energy
   7. Feelings of worthlessness or inappropriate guilt
   8. Diminshed ability to think or concentrate
   9. Recurrent thoughts of death or suicide
B. Not a mixed episode
C. Causes significant distress or impairs function
D. Not attributable to medical condition or substance abuse
E. Not attributable to bereavement

A mnemonic may be useful to recall these criteria: **D**epression **i**s **w**orth **s**eriously **m**emorizing **e**xtremely **g**ruesome **c**riteria, **s**orry (DIWS MEGCS). These initials stand for: **D**epressed mood, **I**nterest, **W**eight, **S**leep, **M**otor activity, **E**nergy, **G**uilt, **C**oncentration, and **S**uicide.[8]

Source: Adapted from American Psychiatric Association.[1] With permission.

Bipolar disorders are divided into types I and II, the former characterized by at least one manic (Table 23.4) or mixed episode, the latter by at least one hypomanic episode and major depressive episodes. Mania is distinguished from hypomania by the longer duration and presence of marked impairment in social or occupational functioning or the need for admission to a hospital because of danger to self or others. A mixed episode is defined as fitting criteria for major depressive and manic episodes together for 1 week.

TABLE 23.3. *DSM-IV* diagnostic criteria for dysthymic disorder

A. Depressed mood for at least 2 years
B. Two of the following six symptoms
   1. Poor appetite or overeating
   2. Insomnia or hypersomnia
   3. Low energy or fatigue
   4. Low self-esteem
   5. Poor concentration or difficulty making decisions
   6. Feelings of hopelessness
C. Never interrupted for more than 2 months at a time
D. No major depression during the first 2 years
E. Never had a manic episode
F. Not superimposed on a psychotic disorder
G. Not attributable to medical conditions or substance abuse
H. Causes significant distress or impairment

Source: Adapted from American Psychiatric Association.[1] With permission.

TABLE 23.4. *DSM-IV* diagnostic criteria for a manic episode

A. Distinct period of elevated, expansive, or irritable mood for 1 week
B. Three of the following seven symptoms (four if the mood is only irritable)
   1. Inflated self-esteem or grandiosity
   2. Decreased need for sleep
   3. More talkative than usual or pressure to keep talking
   4. Flight of ideas or experience of racing thoughts
   5. Distractibility
   6. Increased goal-directed activity or psychomotor agitation
   7. Excessive involvement with pleasurable activities with potential painful consequences
C. Not a mixed episode
D. Disturbance sufficiently severe to cause marked impairment
E. Not based on medical conditions or substance abuse

Source: Adapted from American Psychiatric Association.[1] With permission.

Analogous to dysthymia, *cyclothymia* is a disorder characterized by hypomanic and depressed episodes over 2 years, never without affective symptoms for longer than 2 months. Mood disorders caused by general medical conditions and substance-induced mood disorders are now included within the group of affective disorders, and atypical disorders are divided into three "not otherwise specified" categories.

In all cases, an organic basis for the disturbance must be ruled out. The condition should also not be attributable to a primary psychotic disorder. Depressive disorders can be linked in a diagnostic algorithm (Fig. 23.1). The important role of early detection of a possible manic episode is emphasized by its placement near the top of the sequence.

Related Diagnoses

Several other disorders present with dysphoria as the chief complaint or prominent feature. They should be considered as part of a differential diagnosis (Fig. 23.2).

COGNITIVE DISORDERS

Cognitive mood disorders may include both depressed and manic presentations together with indication of an underlying medical disorder in the physical, mental status, or laboratory examination. In particular, abnormalities in cognitive testing, such as disorientation, memory deficits, attention, and concentration difficulties should raise the concern of a cognitive disorder.

Delirium and dementia may have prominent affective symptoms. *Delirium,* characterized by inability to sustain attention, is more likely in elderly or medically ill patients. It is often acute in onset and shows fluctuation. *Dementia* begins insidiously. Affective lability, periods of apathy, and concentration and memory problems are prominent. Dif-

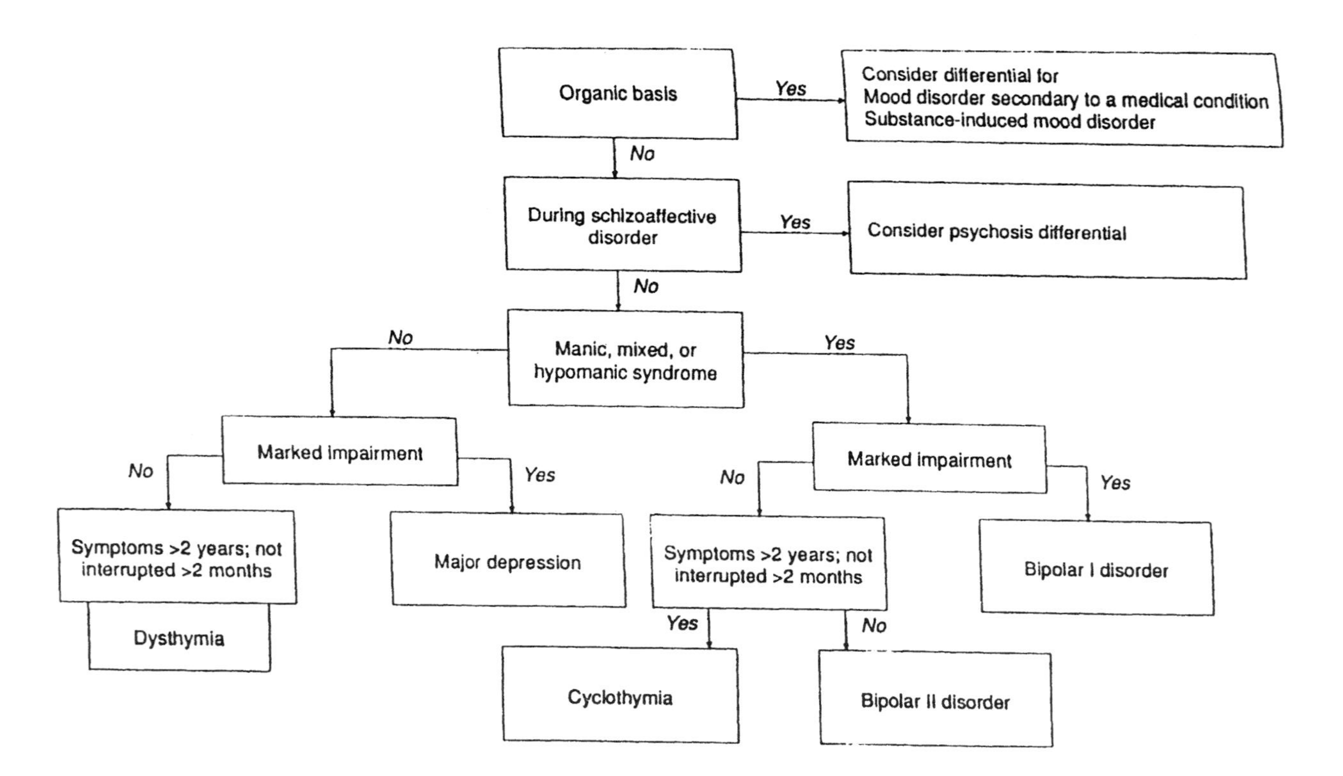

FIGURE 23.1. Differential diagnostic algorithm of affective disorders.

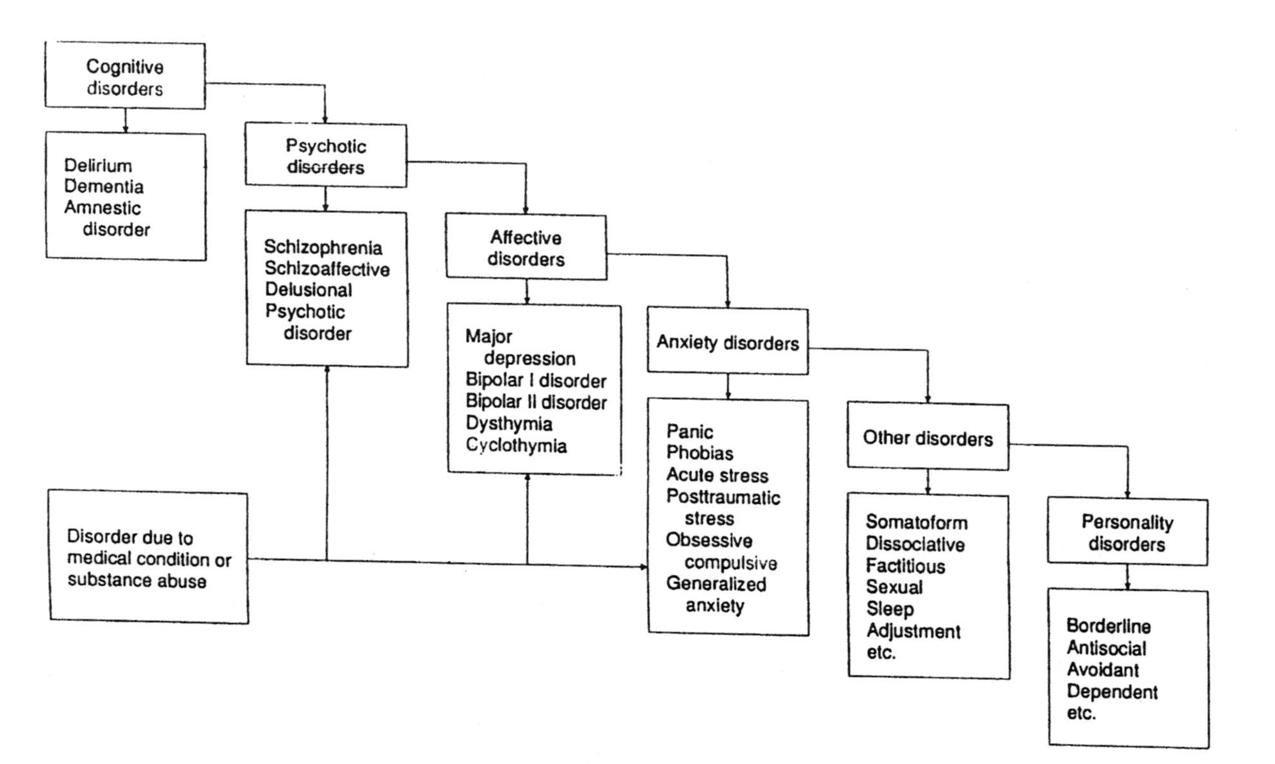

FIGURE 23.2. Implied differential diagnostic cascade of psychiatric disorders.

ferentiation from the "pseudodementia of depression" may be difficult, and treatment may have to be directed at an affective disorder to clarify the diagnosis. Alcohol and drug abuse and dependence disorders fall into the category of substance-related mental disorders. The classification of the psychiatric disorders induced by substances into each category emphasizes the importance of distinguishing them as a first priority.

PSYCHOTIC DISORDERS

Psychotic disorders are characterized by loss of reality contact. When the affective symptoms meeting criteria for a major depressive episode or for mania are present as well, a diagnosis of a schizoaffective disorder is assigned. Differentiation from the affective disorders with psychotic features is possible when there is a 2-week history of psychosis in the absence of affective symptoms. Occasionally, treatment for both disorders over time is required to clarify the underlying diagnosis.

ANXIETY DISORDERS

Anxiety disorders, in particular panic and posttraumatic stress disorder, may have severe dysphoria as the presenting complaint. The prominence of anxiety and vegetative signs characteristic of depression may help define the diagnosis.

SOMATOFORM DISORDERS

With somatoform disorders, such as chronic pain (somatoform pain disorder) and hypochondriasis, a patient who meets criteria for the affective disorder should be assigned this diagnosis in addition to the somatoform diagnosis.

PERSONALITY DISORDERS

Personality disorders are characterized by long-standing, pervasive, maladaptive personality traits; they therefore also often include significant dysphoria. The presence of a personality disorder should not obviate the diagnosis of a major affective disorder. However, a patient who has suffered from intense constant depression since adolescence is much less likely to respond to biologic treatments than a patient with major depression alone.

BEREAVEMENT

Grief, though intense, must be seen within its cultural context. The duration may be variable, though morbid preoccupation with worthlessness, prolonged and marked functional impairment, and marked psychomotor retardation may raise the concern that the patient is suffering from a major depression.

Evaluation

A clear series of diagnostic and therapeutic steps allows differentiation of disorders and logical treatment choice. Practice guidelines may help to focus this workup.[9]

1. *History.* A thorough evaluation should include safety, current history and review of systems, prior episodes of depression (including psychosis, suicide ideations and attempts), treatments, prior medical problems, childhood and developmental difficulties, and family and social histories. The question of suicidal risk is the initial overriding concern. Together with this consideration the degree of the patient's competence to participate in treatment planning must be assessed.[10] History of a previous manic episodes must be investigated. Vegetative signs, including changes in sleep, appetite, weight, and sexual functioning, should be explored because of their relevance for medication choice.
2. *Mental status examination.* The general appearance of the patient must be noted. Abnormalities in the patient's cognitive function should raise the suspicion of an organic etiology. Loose associations, flight of ideas, or loss of reality contact point toward psychosis. Abnormal emotional states are the hallmark of affective disorders. Irritability and euphoria may speak for mania. Rating scales such as the Mini-Mental Status Examination or the Beck Depression Inventory may be helpful for objectifying this examination.
3. *Laboratory evaluation.* Laboratory workup of depression should include basic chemistries, complete blood count, and thyroid studies. Patients evaluated for depression are at increased risk for physical disorders.
4. *Consultation.* Each family physician must define when to refer a patient. Physician variables regarding consultation include experience with particular drugs, comfort with psychotherapeutic modalities, and availability of reliable consultants. Patient variables include trust in the physician, openness to referral, specific diagnostic characteristics such as psychosis, or treatment failure. Admission of a suicidal patient or treatment with electroconvulsive therapy (ECT) generally requires psychiatric consultation.

Treatment Principles

The patient's safety must be established. Voluntary or involuntary hospitalization must be offered when such safety is in doubt. No-harm contracts may be useful for assessing the risk to the patient; their therapeutic value is unclear. Biologic, psychological, and social interventions must be prioritized. A return visit for more extended evaluation and treatment planning may be necessary.

In the context of depression several basic rules have been formulated to guide treatment.

1. Treat medical disorders that underlie the depression first.
2. Address alcohol and drug abuse before attempting other interventions.
3. When a patient meets criteria for major depression, make the diagnosis and provide medical treatment.
4. When a patient does not fully meet these criteria, a treatment trial with antidepressants may be reasonable.
5. A 6-week treatment period, with at least 3 weeks at the highest tolerated safe dose can be considered an adequate treatment trial.
6. Psychotherapy should be provided in addition to biologic treatments.

When a patient does not respond to the initial treatment strategy, the history is reviewed for hidden alcohol or drug abuse, unrecognized underlying medical problems, or subtle psychotic symptoms. Patient compliance and determination of antidepressant blood levels are considered. The treatment plan is reviewed and revised as appropriate. Strategies used when there has been no response include changing to another antidepressant, such as tricyclics or even monoamine oxidase inhibitors (MAOIs), or augmentation with lithium or thyroid. Finally, ECT or combinations of tricyclic antidepressants, even with MAOIs, have been advocated but require special precautions.

Treatment

Biologic Therapies

Differentiation of unipolar from bipolar affective disorders is crucial because the basic treatment strategies differ. The mainstay of therapy for major depression is the antidepressant, although mood stabilizers and neuroleptics are used adjunctively. Conversely, the main treatment for bipolar disorders is a mood stabilizer, and adjunctive use of neuroleptics and antidepressants may be required.

When major depression is present, treatment with antidepressants should (and in some cases of dysthymia may) be offered. The compounds differ little in their antidepressant efficacy, but their side effect profiles are diverse. Choice is dictated by the desire to achieve or avoid certain side effects. Obviously, cost is also an important consideration, highlighted by managed care. Tables 23.5 and 23.6 outline specifics on the pharmacology and side effects of available preparations. Use of antidepressants in patients with bipolar disorders may increase the number of cycles per year and may provoke a manic episode.

TABLE 23.5. Effects and side effects of common antidepressants

Generic and trade names	Chemical type	Mean $t_{1/2}$ (hours)	Seda-tion	Anticho-linergic	Ortho-stasis	Usual dosage[a] (mg/day)	Cost[b] ($/month)	Watch for
Amitriptyline	Tricyclic tertiary amine	35	+++	+++	+++	75–300	5.30	
Elavil							47.99	
Endep							44.36	
Amoxapine	Dibenzoxapine	8	++	+++	+	100–300		EPS
Asendin							180.81	
Buproprion	Aminoketone	15	+	+	+	75–450		Seizures, agitation
Wellbutrin							67.60	
Clomipramine	Tricyclic tertiary amine	25	+++	+++	++	75–200		
Anafranil							98.10	
Desipramine	Tricyclic secondary amine	20	+	+	+	75–200	53.36	
Norpramin							105.62	
Pertofrane								
Doxepin	Tricyclic tertiary amine	15	+++	++	++	75–200	16.94	
Sinequan							57.27	
Adapin							48.20	
Fluoxitine	SSRI	100	0	0	0	20–60	64.75	Insomnia, anxiety
Prozac								
Fluvoxamin (Luvox)	Aralkylketone	15	+/–	0	0	50–300	121.00	Nausea
Imipramine	Tricyclic tertiary amine	20	++	++	+++	75–200	5.40	
Tofranil							88.94	
Janimine								
Maprotiline	Tetracyclic	25	++	++	++	75–225[c]	64.37	Seizures, rash
Ludiomil							81.15	
Mirtazepine (Remeron)	Piperazinoazepine	30	+/–	++	+/–	15–45	29.10	Weight gain
Nefazodone	Phenylpiperazine	3	+/–	+/–	0	200–600	53.10	Headache, nausea
Serzone								

(*Table continues on next page*)

TABLE 23.5. Effects and side effects of common antidepressants

Generic and trade names	Chemical type	Mean $t_{1/2}$ (hours)	Sedation	Anticholinergic	Orthostasis	Usual dosage[a] (mg/day)	Cost[b] ($/month)	Watch for
Nortriptyline	Tricyclic secondary amine	35	+	+	+	50–150	60.51	
Pamelor							78.43	
Aventyl							74.92	
Paroxetine	SSRI	20	+/–	+/–	0	20–50		
Paxil							54.60	Headache, nausea
Protriptyline	Tricyclic secondary amine	80	+	+++	++	15–40		
Vivactyl							83.82	
Sertraline	SSRI	25	+/–	0	0	50–200		
Zoloft							58.23	
Trazodone	Triazolo-pyridine	7	+++	+/–	++	100–400	34.37	Priapism
Desyrel							99.02	
Trimipramine	Tricyclic tertiary amine	20	+++	++	++	75–200	67.74	
Surmontil								
Venlafaxine	Cyclohexanol	5	+/–	0	0	75–300	32.42	Headache, nausea
Effexor								

Treat the elderly with approximately half the recommended dosage of each of these medications.
+++ = marked; ++ = moderate; + = mild; +/– = equivocal; 0 = none.
SSRI = selective serotonin reuptake inhibitor; EPS = extrapyramidal symptoms.
[a]Dosage: usual daily maintenance dose.
[b]Based on wholesale price listings, 1995.
[c]Maprotiline: ceiling dose due to possible seizures.

TABLE 23.6. Preferred use for antidepressants

Target symptom	Suggested choices[a]
Insomnia	Amitryptyline, doxepin
Hypersomnia	SSRI
Anorexia	Tricyclic
Hyperphagia	SSRI
Obsessions/compulsions	SSRI, clomipramine
Anxiety	SSRI, nefazodone, venlafaxine, imipramine
Panic	SSRI, imipramine, MAOIs
Elderly/frail	SSRI, desipramine, trazodone, buproprion
Cardiovascular disorders	Maprotiline,
Chronic pain	Amitriptyline, doxepin, nortriptyline
Peptic ulcer	Amitriptyline, imipramine
Pregnancy	Amitriptyline

[a]These suggestions are meant only as examples; the overall clinical picture guides choice.
SSRI = selective serotonin reuptake inhibitor

TRICYCLIC AND RELATED ANTIDEPRESSANTS

These classic antidepressants include, for example, amitriptyline, imipramine, nortriptyline, and desipramine (from most sedating to least). They are well studied, effective, and generally the most expensive.

Once a medication is chosen, a low starting dose is generally initiated. Incremental increases are made until the expected target range is reached, a clinical response is noted, or unacceptable side effects occur. Such dosage increases are often tolerated every 3 or 4 days. The patients should understand that a full therapeutic effect on their mood and energy can be expected after approximately 4 weeks. Sleep may improve within a few days, a desirable feature for patients suffering from associated insomnia. The patient may experience increased energy before mood and depressive thought patterns are reversed. Thus the early treatment phase is potentially more dangerous for a patient with suicidal thoughts. Because beneficial effects and side effects vary greatly in individual patients, frequent visits, initially weekly or even more often, are required until the depression has been alleviated.

When the patient has achieved remission of the depression, the medication should be continued for a minimum of 4 to 5 months. In cases of recurring or severe depression, continued medication for longer, possibly years, may be best. Once the decision to stop treatment has been made, dosage should be reduced slowly over several weeks while observing for any signs of relapse for several months.

SEROTONIN AGENTS

Newer antidepressants, (e.g., fluoxetine, fluvoxamine, nefazodone, sertraline), with almost exclusive serotonin activity (selective serotonin reuptake inhibitors, SSRIs), have favorable side effect profiles which may allow initiation at an effective antidepressant dose. Side effects at the beginning should prompt more gradual dosage increase; lack of response at the initial dose should prompt reevaluation for possible increase. Sexual side effects, such as decreased libido, premature ejaculation or anorgasmia may require additional treatments, such as addition of buproprion or a tricyclic, or medication change.

Combined serotonin and norepinephrine antidepressants, (e.g., nefazodone, venlafaxine), may be particularly useful in depression with comorbid anxiety. "Flu-like" symptoms may accompany their rapid discontinuation.[11]

MONOAMINE OXIDASE INHIBITORS

Monoamine oxidase inhibitors (MAOIs), e.g., phenelzine and tranylcypromine, have largely been replaced by newer antidepressants. They remain effective and are often used with psychiatric consultation. The risk of a hypertensive crisis can be avoided with dietary restrictions, excluding foods high in tyramine. Postural hypotension is likely to be the main side effect.

ELECTROCONVULSIVE THERAPY

Electroconvulsive therapy is a useful, effective procedure for treatment of severe depression and mania. Studies have shown it to be as effective or superior to other antidepressant treatments. It is contraindicated in patients with recent stroke, space-occupying intracranial lesions, or recent myocardial infarction. There are no scientifically valid studies showing longer-term memory loss or disturbances in the ability to learn new information. Maintenance antidepressant treatment should follow to prevent relapse.[12]

LITHIUM

Bipolar disorder is most commonly treated with lithium, one of the most effective mood stabilizers. It has antidepressant properties for the bipolar patient with depression as well as antimanic properties for the patient with elevated mood; it works best when used prophylactically.

It is excreted renally, so changes in fluid balance or dietary salt intake can dramatically affect the lithium level and produce toxicity. Dose-dependent side effects include gastrointestinal disturbances such as diarrhea and a fine hand tremor. Hypothyroidism occurs in up to 20% of patients. Thyroid levels must be checked before and every 6 months during treatment. Nephrogenic diabetes insipidus is infrequent, though up to 60% of patients on lithium complain of increased urination. Less frequent side effects seen at high lithium levels include vomiting and abdominal pain, nystagmus, slurred speech, weakness, dizziness, ataxia.

After a patient has reached stability, levels are rechecked every 3 to 6 months. Carbamazepine and valproate represent alternatives to lithium in nonresponsive patients.[13]

Psychological Therapies

Although biologic and, more controversially, psychoanalysis were the main treatments for depression in the past, studies since the 1970s have examined the usefulness of several psychotherapeutic modalities. For mild cases of major depression, interpersonal and cognitive-behavioral treatments should be used first. Combination of psychotherapy with antidepressants may be particularly indicated in patients maintained on medications, patients with severe neurotic character problems, and in the context of marital conflict.[14] There may be significant differences in the usefulness of these therapies for the short-term versus the long-term treatment of depression. Particularly when both biologic and psychological treatments are suggested, clear agreements, possibly contractual, between collaborating providers regarding who is responsible for care are necessary.

Social Treatments

Implications of the depression for marital, family, job, and social functioning must be considered and addressed. The patient's support network must be explored. Expectations regarding length of complete or partial disability should be discussed early. Social work interventions can hasten full recovery, which may otherwise be delayed or even made impossible.

Special Populations

Children

Social withdrawal, poor school performance, a phobia, aggression or self-deprecation, and somatic complaints may herald depression, in which case standardized testing of children may be helpful (see Chapter 22). Biologic treatments are generally considered to be effective for major depression in children and adolescents. The dosage of medications must take into consideration the lower fat/muscle ratio, which leads to a decreased volume for distribution of the drug. The relatively larger liver in children leads to more rapid metabolism of the tricyclic agents than in adults. Prepubertal children can have more dramatic swings in blood levels; therefore doses should be divided three times daily, a practice that can likely be discontinued in the adolescent.[15] Psychotherapy is frequently necessary, at times with inclusion of the whole family in treatment.

Elderly Population

Distinction between somatic (vegetative) symptoms of depression and physical problems is a common problem in the elderly (see Chapter 5). Vague somatic discomforts may herald depression. Psychotic symptoms may be subtle and focus on somatic complaints. When symptoms of cognitive impairment accompany depression, three main disorders must be distinguished: delirium, pseudodementia of depression, and depression in dementia. Delirium is characterized by its course, but the latter two diagnoses may be more difficult to delineate. A family history of affective disorder, concern about the deficits, and an inability to try hard at cognitive tasks all speak for depression.

A treatment trial with antidepressants to influence the reversible portion of the patient's dysfunction may be helpful. Side effects require particular attention. Of most concern are excess sedation, cardiac arrhythmias, orthostatic hypotension, and anticholinergic syndromes. Medications are usually begun at half the normal dosages for the average adult patient, and changes are made less frequently. Side effects should be monitored carefully and levels determined when questions arise. ECT may be useful in elderly patients with refractory depression, psychotic symptoms, medication intolerance, or medical compromise, as rapid progression to severe nutritional depletion is not uncommon.

References

1. American Psychiatric Association. Diagnostic and statistical manual of mental disorders. 4th rev ed. Washington, DC: APA, 1994.
2. Schurman R, Kramer P, Mitchell J. The hidden mental health network. Arch Gen Psychiatry 1985;42:89–94.
3. Williamson PS, Yates WR. The initial presentation of depression in the family practice and psychiatric outpatients. Arch Gen Psychiatry 1989;11: 188–93.
4. Engel G. The clinical application of the biopsychosocial model. Am J Psychiatry 1980;137:535–44.
5. Torgersen S. Genetic factors in moderately severe and mild affective disorders. Arch Gen Psychiatry 1986;43:222–6.
6. Lewinsohn PM. A behavioral approach to depression. In: Friedman R, editor. The psychology of depression: contemporary theory and research. New York: Wiley, 1974:157–85.
7. Beck AT. Depression: causes and treatment. Philadelphia: University of Pennsylvania Press, 1972.
8. Andreasen NC, Black DW. Introductory textbook of psychiatry. Washington, DC: American Psychiatric Press, 1990:191.
9. Depression Guideline Panel: Depression in Primary Care: Vol 1.: Diagnosis and Detection; Vol. 2.: Treatment of Major Depression. Clinical Practice Guideline No. 5. Rockville, M.D.: U.S. Department of Health and Human

Services, Public Health Service, Agency for Health Care Policy and Research, 1993; AHCPR Publications No.: 93-0550 and 93-0551.
10. Gutheil TG, Bursztajn H, Brodsky A. The multidimensional assessment of dangerousness: confidence assessment in patient care and liability prevention. Bull Am Acad Psychiatr Law 1986;14:123–9.
11. Wolfe R: Antidepressant withdrawal reactions. Am Fam Physician 1997;56: 455–462
12. Electroconvulsive therapy: consensus conference. JAMA 1985; 254(15):2103–8.
13. Janicak PG, Boshes RA. Advances in the treatment of mania and other acute psychotic disorders. Psychiatr Ann 1987;17: 145–9.
14. Scott WC. Treatment of depression by primary care physicians: psychotherapeutic treatments for depression. In: Informational report of the Council on Scientific Affairs, American Medical Association. Chicago: AMA, 1991.
15. Puig-Antich J, Ryan ND, Rabinovitch H. Affective disorders in childhood and adolescence. In: Weiner JM, editor. Diagnosis and psychopharmacology of childhood and adolescent disorders. New York: Wiley, 1985.

CASE PRESENTATION

Subjective

PATIENT PROFILE

Mary Nelson is a 71-year-old married white female retired teacher.

PRESENTING PROBLEM

"No energy and sleeping poorly."

PRESENT ILLNESS

For the past 2 months, Mrs. Nelson has noted tiredness and disturbed sleep. She lacks energy all day, yet sleeps for only short periods at night and wakes each morning about 4 a.m. unable to fall asleep again. Her appetite is poor, and she sometimes cries inappropriately. She has had several similar episodes in the past treated with antidepressants. Her last visit, about 8 months ago, focused on management of her hypertension (see Chapter 8).

PAST MEDICAL HISTORY

She is hypertensive on hydrochlorothiazide for 10 years, with a calcium channel blocker added 8 months ago.

SOCIAL HISTORY, HABITS, AND FAMILY HISTORY

All are unchanged since her previous visit.

REVIEW OF SYSTEMS

She occasionally notes flushed skin, especially during the afternoon. She believes she has lost some weight recently.

- What additional medical history might help clarify the problem?
- How might you inquire about life events that could be contributing to Mrs. Nelson's problem?
- What might have prompted the visit today? How would you elicit this information?
- What more might you like to know about the flushed skin?

Objective

VITAL SIGNS

Weight, 119 lb (decrease of 3 lb since her previous visit 8 months ago); blood pressure, 142/76; pulse, 70.

EXAMINATION

The patient has a flat affect, speaks slowly, and becomes tearful several times during the interview. The eyes, ears, nose, and throat are normal. There are no abnormalities of the neck and thyroid. The hands are warm, and there is no tremor.

- What additional data—if any—might you obtain from the physical examination? Why?
- What physical diseases—if any—might account for today's symptoms? How would you examine for these possibilities?
- What—if any—laboratory tests would you obtain today?
- What physical findings—if present—would suggest that the problem is other than a primary affective disorder? Explain.

Assessment

- What is your diagnostic assessment? How would you explain this to the patient?
- How might the family be contributing to the illness?
- How might you assess the possibility of suicidal intent? Describe how you would frame this inquiry.
- What is likely to be the meaning of this illness to the patient? To the family?

Plan

- Describe your specific recommendations. How would you present these to Mrs. Nelson?
- What community resources—if any—might be useful in caring for this patient's problem? How would you gain involvement of these other professionals?
- If Mrs. Nelson indicated that she had thoughts of suicide, what would you do?
- What continuing care would you advise?

24

Care of Acute Lacerations

Bryan Campbell and George F. Snell

The optimum management of lacerations requires knowledge of skin anatomy and the physiology of wound healing. Such knowledge facilitates proper management of wounds of varying depth and complexity. By understanding the healing process the family physician can maximize the options for repair and minimize the dangers of dehiscence and infection. The goals of primary closure are to stop bleeding, prevent infection, preserve function, and restore appearance. The patient always benefits from a physician who treats the patient gently, handles the tissue carefully, understands anatomy, and appreciates the healing process.[1,2]

Skin Anatomy

Figure 24.1 represents a model of the skin and the underlying tissue down to structures such as bone or muscle. Two additional features of skin anatomy that affect the repair of injuries are cleavage lines and wrinkles. Lines of cleavage are also known as Langer's lines. These lines (Fig. 24.2) are formed by the collagen bundles that lie parallel in the dermis. An incision or repair along these lines lessens disruption of collagen bundles and decreases new collagen formation and therefore causes less scarring. Wrinkle lines are not always consistent with Langer's lines. If a laceration is not in an area of apparent wrinkling, following the basic outline of Langer's lines results in the best repair.

Wound Healing

Phase One: Inflammatory Phase

The substrate, or inflammatory, phase occurs during the first 5 to 6 days after injury. Leukocytes, histamines, prostaglandins, and fibrinogen, delivered to the injury site via blood and lymphatic channels, attempt to neutralize bacteria and foreign material. The amount of inflammation

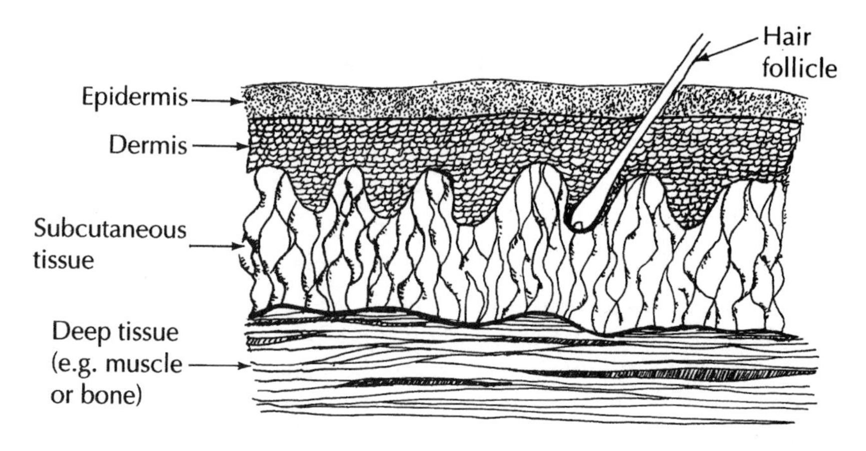

FIGURE 24.1. Model of skin and subcutaneous tissue.

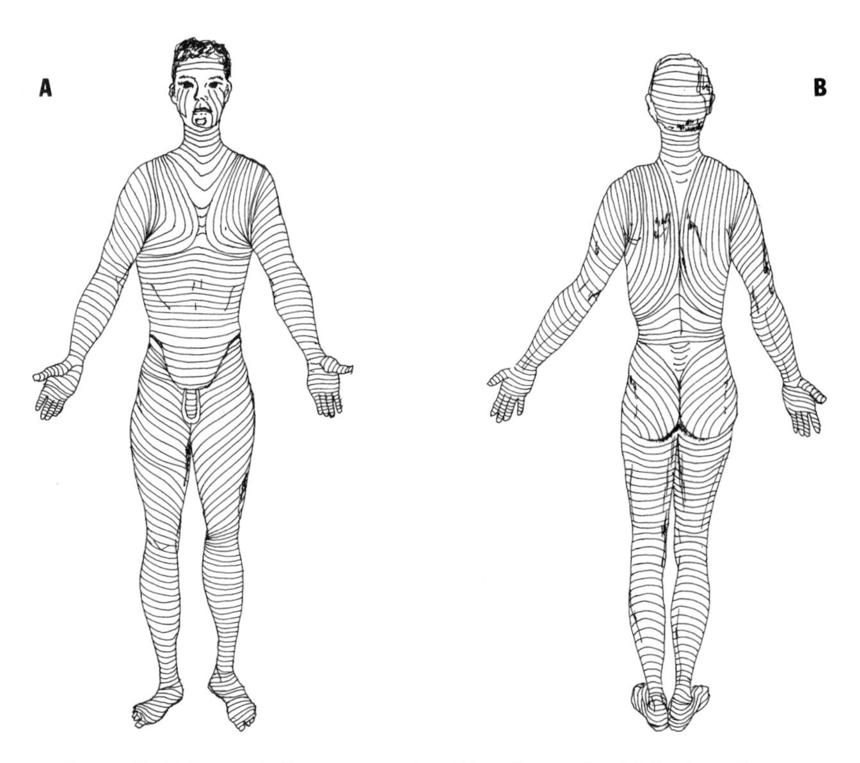

FIGURE 24.2. Langer's lines on anterior (A) and posterior (B) body surfaces.

present in a wound is related to the presence of necrotic tissue, which is increased by deadspace and impaired circulation. Specific measures that reduce the inflammatory response include débridement, removal of foreign material, cleaning, control of bleeding, and precise tissue coaptation.

Phase Two: Fibroblastic Phase

The fibroblastic, or collagen, phase occupies days 6 though 20 after injury. Fibroblasts enter the wound rapidly and begin collagen synthesis, which binds the wound together. As the collagen content rises, the wound strength increases until the supporting ligature can be removed. Compromise of the vascular supply can inhibit the development of collagen synthesis and interfere with healing.

Phase Three: Maturation (Remodeling) Phase

The wound continues to undergo remodeling for 18 to 24 months, during which time collagen synthesis continues and retraction occurs. Normally during this time the scar becomes softer and less conspicuous. The prominent color of the scar gradually fades, resulting in a hue consistent with the surrounding skin. Aberrations of the maturation process can result in an unsightly scar such as a keloid. Such scars are due to a combination of inherited tendencies and extrinsic factors of the wound. Proper technique in wound care and repair minimizes the extrinsic contribution to keloid formation. If it is necessary to revise an unsightly scar, the ideal delay is 18 months or more after the initial repair.

Anesthesia

Under most circumstances it is preferable to anesthetize the wound prior to preparation for closure. Before anesthesia a wound is inspected using a slow, gentle, aseptic technique to ascertain the extent of injury including an assessment of the neurovascular supply. At this time a decision is made to refer the patient if the complexity of the wound warrants consultation.

Topical Agents

When appropriate, topical anesthesia is ideal, as pain can be relieved without causing more discomfort or anxiety. Small lacerations may be closed without additional medications.

PAC (Pontocaine/Adrenaline/Cocaine) and TAC (Tetracaine/Adrenaline/Cocaine)

Pontocaine or tetracaine 2%/aqueous epinephrine (adrenaline) 1:1000/ cocaine (PAC) is the most commonly used topical agent.[3,4] It may be prepared in a 100 ml volume by mixing 25 ml of 2% tetracaine, 50 ml of 1:1000 aqueous epinephrine, 11.8 g of cocaine, and sterile normal saline to a volume of 100 ml.

Placing a saturated pledget over the wound for 5 to 15 minutes often provides adequate local anesthesia. Blanching of the skin beyond the margin of the wound allows an estimation of adequate anesthesia. Further anesthesia may be applied by injection if necessary.

Emla

Emla is a commercially available preparation of 2.5% lidocaine/2.5% prilocaine in a buffered vehicle. It is squeezed onto the skin surface and covered with an occlusive dressing. Its efficacy is similar to that of TAC, but it takes nearly twice as long to anesthetize the skin (30 minutes). The same guideline of skin blanching applies to the use of Emla.

Ethyl Chloride

A highly volatile fluid, ethyl chloride comes in commercially prepared glass bottles with a sprayer lid. This fluid can be sprayed onto the skin surface by inverting the bottle and pressing the lid. The flammable fluid chills the skin rapidly. The agent may be applied until skin frosting occurs. It provides brief anesthesia, allowing immediate placement of a needle without causing additional pain.

Injectable Agents

Lidocaine

Lidocaine produces moderate duration of anesthesia (about 1–2 hours) when used in a 1% or 2% solution. When mixed with 1:100,000 aqueous epinephrine, the anesthetic effect is prolonged (2–6 hours), and there is a local vasoconstrictive effect. Any anesthetic mixed with epinephrine should be used with caution on fingers, toes, or the penis to avoid risk of ischemia and subsequent necrosis. Occasional toxicity occurs with lidocaine, but most reactions are due to inadvertent intravascular injection. Manifestations of toxicity include tinnitus, numbness, confusion, and rarely, progression to coma. True allergic reactions are unusual.

It is possible to reduce the discomfort of lidocaine injection by buffering the solution with the addition of sterile sodium bicarbonate.[5–8] A solution of 9 ml of lidocaine plus 1 ml of sodium bicarbonate (44 mEq/50 ml) is less painful to inject but provides the same level of anesthesia as the unbuffered solution. It is also possible to buffer other injectable agents including those with epinephrine. However, epinephrine is unstable at a pH above 5.5 and is commercially prepared in solutions below that pH. Therefore any buffered local anesthetic with epinephrine must be used within a short time of preparation.[9] Warming a buffered solution to body temperature provides additional reduction of the pain of injection. Buffering also appears to increase the antibacterial properties of anesthetic solutions.[10]

Additional Agents

Mepivacaine (Carbocaine) produces longer anesthesia than lidocaine (about 45–90 minutes). It is not used with epinephrine. Reactions are similar to those seen with lidocaine. Procaine (Novocain) works quickly but has a short duration (usually less than 30–45 minutes). It has a wide safety margin and may be used with epinephrine. Bupivacaine (Marcaine) is the longest-acting local anesthetic (approximately 6–8 hours). It is often used for nerve blocks or may be mixed with lidocaine for problems that take longer to repair. It is also useful for injecting into a wound to provide postprocedural pain relief. It may be mixed with epinephrine and is available in 0.25%, 0.50%, and 0.75% solutions.

Diphenhydramine

Diphenhydramine (Benadryl) may also be used as an injectable anesthetic.[11] It is somewhat more painful to inject than lidocaine but has an efficacy similar to that of lidocaine. Diphenhydramine may be prepared in a 0.5% solution by mixing a 1 ml vial of 50 mg diphenhydramine with 9 ml of saline. This solution is useful when a patient claims an allergy to all injectable anesthetics.

Anesthetic Methods

Infiltration Blocks

Infiltration blocks are useful for most laceration repairs. The wound is infiltrated by multiple injections into the skin and subcutaneous tissue. Using a long needle and a fan technique decreases the number of injection sites and therefore decreases the pain to the patient. Using a 27-gauge or smaller needle to inject through the open wound margin also minimizes the patient's discomfort, as does moving from an anesthetized area slowly toward the unanesthetized tissue.

Field Blocks

Field blocks result in similar pain control but may distort the wound margin less and are useful where accurate wound approximation is necessary (e.g., the vermillion border). The area around the wound is injected in a series of wheals completely around the wound, thereby blocking the cutaneous nerve supply to the laceration. This technique is more time-consuming but produces longer-lasting anesthesia. Another option to reduce the initial pain of the injection is to produce a small wheal using buffered sterile water and then injecting the anesthetic through the wheal. The buffered water has a brief anesthetic action.

NERVE BLOCKS

Nerve blocks are most commonly effected by injecting a nerve proximal to the injury site. The most frequent use of this technique is the digital block performed by injecting anesthetic into the webbing between the digits at the metacarpophalangeal joint on each side of the digit (Fig. 24.3). Mouth and tongue lacerations are repairable using dental blocks. It is useful to receive practical instruction in such blocks from a willing dental colleague.

Sedation

The Task Force on Sedation and Analgesia by Non-Anesthesiologists[12] provides excellent protocols for sedative use by family physicians. Under adequate observation sedative agents can help the doctor deal with

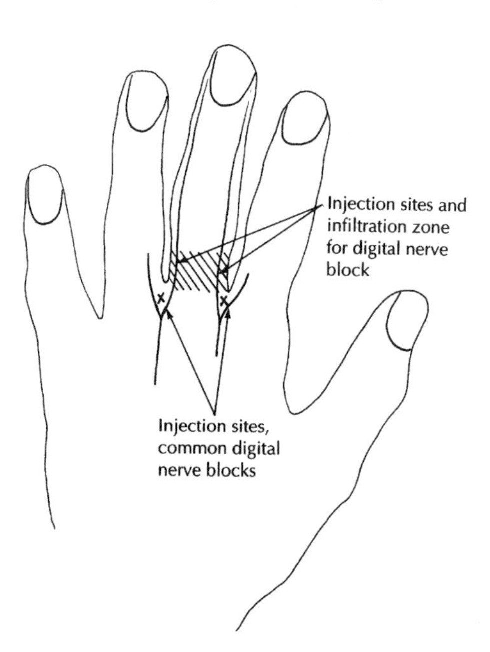

FIGURE 24.3. Digital nerve block.

difficult patients. For all agents described herein it is imperative that there be appropriate monitoring and that adequate resuscitation equipment be readily available. The welfare of the patient is of prime concern, and such medications should not be used solely for the provider's convenience.

Ketamine

Ketamine is a phencyclidine derivative. It provides a dissociative state resulting in a trance-like condition and may provide amnesia for the procedure. Ketamine can be administered by many routes, but the most practical for laceration repair is the oral method. It usually results in significant analgesia without hypotension, decreased heart rate, or decreased respiratory drive. The use of proper monitoring and the availability of resuscitation equipment is mandatory. Oral ketamine can be prepared by adding 2.5 ml of ketamine hydrochloride injection (100 mg/ml) to 7.5 ml of flavored syrup. It is then given at a dose of 10 mg/kg. Sedation occurs over 20 to 45 minutes after ingestion. The most common side effects include nystagmus, random extremity movements, and vomiting during the recovery stage.[13]

Midazolam (Versed)

Midazolam is a benzodiazepine with typical class effects of hypnosis, amnesia, and anxiety reduction. It is readily absorbed and has a short elimination half-life. It may be given as a single dose via the nasal, oral, rectal, or parenteral route. The rectal route is useful when the patient is combative. A cooperative patient prefers oral or nasal administration (oral dose 0.5 mg/kg; nasal dose 0.25 mg/kg, by nasal drops). Injectable midazolam is used to make a solution that may be given orally or nasally. The drug should be made into a 5 mg/ml solution. For oral use it may be added to punch or apple juice to improve the taste. The maximum dose for children by any route is 8 mg.

For rectal administration, a 6F feeding tube is attached to an angiocath connected to a 5 ml syringe. The lubricated catheter is then inserted into the rectum and the drug injected followed by a syringe full of air to propel the medication into the rectum. The tube is then withdrawn and the patient's buttocks are held together for approximately 1 minute. The dose is 0.45 mg/kg by this route. The medication may begin to work as soon as 10 minutes after administration. Side effects may be delayed, so the patient should be observed for at least an hour as the duration of a single dose lasts about an hour. Some burning can occur when the nasal route is used. Inconsolable agitation may appear regardless of the route of administration. This side effect of agitated crying resolves after several hours. Vomiting may also occur.[12,14,15]

Fentanyl

Fentanyl is a powerful synthetic opioid that produces rapid, short-lasting sedation and analgesia. Like other opioids, its effects are reversible, and it has limited cardiovascular effects. Although it can be given in many forms, oral transmucosal fentanyl citrate (OTFC) is available commercially in a lollipop (Fentanyl Oralet). This drug, commonly used as an preanesthetic medication, is available in three dosage forms (200, 300, and 400 μg). The dose for adults is 5 μg/kg to a maximum of 400 μg regardless of weight. Pediatric dosages begin at 5 μg/kg to a maximum of 15 μg/kg or 400 μg (whichever is less). Children weighing less than 15 kg should not receive fentanyl. OTFC effects are apparent 5 to 10 minutes after sucking the Oralet. The maximum effect is usually achieved about 30 minutes after use, but effects may persist for several hours. Side effects are common but usually minor. About half of patients develop transient pruritus, 15% notice dizziness, and at least one-third develop vomiting. The most dangerous effect is hypoventilation, which can be fatal.[12,16,17] Oversedation or respiratory depression responds to naloxone.

Nitrous Oxide

Nitrous oxide is a rapid-acting anesthetic that works within 3 to 5 minutes with a similar duration after cessation of administration.[18] Commercial equipment is available to deliver a mixture of nitrous oxide and oxygen at various ratios (usually 30–50% N_2O/50–70% O_2). Side effects include nausea in about 10% to 15% of patients with occasional emesis. The efficacy of nitrous oxide is known to be variable. Although some patients object to the use of the mask, many patients prefer using a specially designed self-administration mask. Nitrous oxide can cause expansion of gas-filled body pockets, and for that reason it should not be used in patients with head injuries, pneumothoraces, bowel obstructions, or middle ear effusions.

Wound Preparation

Proper preparation of a wound can improve the success of esthetically acceptable healing. The wound should be closed as soon as possible, although most lacerations heal well if closed within 24 hours after the injury. After anesthesia, proper cleansing should be accomplished by wiping, scrubbing, and irrigating with antiseptic soaps such as hexachlorophene (pHisoHex), chlorhexidine gluconate (Hibiclens), or povidone-iodine (Betadine). Irrigating the wound with normal saline using a syringe with a 22-gauge needle produces enough velocity to clean most wounds. Sterile scrub brushes may be useful for cleaning grossly contaminated lesions.

After washing and irrigation, the area is draped with sterile towels to create a clean field. The wound is then explored using sterile technique to confirm the depth of injury, ascertain whether injury to underlying tissue has occurred, rule out the presence of any foreign body, and determine the adequacy of anesthesia. After examination débridement is performed if necessary.

Débridement is the process of converting an irregular dirty wound to a clean one with smooth edges. Wound margins that are crushed, mangled, or devitalized are excised unless it is unwise to do so. Tissue in areas such as the lip or eyelid is removed with extreme caution. It is pointless to increase the deformity when a somewhat imperfect scar can provide a more functional result. If a considerable amount of tissue has been crushed, initial removal of all the damaged tissue may result in undesirable function (such as would occur if the skin over a joint was removed). Such injuries should be closed loosely using subcutaneous absorbable sutures. The scar can be revised later if necessary.

The initial incision is made with a scalpel followed by excision with a pair of sharp tissue scissors. The edges should be perpendicular to the skin surface or even slightly undercut to facilitate eversion of the skin margins (Fig. 24.4). In hairy areas incisions should parallel the hair shafts to minimize the likelihood of hairless areas around the healed wound (Fig. 24.5).

After débridement the skin edges are held together to see if it is possible to approximate them with minimal tension. Generally, it is necessary to undermine the skin to achieve greater mobility of the surface by releasing some of the subcutaneous skin attachments that

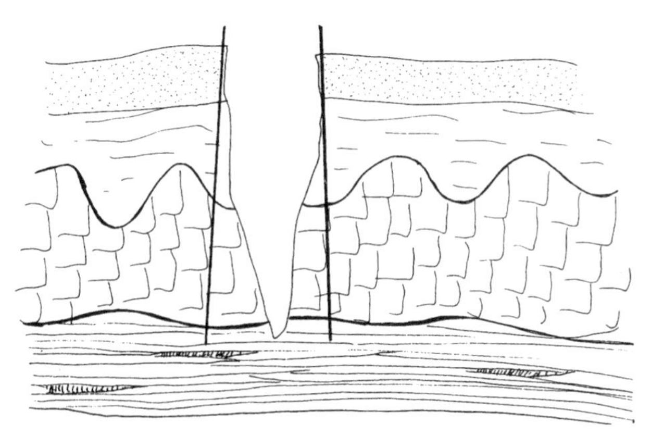

FIGURE 24.4. Slight undercutting of the wound edges facilitates slight eversion of the wound edge.

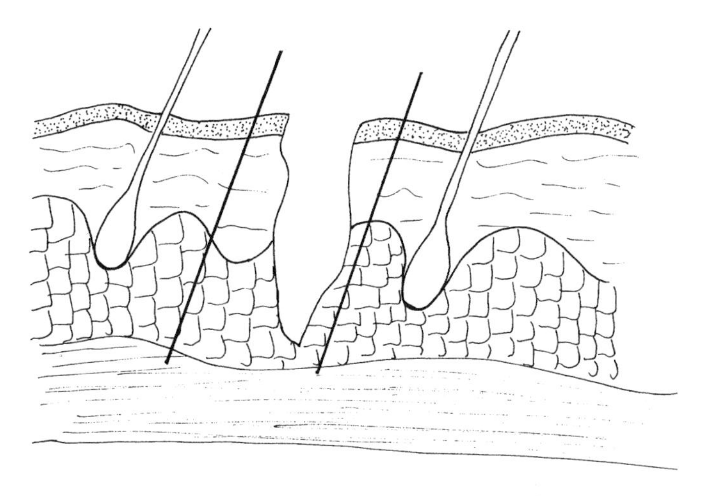

Figure 24.5. Parallel débridement in a hairy area avoids damaging hair follicles.

prevent the skin from sliding (Fig. 24.6). This step takes place in the subcutaneous layer and can be done with a scalpel or scissors. The wound is then undermined circumferentially about 4 to 5 mm from the edge of the margin. The undermining should be equal across the wound and widest where the skin needs to move the most, usually the center of the cut.

Hemostasis can be accomplished most easily by simple pressure on the wound site for 5 to 10 minutes. If pressure is unsuccessful, bleeders may be carefully cauterized or ligated. Cautery or ligation can hinder healing if large amounts of tissue are damaged. Small vessels can be controlled with absorbable suture if necessary, but large-arterial bleeders may need to be controlled with permanent ligature if it is possible to do so without

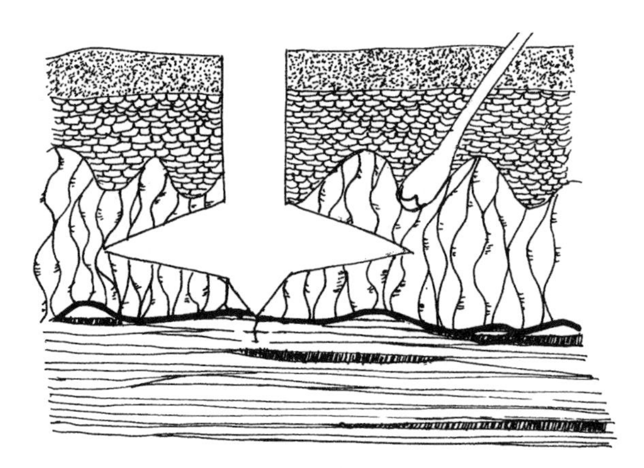

Figure 24.6. Undermining the subdermal layer facilitates closure.

compromising the distal circulation. If oozing persists, the wound is closed with a drain (e.g., a sterile rubber band or Penrose drain) left in the wound several days. An overlying pressure dressing minimizes bleeding. Advancing the drain every other day permits healing with minimal hematoma formation.

Wound Closure

Suture options are noted in Table 24.1. Absorbable materials are gradually broken down and absorbed by tissue; nonabsorbable sutures are made from chemicals that are encapsulated by the body and thus isolated from tissue. Monofilament sutures are less irritating to tissue but are more difficult to handle and require more knots than braided sutures. Stitches placed through the epidermis are done with nonabsorbable materials to minimize the tissue reactivity that occurs with absorbable stitches. Reverse cutting needles in a three-eighths or one-half circle design are available in various sizes for each type of suture.

TABLE 24.1. Common suture materials

Suture	Advantages	Disadvantages
Absorbable		
Catgut	Inexpensive	Low tensile strength Strength lasts 4–5 days High tissue reactivity
Chromic catgut	Inexpensive	Moderate tensile strength and reactivity
Polyglycolic acid (Dexon)	Low tissue reactivity	Moderately difficult to handle
Polyglactic acid (Vicryl)	Easy handling Good tensile strength	Occasional "spitting" of suture due to absorption delay
Polyglyconate (Maxon)	Easy handling Good tensile strength	Expensive
Nonabsorbable		
Silk	Handles well Moderately inexpensive	Low tensile strength High tissue reactivity Increased infection rate
Nylon (Ethilon, Dermilon)	High tensile strength Minimal tissue rectivity Inexpensive	Difficult to handle; slippery, so many knots needed
Polypropylene (Proline, SurgiPro)	No tissue reaction Stretches, accommodates swelling	Expensive
Braided polyester (Mersilene, Ethiflex)	Handles well Knots secure	Tissue drag if uncoated Expensive
Polybutester (Novafil)	Elastic, accommodates swelling and retraction	Expensive

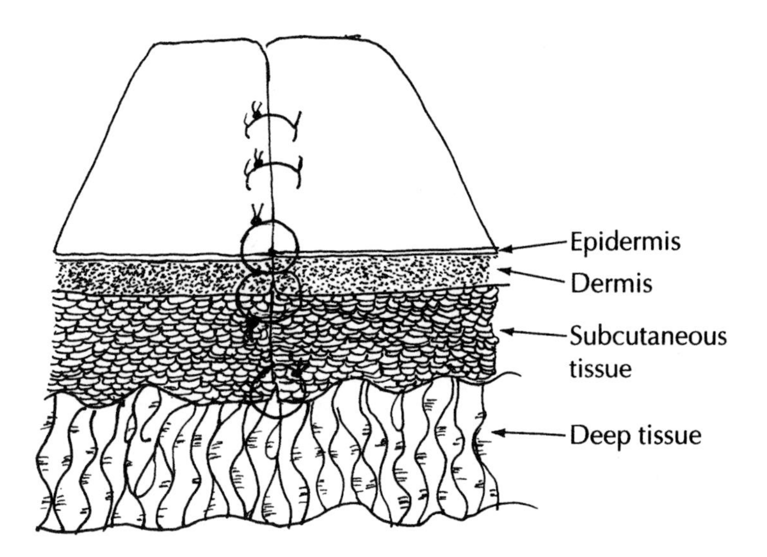

FIGURE 24.7. Layer closure showing sutures in the epidermis, at the dermal–epidermal junction, and at the dermal–fat junction.

A well-closed wound has three characteristics: The margins are approximated without tension; the tissue layers are accurately aligned; and deadspace is eliminated. Deep stitches are placed in layers that hold the suture, such as the fat–fascial junction or the derma–fat junction. A buried knot technique is the preferred method for placing deep sutures. Deep sutures provide most of the strength of the repair; and skin sutures approximate the skin margins and improve the cosmetic result (Fig. 24.7).

Suture Techniques

Simple Interrupted Stitch

A simple interrupted stitch is placed by passing the needle through the skin surface at right angles, placing the suture as wide as it is deep. The goal is to place sutures that slightly evert the edge of the wound (Fig. 24.8). This maneuver produces a slightly raised scar that recedes during the remodeling stage of healing and leaves a smooth scar. The opposite margin is approximated using a mirror image of the first placement. Following the natural radius of the curved needle places the suture in such a way as to evert the wound margin. It can be modified to correctly approximate the margins when the wound edges are asymmetric[1] (Fig. 24.9). Occasionally a wound exhibits excessively everted margins.

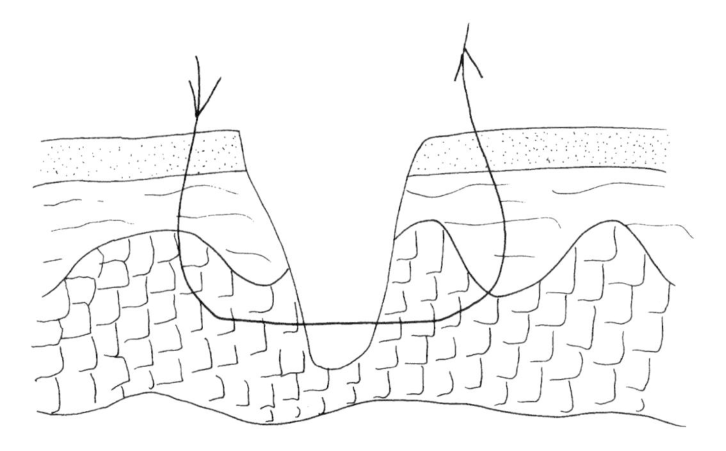

FIGURE 24.8. Simple interrupted suture with placement to facilitate wound eversion.

By reversing the usual approach and taking a stitch that is wider at the top than at the base, the wound can be inverted, improving the cosmetic appearance (Fig. 24.10). A useful general rule is that the entrance and exit points should be 2 mm from the margin for facial wounds but may be farther apart on other surfaces.[1,2] The open-loop knot (Fig. 24.11) avoids placing the suture under excessive tension and facilitates removal of the stitch. The first throw of the knot with two loops ("surgeon's knot") is placed with just enough tension to approximate the wound margin. The

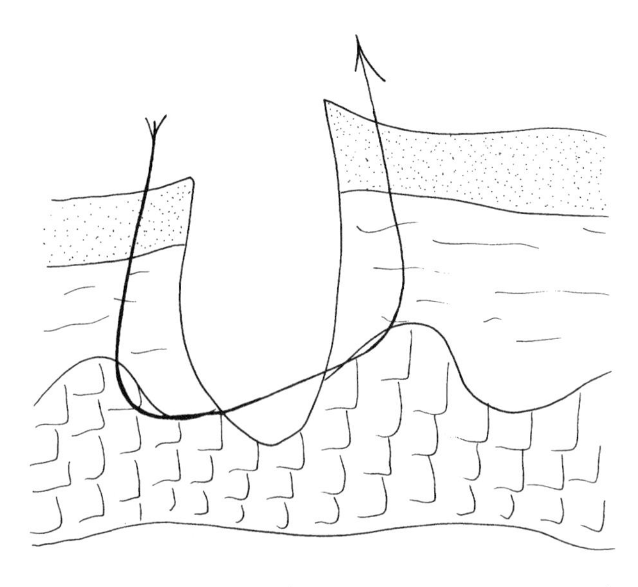

FIGURE 24.9. Placement of suture in an asymmetric wound.

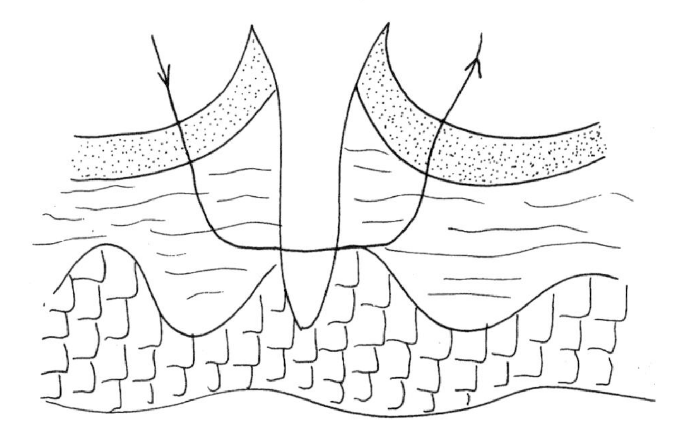

FIGURE 24.10. Suture placement in a wound with everted edges.

second throw, a single loop, is tied, leaving a little space so no additional tension is place on the first loop. Subsequent throws can be tightened snugly without increasing tension on the wound edge. Pulling all the knots to the same side of the wound makes suture removal easier and improves the aesthetics of the repair. As a rule of thumb one should put at least the same number of knots of a monofilament suture as the size of the ligature (e.g., five knots with 5-0 suture).

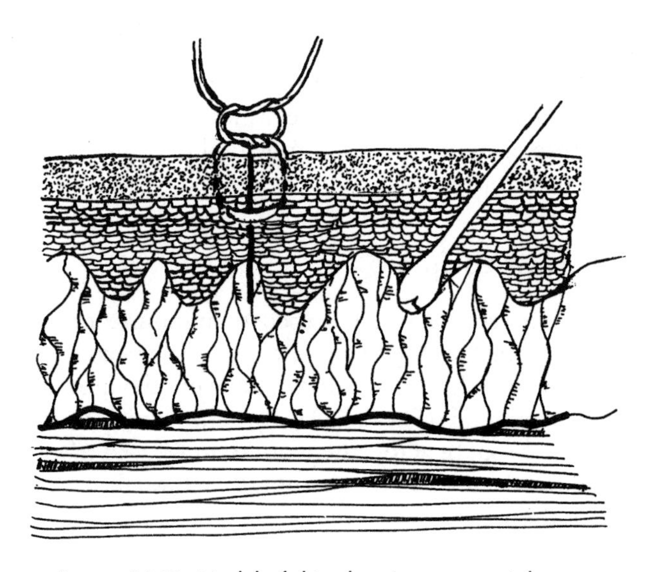

FIGURE 24.11. Model of skin showing surgeon's knot.

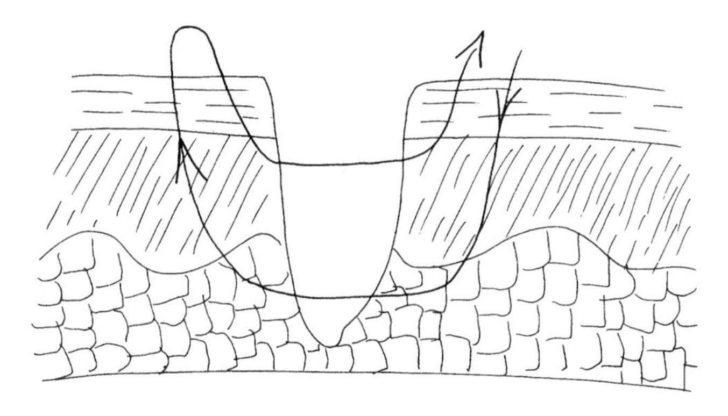

FIGURE 24.12. Vertical mattress suture.

Vertical Mattress Suture

The vertical mattress suture promotes eversion and is useful where thick layers are encountered or tension exists. Two techniques may be used. The classic method first places the deep stitch and closes with the superficial stitch (Fig. 24.12). The short-hand method[22] is performed by placing the shallow stitch first, pulling up on the suture (tenting the skin), and then placing the deeper stitch.

Intracuticular Running Suture

The intracuticular running suture, utilizing a nonabsorbable suture, can be used where there is minimal skin tension. It results in minimal scarring without suture marks. Controlled tissue apposition is difficult with this method, but it is a popular technique because of the cosmetic result. The suture ends do not need to be tied but can be taped in place under slight tension (Fig. 24.13).

Three-Point Mattress Suture

The three-point or corner stitch is used to minimize the possibility of vascular necrosis of the tip of a V-shaped wound. The needle is inserted into the skin of the wound edge on one side of the wound opposite the flap near the apex of the wound (Fig. 24.14A,B). The suture is placed at the mid-dermis level, brought across the wound, and placed transversely at the same level through the apex of the flap. It is then brought across the wound and returned at the same level on the opposite side of the V parallel to the point of entry. The suture is then tied, drawing the tip of the wound into position without compromising the blood supply (Fig. 24.14C). This

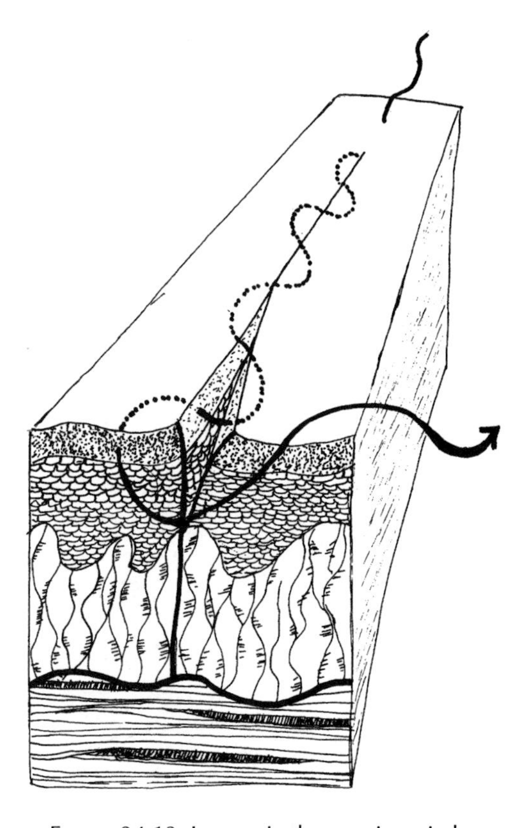

FIGURE 24.13. Intracuticular running stitch.

method can also be used for stellate injuries where multiple tips can be approximated in purse-string fashion.

Running or Continuous Stitch

The running stitch is useful in situations where speed is important (e.g., a field emergency) because individual knots do not have to be tied. It is appropriate for use on scalp lacerations especially because it is good for hemostasis. The continuous method does not allow fine control of wound margins (Fig. 24.15).

Specific Circumstances

Lacerations Across a Landmark

Lacerations that involve prominent anatomic features or landmarks, such as the vermilion border of the lip or the eyebrow, require special

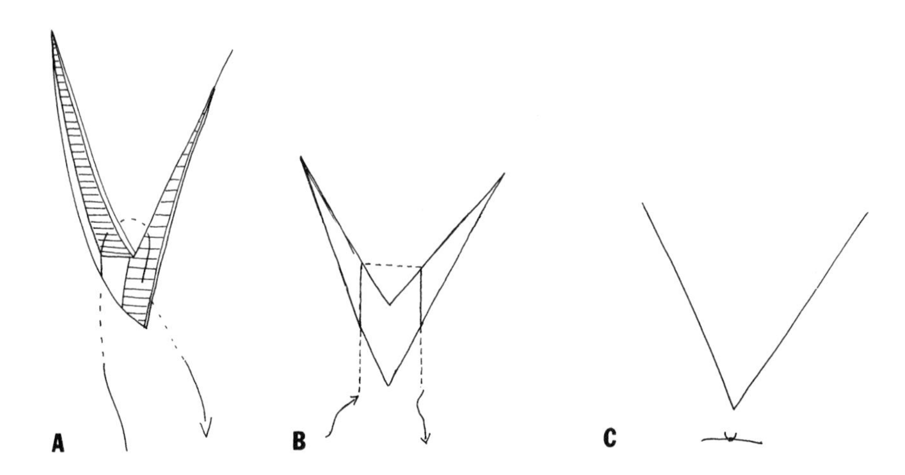

FIGURE 24.14. Three-point stitch. (A) Three-dimensional view showing suture placement. (B) Schematic view. (C) Finished stitch.

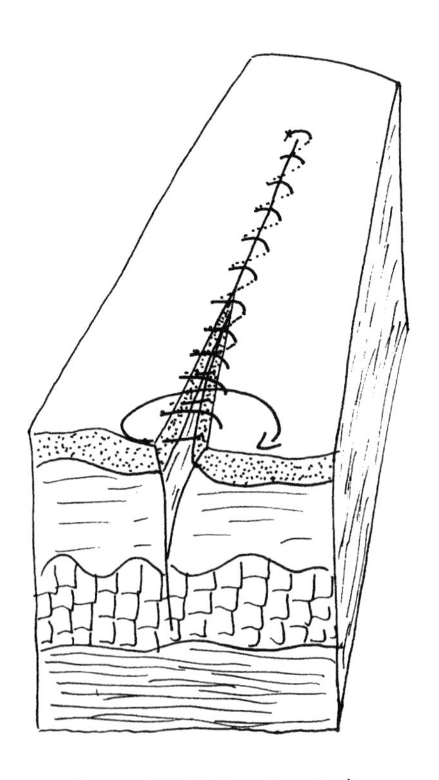

FIGURE 24.15. Running stitch

consideration. Commonly a laceration is closed from one end to the other, but in special situations it is advisable to place a retention stitch (a simple or vertical mattress stitch) to reapproximate the landmark border accurately. The remainder of the wound can then be closed by an appropriate method. If the retention stitch is under significant tension when the repair seems complete, it should be removed and replaced.

Beveled Lacerations

A frequently seen injury, the beveled laceration, tempts the physician to close it as it is; but the undercut flap may not heal well owing to disruption of the blood supply. The margins of the wound should be modified, as shown in Figure 24.16. The edges are squared, undermined, and closed in layers.

"Dog Ear" Lacerations

Dog ears, a common problem, results from wound closure where the sides of the laceration are unequal. One side bunches up, and a mound of skin occurs. It also occurs when an elliptical wound is closed in the center, leaving excess tissue at each end. To correct the problem, the dog ear is tented up with a skin hook, and a linear incision is made along one side. The excess triangle is then grasped at the tip and a second linear incision is made (Fig. 24.17). This maneuver allows closure in a single line.

Complex Lacerations

A wound may occur with unequal sides with a hump of tissue on one side. This lump of tissue may be excised using the technique described above for removal of dog ears. The triangular defect is then closed using a modification of the three-point mattress suture, the four-point technique shown in Figure 24.18. The resulting closure forms a T-shaped repair.

Finger Injuries

AMPUTATED FINGERTIP

If the area of the fingertip amputation is less than 1 cm^2, the wound can be handled by careful cleansing, proper dressings, and subsequent healing by secondary intention. If the wound is larger, the complexity of treatment increases. If the amputation is beveled dorsally and distally, a conservative approach without suturing or grafting usually results in

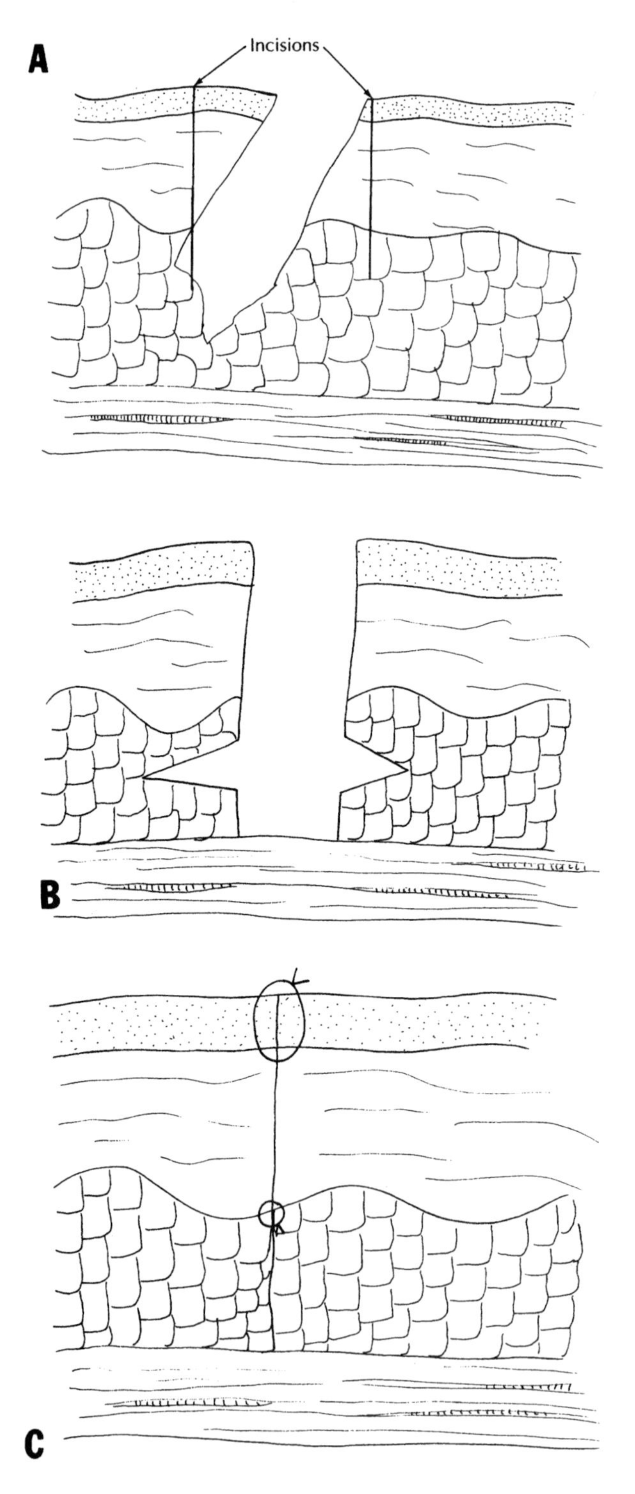

FIGURE 24.16. Closure of beveled wound. (A) Squaring beveled edges. (B) Undermining the fat layer. (C) Layered closure.

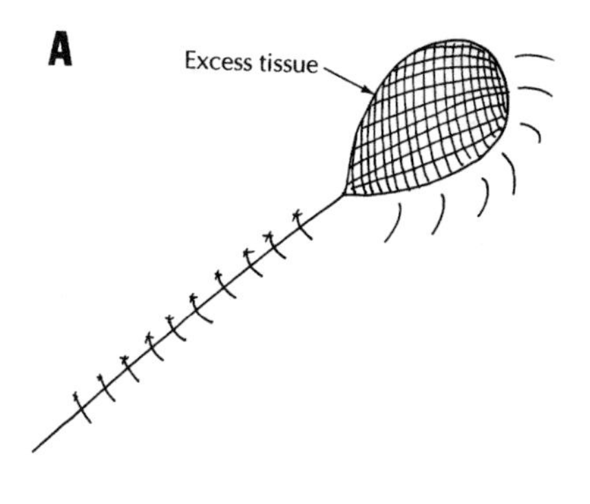

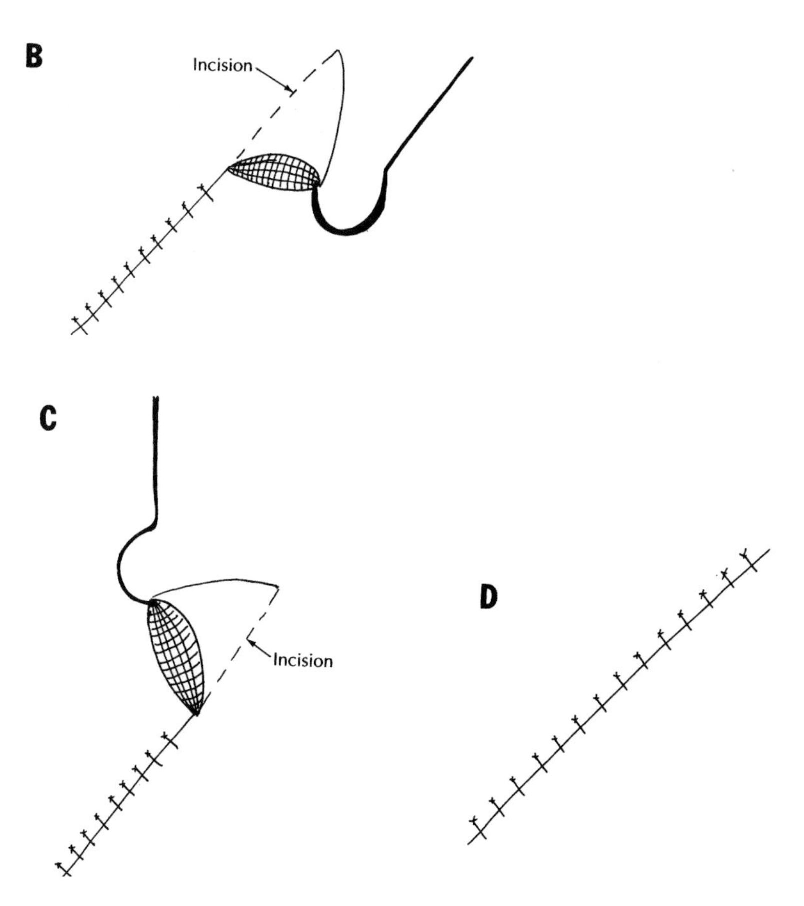

FIGURE 24.17. Correction of "dog ear." (A) Excess tissue at end of repair. (B) Tenting the dog ear and first incision. (C) Pulling flap across initial incision and position of second incision. (D) Appearance of final closure.

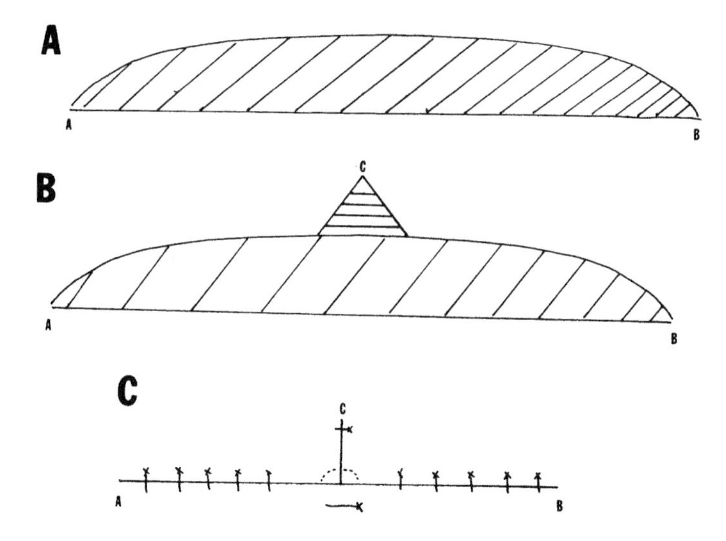

FIGURE 24.18. Unequal wound closure. (A) Sides of laceration are unequal. (B) Excise triangle of tissue on longer side. (C) T-Closure showing four-point suture.

good healing. An unfavorable angle requires more extensive repair.[23] Referral to a plastic or hand surgeon may be warranted.

NAIL BED INJURIES

Nail bed injuries can be managed by saving the nail and reapproximating nail matrix lacerations with fine absorbable sutures. It may be necessary to remove the nail to repair an underlying nail bed tear. The nail may then be replaced and held in position with several sutures, allowing the nail to act as a splint.

Alternatives to Suturing

Suturing has been an effective method for closing wounds for centuries, but options for skin suturing are now available. They may even represent more cost-effective methods of wound closure.

Staples

One option is the use of skin staples, which have been used for years in the operating room as the final closure for a variety of incisions. Typically, staples are used on the skin in wounds that would be closed in a straight line. The skin is closed with staples after other layers are closed by suturing. The most significant advantage to the use of staples is the decreased time necessary to close the skin. An assistant may be required to position the skin properly.[24]

Adhesives

The most commonly used tissue glues are related to cyanoacrylate ester known as Super Glue. Tissue glues for superficial wounds have the advantage of rapid closure, minimal physical and emotional trauma to the patient, and absence of a foreign body in the wound.[25,26] They may also be less expensive to use than traditional methods of closure.

Histoacryl Blue has been commercially available in Canada since 1975. It appears to be a safe alternative to suturing.[27–29] Hemostasis must be achieved before applying the glue. Layered closure may be accomplished using deep sutures combined with surface adhesive.

Postrepair Management

Most wounds should be protected during the first 1 to 2 days after repair. Frequently a commercial bandage may be used; but when the wound is still oozing, a pressure dressing is applied. The initial layer is a nonstick gauze dressing available in sterile packages, such as Adaptic, Telfa, or Xeroderm. A gauze pad is then placed and held in place by roller gauze, elastic wrap, or elastic tape. Dressings are removed and the wound reexamined at 48 to 72 hours. If a drain has been placed, it should be advanced every 24 to 48 hours. If the wound is under significant tension, additional support can be achieved by using steristrips or bulky supportive dressings, including splints that are commercially available or custom-made from plaster or fiberglass.

Most wounds can be left open after the first 24 to 48 hours. It is important to remove wet dressings from a repair because the skin maceration that results from them may prolong healing and increase the risk of infection. Initial epithelialization takes place during the first 24 hours, and thereafter it is permissible to wash the wound briefly. Lacerations on the scalp and face may be impractical to bandage.

Wounds should be reexamined for infection or hematoma formation after 2 to 3 days if there is any concern at the time of repair. Contaminated wounds and wounds that have been open longer than 24 hours have a greater likelihood of infection.

Timing of suture removal should be individualized, based on wound location, the mechanical stress placed on the repair, and the tension of the closure. Facial sutures should be removed within 3 to 5 days to minimize the possibility of suture tracks. Supporting the repair with steristrips may

TABLE 24.2. Instructions for patients

1. Keep wound dressings clean and dry. Protect dressings from moisture when bathing.
2. If the dressing gets wet, remove it and reapply a clean, dry dressing.
3. Remove the dressing after 2 days and reapply every 2 days unless instructed otherwise.
4. If any of the following signs appears, contact your physician or clinic immediately.
   A. Wound becomes red, warm, swollen, or tender.
   B. Wound begins to drain.
   C. Red streaks appear near the wound or up the arm or leg.
   D. Tender lumps appear in the armpit or groin.
   E. Chills or fever occur.
5. Because of your particular injury the doctor would like your wound checked in ____ days.
6. Please return for removal of your stitches in ______ days.
7. You received the following vaccinations.
   A. Tetanus toxoid ________________
   B. Td (tetanus/diphtheria) ___________
   C. DPT (diphtheria/pertussis/tetanus) _______________

decrease the likelihood of dehiscence. In skin areas that are not highly mobile (e.g., the back or extremities) sutures are left in place for 7 to 10 days. On fingers, palms, soles, and over joints the sutures remain in place at least 10 to 14 days and sometimes longer. Table 24.2 is a sample instruction sheet for patients.

Concurrent Therapy

Preventing infection is an important aspect of laceration treatment. Puncture wounds and bites usually should not be closed because the risk of infection negates the advantage of closure. Sometimes a gaping puncture wound on the face requires closure for cosmetic reasons despite the risk of infection.

Antibiotic Usage

Antibiotic prophylaxis is probably not helpful in most circumstances unless given in sufficient quantity to obtain good tissue levels while the wound is still open. If extensive repair is necessary, intravenous antibiotics should be started during wound closure. Animal and human bite wounds are often treated by postclosure antibiotics. The efficacy of this practice remains controversial, but antibiotics are often given because of the extensive contamination that occurs with bite wounds. Amoxicillin-clavulanate covers the typical bacteria of bite wounds. Doxycycline and ceftriaxone are alternative medications.[29]

TABLE 24.3. Guide to tetanus prophylaxis during routine wound management

History of adsorbed tetanus toxoid (doses)	Clean, minor wounds		All other wounds[a]	
	Td[b]	TIg	Td[b]	TIg
Unknown or < 3	Yes	No	Yes	Yes
≥ Three[c]	No[d]	No	No[e]	No

[a]Such as, but not limited to, wounds contaminated with dirt, feces, soil, and saliva; puncture wounds; avulsions; and wounds resulting from missiles, crushing, burns, and frostbite.
[b]For children < 7 years old; DPT (DT if pertussis vaccine is contraindicated) is preferred to tetanus toxoid alone. For persons ≥ 7 years of age Td is preferred to tetanus toxoid alone.
[c]If only three doses of *fluid* toxoid have been received, a fourth dose of toxoid, preferably an adsorbed toxoid, is given.
[d]Yes, if > 10 years since last dose.
[e]Yes, if > 5 years since last dose. (More frequent boosters are not needed and can accentuate side effects.)

Tetanus Prophylaxis

Tetanus prophylaxis is a crucial part of the care of the lacerated patient; it is imperative that the immunization status of the patient be documented. Patients most likely to be inadequately immunized are the elderly, who may have never received a primary series. Table 24.3 is a summary of the guide published by the Centers for Disease Control in 1991. Whenever passive immunity is required, human tetanus immune globulin (TIg) is preferred. The usual dose of TIg is 500 units IM. Tetanus toxoid and TIg should be given through separate needles at separate sites.[30,31]

References

1. Brietenbach KL, Bergera JJ. Principles and techniques of primary wound closure. Prim Care 1986;13:411–31.
2. Snell G. Laceration repair. In: Pfenninger JL, Fowler GC, editors. Procedures for primary care physicians. St. Louis: Mosby, 1994:12–19.
3. Bonadio WA, Wagner V. Efficacy of TAC topical anesthetic for repair of pediatric lacerations. Am J Dis Child 1988; 142:203–5.
4. Hegenbarth MA, Altieri MF, Hawk WH, Green A, Ochsenschlager DW, et al. Comparison of topical tetracaine, adrenaline, and cocaine anesthesia with lidocaine infiltration for repair of lacerations in children. Ann Emerg Med 1990;19:63–7.
5. Matsumoto AH, Reifsnyder AC, Hartwell GD, Angle JF, et al. Reducing the discomfort of lidocaine administration through pH buffering. J Vasc Interv Radiol 1994;5:171–5.
6. Bartfield JM, Ford DT, Homer PJ. Buffered versus plain lidocaine for digital nerve blocks. Ann Emerg Med 1993;22:216–19.
7. Mader TJ, Playe SJ, Garb JL. Reducing the pain of local anesthetic infiltration: warming and buffering have a synergistic effect. Ann Emerg Med 1994;23:550–4.

8. Brogan BX Jr, Giarrusso E, Hollander JE, et al. Comparison of plain, warmed, and buffered lidocaine for anesthesia of traumatic wounds. Ann Emerg Med 1995;26:121–5.
9. Murakami CS, Odland PB, Ross BK. Buffered local anesthetics and epinephrine degradation. J Dermatol Surg Oncol 1994;20:192–5.
10. Thompson KD, Welykyj S, Massa MC. Antibacterial activity of lidocaine in combination with a bicarbonate buffer. J Dermatol Surg Oncol 1993; 19:216–20.
11. Ernst AA, Marvez-Valls E, Mall G, et al. 1% Lidocaine versus 0.5% diphenhydramine for local anesthesia in minor laceration repair. Ann Emerg Med 1994; 23:1328–32.
12. Task Force on Sedation and Analgesia by Non-Anesthesiologists. Practical guidelines for sedation and analgesia by non-anesthesiologists. Anesthesiology 1996;84:459–71.
13. Qureshi FA, Mellis PT, McFadden MA. Efficacy of oral ketamine for providing sedation and analgesia to children requiring laceration repair. Pediatr Emerg Care 1995;11: 93–7.
14. Connors K, Terndrup TE. Nasal versus oral midazolam for sedation of anxious children undergoing laceration repair. Ann Emerg Med 1994;24: 1074–9.
15. Shane SA, Fuchs SM, Khine H. Efficacy of rectal midazolam for the sedation of preschool children undergoing laceration repair. Ann Emerg Med 1994;24:1065–73.
16. Schutzman SA, Burg J, Liebelt E, et al. Oral transmucosal fentanyl citrate for the premedication of children undergoing laceration repair. Ann Emerg Med 1994;24:1059–64.
17. Clinical considerations in the use of fentanyl oralet. North Chicago, IL: Abbott Laboratories, 1995:1–16.
18. Gamis AS, Knapp JF, Glenski JA. Nitrous oxide analgesia in a pediatric emergency department. Ann Emerg Med 1989;18: 177–81.
19. Moy RL, Lee A, Zolka A. Commonly used suture materials in skin surgery. Am Fam Physician 1991;44:2123–8.
20. Epperson WJ. Suture selection. In: Pfenninger JL, Fowler GC, editors. Procedures for primary care physicians. St. Louis: Mosby, 1994:3–6.
21. Moy RL, Waldman B, Hein DW. A review of sutures and suturing techniques. J Dermatol Surg Oncol 1992;18:785–95.
22. Jones JS, Gartner M, Drew G, Pack S. The shorthand vertical mattress stitch: evaluation of a new suture technique. Am J Emerg Med 1993;11:483–5.
23. Ditmars DM Jr. Finger tip and nail bed injuries. Occup Med 1989;4:449–61.
24. Edlich RF, Thacker JG, Silloway RF, et al. Scientific basis of skin staple closure. In: Haval Mutaz B, editor. Advances in plastic and reconstructive surgery. Chicago: Year Book, 1986:233–71.
25. Osmond MH, Klassen TP, Quinn JV. Economic comparison of a tissue adhesive and suturing in the repair of pediatric facial lacerations. J Pediatr 1995;126(6):892–5.
26. Quinn JV, Drzewiecki A, Li MM, et al. A randomized, controlled trial comparing tissue adhesive with suturing in the repair of pediatric facial lacerations. Ann Emerg Med 1993;22: 1130–5.

27. Applebaum JS, Zalut T, Applebaum D. The use of tissue adhesive for traumatic laceration repair in the emergency department. Ann Emerg Med 1993;22:1190–2.
28. Fisher AA. Reactions to cyanoacrylate adhesives: "instant glue." Cutis 1995:18–22, 46, 58.
29. Lewis KT, Stiles M. Management of cat and dog bites. Am Fam Physician 1995;52:479–85.
30. Centers for Disease Control. Morb Mortal Wkly Rep MMWR 1991 Aug 8;40(RR-10):1–28.
31. Richardson JP, Knight AL. The management and prevention of tetanus. J Emerg Med 1993;11:737–42.

CASE PRESENTATION

You are called by the hospital emergency department staff at 6 p.m. One of your patients is there with a hand laceration. You go there to meet him.

Subjective

PATIENT PROFILE

Ken Nelson is a 47-year-old married white male home builder.

PRESENTING PROBLEM

"I cut my hand today."

PRESENT ILLNESS

Five hours ago, the patient cut his right hand on sheet metal at work. He finished his work shift and now presents at the end of the day for treatment.

PAST MEDICAL HISTORY

No serious illness or hospitalization.

SOCIAL HISTORY

Ken Nelson is a self-employed building contractor who lives with his wife and 16-year-old daughter.

HABITS

He does not use tobacco or alcohol. He drinks one thermos of coffee per day.

FAMILY HISTORY

Not recorded because of the limited nature of today's problem.

- What more would you like to know about the injury? Why might this information be important?
- What do you need to know about his tetanus immunizations status?
- What are pertinent safety issues that should be elicited?
- What might be the significance of the 5-hour delay in seeking care? How would you inquire about this?

Objective

VITAL SIGNS

Blood pressure, 132/86; pulse, 66.

EXAMINATION

There is a 4-cm-long linear laceration of the lateral right hand; the wound extends into the subcutaneous tissues. The patient has full active and passive motion of the hand and fingers. There is no loss of neurologic function.

- What further information—if any—regarding the physical examination might be important?
- What are some concerns regarding hand injuries, and how would you examine to address these possibilities?
- How can you determine that neurologic function is intact?
- In what circumstances would you obtain laboratory testing or diagnostic imaging?

Assessment

- What are some concerns regarding this injury? How would you describe these concerns to the patient?
- If the patient had lost sensory perception to one of his fingers, what would you do?
- Is this a teachable moment for accident prevention? How would you approach this issue with the patient?
- What are pertinent insurance issues in regard to this injury?

Plan

- How would you prepare the wound for suturing, and what suture material would you use? Describe special considerations in suture technique for hand lacerations.
- What would be your recommendation regarding tetanus prophylaxis?
- Mr. Nelson asks about returning to work. How would you respond?
- What aftercare would you recommend for this injury?

25

Athletic Injuries

Michael L. Tuggy and Cora Collette Breuner

Family physicians invariably treat many athletic injuries during their routine clinical practice. With the increased interest in fitness in the general population, the number of people resuming active exercise as they age is increasing. Injuries sustained during childhood or adolescence frequently have lifelong effects that can hamper later attempts at physical activity.[1] Elderly patients are commonly afraid of exercise for fear of injury or exacerbation of degenerative joint disease. For patients at all ages, proper training and prevention can lead to lifelong athletic activities that reduce significantly the risks of cardiovascular disease, osteoporosis, and complications from falls by the elderly.

Most sports injuries are related to overuse injuries and often are not brought to the attention of the family physician until the symptoms are advanced. Traumatic injuries are readily diagnosed but may have serious long-term sequelae for the life of the athlete. Sport selection has a great impact on the risk of injury. The adolescent athlete is probably at highest risk for injury due to sport selection, the presence of immature growth cartilage at the growth plates and joint surfaces, and lack of experience.[2] Many sports selected by young adults also have higher degrees of risk, which can be modified by training and education. Table 25.1 lists common sports activities and their relative injury rates.

Mechanisms of Injury

Traumatic injuries are generally caused by a combination of forces. Deceleration injuries are the most common form of serious injury, resulting in significant blunt trauma or joint injury. The athlete's momentum, enhanced by self-generated speed, gravity, and equipment, is translated into energy when impact occurs. This energy is then absorbed by the body in the form of blunt trauma, torsion of joints, or transfer of stress within the skeleton.

TABLE 25.1. Common sports injuries and injury rates

Sports activity	Common injuries	Injury rate (per 1000 exposures)
Running	Tibial periostitis, stress fracture Metatarsal stress fractures	14
Football	ACL/MCL tears Shoulder dislocation/separation Ankle sprain	13
Wrestling	Shoulder dislocation MCL, LCL tears	12
Gymnastics	Spondylolysis/spondylolisthesis Ankle sprains	10
Alpine/telemark skiing	ACL/MCL tears Skier's thumb Shoulder dislocation	10
Basketball	Ankle sprains Shoulder dislocation/separation	4
Baseball	Lateral epicondylitis Rotator cuff tear	4
Cross-country skiing	Ankle sprains Lateral epicondylitis	3

ACL = anterior cruciate ligament (knee); MCL = medial collateral ligament (knee); LCL = lateral collateral ligament (knee).

Collision sports, such as football or rugby, and high-velocity sports, such as alpine skiing, have much higher rates of significant musculoskeletal injury due to the combination of speed and mass effect on impact. Factors that affect the extent of injury include the tensile strength of the ligaments and tendons of affected joints, bony strength, flexibility, and ability of the athlete to reduce the impact. Appropriate conditioning for a sport reduces injury risk. Not only are endurance and strength training important, but practicing falls and recovery from falls can help the athlete diffuse the energy of the fall or impact. Athletes should be encouraged to use the appropriate safety equipment and to train comprehensively for their sport.

Overuse injuries constitute the most common form of sports injuries seen by the family physician. These injuries are induced by repetitive motion leading to microscopic disruption of a bone–tendon or bone–synovium interface. This microtrauma initiates an inflammatory response. If the inflammatory response is not modulated by a rest phase or is excessive owing to mechanical factors, degradation of the tendon or bone may occur. Predisposing factors that lead to overuse injuries include poor flexibility, an imbalance of strength of opposing muscle groups, mechanical deformity (i.e., pes planus), inadequate rest between exercise periods, and faulty equipment.[3] Adolescent athletes are especially vulnerable to such injuries, especially in areas where growth cartilage is present in the epiphyseal or apophyseal attachments of major muscle groups. Elderly athletes also are at higher risk because of preexisting degenerative joint disease and poor flexibility.

Most overuse injuries are seen at later stages (stage 3 or 4) by physicians and require significant alteration in training schedules to allow healing of the injury. Progressive inflammation due to overuse can eventually lead to tendon disruption, periostitis (stress reaction), true stress fractures, or cartilaginous degeneration. Early periostitis may appear as a "fluffiness" of the cortical margin with compensatory cortical thickening underlying it (Fig. 25.1). In more advanced cases, the margin is clearly blurred and the cortex significantly thickened. If symptoms suggest a significant stress reaction but radiographs are negative, a bone scan is indicated. True stress fractures can be visualized on plain films, whereas stress reactions (periostitis) are best seen on bone scans. Because stress fractures are inflammatory in nature, the complication rates due to delayed union or nonunion are higher than those with traumatic fractures.[4] The results of

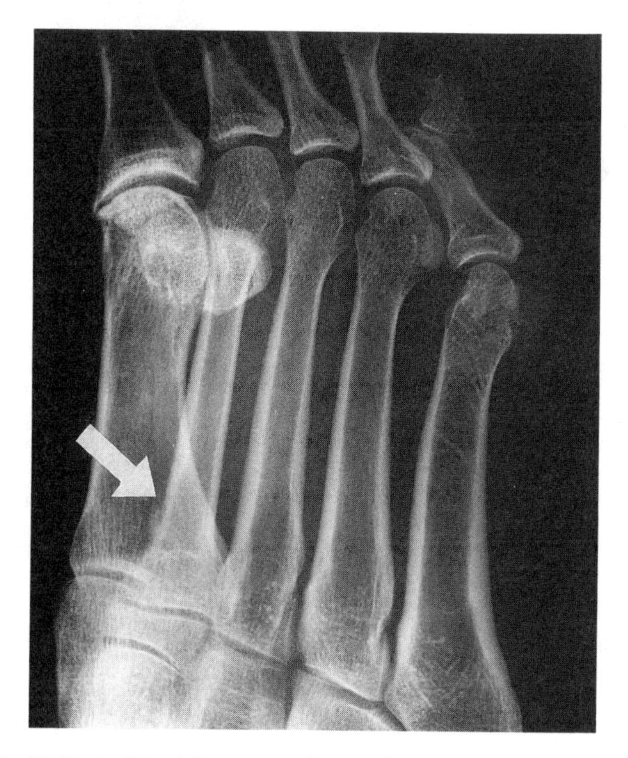

FIGURE 25.1. **(A)** Periostitis of the proximal second metatarsal characterized by thickening of the cortex and "fluffy" appearance of the medial margin of the cortex.

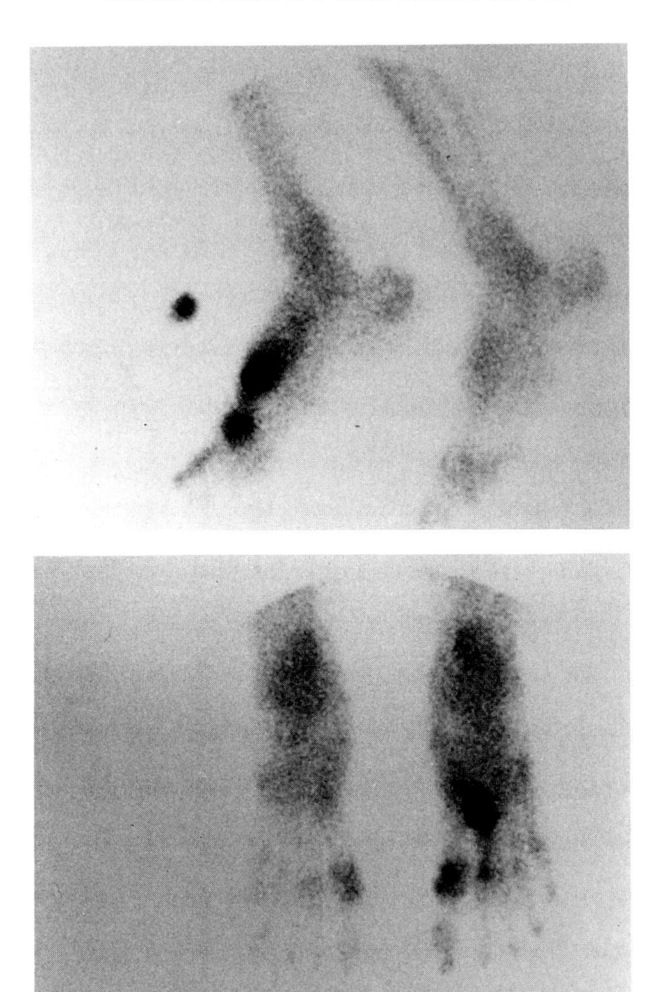

FIGURE 25.1. (*continued*) **(B)** Confirmatory bone scan identified two areas of significant inflammation of the second metatarsal.

improper treatment of these injuries can be severe, resulting in permanent degenerative changes or deformity. The primary care provider plays an important role, not only in diagnosing the injury early (and thus shortening the rehabilitation period), but also in stressing prevention with proper training guidance and timely intervention.

Traumatic Injuries

Physicians providing coverage for athletic events must recognize high-risk situations for serious injuries and evaluate the safety of the sports environment. Asking the following questions when first evaluating a patient with a traumatic injury helps to suggest the correct diagnosis and focus the physical examination: During what sport did the injury occur? How did the injury occur? Where does it hurt? What aggravates the pain? Did other symptoms accompany the injury? Did swelling occur and, if so, how soon? How old is the athlete? Has the athlete been injured before? Once these questions are answered, the physician performs a focused musculoskeletal and neurovascular examination.

Ankle Injuries

Ankle injuries are ubiquitous and constitute the most common acute musculoskeletal injury affecting the entire spectrum of professional to grade school athletes. It is estimated that 1 million people present with ankle injuries each year, with an average cost of $300 to $900 for diagnosis and rehabilitation that requires 36 to 72 days to be complete. Basketball players have the highest rate of ankle injuries, followed by football players and cross-country runners.[5]

Eighty-five percent of athletes with ankle sprains have inversion injuries. The most common structures injured with inversion are the three lateral ligaments that support the ankle joint: the anterior and posterior talofibular ligaments and the calcaneofibular ligament (Fig. 25.2). The

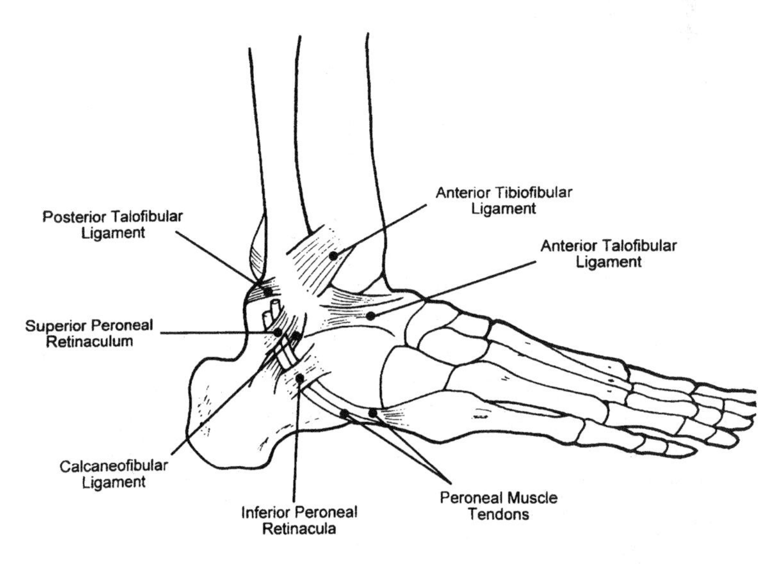

FIGURE 25.2. Lateral view of major ankle ligaments and structures.

other primary mechanism of ankle sprains is eversion, accounting for 15% of ankle injuries. In general, these injuries are more severe than inversion injuries because of a higher rate of fractures and disruptions of the ankle mortise, leading to instability. The deltoid ligament is the most common ligament to be injured in eversion injuries. Fifteen percent of all complete ligament tears are associated with avulsion fractures of the tibia, fibula, talus, or the base of the fifth metatarsal. Epiphyseal growth plate injuries may be present in the young athlete who sustains an ankle injury. Clinical evidence for an epiphyseal injury of the distal fibula or tibia is bony tenderness about two fingerbreadths proximal to the tip of the malleolus.[6]

DIAGNOSIS

Examination during the immediate postinjury period may be limited by swelling, pain, and muscle spasm. Inspection should focus on the presence of an obvious deformity and vascular integrity. Ankle radiographs are necessary only if there is inability to bear weight for four steps at the scene and in the emergency department or the presence of bony tenderness at the posterior edge or tip of either malleolus.[7] When swelling has subsided, the patient should be reexamined, as the second examination may be more useful for pinpointing areas of tenderness. Pain-free passive and active range of motion of the ankle should be determined for all aspects of movement. One should also try to assess for joint instability using the anterior drawer test. A positive test (palpable and visible displacement of the foot more than 4 mm out of the mortise) is consistent with a tear of the anterior talofibular ligament and the anterior joint capsule.[8] Injuries to the lateral ligament complex are graded depending on the amount of effusion, laxity, and functional disability.

MANAGEMENT

Immediate treatment is applied according to the RICE (*r*est, *i*ce, *c*ompression, *e*levation) mnemonic. *Rest:* the athlete can exercise so long as the swelling and pain are not worse within 24 hours. Exercise includes simple weight-bearing. If there is pain with walking, crutches are required with appropriate instructions on use until the athlete is able to walk without pain. *Ice* is applied directly to the ankle for 20 minutes at a time every 2 hours, if possible, during the first 1 to 2 days. Icing continues until the swelling has stopped. *Compression* can be applied in the form of a horseshoe-shaped felt adhesive (0.625 cm thick). An elastic wrap can be used but is not optimal. The compression dressing is worn for 2 to 3 days. Air stirrups are recommended and effectively eliminate inversion and eversion but allow dorsiflexion and plantar flexion. Casting for 10 to 14 days may be the second option. The leg is *elevated* as much as possible until the swelling has stabilized.

Indications for orthopedic referral include the following factors: fracture, dislocation, evidence of neurovascular compromise, penetrating wound into the joint space, and grade 3 sprain with tendon rupture. All patients with ankle injuries should begin rehabilitation exercises immediately.

Knee Injuries

It has been estimated that during each week of the fall football season at least 6000 high school and college players injure their knees, 10% of whom require surgery. Even more discouraging are the results of a 20-year follow-up study of men who had sustained a knee injury in high school. The investigators found that 39% of the men continued to have significant symptoms, 50% of whom had radiographic abnormalities.[9] Knee braces, though popular, have not been proved to be effective in preventing knee ligament injuries. The best time to evaluate the knee is immediately after the injury. Within an hour of a knee injury, protective muscle spasm can prevent reliable assessment of the joint instability. The following day there may be enough joint effusion to preclude a satisfactory examination. When evaluating knee injuries, compare the injured knee to the uninjured knee. When an effusion is present, radiographs are necessary to rule out tibial tubercle avulsion fractures, epiphyseal fractures, and osteochondral fractures. Finally, evaluation of the neurovascular status of the leg and foot is mandatory.

Meniscal Injuries

Meniscal injuries result from twisting or rotating the knee along with deep flexion and hyperextension. Symptoms include pain, recurrent effusions, and clicking and are associated with limited range of motion. Meniscal flaps may become entrapped within the joint space, resulting in locking or the knee "giving out."

Diagnosis

Classically, meniscal tears are characterized by tenderness or pain over the medial or lateral joint line in hyperflexion or hyperextension. This injury must be differentiated from tenderness along the entire medial collateral ligament elicited when that ligament is sprained. When the lower leg is rotated with the knee flexed about 90 degrees, pain during external rotation indicates a medial meniscus injury (McMurray's test).

Management

After a meniscal injury, the athlete should follow the RICE protocol. Crutch usage should be insisted on to avoid weight-bearing until the pain and edema have diminished. For most athletes an orthopedic referral should be considered for arthroscopy to repair the damaged meniscus. Follow-up is planned to initiate a rehabilitative program and return to sports.

Medial Collateral Ligament Sprain

The medial collateral ligament (MCL) is the medial stabilizer of the knee, and it is usually injured by excessive valgus stress on the knee. The result is a first, second, or third degree sprain. MCL tears are often associated with medial meniscus injury. Lateral collateral ligament tears are unusual and are caused by an inwardly directed blow (varus force) to the inside of the knee.

DIAGNOSIS

The player is usually able to bear some weight on the leg immediately after the injury. Medial knee pain is generally felt at the time of the injury, and the knee may feel "wobbly" while the player walks afterward. Examination reveals acute tenderness somewhere over the course of the MCL usually at or above the joint line. The integrity of the MCL is assessed by applying valgus stress by holding the tibia about one-third of the way down and forcing it gently laterally while holding the distal femur in place. Tears are graded based on the degree of laxity and the presence or absence of an endpoint on the examination. Grade 1 tears have minimal laxity with a solid endpoint; grade 2 tears have moderate laxity with an intact endpoint. A patient with a partial tear of the MCL has marked discomfort with valgus and varus testing. The athlete with a complete (grade 3) tear of the MCL may have surprisingly little pain on testing but remarkably increased laxity of the ligament without a definable endpoint. Swelling, ecchymosis over the ligament, or joint effusion usually develops within several hours of the injury.

MANAGEMENT

A first-degree sprain is treated with RICE. Running is restricted until the athlete is pain-free in knee flexion. There is complete recovery generally within 5 to 10 days; and with physician clearance the player can resume full activity. The management of more serious sprains should be directed by an orthopedist.

Anterior Cruciate Ligament Injuries

Anterior cruciate ligament (ACL) injury is the most frequent, most severe ligamentous injury to the knee. The injury usually occurs without a direct blow to the knee; rather, it results from torsional stress coupled with a deceleration injury. These injuries are seen when an athlete changes direction while running and the knee suddenly "gives out."

Diagnosis

A "pop" is often felt during the injury. The player falls down on the field in extreme pain and is unable to continue participating. A bloody effusion develops in 60% to 70% of athletes within the next 24 hours. One of three tests can be employed to test for ACL injury: the anterior drawer test, the Lachman maneuver, or the pivot shift test.

The *anterior drawer test* is performed with the knee in 30 degrees of flexion. The injured leg is externally rotated slightly to relax the hamstrings and adductor muscles. The examiner kneels lateral to the injured leg, stabilizes the femur with one hand, and directs a gentle but firm upward force with the other hand on the proximal tibia. If the tibia moves anteriorly, the ACL has been torn.

The *Lachman test* is performed with the hamstrings relaxed and the knee placed in 15 degrees of flexion. With one hand on the femur just above the knee to stabilize it, the tibia is pulled forward with the opposite hand placed over the tibial tuberosity. If the ACL is intact, the tibia comes to a firm stop. If the ligament is torn, the tibia continues forward sluggishly.

A *pivot shift test* is performed with the ankle and leg held under the examiner's arm. The leg is abducted and the knee extended. The hands are under the proximal tibia applying gentle anterior and internal rotation force. The tibia subluxes forward; and as pressure is applied in line with the leg, the tibia reduces.

Posterior cruciate ligament injuries are caused by a direct blow to the upper anterior tibia. For example, a karate player is kicked in the area of the tibial tuberosity while the foot is firmly on the ground, or someone else falls forward onto a flexed knee. Posterior cruciate tears are detected by posterior displacement of the tibial tuberosity (sag sign) when the leg is held by the heel with the hip and knee flexed.

MANAGEMENT

Initial management of ACL tears follows RICE principles along with immobilization or crutches with instructions on their use. Rehabilitation requires early initiation of quadriceps contractions to prevent atrophy and promote strengthening. Protective bracing with a hinged knee brace is appropriate for certain athletes. Referral to an orthopedist should be made immediately if there is radiographic evidence of an avulsion fracture of the ACL attachments; referral may be made later for possible arthroscopic repair if there is joint laxity.

Patellar Dislocation

Patellar dislocation can result from a blow to the patella or when an athlete changes direction and then straightens the leg. It is most common in adolescents and athletes with significant valgus deformity of the knee joint.

DIAGNOSIS

The dislocation usually occurs laterally, but the medial joint capsule and retinaculum may also be torn, sometimes simulating or associated with an MCL sprain. The dislocation usually reduces spontaneously, and the athlete has a painful swollen knee due to hemarthrosis and tenderness at the medial capsule. Lateral pressure on the patella while gently extending the knee is met with obvious anxiety and resistance.

MANAGEMENT

If there is no obvious evidence of fracture, reduction of the dislocation may be attempted by first extending the knee. It can be helpful to massage the hamstring muscle and ask the athlete to relax it. As the patient allows more knee extension, exert gentle midline-directed pressure to the lateral aspect of the patella. The patella should relocate within seconds to minutes. Difficulty with this maneuver suggests a fracture or displaced chondral fragment; the next step is to splint the knee and refer the athlete to an emergency room for radiographs and reduction. Postreduction management follows RICE principles with crutch use for those who cannot bear weight. The leg must be elevated for as long as the edema persists, with immediate quadriceps strengthening exercises to prevent atrophy.

Neck Injuries

Injuries to the head and neck are the most frequent catastrophic sports injury. The four common school sports with the highest risk of head and spine injury are football, gymnastics, ice hockey, and wrestling.[10] Fortunately, many neck injuries are minimal strains, diagnosed after a quick history and physical examination. Axial loading is the most common mechanism for serious neck injury. Classic examples include the football player "spearing" or tackling head-first and the hockey player sliding head-first into the boards. Axial loading can produce spinal fracture, dislocation, and quadriplegia at low-impact velocities.

Extension spinal injuries are more serious than flexion injuries. With extension spine injury (whiplash), the anterior elements are disrupted and the posterior elements compressed. With flexion injury the anterior elements are compressed, causing anterior vertebral body fracture, chip fracture, and occasionally anterior dislocation.

DIAGNOSIS

When an athlete is unconscious and motionless, an initial assessment is mandatory. Athletes with focal neurologic deficits or marked neck pain should be suspected of having cervical spine injury until cleared by radiographic examination.

MANAGEMENT

The patient's airway, breathing, and circulation are assessed rapidly followed by neck stabilization and initiation of emergency transport. Cervical spine injury is assumed until proved otherwise. Proper stabilization precautions must be carried out while the athlete is removed from the playing field or injury site. If the athlete is wearing a helmet, it should not be removed until in the emergency room.

Closed Head Injuries

A definition of concussion is "a clinical syndrome characterized by immediate and transient posttraumatic impairment of neural function, such as the alteration of consciousness, disturbance of vision, equilibrium etc., due to brainstem involvement."[11] There is also a complication of concussion called a "second impact syndrome" in which fatal intracerebral edema is precipitated by a second blow to the head of an athlete who has symptoms persisting from an earlier concussion.[12] Fortunately, this syndrome is rare. If the athlete has any persisting symptoms from any degree of concussion, he or she should not be allowed to play. Postconcussion syndrome consists of headache (especially with exertion), labyrinthine disturbance, fatigue, irritability, and impaired memory and concentration. These symptoms can persist for weeks or even months.

Epidural hematoma results when the middle meningeal artery, which is embedded in a bony groove in the skull, tears as a result of a skull fracture crossing this groove. Because the bleeding is arterial, accumulation of clot continues under high pressure, and serious brain injury can result. Subdural hematomas are caused by shearing forces applied to the bridging arachnoid veins that surround the brain.

DIAGNOSIS

Table 25.2 describes how the recognition and classification of concussion can simplify its management. The classic signs of an epidural hematoma are loss of consciousness for a variable period and then recovery of consciousness after which the patient is lucid. This phase is followed by the onset of increasingly severe headache, decreased level of consciousness, dilation of one pupil (usually on the same side as the clot), and decerebrate posturing and weakness (usually on the side opposite the hematoma). Patients with acute subdural hematoma are more likely to have a prolonged lucid interval following their injury and less likely to be unconsciousness at admission than patients with epidural hematomas.

TABLE 25.2. Guide to concussion

Grade	Symptoms	Resolution	Return to Play
1: Mild	No loss of consciousness Momentary confusion Mild dizziness Headache Posttraumatic amnesia (< 30 minutes)	Athlete normally recovers quickly but should be watched for changing symptoms.	May return following complete return of cognition, if symptom-free and if has normal neurologic examination. Observation still necessary
2: Moderate	Loss of consciousness < 5 minutes Posttraumatic amnesia (30 minutes or more but < 24 hours) Confusion Severe dizziness Blurred or double vision Loss of balance/ coordination Nausea Tinnitus	Symptoms usually subside somewhat in 30–60 minutes but usually do not completely disappear for a few days. Some linger up to a week. Athlete should be observed for at least 24 hours for changing symptoms.	Return to play after asymptomatic for 1 week. Terminate season if more than two concussions.
3: Severe	Loss of consciousness ≥ 5 minutes Posttraumatic amnesia ≥ 24 hours Severe confusion Loss of balance/ coordination Severely altered vision Nausea	Recovery takes several days, and some symptoms can linger for weeks. Athlete should be referred to a neurologist, watched for 48 hours, and checked periodically for several weeks.	Minimum of 1 month without play. Terminate if more than one concussion.

MANAGEMENT

Patients with closed head injuries require a thorough neurologic evaluation, usually including computed tomography (CT) or magnetic resonance imaging (MRI). Return to competition should be deferred until all symptoms have abated and guidelines are followed as described in Table 25.2.

Shoulder Dislocation

Shoulder dislocation may occur when sufficient impact tears the anterior joint capsule of the glenohumeral joint, resulting in slippage of the humeral head out of the glenoid fossa. There are two mechanisms of injury for anterior glenohumeral dislocation: a fall onto an outstretched hand or a collision with a player or object with the shoulder abducted to 90 degrees and externally rotated. The shoulder may dislocate posteriorly, but an anteroinferior dislocation is the most common.

Diagnosis

Athletes who have anterior shoulder dislocation often state that the shoulder has "popped out" and describe excruciating pain. The athlete is unable to rotate the arm and has a hollow region just inferior to the acromion with an anterior bulge caused by forward displacement of the humeral head. Subluxation of the shoulder may occur when the humerus slips out of the glenohumeral socket and then spontaneously relocates. Posterior subluxations are seen more commonly in athletes who use repetitive overhand motions, such as swimmers and baseball and tennis players.

Management

Anterior dislocation is the only shoulder injury that requires prompt manipulation. The Rockwood technique requires an assistant who applies a long, folded towel around the ipsilateral axilla, crossing the upper anteroposterior chest. Gentle traction is applied while the physician applies in-line traction on the injured extremity. Traction is gradually increased over several minutes. Successful reduction manifests as a "thunk" when the humerus relocates in the glenoid cavity. If relocation is attempted immediately, the dislocation should be reducible within 2 to 3 minutes. Postreduction radiographs are required.

With the Stimson technique, the patient lies prone on a flat surface with the arm hanging down. A 5-pound weight is tied to the distal forearm. The reduction usually take place within 20 minutes.[13] If these attempts at early reduction are unsuccessful, reduction using analgesia or anesthesia can be attempted in the emergency room. For the patient who is experiencing dislocation for the first time, the shoulder is immobilized for 2 to 3 weeks. Rehabilitation may reduce the rate of recurrence, with goals being the restoration of full shoulder abduction and strengthening of the rotator cuff muscles.[14]

Acromioclavicular Separation

Acromioclavicular (AC) separation may be caused by a direct blow to the lateral aspect of the shoulder or a fall on an outstretched arm. AC separations are classified as grade 1, 2, or 3, as determined by the involvement of the AC or coracoclavicular ligament.

Diagnosis

Discrete tenderness is felt at the AC joint. With grade 1 AC separation, there is tenderness to palpation at the AC joint but no visible defect. Grade 2 or 3 AC separation causes a visible gap between the acromion and the clavicle. Grade 2 separation involves partial tear of the AC ligaments, and grade 3 separation is due to complete tear of the AC ligaments. When a grade 2 or 3 separation is suspected, a radiograph is obtained of both shoulders to rule out fracture and to delineate the grade of separation. With grade 2 injuries, the clavicle is elevated by one-half the width of the AC joint owing to disruption of the AC joint. With grade 3 injuries, both the AC and coracoclavicular ligaments are disrupted, with resultant dislocation of the AC joint and superior migration of the clavicle.

MANAGEMENT

Initial management of AC separations requires the shoulder to be immobilized in a sling. The medical intervention is determined by the grade of the injury. Those with grade 1 and 2 injuries may be treated conservatively with sling immobilization for 7 to 14 days. When symptoms subside, controlled remobilization and strengthening of the shoulder should begin. There is ongoing controversy regarding conservative versus operative management of the grade 3 injury. An orthopedic referral is made for these athletes.

Brachial Plexus Injury

A brachial plexus injury, or "burner" or "stinger," is a temporary dysfunction of the neural structures in the brachial plexus after a blow to the head, neck, or shoulder. Burners are reported in football, wrestling, ice hockey, skiing, motocross, soccer, hiking, and equestrian sports.[15] Several mechanisms probably contribute to injuries to the brachial plexus: pure lateral flexion of the cervical spine, lateral flexion with rotation and extension, shoulder depression, or a direct blow to the cervicobrachial area.[16]

DIAGNOSIS

Typically, the player experiences a sharp, burning pain in the shoulder with paresthesia or dysesthesia radiating into the arm and hand. There may also be associated sensory deficits, decreased reflexes, and weakness of the deltoid, biceps, supraspinatus, or infraspinatus muscles.

MANAGEMENT

If the neurologic findings return to normal within a few minutes, the athlete may return to play. In 5% to 10% of patients, signs and symptoms persist, requiring referral to a neurologist or physiatrist.

Thumb and Finger Injuries

Extensor injuries of the distal phalangeal joints occur when there is avulsion of the extensor tendon from the distal phalanx with or without a fracture. It results in a "mallet" or "drop" finger. Proximal phalangeal joint injuries occur when there is avulsion of the central slip of the distal phalanx resulting in a flexion "boutonniere" deformity. Metacarpophalangeal (MCP) joint sprain of the thumb (gamekeeper's thumb) is caused by a fall on an outstretched hand, causing forced abduction of the thumb.

Diagnosis

The phalangeal joints are flexed and lack active extension with extensor tendon ruptures. Gamekeeper's thumb causes pain and swelling over the ulnar aspect of the MCP joint and is made worse by abducting or extending the thumb. Complete tear of the ulnar collateral ligament is demonstrated by marked laxity in full extension.

Management

A radiograph is obtained for all of the above injuries to rule out intraarticular fractures or avulsions, which would require orthopedic referral. For extensor tendon injuries, continued splinting of the distal finger joint in extension for at least 6 weeks is necessary. Treatment for a gamekeeper's thumb requires a thumb spica cast or splint protection for 4 to 6 weeks. During activity the thumb can be protected by taping it to the index finger to prevent excessive abduction. A complete tear of the ulnar collateral ligament requires orthopedic referral for surgical repair.[17] Minor sprains can be rehabilitated within 3 to 4 weeks.

Specific Overuse Injuries

Shoulder Impingement Syndromes

Overuse injuries of the shoulder are most common in individuals participating in swimming, throwing, or racquet sports. Swimmers almost uniformly develop symptoms of this injury to varying degrees, especially those who perform the butterfly stroke regularly. Repetitive motions that abduct and retract the arm followed by antegrade (overhand) rotation of the glenohumeral joint can lead to impingement of the subacromial bursa and the supraspinatus tendon. Early in its course only the subacromial bursa may be inflamed, but with progressive injury supraspinatus tendonitis develops and may become calcified. Other muscles that make up the rotator cuff can also be strained with this motion and eventually can lead to rotator cuff tears.

Diagnosis

Patients with impingement complain of pain with abduction to varying degrees and especially with attempts to raise the arm above the level of the shoulder. The pain radiates deep from the subacromial space to the deltoid region and may be vague and not well localized. Palpation of the subacromial bursa under the coracoacromial ligament often elicits pain deep to the acromion as does internal rotation of the arm when abducted at 90 degrees with the elbow also flexed at 90 degrees. A second maneuver to detect impingement is to extend the arm forward so it is parallel to the ground, then internally rotate and abduct the arm across the chest while stabilizing the shoulder with the examiner's hand. Both maneuvers narrow the subacromial space to elicit symptoms. The "painful arc"—pain only within a limited range of abduction—may indicate an advanced calcific tendonitis of the supraspinatus tendon. Radiographic imaging may be useful if this finding is present, as calcific tendonitis may require more invasive treatment.

MANAGEMENT

Modification of shoulder activity and antiinflammatory measures, such as RICE and nonsteroidal antiinflammatory drugs (NSAIDs), are instituted early. Swimmers must alter the strokes during their training periods and reduce the distance they swim to the point that the pain is decreasing daily. Rehabilitation exercises consist of aggressive shoulder stretching to lengthen the coracoacromial ligament and improve range of motion. The use of an upper arm counterforce brace can alter the fulcrum of the biceps in such a way as to depress the humeral head further. Strength training of the supraspinatus and biceps internal and external rotator muscles can be performed to aid in depressing the humeral head when stressed, thereby increasing the subacromial space. With advanced calcific tendonitis, steroid injection into the subacromial bursa or surgical removal of the calcific tendon may be required.[18]

Tennis Elbow (Lateral Epicondylitis)

Lateral epicondylitis is characterized by point tenderness of the lateral epicondyle at the attachment of the extensor carpi radialis brevis. The most common sports that cause this syndrome are tennis, racquetball, and cross-country skiing.[19] The mechanism of injury in all of the sports is repetitive extension of the wrist against resistance. Adolescent or preadolescent athletes are at highest risk of significant injury if the growth plate that underlies the lateral epicondyle is not yet closed. If the inflammation of the epicondyle is not arrested, the soft growth cartilage can fracture and rotate the bony attachment of the extensor ligaments, requiring surgical reimplantation of the epicondyle. Without surgery a permanent deformity of the elbow results.

Diagnosis

Patients complain of pain with active extension of the wrist localized to the upper forearm and lateral epicondyle. There is usually marked tenderness of the epicondyle itself. Pain upon grasping a weighted cup (Canard's test) or resisted dorsiflexion is also diagnostic. Radiographs are not necessary but may show calcific changes to the extensor aponeurosis in chronic cases. Comparison views of the unaffected elbow may be helpful in the adolescent in whom a stress fracture is suspected and the growth plate is not yet closed. Stress fractures of the lateral epicondyle are best diagnosed with a technetium 99 bone scan.

Management

Rest, NSAIDs, and ice on the area constitute the initial treatment. Modification of the gripped object (racquet or ski pole) with a thicker grip reduces the stress on the extensors. A counterforce brace worn over the belly of the forearm extensors or a volar cock-up splint can be used to relieve symptoms and alter the dynamic fulcrum of the muscles. Steroid injections superficial to the aponeurosis can be used for more refractory cases but should be limited to three.[20] Steroids should not be used in patients who may have a stress fracture or if the growth plates have not yet closed. Gradual return to the sport may begin immediately with grade 1 or 2 injuries or, with higher-grade injuries, as soon as the tenderness has resolved.

Lumbar Spondylolysis/Spondylolisthesis

Spondylolysis (fracture of the pars interarticularis) of the vertebrae results from repeated forced hyperextension of the spine. Spondylolisthesis (slippage of one vertebra over another) may result from facet joint degeneration induced by spondylolysis. Preadolescent gymnasts are at highest risk for developing spondylolysis, but it is also seen in weight lifters, runners, swimmers who perform the butterfly stroke, divers, and football players.[21] In one large study, up to 10% of adolescent female gymnasts had spondylolysis.[22] Spondylolisthesis usually occurs in older teens and develops primarily at the L5–S1 joint. Their prognosis is worse than those with isolated spondylolysis.

Diagnosis

The athlete usually complains of unilateral back pain that worsens with rotation of the trunk. There is usually regional spasm of the paraspinous musculature and the hamstrings. Pain from spondylolisthesis may cause radicular symptoms in the L5–S1 distribution. Lateral and anteroposterior radiographs of the spine may not reveal pars interarticularis pathology, so oblique films should be added. Even if the radiographs are normal, if the diagnosis is suspected, activity restriction is necessary until repeat films are obtained in 4 to 6 weeks. A technetium 99 bone scan is a sensitive test for detecting pars interarticularis fractures or stress reactions.

MANAGEMENT

Rest is essential with both of these conditions. Bone scans can be used to follow the healing process, but the cost may be prohibitive; and resolution of symptoms is an adequate indicator of healing. The athlete may continue to train in sports that do not result in hyperextension or rotation of the spine (e.g., cycling, stair-climbing) so long as the back symptoms are improving. Referral to a physical therapist for neutral spine stability exercises is warranted.

Low-grade spondylolisthesis can be managed conservatively by restricting activity until the pain has resolved. Serial radiographs every 4 to 6 months can be used to monitor for progression in athletes who returned to their sport after the symptoms resolved. High-grade spondylolisthesis (> 25% displacement of the vertebral body) can also be managed conservatively, but the patient must be permanently restricted from contact or collision sports. Bracing or surgical repair of spondylolisthesis may be required if the pain is severe or persistent nerve root irritation is present.[23]

Retropatellar (Patellofemoral) Pain Syndrome

Retropatellar pain syndrome (RPPS) is most commonly found in patients who run, hike, or cycle. The symptoms probably represent most of the knee pain complaints by athletes. Retropatellar pain is caused by repetitive glide of the patella over the femoral condyles, which can lead to inflammation of the retropatellar synovium or of the cartilage itself. The glide of the patella is usually laterally displaced in athletes who have recurrent symptoms. Factors that increase this friction are instability of the knee from previous injury, valgus deformity of the knee, deficient vastus medialis obliquus muscle strength, patella alta, or a recent increase in the running program. Relative valgus stress on the knee is created in patients with abnormal Q angles, pes planus, femoral anteversion, or external tibial torsion causing lateral displacement of the patella. If progressive, RPPS can progress to chondromalacia patellae with destruction of the retropatellar cartilage.

DIAGNOSIS

Patients with RPPS present with vague retropatellar or peripatellar pain, which is usually most significant several hours after exercise. Walking downhill or downstairs, bending at the knees, and kneeling can exacerbate the pain. With more advanced cases, the pain can be constant, occurring during and after exercise. Oddly, patients often experience pain if the knee is not moved enough; that is, if the knee remains flexed for several minutes, pain develops.

Examination of the knee first involves inspection of the patient's entire leg, feet, and hips to assess for a significant Q angle, torsional deformities, leg length discrepancy, or pes planus. When palpating the knee, the lateral posterior margins of the patella are palpated with the patella deviated laterally to detect tenderness of the retropatellar surface. This maneuver is repeated on the medial aspect of the patella with medial deviation. Effusions are usually absent in patients with RPPS. A compression test of the patella is performed with the patient relaxing and then flexing the quadriceps group while the patella is displaced distally by the examiner. Fine crepitus with this test may indicate synovial inflammation, but it is not a specific sign. Coarse crepitus or popping with significant pain is indicative of chondromalacia. Sunrise views of the knees may reveal radiographic evidence of retropatellar degeneration; but usually these findings are present only in advanced cases, and they are not necessary for diagnosis.[24]

Management

For athletes with symptoms only at high training levels, reduction of the exacerbating activity and NSAID use are the first steps. If the patient has a grade 3 or 4 injury, cessation of the exacerbating activity for 2 to 4 weeks until the pain is no longer present at rest is necessary. Selective strengthening of the vastus medialis obliquus (VMO), orthotics, and alteration of mechanical forces when pedaling (cyclists) can also relieve symptoms. Lateral deviation of the foot while extending the knee allows more medial tracking of the patella during exercise and forces the VMO to perform more of the quadriceps' function. Stretching to reduce both hamstring and quadriceps tension is an important component of rehabilitation for RPPS. As with all overuse injuries, a graduated increase in exercise duration at a rate of 10% per week, with relative rest periods every 3 to 4 weeks, may prevent recurrence of the symptoms.

Tibial Periostitis ("Shin Splints")

Tibial periostitis is the most common overuse injury in recreational runners and is often confused with other lower leg pain syndromes.[25] Any pain in the tibial area is often labeled "shin splints," but must be differentiated from anterior compartment syndrome, patellar tendonitis, or a simple muscular strain. The primary cause of tibial periostitis is mechanical; the attachment of a calf muscle is strained because of the pounding of running on a mechanically deficient foot. A recent increase in duration of running often triggers shin splints if the increase is too rapid and there is no rest phase. Over 4 to 8 weeks after such increases in training, the problem progresses to involve the bone by disrupting the periosteum and cortex.

DIAGNOSIS

Most patients with this syndrome have pes planus, which results in tibialis posterior tendonitis initially. Their pain is localized to the lower third of the medial aspect of the tibia. Patients with pes cavus have anterior tibialis tendonitis with pain localized laterally on the middle or upper tibia. If other calf flexors are involved, the pain may be deep in the calf, resembling a deep vein thrombosis. Homan's sign may be positive in these patients because the posterior aspect of the tibia is inflamed. If point tenderness is present, radiographic studies are indicated, with careful attention paid to subtle changes in the cortical margin in the area of pain.

MANAGEMENT

Table 25.3 delineates rehabilitation strategies for this injury. The importance of adequate rest and graduated resumption of exercise with cycled rest phases cannot be overemphasized.[26] Aggressive stretching of the calf muscles, twice-daily icing of the affected area, and NSAIDs are essential adjuncts to adjustments in the training program. Corrective arch supports for those with either pes planus or pes cavus are necessary if these conditions

TABLE 25.3. Overuse injuries: staging and rehabilitation

Stage	Symptoms	Rehabilitation
Grade 1	Pain with maximal exertion, resolves after event Nonfocal examination	Decrease activity to 50–70%, ice, NSAIDs for 7 days. Every-other-day training.
Grade 2	Pain with minimal exertion, resolves in < 24 hours Minimal tenderness	Decrease activity to 50%, ice, NSAIDs for 10–14 days. Every-other-day training.
Grade 3	Pain despite rest, not resolved within 48 hours Tender on examination, mild swelling of tendon	Stop activity 2–4 weeks or until pain-free. Ice, NSAIDs. Resume training at 50%, increase by 10% per week. Every 4 weeks reduce to 50%.
Grade 4	Continual pain, stress fracture, point tenderness and swelling	Immobilize if indicated. Rest 4–6 weeks until pain-free. Ice, NSAIDs. Resume training at 50%, increase by 10% per week. Every 4 weeks reduce to 50%.

are present. Combining strength training with resumption of running enhances tendon healing and adaptive cortical thickening.

Jones' Fractures (Proximal Fifth Metatarsal Fractures)

Overuse injuries of the foot can occur at multiple sites including the metatarsal, tarsal, and sesamoid bones. Jones' and sesamoid bone fractures have high rates of nonunion (50–90%).[27] These stress fractures must be detected and treated early to prevent this complication. Jones' fractures are primarily seen in distance runners, especially those with a recent increase in activity. There is usually a history of antecedent pain for several weeks where the peroneus brevis tendon attaches to the proximal fifth metatarsal.

Diagnosis

Pain and tenderness at the site are universal. Inversion of the ankle, causing stress of the peroneus brevis tendon, or attempts to evert the foot against stress also localize pain to the proximal head of the fifth metatarsal. Radiographs may show evidence of cortical thickening, sclerotic changes within the medullary bone, or a true fracture line. The more proximal the fracture, the higher the risk of delayed union. If the radiographs are negative, but there is significant tenderness, a bone scan should be performed because of the high rate of false-negative radiographs for this fracture.

Management

All athletes with evidence of stress fracture on bone scans or sclerotic changes on radiographs should be referred for possible screw placement.[28] If there is evidence only of a periosteal reaction, without visible fracture or medullary sclerosis, the foot is placed in a non-weight-bearing short leg cast for 4 to 6 weeks; follow-up films are obtained when the patient is pain-free to ensure that healing is complete. Despite appropriate care, avascular necrosis may occur, requiring bone grafting. After the fracture is healed, the athlete may gradually return to the activity with close follow-up to prevent recurrence of symptoms.

Prevention of Injuries

The primary focus of injury prevention stems from understanding the mechanisms of injury. With contact or collision sports, appropriate protective equipment is essential for reducing the severity of injuries sustained by the participants. Wearing protective helmets substantially reduces the risk of head injuries in many collision sports. In sports where the risk of falls is prominent, use of wrist guards and knee pads can reduce injuries to these joints. Alpine skiers must use releasable bindings that are adjusted appropriately for their weight and skill level to reduce the risk of ligamentous knee injuries. Overuse injuries can be prevented by developing graded training programs that allow time for compensatory changes in tendons and bones to prevent inflammation. Orthotics and focused training of muscle groups can correct mechanical problems that could lead to overuse injuries.

The second aspect of injury prevention is maximizing the strength, proprioceptive skills, and flexibility of the athlete. Appropriate off-season and preseason training of athletes, coaches, and trainers can substantially reduce injuries during the regular season.

References

1. Cook PC, Leit ME. Issues in the pediatric athlete. Orthop Clin North Am 1995;26:453–64.
2. Dalton SE. Overuse injuries in the adolescent athlete. Sports Med 1992;13: 58–70.
3. Brody DM. Running injuries. Clin Symp 1987;39:23–5.
4. Hulkko A, Orava S. Stress fractures in athletes. Int J Sports Med 1987; 8:221–6.
5. Hergenroeder AC. Diagnosis and treatment of ankle sprains. Am J Dis Child 1990;144:809–14.
6. Brostrom L. Sprained ankles, I. Anatomic lesions in recent sprains. Acta Chir Scand 1964;128:483–95.
7. Stiell IG, Greenberg GH, Mcknight D, et al. Decision rules for the use of radiography in acute ankle injuries. JAMA 1993;269:1127–32.
8. Perlman M, Leveille D, DeLeonibus J, et al. Inversion lateral ankle trauma: differential diagnosis, review of the literature and prospective study. J Foot Surg 1987;26:95–135.
9. Dyment PG. Athletic injuries. Pediatr Rev 1989;10(10):1–13.
10. Cantu RC. Head and spine injuries in youth sports. Clin Sports Med 1995;14:517–31.
11. Committee on Head Injury Nomenclature of the Congress of Neurological Surgeons. Glossary of head injury including some definitions of injury to the cervical spine. Clin Neurosurg 1966;12:386.
12. Saunders RL, Harbaugh RE. The second impact in catastrophic contact sports head trauma. JAMA 1984;252:538–9.
13. Hergengroeder AC. Acute shoulder, knee and ankle injuries. I. Diagnosis and management. Adolesc Health Update 1996;8(2):1–8.
14. Aronen JC, Regan K. Decreasing the incidence of recurrence of first time anterior shoulder dislocations with rehabilitation. Am J Sports Med 1984; 12:283–91.
15. Archambault JL. Brachial plexus stretch injury. J Am Coll Health 1983; 31:256–260.

16. Vereschagin KS, Weins JJ, Fanton GS, Dillingham MF. Burners, don't overlook or underestimate them. Phys Sportsmed 1991;19(9):96–106.
17. Kahler DM, McLue FC. Metacarpophalangeal and proximal interphalangeal joint injuries of the hand, including the thumb. Clin Sports Med 1992;11:5–76.
18. Smith DL, Campbell SM. Painful shoulder syndromes: diagnosis and management. J Gen Intern Med 1992;7:328–39.
19. Safran MR. Elbow injuries in athletes: a review. Clin Orthop 1995;310: 257–77.
20. Mehlhoff TL, Bennett B. The elbow. In: Mellion MB, Walsh WM, Shelton GL, editors. The team physician handbook. Philadelphia: Hanley & Belfus, 1990.
21. Wilhite J, Huurman WW. The thoracic and lumbar spine. In: Mellion MB, Walsh WM, Shelton GL, editors. The team physician handbook. Philadelphia: Hanley & Belfus, 1990.
22. Jackson DW, Wiltse LL. Low back pain in young athletes. Phys Sportsmed 1974;2:53–60.
23. Kuland DN. The injured athlete. 2nd ed. Philadelphia: Lippincott, 1988: 418–20.
24. Davidson K. Patellofemoral pain syndrome. Am Fam Physician 1993;48: 1254–62.
25. Batt ME. Shin splints—a review of terminology. Clin J Sports Med 1995;5: 53–7.
26. Stanitski CL. Common injuries in preadolescent and adolescent athletes. Sports Med 1989;7:32–41.
27. Orava S, Hulkko A. Delayed unions and nonunions of stress fractures in athletes. Am J Sports Med 1988;16:378–82.
28. Lawrence SJ, Bolte MJ. Jones' fractures and related fractures of the fifth metatarsal. Foot Ankle 1993;14:358–65.

CASE PRESENTATION

Subjective

PATIENT PROFILE

Kendra Nelson is a 16-year-old white female high school sophomore.

PRESENTING PROBLEM

"Ankle injury."

PRESENT ILLNESS

Three hours ago, Kendra twisted her left ankle while playing basketball in the high school gym. She noted immediate pain and swelling, and she can bear almost no weight on the ankle. However, she states that "the pain is not really bad."

PAST MEDICAL HISTORY

Kendra had a similar ankle sprain about 4 months ago.

SOCIAL HISTORY, HABITS, AND FAMILY HISTORY

These are unchanged since her last office visit for viral influenza 7 months ago (see Chapter 10).

- What additional history regarding the injury might be helpful?
- How might today's problem relate to the injury 4 months ago?
- What might be significant regarding Kendra's assessment of the pain?
- What might be the meaning of this injury to Kendra? How would you inquire about this?

Objective

GENERAL

The patient hops, rather than walks, to the examination room using the left lower extremity only for balance.

VITAL SIGNS

Blood pressure, 102/64; pulse, 74.

EXAMINATION

The left ankle is swollen and ecchymotic. It is tender laterally, and there is limited range of motion. The dorsalis pedis pulse is normal.

LABORATORY

An office x-ray with routine views of the ankle reveals soft tissue injury with swelling most prominent laterally. There are no bony abnormalities, and the ankle mortise is intact.

- What more would you include in the physical examination?
- What would be evidence on physical examination to help differentiate between soft tissue injury and fracture?
- Have you seen other patients with similar findings? If so, what was the diagnostic assessment and outcome of therapy?
- What are possible complications of this injury, and how would you examine for these?

Assessment

- Based on the findings described above, what is your diagnosis? How would you explain this to Kendra?
- Describe the tissue and pathologic changes involved in this injury.
- What are the implications of this injury for the family and the school?
- If the ankle mortise seemed unstable, what would you do differently?

Plan

- What would be your therapy of this injury? How would you explain your plan to Kendra and her parents?
- Kendra asks about weight-bearing, return to school, and participation in sports. What would you advise?
- What should you tell the school about the injury? How will you communicate this information?
- What follow-up would you advise?

26

Care of the Dying Patient

FRANK S. CELESTINO

Family physicians have traditionally prided themselves on comprehensive and continuous provision of care throughout the human life cycle. When managing the terminal phases of illness, however, most clinicians have had little formal education directed at the experience of human suffering and dying. For many physicians the task and challenge of caring for a dying patient can seem overwhelming. The aging of America, development and widespread use of life-prolonging technologies, the ascendency of managed care emphasizing the central role of the primary care physician, media attention, growing discomfort with futile treatment, and the public's demand for better palliation have all fueled a growing need for physicians to master the art and science of helping patients achieve death with dignity.

This chapter reviews the key components of a comprehensive care program for terminally ill patients (Table 26.1). The focus is on optimum care of patients who experience prolonged but predictable dying. Classically, these individuals have had disseminated cancer. It is now recognized that a much broader array of dying patients—those with acquired immunodeficiency syndrome (AIDS), end-stage renal or cardiac disease, emphysema, and degenerative neurologic diseases—deserve such comprehensive palliative care. For a more detailed discussion of the topics covered in this chapter, the reader can consult two monographs[1,2] that exhaustively review the cultural, spiritual, political, ethical, economic, social, and medical aspects of terminal care.

Cultural Context of Dying and Suffering

The last 50 years have witnessed the increasing medicalization of death in the United States, with most patients now dying in hospitals instead of at home. Contemporary American culture has refused to accept "the naturalness of dying"[3] and seems unusual among developed countries in its passion to conquer death, often acting as if death were simply one more disease to overcome.

TABLE 26.1. Components of a comprehensive care plan for dying patients

Components
Compassionate and professional communication of diagnosis, treatment options, and prognosis
Psychosocial support of the patient and family
Includes developing an understanding of the cultural and religious (spiritual) meaning of suffering and death for the patient and family
Implementation of a comprehensive palliative care program
Multidisciplinary in nature (physicians, nurses, clergy, social workers, pharmacists, nutritionists, lawyers, patient advocates)
Hospice involvement
Establishment and clarification of advance care directives (living wills, durable power of attorney for health care, autopsy and organ donation wishes, dying in hospital versus at home), and attitudes toward physician-assisted suicide
Pain management (WHO and AHCPR guidelines)
Nonpain symptom treatment (including behavioral/ psychiatric issues)
Nutritional support
Acknowledgement and management of financial and reimbursement issues
Bereavement management

WHO = World Health Organization; AHCPR = Agency for Health Care Policy and Research.

Daniel Callahan, a noted bioethicist with the Hastings Center, has presented a perceptive, profound exploration of the difficulty of pursuing a peaceful and dignified death.[4,5] He reflected that physicians have not come to grips with their own mortality, and that "a powerful attraction to technology, a fear of malpractice litigation, and a fundamental ambivalence about the response they should have to death help explain why the care of dying patients has been so difficult, so controversial, and so troubling to both the medical and lay communities."[5]

The Council on Scientific Affairs of the American Medical Association (AMA), after an extensive literature review, echoed similar concerns, commenting that "in the current system of care, many dying patients suffer needlessly, burden their families, and die isolated from families and community."[6] Both Callahan and the AMA Council cited the advance directives movement, rising public enthusiasm for euthanasia and physician-assisted suicide, popularity of the hospice, sensationalized court cases, and establishment of organizations such as Concern for Dying and the Hemlock Society as evidence of increasing uneasiness with medicine's response to dying. They call for acceptance of dying as a normal part of the human life cycle, expanded research into terminal care, educational programs for all health professionals, and better reimbursement for terminal care.[5,6]

Communication of Diagnosis, Therapy Plans, and Prognosis

A common practice in the past has been to maintain a conspiracy of silence in which the patient's physician, in collusion with family members, has covered up the diagnosis of a terminal illness supposedly to protect the patient from emotional shock. Such a practice is now recognized to be counterproductive in most cases, making effective management of dying an impossibility.[7] Not only has the primacy of patient autonomy in modern medicine encouraged truth telling, but studies reveal that patients greatly prefer open, honest communication.[8] Occasionally a patient is inclined toward denial, giving clear signals that he or she does not want to know all of the details of the unpleasant truth. In such cases one initially must respect those wishes. Almost always, however, these patients come to know the gravity of their situations through other means.

Buckman,[9] a medical oncologist, examined a number of sources of communication difficulties with dying patients, including social factors, patient and family barriers, and issues specific to physicians. After reviewing basic active listening skills, he addressed two specific tasks of communication in terminal care: breaking bad news and engaging in therapeutic dialogue. His six-step protocol is a useful paradigm for all health care practitioners: (1) getting started, which includes such issues as location, eye contact, personal touch, timing, and participants; (2) finding out how much the patient already knows and understands; (3) learning how much the patient wants to know; (4) sharing appropriate amounts of information, with attention to aligning and educating; (5) responding to the patient's and family's feelings; and (6) planning ongoing care and follow-through.

There is usually no reason to provide detailed answers to questions the patient has not yet asked. The concept of gradualism—revealing the total truth in small doses as the illness unfolds—allows the patient the opportunity to develop appropriate coping strategies. However, it is important not to use euphemisms (such as swelling or lump), but to acknowledge the presence of cancer when confirmation is in hand. One must also realize that many patients "do not hear" the bad news accurately when it is first presented, and reexplanation is often needed.

Overall, the drive for disclosure must be counterbalanced by the realization that the terminally ill patient struggles to maintain a sense of hope in the face of an increasingly ominous medical situation. Clinicians must continue to nurture hope in their dying patients through appropriate optimism around aspects of treatment, achievable goals, and prognosis, combined with timely praise for the patient and family's efforts to achieve spiritual healing and death with dignity. When physicians apply good communication skills (including attending to both verbal and nonverbal signals, exploring incongruent affect, and empathically eliciting patients' perspectives) and actively work to reduce barriers to mutual understanding, patients experience a reduction in both physical and psychological aspects of suffering.

Regarding prognosis, one of the most difficult tasks is predicting how long the patient will live. Until recently, all physicians had to offer for prognostication were descriptions of the average survival experience of a large group of persons defined by having the same diagnosis or stage of illness, with no attention to individual patient characteristics. Now with the introduction of improved computing and statistical tools, more accurate objective estimates of survival are often available.[10] Despite these computer-generated indexes and models,[10,11] prognostication for many patients remains an imperfect science. Perhaps the best approach in most cases is to provide a conservative, mildly optimistic estimate that allows the patient and family to feel proud about "beating the odds" and exceeding expectations.

Psychosocial Support of the Patient and Family

One of the greatest challenges facing clinicians is to adequately address the multitude of psychosocial needs of dying patients and their families. They must not only continually assess and reconfirm the physiologic stage of dying but, more important, attend to the patient's psychological state.

Kubler-Ross was one of the first to study and popularize the notion that terminally ill individuals often experience *predictable* stages of emotional adaptation and response to the dying process.[12] The five stages were characterized as shock and denial, anger, bargaining, depression, and acceptance. It is now recognized that the duration of these stages and the intensity and sequencing with which they are experienced are highly variable from one individual to the next. Nonetheless, accurate recognition of the patient's psychological stage allows the clinician to optimize communication, support, and empathy to meet new needs as they arise.

In addition to the needs delineated in Table 26.1, and the desire for truth telling and a sense of hopefulness, dying patients above almost all else want assurance that the physician (and others) will not abandon them. There is often great fear of dying alone in a medical environment separated from loved ones and worry about being repulsive to others because of loss of control over bodily functions and hygiene. Terminally ill patients often seek physical expressions of caring: touching, hugging, kissing. Regardless of their formal involvement with organized religion, they also often seek closure on the spiritual issues of their lives. Many individuals find great solace in life review: the pleasures, pains, accomplishments, and regrets. Most desire to have some input into making decisions about their care. Interestingly, the above list of concerns applies as much to the family as to the patient.

Although in many circumstances family members are critical to the success of terminal care, one must be vigilant in recognizing not only depression and burnout but also dysfunctional family relationships that impede successful physician management. In families with preexisting psychiatric problems, substance abuse patterns, and poor family dynamics, physicians may have to be proactive to protect the dying patient from unnecessary conflict and added emotional stress.

An often underappreciated aspect of successful supportive care is to develop insight into and understanding of the symbolic meaning of suffering and dying for the individual patient. Experiences of illness and death and beliefs about the appropriate role of healers are profoundly influenced by a patient's cultural background. Efforts to use racial or ethnic background alone as simplistic, straightforward predictors of beliefs or behaviors may lead to harmful stereotyping of patients and culturally insensitive care for the dying. Koenig and Gates-Williams suggested a protocol to assess the impact of culture.[13] They recommended assessing, in addition to ethnicity: (1) the vocabulary most appropriate for discussing the illness and death; (2) who has decision-making power—the patient or the larger family unit; (3) the relevance of religious beliefs (death, afterlife, miracles, sin); (4) the attitude toward dead bodies; (5) issues of age, gender, and power relationships within both the family and the health care team; and (6) the patient's political and historical context (e.g., poverty, immigrant status, past discrimination, and lack of access to care).

Comprehensive Palliative Care

At some point in the course of a chronic illness, it becomes clear that further therapeutic efforts directed at cure or stabilization are futile. Emphasis then shifts from curative to palliative care with an enhanced focus on optimal function and quality of life. According to the World Health Organization (WHO), palliative care "affirms life, regards dying as a normal process, neither hastens nor postpones death, provides relief from pain and other distressing symptoms, integrates the psychological and spiritual aspects of care, offers a support system to help patients live as actively as possible until death and provides support to help the family cope during the patient's illness and in their own bereavement."[14]

Hospice

In the United States, palliative care is most effectively provided by the now more than 2000 hospice organizations that coordinate the provision of high-quality, interdisciplinary care to patients and families much more effectively and efficiently than most physicians could do on their own. The first hospice was opened in South London by Dr. Cicely Saunders in 1967, with the concept first appearing in America by 1974.[15] Philosophically, the objectives of hospice and palliative care are the same with the addition that hospice care is provided regardless of ability to pay. In just over 20 years of existence, the hospice has grown from an alternative health care movement to an accepted part of the American health care system, with Medicare reimbursement beginning in 1982. Hospice organizations provide a highly qualified, specially trained interdisciplinary team of professionals (nurses, pharmacists, counselors, pastoral care, patient care coordinators, volunteers) who work together to meet the physiologic, psychological, social, spiritual, and economic needs of patients and families facing terminal illness.[16] Classically, more than 80% of hospice patients have had disseminated cancer, but in recent years patients with chronic diseases that are deemed inevitably terminal within 6 months have become eligible as well. The hospice team collaborates continuously with the patient's attending physician (who must certify the terminal condition) to develop and maintain a patient-centered, individualized plan of care.

Hospice medical services and consultation are available 24 hours a day, 7 days a week, though minute-to-minute personal care of the patient by the hospice team is not feasible and must be provided by family or volunteers. Hospice care, though aimed at allowing the patient to remain at home if desired, continues uninterrupted should the patient need acute hospital care or a hospice inpatient unit.

Advance Directives

Some argue that modern medicine has made prolonged dying an art form. It is now possible to keep sick patients alive longer at greater cost with poorer quality of life. Because of this stark reality, patients and physicians have welcomed the emphasis on advance directives planning, though both parties hope that the other will initiate such discussions. Advance directive is an "umbrella" term that refers to any directive for health care made in advance of serious illness that causes cognitive impairment and robs the patient of decision-making capability.

Two general types of directive are widely recognized.[17] With the instructional type the patient specifies in writing certain circumstances and, in advance, declines or accepts specific treatments. Beginning in

1976 with California's Natural Death Act, legislation has been enacted in all 50 states recognizing "living wills" and similar instructional documents. The second type involves appointment of a health care agent, a person to whom is delegated all authority about medical decisions. Many states now also legislatively support this form of advance directive. Each type of directive has its strengths and drawbacks, and they should be seen as complementary, not competitive.

The advance directives movement seems to fit well with an emphasis on patient autonomy and the economic reality of needing to conserve health costs. Unfortunately, studies have revealed that advance directives may make little difference in the way patients are treated at the end of life and reduce costs only modestly.[18–20] Similar drawbacks have applied to the Patient Self-Determination Act,[21] which when implemented in 1991 was designed to encourage competent adults to complete advance directives and to help identify those patients who previously had executed such documents on admission to acute or long-term facilities.[22] Nonetheless, in practice the discussions among physician, patient, and family leading up to establishment of a formal directive are often of greater importance than the documents themselves. When a terminally ill patient calmly discusses foreseeable events and choices leading up to death, the effect on anxious family members can be dramatic and salutary. Such discussions ideally occur relatively early after a terminal illness is diagnosed so as to avoid a crisis situation in which the patient becomes incapacitated and the family must assume responsibility for clinical decisions in the absence of knowledge about their loved one's preferences. States vary widely in the authority granted to close friends or family members in the common situation where an incapacitated person has left no advance directives.

Physicians must realize that most dying patients at some point contemplate suicide and that a small but significant number, in one way or another, will ask their physicians to help hasten death.[23] With the publicity surrounding doctor-aided suicides in Michigan and the onslaught of state and federal judicial and legislative activity concerning physician-assisted suicide, clinicians caring for dying patients must explore their own moral stance in this challenging area so as to deal more effectively with patient suffering.

Inherent in any discussion of advance directives is the concept of the loss of "decision-making capacity." This catch-phrase obscures the fact that in common practice decisional capacity is difficult to assess for most physicians. The elements of capacity seem straightforward: Can the person indicate a choice and do so free of coercion? Can the person manipulate relevant information meaningfully and understand the consequences of choosing each of the options? Searight[24] published a helpful, clinically relevant interview framework for assessing patient medical decision-making capacity.

Pain Management

Symptom management, especially achieving pain relief, remains the first priority for the attending physician and palliative care team.[25] Without effective control of pain and other sources of physical distress, quality of life for the dying patient is unacceptable, and progress on the psychological work of dying is aborted. The very prospect of pain induces fear in the patient; and frustration, anxiety, fatigue, insomnia, boredom, and anger contribute to a lowered threshold for pain.[26] Thus treatment of the *entire* patient contributes to pain control.

Despite several decades of evidence that physicians can and should be successful in controlling cancer pain, studies continue to reveal undertreatment[18,25–28] and multiple barriers to effective cancer pain management.[26] Physicians have been guilty of inadequate knowledge of pain therapies, poor pain assessment, overconcern about controlled substances regulations, and fear of patient addiction and tolerance. On the other hand, patients may be reluctant to report pain or to take medication correctly. The health care system also presents impediments by giving cancer pain treatment low priority and inadequate reimbursement, in conjunction with restrictive regulation of controlled substances.

Pain during terminal illness and with cancer may be of two types: (1) nociceptive (somatic/visceral) and (2) neuropathic.[25–27] Somatic/visceral pain arises from direct stimulation of afferent nerves due to tumor infiltration of skin, soft tissue, or viscera. Somatic pain is often described as dull or aching and is well localized. Bone and soft-tissue metastases are examples of somatic pain. Visceral pain tends to be poorly localized and is often referred to dermatomal sites distant from the source of the pain.

Neuropathic pain results from injury to some element of the nervous system because of the direct effect of the tumor or as a result of cancer therapy (surgery, irradiation, chemotherapy). Examples include brachial or lumbosacral plexus invasion, spinal nerve root compression, or neuropathic complications of drugs such as vincristine. Neuropathic pain is described as sharp, shooting, shock-like, or burning and is often associated with dysesthesias. Unlike somatic/visceral pain, neuropathic pain may be relatively less responsive to opioids, whereas antidepressants, anticonvulsants, or local anesthetics may have good efficacy.

An optimum pain management program includes assessment of the pathophysiology of the patient's pain, taking a pain history, noting response to prior therapies, discussing the patient's goals for pain control, assessing psychosocial contributors to pain, and frequently reevaluating the patient after changes in treatment. Use of a visual analog scale, where the patient notes the level of pain anywhere along a continuous line, is a particularly useful tool for the initial assessment and follow-up of patients.

Classically, the management of pain in terminally ill patients has involved multiple modalities: analgesic drugs, psychosocial and emotional support, palliative irradiation and surgery, and anesthesia-related techniques, such as nerve blocks, which can be both diagnostic and therapeutic.[25–28] Sometimes chemotherapy or hormonal therapies are of some help with cancer pain.

Analgesics are the mainstay for management of cancer and terminal illness pain. Traditionally, they have been classified into three broad categories: nonopioids (aspirin, acetaminophen, nonsteroidal anti-inflammatory agents), opioids (with morphine the prototype), and adjuvant analgesics (antidepressants, anticonvulsants, local anesthetics, capsacin, corticosteroids, and neuroleptics). The recent availability of tramadol, a "binary" noncontrolled analgesic with both serotonergic and weak opioid actions, perhaps adds a fourth class.

Because patients with advanced disease often have mixed types of pain, drugs from different classes are often combined to achieve optimal pain relief. This concept, together with the principle of using the simplest dosing schedule and the least-invasive modalities first, form the basis for WHO's "analgesic ladder" approach to pain management.[14] This approach, which has been validated in clinical trials worldwide and championed by other agencies,[26] recommends nonopioids (with or without tramadol) for mild to moderate pain (step 1), adding opioids for persistent or increasing pain (step 2), and finally increasing the opioid potency or dose as the pain escalates (step 3). At each step, adjuvant medications are considered based on the underlying causes of the pain. The ladder-based protocol should not be seen as rigid, as therapy must always be individualized, with doses and intervals carefully adjusted to provide optimal relief of pain with minimal side effects.

Although many opioid analgesics exist, morphine remains the gold standard, as no other narcotic is more effective. Morphine has a simple metabolic route with no accumulation of clinically significant active metabolites. There are a wide variety of preparations, making it easy to titrate or change routes of administration. When switching narcotics or routes of administration, physicians must be familiar with the well publicized charts of equianalgesic dosing equivalents.[14,26,27]

Regardless of the choice of specific drug, doses should be given on a regular schedule, by the clock, to maintain steady blood levels. Additional doses can be superimposed as needed on the baseline regimen. Transdermal fentanyl has been another option for achieving steady-state blood levels.

There is no ceiling effect for morphine dosing. The hallmark of tolerance development is shortening of the duration of analgesic action. Physical dependence is expected, and addiction is rare. Sharp increases in dosage requirements usually imply worsening of the underlying disease. Opioid side effects—constipation, nausea, vomiting, mental clouding, sedation, respiratory depression—are watched for vigilantly, anticipated, and prevented if possible. Constipation is so pervasive a problem that all patients on opioids should be started on a bowel management regimen that may include fluid, fiber, stool softeners, stimulant or osmotic laxatives, periodic enemas, or lactulose.

Regarding adjuvants, corticosteroids provide a range of effects, including mood elevation, antiinflammatory activity, antiemetic effects, appetite stimulation (helpful with cachexia), and reduction of cerebral and spinal cord edema. They may be helpful for bone and nerve pain. Antidepressants in lower doses (e.g., 10–100 mg of the prototype amitriptyline) help alleviate neuropathic pain and provide innate analgesia as well as potentiation of opioids. In standard doses they are mood elevating, with particularly promising results achieved with the newer selective serotonin reuptake inhibitors. Psychostimulants (e.g., methylphenidate) may be useful for reducing opioid-induced and respiratory depression sedation when dosage adjustment is not feasible. Biphosphonates show early promise for use against bone pain.

Physical and psychosocial modalities can be used with drugs to manage pain during all phases of treatment. Physical modalities include cutaneous stimulation, heat, cold, massage, pressure, gentle exercise, repositioning, biofeedback, transcutaneous electrical nerve stimulation, aroma therapy, acupuncture, and even immobilization (casting). A variety of cognitive-behavioral interventions can also be employed: relaxation, guided imagery, distraction, reframing, psychotherapy, and support groups.

Nonpain Symptom Management

Dying patients struggle with numerous losses and fears that are exacerbated by debilitating and often demeaning nonpain symptoms, including nausea, vomiting, anorexia, diarrhea, bowel impaction, depression, anxiety, cough, dyspnea, visceral or bladder spasms, hiccups, decubiti, and xerostomia. To preclude unnecessary suffering, clinicians must utilize diverse methods[29] to optimize palliative care and provide a relatively symptom-free death. The key is to search for reversible causes of these diverse symptom complexes before resorting to medication management.

Anorexia with decreased intake is distressing to families. In addition, concerns about providing adequate nutrition and hydration have arisen on both a moral and symptom relief basis. Studies have revealed that hunger is a rare symptom, and that thirst and dry mouth are usually easily managed with local mouth care and sips.[30] Thus food and fluid administration are now thought not to play a significant role in providing comfort to terminally ill patients, nor is such provision thought to be morally mandated (though the symbolic meaning of feeding efforts should not be overlooked). Finally, force feeding and total parenteral nutrition have been repeatedly shown to shorten survival.[31]

Bereavement and Grief

Most family members suffer psychologically during the dying of a loved one and then go through an expected process of bereavement. A multitude of feelings—shock, disbelief, a general numbing of all affect, protest, relief, guilt, anguish, emotional lability, tearfulness—accompany the first days to weeks of grieving, eventually giving way to less intense feelings that in normal circumstances are largely resolved within 1 year. The mourning period is a time of physical vulnerability, with bereaved persons likely to suffer impaired immune status and behavioral problems.[32]

The family physician is often best situated to provide ongoing bereavement services. The 13-month bereavement support offered by hospice agencies[16] and community grief support groups can be utilized. Key tasks for the physician who is providing care to the bereaved include validating and normalizing feelings, not medicating emotions simply because they are intense, assessing the progress of the family's grief work, identifying and intervening in abnormal grief, and using age-appropriate models and interactional styles.[33] Short-acting benzodiazepines can be helpful during the first 1 to 2 weeks if family members need relief from sleeplessness and extreme tearfulness.

Special Needs of Dying Children

Although most of the previously mentioned principles of comprehensive terminal care apply equally well to dying children, several additional considerations should be emphasized.[34–37] Communication must include age and developmentally appropriate vocabulary. Although most children do not develop an accurate understanding of dying until age 7 to 8, those as young as 4 to 5 recognize that they are gravely ill. Physicians should openly discuss with parents what role they wish to play in discussions of diagnosis, prognosis, and death.

Multidisciplinary hospice involvement may be even more important for children than adults. Likewise, studies have verified[36] that most terminally ill children, as well as their families, fare better when the caring and dying occur at home. The parents must be continually supported in their efforts to make the child's remaining time meaningful and memorable. Clinicians must remain cognizant of sibling issues such as feelings of neglect or jealousy. Siblings may need reassurance that they are not in some way responsible for the child's dying. In general, siblings should be encouraged to participate in the care of their dying loved one. Lastly, physicians can recognize and support family members' differing styles of bereavement, which may encompass "getting over it," "filling the emptiness," or "keeping the connection."[36]

Conclusion

The challenge in providing terminal care is to form an accurate understanding of the needs and preferences of the dying patient and to fit the delivery of care to those needs.[38] The fundamental rule here is that good care involves giving patients options and some sense of control. Physicians should realize and accept that patients' needs are shaped in unusual ways by factors (cultural and religious) that fall outside the comfortable biomedical domain. The medical profession, and physicians in particular, will increasingly be held accountable for keeping abreast of advances in terminal care that will ensure optimum care of dying patients.[39,40]

References

1. Schonwetter RS, editor. Care of the terminally ill patient. Clin Geriatr Med 1996;12:237–433.
2. Cassel CK, Omenn GS, editors. Special issue: caring for patients at the end of life. West J Med 1995;163:224–305.
3. McCue JD. The naturalness of dying. JAMA 1995;273:1039–43.
4. Callahan D. The troubled dream of life: living with mortality. New York: Simon & Schuster, 1993.
5. Callahan D. Frustrated mastery: the cultural context of death in America. West J Med 1995;163:226–30.
6. Council on Scientific Affairs, American Medical Association. Good care of the dying patient. JAMA 1996;275:474–78.
7. Wanzer SH, Federman DD, Adelstein SJ, et al. The physician's responsibility towards hopelessly ill patients. N Engl J Med 1989;320:844–9.
8. Waitzkin H. Doctor-patient communication—clinical implications of social scientific research. JAMA 1984;252: 2441–6.
9. Buckman R. How to break bad news: a guide for health care professionals. Baltimore: Johns Hopkins University Press, 1992.
10. Lynn J, Teno JM, Harrell FE. Accurate prognostication of death: opportunities and challenges for clinicians. West J Med 1995;163:250–7.
11. Evans C, McCarthy M. Prognostic uncertainty in terminal care: can the Karnofsky index help? Lancet 1985;1:1204–8.
12. Kubler-Ross E. On death and dying. New York: Macmillan, 1969.
13. Koenig BA, Gates-Williams J. Understanding cultural differences in caring for dying patients. West J Med 1995; 163:244–9.
14. World Health Organization. Cancer pain relief and palliative care. Geneva: WHO, 1990. Technical Report Series 804.
15. Berry ZS, Lynn J. Hospice medicine. JAMA 1993;270:220–3.
16. National Hospice Organization. Standards of hospice program of care. Arlington, VA: NHO, 1993.
17. Finucane TE, Harper M. Ethical decision-making near the end of life. Clin Geriatr Med 1996;12:369–77.

18. Support Principal Investigators. A controlled trial to improve care for seriously ill hospitalized patients—the Study to Understand Prognoses and Preferences for Outcomes and Risks of Treatments (SUPPORT). JAMA 1995;274:1591–8.
19. Emanuel EJ. Cost savings at the end of life: what do the data show? JAMA 1996;275:1907–14.
20. Morrison RS, Olson E, Mertz KR, Meier DE. The inaccessability of advance directives on transfer from ambulatory to acute care settings. JAMA 1995;274:478–82.
21. The Patient Self-Determination Act of 1990, §§ 4206, 4751 of the Omnibus Reconciliation Act of 1990, Pub L No. 101-508, November 5, 1990.
22. Lynn J, Teno JM. After the Patient Self-Determination Act: the need for empirical research on formal advance directives. Hastings Cent Rep 1993; 23:20–4.
23. Task Force on Physician-Assisted Suicide of the Society for Health and Human Values. Physician-assisted suicide: toward a comprehensive understanding. Acad Med 1995;70: 583–90.
24. Searight HR. Assessing patient competence for medical decision making. Am Fam Physician 1992;45:751–9.
25. American Geriatrics Society Clinical Practice Committee. Clinical Practrice Guideline: Management of cancer pain in older patients. JAGS 1997;45:1273–76.
26. Jacox AK, Carr DB, Payne R, et al. Management of cancer pain: clinical practice guidelines #9. Rockville, MD: Agency for Health Care Policy and Research, 1994. AHCPR Publ. No. 94-0592.
27. American Pain Society. Principles of analgesic use in the treatment of acute pain and cancer pain. 3rd ed. Skokie, IL: APS, 1992.
28. Cleeland CS, Gonin R, Hatfield A, et al. Pain and its treatment in outpatients with metastatic cancer. N Engl J Med 1994;330:592–6.
29. Rousseau P. Non-pain symptom management in terminal care. Clin Geriatr Med 1996;12:313–28.
30. McCann RN, Hall WJ, Groth-Juncker A. Comfort care for terminally ill patients—the appropriate use of nutrition and hydration. JAMA 1994; 272:1263–6.
31. American College of Physicians. Position paper: parenteral nutrition in patients receiving cancer chemotherapy. Ann Intern Med 1989;110:734–6.
32. Spratt ML, Denney DR. Immune variables, depression, and plasma cortisol over time in suddenly bereaved parents. J Neuropsychiatry Clin Neurosci 1991;3:299–306.
33. Ogle KS, Plumb JD. The role of the primary care physician in the care of the terminally ill. Clin Geriatr Med 1996;12:267–78.
34. Foley G, Whittam EH. Care of the child dying of cancer: Part I. CA 1990;40:327–54.
35. Foley G, Whittam EH. Care of the child dying of cancer: Part II. CA 1991;41:52–60.
36. Martinson IM. Improving the care of dying children. West J Med 1995; 163:258–62.

37. Carr-Gregg MR, Sawyer SM, Clarke CF, Bowes G. Caring for the terminally-ill adolescent. Med J Australia 1997;166:255–8.
38. Lynn J. Clinical Crossroads: An 88-year-old woman facing the end of life. JAMA 1997;277:1633–40.
39. Leland JY, Schonwetter RS. Advances in hospice care. Clin Geriatr Med 1997;13:381–401.
40. Rudberg, MA, Teno JM, Lynn J. Developing and implementing measures of quality of care at the end of life: a call to action by the American Geriatrics Society's Ethics Committee. JAGS 1997;45:528–30.

CASE PRESENTATION

Subjective

PATIENT PROFILE

Samuel Nelson is a 48 year old single white male farm worker.

PRESENTING PROBLEM

"Weight loss and shortness of breath"

PRESENT ILLNESS

Samuel Nelson is brought to the office by his mother, who has been concerned about her son's recent loss of some 25 pounds in weight. He has also been coughing more than usual, and the cough has been productive of blood-streaked sputum over the past few weeks. For the past 10 days, he has been unable to work because of weakness.

PAST MEDICAL HISTORY

Mr. Nelson is a heavy smoker and has had chronic obstructive pulmonary disease for more than 5 years. He had pneumonia treated as an outpatient 3 years ago.

SOCIAL HISTORY, HABITS, AND FAMILY HISTORY

These were recorded at his last visit about 7 months ago (See Chapter 13) and there has been no change since that time.

- What are the diagnostic possibilities at this stage of the visit?
- What additional data might help clarify what is wrong with this patient?
- What might be the significance of the patient being unable to work?
- What might be the relevance of the mother accompanying her adult son to this office visit?

Objective

VITAL SIGNS

Height, 5 ft, 10 in; weight, 154 lb; blood pressure, 110/62; pulse, 92; respirations, 36; temperature, 37.2°C.

EXAMINATION

The patient is sitting on the edge of the examination table, pale and short of breath. He appears chronically ill, with evidence of recent weight loss. The eyes appear sunken and the oral cavity is slightly dry. There is a palpable left supraclavicular lymph node with a diameter of approximately 3 cm. Breathing is labored; on examination of the chest, there are decreased breath sounds and dullness to percussion at the apex posteriorly and at the left lung base. The heart rate is 90–94 per minute with a regular sinus rhythm and no murmur audible. The liver is enlarged 2 to 3 centimeters below the right costal margin.

LABORATORY AND DIAGNOSTIC IMAGING

A chest roentgenogram performed in the office reveals a 6 by 8 centimeter mass in the left lung apex, with prominent hilar adenopathy and a pleural effusion at the left costophrenic sulcus. An office hemoglobin level is 9.4 grams/dl.

- What more—if anything—should be recorded in the physical examination? Why?
- What further diagnostic tests should be performed?
- What are the likely implications of these findings and what would you tell the patient and his mother today?
- What would you do next?

CONTINUING CARE

Upon your referral, Mr. Nelson was examined and treated at the regional medical center. Extensive testing, including needle biopsy of the lung lesion, revealed adenocarcinoma of the left lung with pleural effusion and widespread metastasis including bone, liver and brain. Following a course of palliative therapy, the patient has been returned to you for terminal care.

Assessment

- The patient and his family ask about the outlook for the weeks and months ahead. How would you respond?
- Mr. Nelson's sister, a paralegal employed by a local legal firm, asks about the relationship between the patient's lung cancer and his exposure to pesticides and other chemicals in his work. How would you respond?
- What are some of the implications of this disease for the family?
- What are some symptoms or physical findings—if they develop—that you would consider especially worrisome? Explain.

Plan

- You sense that the patient and family are concerned that they will be somehow left on their own to deal with the illness and eventual death. How can you reassure them?
- Mr. Nelson reports that he has pain in the mid-back that has awakened him from sleep the past few nights. How would you deal with this problem?
- How would you address the issue of advance directives with this patient and family?
- What might be the role of hospice in the care of this patient? When and how would you discuss this with the family?
- When this patient eventually dies, how do you believe you will feel and how will you deal with your feelings?

Index